2nd edition

neuroanatomy

The National Medical Series for Independent Study

2nd edition
neuroanatomy

William DeMyer, M.D.

Professor of Child Neurology
Indiana University School of Medicine
Indianapolis, Indiana

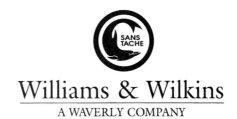

Williams & Wilkins
A WAVERLY COMPANY

BALTIMORE • PHILADELPHIA • LONDON • PARIS • BANGKOK
BUENOS AIRES • HONG KONG • MUNICH • SYDNEY • TOKYO • WROCLAW

Editor: Elizabeth Nieginski
Managing Editor: Darrin Kiessling
Marketing Manager: Rebecca Himmelheber
Production Coordinator: Peter J. Carley
Illustration Planner: Peter J. Carley
Cover Designer: Cotter Visual Communications
Typesetter and Digitized Illustrations: Graphic World, Inc.
Printer/Binder: Port City Press, Inc.

351 West Camden Street
Baltimore, Maryland 21201-2436 USA

Rose Tree Corporate Center
1400 North Providence Road
Building II, Suite 5025
Media, Pennsylvania 19063-2043 USA

Accurate indications, adverse reactions and dosage schedules for drugs are provided in this book, but it is possible that they may change. The reader is urged to review the package information data of the manufacturers of the medications mentioned.

Printed in the United States of America

First Edition, 1988

Library of Congress Cataloging-in-Publication Data
DeMyer, William, 1924–
   NMS neuroanatomy / William DeMyer. —2nd ed.
      p.   cm. — (The National medical series for independent study)
   Rev. ed. of: Neuroanatomy / William DeMyer, ©1988.
   Includes bibliographical references and index.
   ISBN 0-683-30075-X
   1. Neuroanatomy—Outlines, syllabi, etc.   2. Neuroanatomy—
Examinations, questions, etc.   I. DeMyer, William, 1924—
Neuroanatomy.   II. Title.   III. Series.
   [DNLM: 1. Neuroanatomy—examination questions.   2. Neuroanatomy—
outlines.   WL 18.2 D389n 1997]
   QM451.D46   1997
   611'.8—dc21
   DNLM/DLC
   for Library of Congress   97-18904
                                                                          CIP

The publishers have made every effort to trace the copyright holders for borrowed material. If they have inadvertently overlooked any, they will be pleased to make the necessary arrangements at the first opportunity.

To purchase additional copies of this book, call our customer service department at **(800) 638-0672** or fax orders to **(800) 447-8438.** For other book services, including chapter reprints and large quantity sales, ask for the Special Sales department.

Canadian customers should call **(800) 665-1148,** or fax **(800) 665-0103.** For all other calls originating outside of the United States, please call **(410) 528-4223** or fax us at **(410) 528-8550.**

Visit Williams & Wilkins on the Internet: http://www.wwilkins.com or contact our customer service department at **custserv@wwilkins.com.** Williams & Wilkins customer service representatives are available from 8:30 am to 6:00 pm, EST, Monday through Friday, for telephone access.

98 99 00
2 3 4 5 6 7 8 9 10

Contents

Preface

In this new edition of the text, I point out where new research has discarded several previous hypotheses and seeming facts. Now, by imaging with radioisotopes, magnetic resonance scans, and electrical recording, we can almost chase a thought through the circuits of the brain. Each advance in functional localization, though, places more demands on knowing the neuroanatomic basis.

As well as glimpsing exciting new vistas, the text must serve the practitioner. Therefore, I have tried to balance the intellectual neuroanatomy required to correlate neurologic function and structure against the practical neuroanatomy required to diagnose the next patient who comes to your office with numbness and tingling in a toe. In addition, more clinical applications throughout the text justify the student's devotion to learning neuroanatomy.

Acknowledgments

As always in manuscript preparation, other persons provided invaluable and appreciated support: Terry Wenzel in secretarial services and Lisa Kiesel in editing.

Chapter 1

Gross Anatomy of the Nervous System

I. **GROSS APPEARANCE OF THE NERVOUS SYSTEM.** Figure 1-1 shows the nervous system as it appears when dissected free from the body.

II. **GROSS SUBDIVISIONS OF THE NERVOUS SYSTEM**

A. The nervous system has **two main parts:**

1. **Central nervous system (CNS)**

2. **Peripheral nervous system (PNS)**
   a. The PNS commences with the **nerve roots.**
   b. To free the CNS from the PNS, we snip the nerve roots just at their attachment to the CNS (Figure 1-2).
   c. The nerve roots combine into **peripheral nerves** to connect the CNS with the rest of the body.

B. **Gross subdivisions of the CNS**

1. The CNS, or neuraxis, consists of **two main subdivisions:**
   a. **Brain** (encephalon)
   b. **Spinal cord** (myelon)

2. To free the brain from the spinal cord, we cut across the CNS at the level of the foramen magnum of the skull (Figure 1-3).

C. **Anatomical definition of the brain and its subdivisions**

1. The brain is that part of the CNS rostral to a cut through the foramen magnum. The spinal cord is caudal to the cut.

2. **Gross subdivisions of the brain** (see Figure 1-3)
   a. **Cerebrum**
   b. **Diencephalon**
   c. **Brain stem**
   d. **Cerebellum**

3. **Historical note on the definition of cerebrum and brain stem.** The original Basle *Nomina Anatomica* (BNA; 1895) defined the diencephalon and midbrain as part of the cerebrum, a practice uncommon today. Later, some authors included the diencephalon or even the basal ganglia with the brain stem. The Mexico City *Nomina Anatomica* (5th edition; 1980) assigns the basal ganglia to the cerebrum. The diencephalon stands separately. The midbrain, pons, and medulla oblongata comprise the brain stem (the truncus encephali).

III. **GROSS ANATOMY OF THE CEREBRAL SURFACE**

A. **Fissures of the cerebrum**

1. The cerebrum consists of mirror-image halves called **cerebral hemispheres,** which are partially separated by an **interhemispheric fissure** (Figures 1-4 and 1-5).

2. Bundles of nerve fibers and neural tissue unite the two hemispheres deep in the interhemispheric fissure (see Figure 1-5).

FIGURE 1-1. Frontal view of the nervous system dissected free from the body. This figure, although extensive, does not include the profusion of finer peripheral branches to the body wall and viscera. (Courtesy of Dr. P. Amenta, Hahnemann University School of Medicine, Philadelphia, Pennsylvania.)

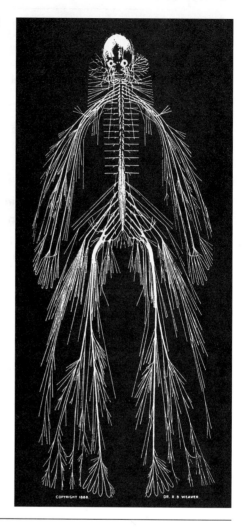

FIGURE 1-2. Frontal view of a transected spinal cord and nerve roots. The scissors' cut, precisely through the attachment of the nerve roots, separates the peripheral nervous system (PNS) from the central nervous system (CNS).

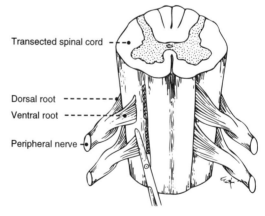

Transected spinal cord

Dorsal root

Ventral root

Peripheral nerve

3. Each cerebral hemisphere has a large fissure, the **sylvian** or **lateral fissure,** seen best on the lateral side (see Figure 1-4A).

B. **Sulci and gyri of the cerebrum**

1. The surface of each cerebral hemisphere displays smaller crevices, called **sulci,** which separate elevations of the surface, called **gyri** (see Figure 1-5).

2. Locate the **central sulcus,** the **calcarine sulcus,** and the **parieto-occipital sulcus** (see Figure 1-4).
   a. The **central sulcus** separates two gyri: a **precentral gyrus** and a **postcentral gyrus.**
   b. The **precentral gyrus** is mainly a **motor area,** which directs volitional movements of the muscles.
   c. The **postcentral gyrus** mediates bodily sensation, such as **touch.**
   d. The gyri around the calcarine sulcus mediate **vision.**
   e. The **transverse temporal** gyri, buried under the posterior part of the sylvian (lateral) fissure, mediate **hearing** (see Figure 13-7).

C. **Lobes of the cerebrum**

1. Fissures, sulci, and certain arbitrary lines divide each cerebral hemisphere into five lobes (see Figure 1-4A):
   a. **Frontal lobe**
   b. **Parietal lobe**
   c. **Temporal lobe**
   d. **Occipital lobe**
   e. **Limbic lobe**

2. On the lateral surface of a hemisphere, notice the following (see Figure 1-4A).
   a. The plane of the **central sulcus** divides the **frontal lobe** from the **parietal lobe.**
   b. The **sylvian fissure** anteriorly divides the **frontal lobe** from the **temporal lobe.** Posteriorly, the sylvian fissure partially divides the **parietal lobe** from the **temporal lobe.**
   c. An arbitrary line drawn laterally from the **superior preoccipital notch** to the **inferior preoccipital notch** divides the **occipital lobe** from the **parietal lobe** and **temporal lobe.**

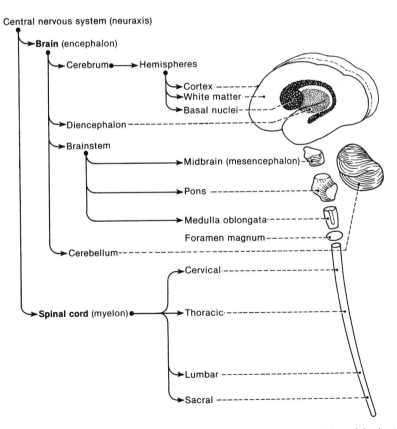

FIGURE 1-3. Lateral view of the central nervous system (CNS), or neuraxis, consisting of the brain, spinal cord, and their subdivisions.

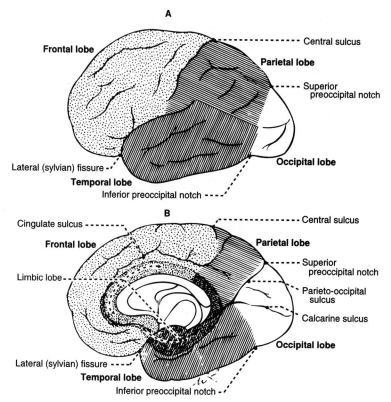

FIGURE 1-4. The two cerebral hemispheres. (A) Lateral view of the left hemisphere. (B) Medial view of the right hemisphere.

      d. An arbitrary line from the midpoint of the foregoing line to the sylvian fissure completes the separation of the **parietal lobe** from the **temporal lobe** posteriorly.

   3. On the medial surface of a hemisphere, notice the following (see Figure 1-4B).
      a. An imaginary extension of the central sulcus divides the **frontal lobe** from the **parietal lobe.**
      b. The **parieto-occipital sulcus** divides the **parietal lobe** from the **occipital lobe.** The parieto-occipital sulcus cuts the superomedial margin of the hemisphere at the superior preoccipital notch.
      c. An arbitrary line extended from the junction of the parieto-occipital sulcus and the calcarine sulcus to the inferior preoccipital notch divides the **temporal lobe** from the **parietal lobe.**

   4. Limbic and olfactory lobes
      a. Some authors list the **limbic lobe,** shown stippled in Figure 1-6, as part of the first four lobes; others list it separately.
      b. The **olfactory lobe** nestles concentrically inside of the limbic lobe, as shown in solid black in Figure 1-6. The circular part of the olfactory lobe extends forward under the frontal lobe as the olfactory bulb and tract.

D. **Cross-sectional anatomy of the cerebrum**

   1. A coronal slice through a cerebral hemisphere discloses the **four gross hemispheric components** (see Figure 1-5):
      a. Superficial, or cortical, gray matter, covering the external surface
      b. White matter

   c. **Deep gray matter**
   d. **Ventricular cavities**

2. **Gray matter.** The gray matter looks gray because it consists of masses of nerve cell bodies that contain pigment and organelles.
   a. The continuous sheet of nerve cell bodies covering the surface of the cerebrum is called the **cerebral cortex.**

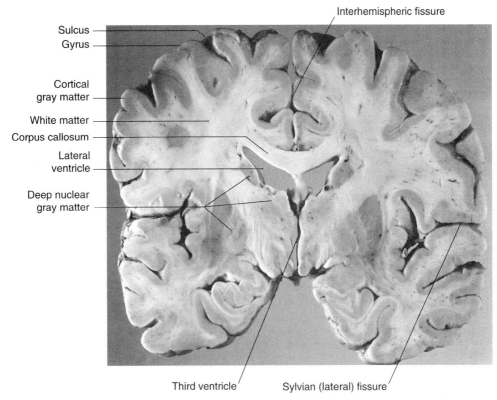

FIGURE 1-5. Gross photograph of an unstained coronal section of the cerebrum showing the two hemispheres with their surface sulci and gyri, gray and white matter, and ventricles. The corpus callosum, a bundle of nerve fibers, connects the two hemispheres across the bottom of the interhemispheric fissure.

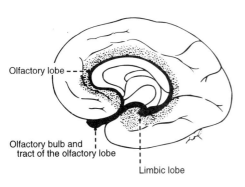

FIGURE 1-6. Medial aspect of the right cerebral hemisphere showing the limbic lobe (stippled) and the olfactory lobe (black).

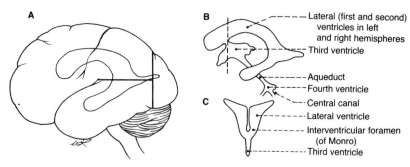

FIGURE 1-7. The cerebral ventricles. (A) Lateral aspect of the left cerebral hemisphere showing the contour of the lateral ventricles and their relation to the cerebral lobes. (B) Lateral outline of the four ventricles. (C) Frontal (coronal) section of the lateral and third ventricles at the level of the dotted line (B), showing their communicating interventricular foramen.

      b. Deep in the hemispheres, the nerve cell bodies accumulate along the wall of the ventricular cavities as masses called **nuclei.**
        (1) A **nucleus** is a fairly compact group of nerve cell bodies, of more or less similar form and function, located **inside the CNS.**
        (2) A **ganglion** is a similar group of nerve cell bodies located **outside the CNS.** The term basal ganglia, used to refer to certain of the deep nuclei, persists from the early days of neuroanatomy. These structures, properly named, are **basal nuclei.**

3. White matter. Gleaming white material called white matter separates the cortex from the deep nuclear masses. It consists of nerve fibers and their coverings, which are called **myelin sheaths.** The myelin is a fatty substance that causes the white appearance, just as fat gives mammalian milk its white color.

4. Cavities of the cerebrum and spinal cord
  a. Although the brain looks solid when viewed externally, it originates embryologically as a tubular structure.
    (1) The original tubular lumen remains as **ventricles,** which circulate **cerebrospinal fluid (CSF).**
    (2) The ventricles conform to the shape of the hemispheres and brain stem (Figure 1-7).
  b. The **ventricular system** consists of (see Figure 1-7B):
    (1) Paired **lateral ventricles** in the cerebral hemispheres
    (2) A slit-like **third ventricle** in the sagittal plane of the diencephalon (see Figure 1-5)
    (3) A narrow tubular **aqueduct,** which runs in the sagittal plane through the midbrain and drains fluid from the third to the fourth ventricle
    (4) An expanded portion called the **fourth ventricle,** which is located in the pons and medulla just ventral to the cerebellum
  c. A small central cavity, called the **central canal,** extends from the fourth ventricle to the caudal tip of the spinal cord.

E. **Cross-sectional anatomy of the brain stem, cerebellum, and spinal cord**

  1. The **brain stem** has a mixture of deep nuclei and white matter (Figure 1-8). Although some neurons are located more superficially, they do not form a surface layer of cortex.

  2. The **cerebellum,** like the cerebrum, has surface cortex and deep nuclear masses, which are separated by white matter (see Figure 1-8B).

  3. The **spinal cord** has a central, H-shaped core of gray matter that consists of nuclei. The spinal cord has no cortex. The periphery of the cord is all white matter (see Figure 6-3).

IV. GROSS ANATOMY OF THE PERIPHERAL NERVOUS SYSTEM

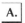

A. **Gross components of a typical peripheral nerve.** Peripheral nerves convey sensory and motor nerve fibers to and from the CNS. Although they differ in fiber ratios and distribution, most peripheral nerves consist of the same gross components, as labeled in Figure 1-9.

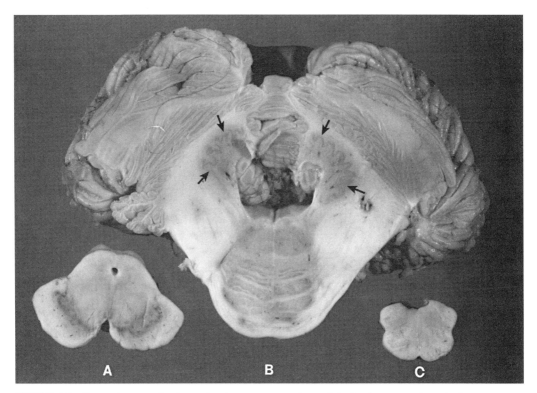

FIGURE 1-8. Gross photograph of unstained transverse sections of the brain stem and cerebellum. (A) Midbrain with aqueduct. (B) Pons connected to the overlying cerebellum by white matter. The cerebellum (B) overlies the pons and has a convoluted cortical surface surrounding its deep white matter. Deep nuclei (arrows) surround the fourth ventricle. (C) Medulla with fourth ventricular cavity dorsally, with the roofing membrane torn away.

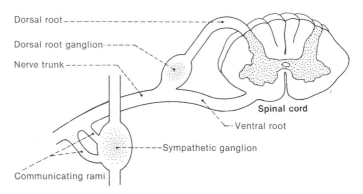

FIGURE 1-9. Gross components of the typical peripheral nerve.

B. **The PNS has three main types of nerves.**

1. All **cranial nerves** attach to the cerebrum or brain stem, except for cranial nerve (CN) XI, which attaches to the rostral part of the spinal cord.

2. All **spinal nerves** attach to the spinal cord.
   a. All spinal nerves have **dorsal** and **ventral roots,** except for the first cervical nerve, which may have no dorsal root.
   b. Spinal nerves innervate skeletal muscles and sensory receptors and, in part, convey visceral nerves.

3. The **autonomic (visceral) nerves** run through the roots of cranial or spinal nerves to ganglia or autonomic plexuses in the walls of the viscera (see Figures 5-1 and 5-2).
   a. The nerves run from the ganglia or plexuses to smooth muscles or glands.
   b. The autonomic nerves return impulses to the CNS from the sensory receptors in the viscera.

V. THE MENINGES AND INTRACRANIAL SPACES

A. **Meninges.** The meninges consist of three distinct sheaths of fibrous connective tissue: the **dura mater, arachnoid,** and **pia mater.** They ensheathe the entire CNS **concentrically** and act as protective coverings for the delicate neural tissue inside (Figure 1-10).

1. The **dura mater,** which is the **outermost** sheath, literally means **hard mother** because it is thick and very tough. It envelopes the arachnoid, which in turn envelopes the pia mater.

2. The **arachnoid,** which is the **intermediate** sheath, literally means **spidery.** The term describes the spidery appearance created by the numerous trabeculae that cross the space beween the arachnoid and pia mater (Figure 1-11).

3. The **pia mater,** which is the **innermost** sheath, literally means **soft mother.** It covers every bump and enters every crevice. In contrast to the thicker, tougher dura mater, the pia mater and the arachnoid together are called the **leptomeninges** (lepto means thin and delicate).

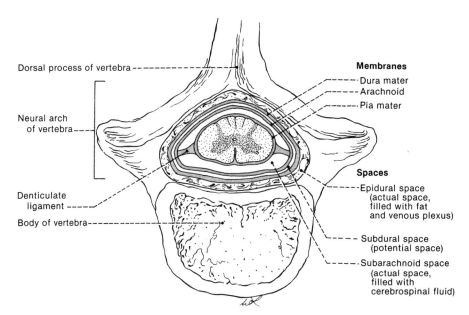

FIGURE 1-10. Cross section through a vertebra showing the vertebral canal with its contained epidural space, meninges, and spinal cord.

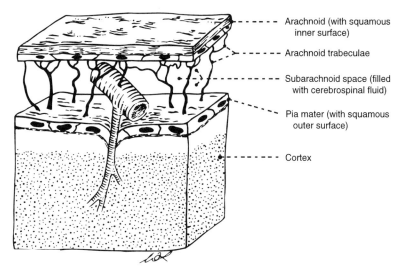

Arachnoid (with squamous
inner surface)

Arachnoid trabeculae

Subarachnoid space (filled
with cerebrospinal fluid)

Pia mater (with squamous
outer surface)

Cortex

FIGURE 1-11. Section through the subarachnoid space, formed between the arachnoid membrane and the pia mater.

B. **Potential and actual dural spaces**

1. Epidural and subdural spaces

  a. The external surface of the dura mater normally adheres to the inner table of the skull, forming the periosteum. However, a **potential epidural space,** like the pleural space, exists between the dura and the inner table. Under pathologic conditions, blood or pus may dissect the dura from the skull, creating an **actual epidural space** from the potential space and compressing the brain (Figure 1-12).

  b. From the level of the foramen magnum, an **actual epidural space** extends caudally along the entire vertebral column. It separates the external dural surface from the vertebral periosteum (see Figure 1-10). Normally, only fat and an epidural plexus of veins occupy this actual epidural space. Pus, blood, or neoplasms may distend the **vertebral epidural space,** compressing the spinal cord.

  c. A **potential subdural space** exists between the dura and the arachnoid membrane. Although it normally contains no free fluid, tissue fluids, blood, or pus may enter this space and compress the brain or spinal cord depending on the site of the lesion.

2. Both subdural and epidural **hematomas** are common complications of head trauma and coagulopathies.

C. **The arachnoid membrane, subarachnoid space, and pia mater**

1. The **arachnoid membrane** ensheaths the pia mater. An **acutal subarachnoid space** separates the **inner** surface of the arachnoid membrane from the **outer** surface of the pia mater (see Figures 1-10 and 1-11).

2. The **subarachnoid space** normally contains **blood vessels** and **CSF.** Numerous fibrous trabeculae bridge the subarachnoid space (see Figure 1-11). In meningitis and encephalitis, pus cells invade the CSF in the subarachnoid space. Neoplastic cells may also disseminate through this space.

  a. After the **blood vessels** for the CNS pierce the dura mater to enter the skull, they ramify in the subarachnoid space, and then must penetrate the pia mater to enter the CNS (see Figure 1-11).

  b. As the blood vessels penetrate the pia mater, they receive a **fibrous connective tissue investment** from the pia mater.

  c. This **connective tissue** forms the external part of the **blood vessel wall.** It is the only fibrous connective tissue central to the pia mater. All remaining connective tissue of the CNS consists of glial cells.

      d. A ruptured blood vessel in the subarachnoid space, as from a ruptured aneurysm, causes **subarachnoid hemorrhage.**

  3. Pia mater
      a. The pia mater is the innermost meningeal sheath (see V A 3).
      b. Because the **end feet** of cells called **astrocytes** adhere tightly to the inner surface of the pia (see Figure 2-12), no actual or potential space exists between the pia mater and the neuraxis.

VI. FOSSAE AND DURAL COMPARTMENTS OF THE SKULL

A. **Fossae of the skull.** The base of the skull displays three hollows, or fossae: the **anterior, middle,** and **posterior** (see Figure 7-23).

  1. Anterior fossa. The orbital plates of the **frontal bone** form the floor of the anterior fossa. The undersurface of the **frontal lobe** rests in the anterior fossa.

  2. Middle fossa. The **temporal bone** forms the floor of the middle fossa. The undersurfaces of the **temporal** and **occipital lobes** rest in the middle fossa.

  3. Posterior fossa. The **temporal** and **occipital bones** form the posterior fossa. The bony floor of the posterior fossa, the **clivus,** underlies the **pons** and **medulla oblongata.**

B. **Dural compartments of the skull.** **Dural folds** called the **cerebral falx** and the **cerebellar tentorium** partition the space within the skull into compartments (Figure 1-13).

  1. The **cerebral falx** is a fold of dura mater in the midsagittal plane, inserted into the interhemispheric fissure. It **separates** the **skull** cavity into **right** and **left** halves.

  2. The **cerebellar tentorium** is a tent-shaped fold of dura inserted between the cerebellum and the inferomedial surfaces of the temporal and occipital lobes. The tentorium separates the skull cavity into a **supratentorial** and an **infratentorial space.**
      a. Anteriorly, the halves of the tentorium separate to form the **tentorial notch.** The midbrain occupies the tentorial notch in its passage from the infratentorial to the supratentorial space (see Figure 1-13).

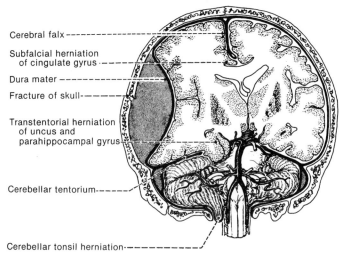

Cerebral falx

Subfalcial herniation of cingulate gyrus

Dura mater

Fracture of skull

Transtentorial herniation of uncus and parahippocampal gyrus

Cerebellar tentorium

Cerebellar tonsil herniation

FIGURE 1-12. Coronal section of the head showing an epidural hematoma causing internal herniation of the cerebrum across the midline and of the cerebellar tonsil down through the foramen magnum. (Adapted with permission from Netter F: *Ciba Symposia,* vol 18, 1966, plate XI.)

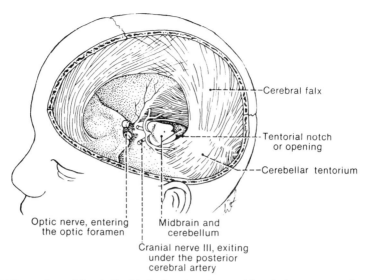

Cerebral falx

Tentorial notch
or opening

Cerebellar tentorium

Optic nerve, entering
the optic foramen

Midbrain and
cerebellum

Cranial nerve III, exiting
under the posterior
cerebral artery

FIGURE 1-13. Oblique view of the skull with the hemicranium and hemispheres removed to show the dural folds called the cerebral falx and cerebellar tentorium.

b. The space **above** the tentorium, the **supratentorial space,** contains the diencephalon and the cerebrum.

c. The space **below** the tentorium, the **infratentorial space** or **posterior fossa,** contains the brain stem and cerebellum.

STUDY QUESTIONS

DIRECTIONS: Each of the numbered items or incomplete statements in this section is followed by answers or by completions of the statement. Select the ONE lettered answer or completion that is BEST in each case.

1. The largest crevice on the lateral surface of the cerebrum that separates the frontal and parietal lobes from the temporal lobe is the

(A) central sulcus
(B) sylvian, or lateral, fissure
(C) superior temporal sulcus
(D) transverse fissure
(E) primary fissure

2. White matter appears white because of

(A) myelin sheaths composed of lipid
(B) profusion of astrocytic processes
(C) axoplasm
(D) large amounts of fluid
(E) numerous blood vessel walls

3. The current definition of the brain stem includes which of the following?

(A) Cerebellum
(B) Deep cerebral white matter
(C) Basal ganglia
(D) Mesencephalon
(E) Diencephalon

4. To reach cerebrospinal fluid (CSF) for withdrawal (i.e., to perform a spinal tap), a needle tip must pass successively through the

(A) pia mater, dura mater, epidural space, and arachnoid membrane
(B) arachnoid membrane, epidural space, dura mater, and subdural space
(C) subdural space, dura mater, epidural space, and arachnoid membrane
(D) arachnoid membrane, subdural space, dura mater, and epidural space
(E) epidural space, dura mater, subdural space, and arachnoid membrane

5. Select the part of the central nervous system (CNS) that occupies the tentorial notch.

(A) Diencephalon
(B) Midbrain
(C) Medulla
(D) Spinal cord
(E) None of the above

DIRECTIONS: Each of the numbered items or incomplete statements in this section is negatively phrased, as indicated by a capitalized word such as NOT, LEAST, or EXCEPT. Select the ONE lettered answer or completion that is BEST in each case.

6. A complete section through the midpoint of the cerebrum either in the horizontal or coronal plane would disclose all of the following EXCEPT

(A) a layer of cortex on the surface
(B) a layer of deep white matter
(C) basal ganglia
(D) lateral ventricles
(E) the occipital lobe

7. All of the following landmarks or lines form an extensive part of some boundary of the parietal lobe EXCEPT

(A) the sylvian fissure
(B) the central sulcus
(C) a line from the superior preoccipital notch to the inferior preoccipital notch
(D) the calcarine sulcus
(E) the limbic lobe

8. Which of the following associations is IN-CORRECT?

(A) Precentral gyrus/motor area
(B) Postcentral gyrus/somatosensory receptive area
(C) Calcarine cortex/visual receptive area
(D) Transverse temporal gyri/auditory receptive area
(E) None of the above

DIRECTIONS: Each set of matching questions in this section consists of a list of four to twenty-six lettered options (some of which may be in figures) followed by several numbered items. For each numbered item, select the ONE lettered option that is most closely associated with it. To avoid spending too much time on matching sets with large numbers of options, it is generally advisable to begin each set by reading the list of options. Then, for each item in the set, try to generate the correct answer and locate it in the option list, rather than evaluating each option individually. Each lettered option may be selected once, more than once, or not at all.

Questions 9–12

For each vernacular or common term, match the correct technical term.

(A) Diencephalon
(B) Truncus encephali
(C) Mesencephalon
(D) Encephalon
(E) Myelon

9. Brain D Encephalon

10. Spinal cord E myelon

11. Midbrain C Mesen

12. Brain stem B Truncus encephali

Questions 13–18

Match the cerebral lobes listed below with the landmarks that completely or partially divide each lobe.

(A) Central sulcus
(B) Lateral (sylvian) fissure
(C) Line from the superior preoccipital notch to the inferior preoccipital notch
(D) Cingulate sulcus
(E) None of the above

13. Separates the frontal lobe from the temporal lobe B

14. Separates the parietal lobe from the temporal lobe B

15. Separates the limbic lobe from the olfactory lobe E

16. Separates the parietal lobe from the occipital lobe laterally C

17. Separates the parietal lobe from the occipital lobe medially E

18. Separates the frontal lobe from the parietal lobe A

ANSWERS AND EXPLANATIONS

1. The answer is B [III A, B; Figure 1-4]. Numerous sulci of varying size and depth appear on the lateral surface of the cerebrum. Sulci are shallower and more numerous and highly branched than fissures. Only one major fissure, the sylvian fissure, appears on the lateral surface. Another major fissure, the interhemispheric fissure, separates the two cerebral hemispheres. Embryologically, fissures arise by a different mechanism than sulci.

2. The answer is A [III D 3]. The white matter of the central nervous system (CNS) appears white because of myelin. Myelin consists of lipid-rich oligodendroglial cell membranes that wrap around the axons. The myelin lipids cause the white color, just as lipids cause the whiteness of mammalian milk.

3. The answer is D [II C 3]. The definition of the brain stem and of the cerebrum itself has changed over the years. Currently, the brain stem is defined as the mesencephalon, pons, and medulla. Some previous authors included the diencephalon and even the basal ganglia with the brain stem. The definition of the brain includes all structures rostral to the level of the cervicomedullary junction at the foramen magnum; thus, it would include the entire brain stem, cerebellum, diencephalon, basal ganglia, white matter, and cerebral cortex. These precise definitions are important because brain death, which is the irreversible loss of all brain function from the cervicomedullary junction rostrally, is the legal definition of death in the United States. Some countries require only brain stem death or cerebral death and do not require proof of death of the entire brain.

4. The answer is E [V; Figures 1-10 and 1-11]. The cerebrospinal fluid (CSF) is in the subarachnoid space between the arachnoid membrane and the pia mater, which is the innermost of the three meningeal sheaths. To reach the CSF, a needle tip passes successively through the epidural space, the dura mater, the subdural space, and the arachnoid membrane. The physician can then collect CSF for diagnostic analysis. The main use of a spinal tap is to diagnose subarachnoid bleeding and infections such as meningitis and encephalitis. The CSF will display inflammatory or neoplastic cells. The invading organism can often be identified by culture, staining, serological tests, or the polymerase chain reaction.

5. The answer is B [VI B 2 a; Figures 1-12 and 1-13]. The midbrain extends through the tentorial notch, from the middle fossa to the posterior fossa. All afferent axonal pathways that reach the cerebrum, diencephalon, or basal nuclei from the body must pass rostrally through the midbrain; all efferent axonal pathways that connect these structures with the rest of the nervous system must pass caudally through the midbrain. Supratentorial masses or cerebral edema may cause herniation of one or both cerebral hemispheres through the tentorial notch. The ensuing midbrain compression interrupts sensory and motor functions and consciousness and may kill the patient.

6. The answer is E [III D 1]. A section through the midpoint of the cerebrum in either the horizontal or coronal plane discloses a thin surface covering of cortex, an adjacent thick layer of deep white matter, basal ganglia, and lateral ventricles. The occipital lobe is too far posterior to appear in a coronal section of the cerebrum through its middle part.

7. The answer is D [III C 2 a–d; Figure 1-4]. The parietal lobe is the "keystone" lobe that contacts all other major lobes of the cerebrum. Knowing the boundaries of the parietal lobe is equivalent to knowing the boundaries of all of the lobes. The central sulcus bounds it anteriorly and the sylvian fissure bounds it inferiorly. Laterally, an arbitrary line from the superior to the inferior preoccipital notches separates the parietal from the occipital lobe. Medially, the parieto-occipital sulcus separates the parietal from the occipital lobe. Neuroanatomists may regard the limbic ring as a separate lobe that borders on the frontal, parietal, and temporal lobes or as composed of continuous segments of the frontal, parietal, and temporal lobes. They may also refer to the limbic ring as the gyrus fornicatus. The calcarine sulcus splits the medial aspect of the occipital lobe into dorsal and ventral parts. Although the calcarine sulcus contacts the narrow isthmus between the parietal and temporal lobes, it does not itself demarcate an extensive boundary of the parietal lobe.

8. The answer is E [III B 2]. Some functions localize to discrete areas of the cerebrum. The areas with the most distinctive localization include the motor area of the precentral gyrus and the respective somatic, visual, and auditory receptive areas. Most other functions localize to some extent; for example, language localizes to the parasylvian area of the left cerebral hemispheres, but not quite as focally or symmetrically as for the motor and sensory areas.

9–11. The answers are: 9-D, 10-E, 11-C, 12-B [II B, C 3; Figure 1-3]. Many parts of the nervous system have two names: a common, or vernacular, name and a technical name. The technical name is usually more precisely used and precisely defined than the vernacular term. In addition, the technical term serves better as a combining form for describing changes in the various parts of the nervous system. For example, the term myelon is the technical term for the spinal cord. To describe inflammation of the spinal cord, one would speak of myelitis rather than spinal corditis. Similarly, the term for brain inflammation would be encephalitis rather than brainitis. To replace the various previous definitions of the brain stem, the present *Nomina Anatomica* uses the term truncus encephali. Because imprecise use of terms has always plagued anatomy, the use of strict technical definitions avoids confusion. Even now, however, we lack universally accepted guiding principles for developing the most descriptive, accurate, and memorable terms.

13–18. The answers are: 13-B, 14-B, 15-E, 16-C, 17-E, 18-A [III C 1, 2, 3; Figure 1-4]. The lobes of the cerebrum were originally named because they underlie the skull bones, which had already received names. The lobes are an arbitrary and artificial subdivision of the cerebrum, but their delineation allows description of normal variations in the regions of the brain as well as the exact sites of lesions and the localization of some functions. The central sulcus separates the largest lobe of the cerebrum, the frontal lobe, from the parietal lobe. This sulcus cuts the crest of the hemisphere just rostral to the ascending ramus of the cingulate gyrus and angles ventrally and somewhat anteriorly along the lateral side of the cerebral wall. It divides the motor cortex of the precentral gyrus from the sensory cortex of the postcentral gyrus.

The sylvian, or lateral, fissure is not a sulcus, but is formed by the evagination of the temporal lobe from the primitive telencephalon. On the lateral surface of the brain, it takes a relatively horizontal course that separates the frontal lobe from the anterior part of the temporal lobe and the parietal lobe from the posterior part of the temporal lobe. Thus, the temporal lobe sits beneath the sylvian fissure, under the posterior inferior part of the frontal lobe, and under the inferior margin of the parietal lobe.

Laterally on a cerebral hemisphere, an arbitrary line from the superior to the inferior preoccipital notch divides the occipital lobe, the smallest of the major lobes, from the parietal and temporal lobes. A bridging vein runs from the site of the superior notch to the superior sagittal sinus and from the inferior preoccipital notch to the transverse sinus. Medially on a cerebral hemisphere, the cingulate sulcus roughly divides the limbic lobe from the parietal and frontal lobes, which occupy the medial hemispheric wall dorsal to the limbic lobe.

Chapter 2

Structure and Function of Neurons and Their Supporting Tissues

I. STRUCTURE OF NEURONS

A. **Neurons are the parenchymal cells of the nervous system.** The supporting cells are glia.

B. **A neuron is a complete cell consisting of** (Figure 2-1):

1. A **nucleus** (karyon)

2. A **cell body** (perikaryon)

3. Typically two **processes:** an **axon** and a **dendrite**
   a. **Axons** are typically long and branch infrequently.
      (1) Axon branches are called **collaterals.**
      (2) Axons and their collaterals terminate as **end feet.**
   b. **Dendrites** are typically much shorter than axons and usually branch extensively, forming dendritic trees.

C. **Morphologic types of neurons**

1. Neurons are classed by the configuration of their processes as **unipolar, bipolar,** or **multipolar** (Figure 2-2).

2. The multipolar neurons in particular differ greatly in shape (Figure 2-3).

3. Neurons are also classified by **axon length.**
   a. **Golgi type I neurons** have long axons (see Figure 2-3). The longest axons in the central nervous system (CNS) of humans extend from the cerebral cortex to the caudal tip of the spinal cord, a distance of 50—70 cm.
   b. **Golgi type II neurons** have short axons (see Figure 2-3). The shortest axons terminate only a few micra from the perikaryon.
   c. **Amacrine neurons,** an unusual neuron type, lack axons.

II. FUNCTION OF NEURONS

A. **Nerve impulses.** Neurons communicate by producing and propagating nerve impulses, much like units linked in an electrical circuit.

1. **Stimuli.** A **stimulus** is any change that elicits nerve impulses. Various stimuli activate impulses in resting neurons; for example, **physical** stimuli, such as heat or light, or **chemical** stimuli, such as aromatic or dissolved chemicals that produce taste or smell.

2. **Resting potential.** At rest, a neuron maintains a difference in potential of approximately -50 mV to -80 mV between the inside and outside of its surface membrane. Thus, the neuronal surface is electrically **polarized** in respect to its interior.

3. **Action potential.** If a stimulus excites a site on the neuronal surface, the negative resting potential at that point drops to zero or even overshoots briefly into the positive range. Then, like a falling row of dominoes, a depolarization wave (action potential) propagates along the surface membrane of the neuron.
   a. The term **nerve impulse** describes all of the **biologic** and **electrical events** involved in the passage of a neuronal message.
   b. The term **action potential** describes only the **electrical component** of the nerve impulse.

FIGURE 2-1. Typical components of a multipolar neuron.

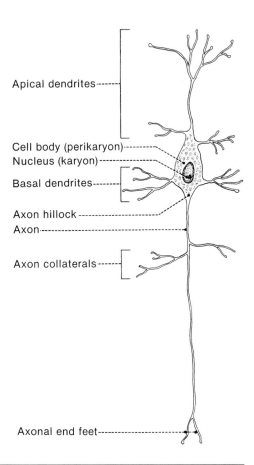

Apical dendrites------

Cell body (perikaryon)---------
Nucleus (karyon)---------
Basal dendrites--------

Axon hillock-----------
Axon------------

Axon collaterals-------

Axonal end feet---------------------

FIGURE 2-2. The three main anatomic types of neurons and their typical locations.

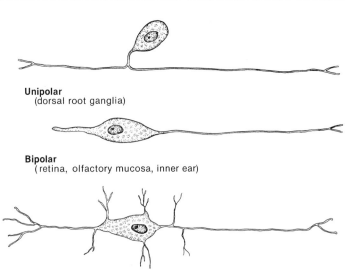

Unipolar
(dorsal root ganglia)

Bipolar
(retina, olfactory mucosa, inner ear)

Multipolar
(CNS and motor ganglia of PNS)

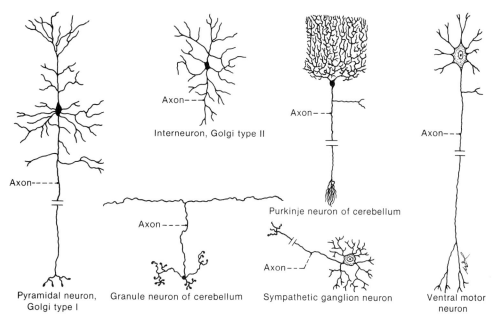

Axon---

Interneuron, Golgi type II

Axon--

Axon--

Axon----

Purkinje neuron of cerebellum

Axon----

Axon--

Pyramidal neuron, Golgi type I

Granule neuron of cerebellum

Sympathetic ganglion neuron

Ventral motor neuron

FIGURE 2-3. Variety of shapes of multipolar neurons.

B. **Directional flow of nerve impulses**

1. Typically, nerve impulses begin **proximally,** with excitation in the dendritic tree or perikaryon of a neuron, and then travel **distally** along the axon to its terminals. Thus, neurons function by **receiving** and **sending** impulses.
   a. **Dendrites** are specialized to **receive** and initiate nerve impulses.
   b. **Axons** are specialized to **convey** nerve impulses **away** from the perikaryon.

2. A single neuron (e.g., a neuron isolated in tissue culture) is functionally useless. To function, a nerve impulse must affect the next cell in line in a circuit.
   a. The next cell in line at the axonal end feet may be another neuron or an effector cell.
   b. **Effector cells** are either:
      (1) Muscle cells (striated, smooth, or cardiac)
      (2) Gland cells

C. **Synapses and neurotransmitters**

1. A **synapse** is the site of functional contact between the axonal membrane of one neuron and the membrane of the neuron or effector cell next in line; thus, synapses are the anatomical basis of interneuronal communication.
   a. **Location and morphologic classification of synapses**
      (1) An axon can synapse on a dendrite of another neuron, on its perikaryon, or less commonly, on its axon hillock or even its axon. Thus, synapses are **axodendritic, axosomatic** (soma means body or perikaryon), and **axoaxonic** (Figure 2-4).
      (2) Some neurons communicate by **dendrodendritic** synapses. This fact tends to blur the classic distinction between axons and dendrites [e.g., the amacrine neurons of the retina (see Figure 9-4) and olfactory bulb lack axons as such].
   b. **Typical synapses** (Figure 2-5) consist of a:
      (1) **Presynaptic membrane** provided by the axonal terminal
      (2) **Synaptic cleft**
      (3) **Postsynaptic membrane** provided by the next cell in line

2. When a nerve impulse arrives at a synapse, it causes the release of a stored chemical into the synaptic cleft (see Figure 2-5).
   a. This chemical unites with chemical **receptors** on the postsynaptic cell and alters the polarity of that cell.

FIGURE 2-4. Axonal end feet on a neuron forming axodendritic, axosomatic (axoperikaryal), and the much rarer axoaxonic synapses.

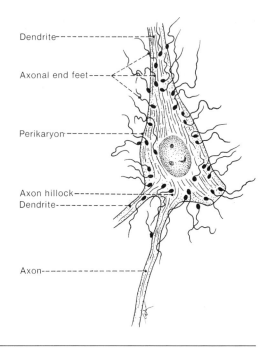

FIGURE 2-5. Diagram of a synapse showing the release of a neurotransmitter; in this case, acetylcholine (ACh).

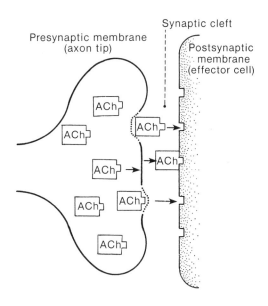

    b. Such chemicals that directly transmit the effect of a stimulus to the next cell are called **neurotransmitters.**

   3. Neurotransmitters are of two types: **excitatory** and **inhibitory.**
    a. Excitatory neurotransmitters tend to excite the next cell by **depolarizing** its membrane. Thus, excitatory neurotransmitters cause a neuron to discharge a nerve impulse or cause an effector, such as a muscle or gland cell, to act.
    b. Inhibitory neurotransmitters tend to **hyperpolarize** the next cell in line. They **inhibit** the production of a new impulse by opposing membrane depolarization. These transmitters cause inhibitory actions, such as slowing of the heart or inhibiting neurons in the CNS that are causing a muscular contraction.

4. CNS neurons, in general, receive thousands of synapses, some excitatory and some inhibitory. Whether a given neuron will generate an impulse or not depends on the algebraic **summation** of the excitatory and inhibitory transmitters acting upon its surface at any particular time.

D. **Polarization of impulse flow**

1. Because dendrites receive impulses and axons send them, nerve impulses normally flow in one direction; that is, to the axonal tip. After a neurotransmitter is released, it acts on the membrane of the next cell, as if the synapse were a one-way valve. This one-way arrangement is called **neuronal polarization** (as contrasted to membrane polarization).

2. Under pathologic or experimental conditions, a neuronal membrane may be **stimulated abnormally;** for example, an experimenter might apply a stimulating electrode halfway along an axon.
   a. A wave of depolarization will sweep in two directions: **distally** toward the axonal tip (orthodromic conduction) and **proximally** toward the perikaryon (antidromic conduction).
   b. The impulse will cross the synapse at the axonal tip but will not cause retrograde stimulation of the synapses on the perikaryon or dendrites made by axons from other neurons. The postsynaptic neuronal membrane at these sites, which is specialized to receive messages, will not release a neurotransmitter to act in the wrong direction.

E. The terms **polar** and **polarization** have been used to:

1. Describe neurons anatomically as **unipolar, bipolar,** or **multipolar**

2. Describe **membrane polarization,** which is the electrical charge across the membrane of the resting neuron (the terms **hyperpolarization** and **depolarization** apply only to membrane polarization)

3. Describe **neuronal polarization** in the sense of the usual one-way transmission of nerve impulses at synapses

F. **Afferent and efferent impulses**

1. The terms **afferent** and **efferent** describe the relative **direction** of impulse flow in neurons and their circuits.
   a. Impulses that flow **from** a designated point on a neuronal membrane or neural circuit are called **efferent.**
   b. Impulses that flow **toward** a designated point on a neuronal membrane or neuronal circuit are called **afferent.**

2. These terms describe nothing about the properties or results of the impulse, only the direction of flow relative to some arbitrarily designated site.

III. FUNCTIONAL CIRCUITS OF NEURONS

A. Based on their **function,** all neurons fall into **three types.**

1. Primary sensory neurons receive stimuli and transmit **afferent** impulses to the CNS.

2. Interneurons (also called internuncial neurons) form **circuits** in the CNS.

3. Primary motoneurons deliver **efferent** impulses from the CNS out through the peripheral nervous system (PNS) to activate effectors.

4. This functional classification reflects the basic plan of the nervous system. Afferent neurons send information into the CNS. In the CNS, countless interneurons integrate the afferent information and ultimately direct the motoneurons to activate **effectors** via the PNS (Figure 2-6).

B. **General characteristics of primary sensory neurons** (afferent neurons)

1. The skin, eyes, ears, tongue, nose, viscera, and skeletomuscular structures contain nerve endings called **receptors,** which are designed to detect various stimuli.

2. The receptor tips may end freely or may become encapsulated by cells to form a sensory **end organ** (see Figure 6-14).

3. **All** primary sensory neurons are **bipolar** or **unipolar** (see Figure 2-2).
   a. **Bipolar** primary sensory neurons occur only in the end organs of the special senses, such as in the retina and in the olfactory, vestibular, and auditory ganglia.
   b. All other primary sensory neurons are **unipolar.**

4. All primary sensory neurons have their **perikarya** located in **ganglia** outside of the CNS, with the major exception of the retina (and a few minor exceptions). Although some specialized CNS cells may respond to internal chemical stimuli, they are not classified as primary sensory neurons.

C. **Characteristics of unipolar primary sensory neurons**

1. The unipolar neurons mediate all general sensation from the **parietes** and **viscera.**

2. The **perikarya** of all unipolar sensory neurons are located in a **dorsal root ganglion** of a spinal nerve or a corresponding ganglion of a cranial nerve.

3. The unipolar process bifurcates into **peripheral** and **central branches.**
   a. The **peripheral** branch runs out through a nerve trunk to the skin, skeletomuscular apparatus, or viscera (Figure 2-7; see Figure 2-2).

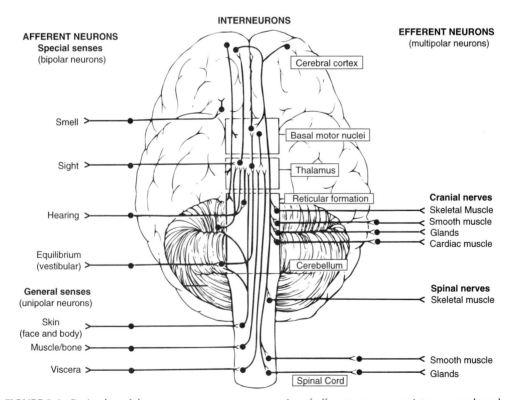

FIGURE 2-6. Basic plan of the nervous system seen as a series of afferent neurons, an interneuronal pool in the brain and spinal cord, and a series of efferent neurons.

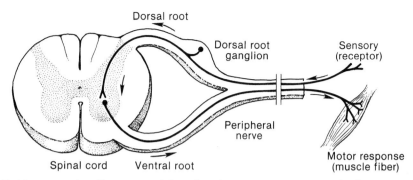

FIGURE 2-7. Monosynaptic reflex arc, consisting of a primary sensory neuron activating a motoneuron by a direct synapse. The motoneuron activates an effector, muscle in this case.

    b. The **central** branch enters the CNS via a dorsal root. It ends on motoneurons, interneurons, or both. Characteristically, the axon branches many times to end on many different CNS neurons.

    c. No primary sensory axon returns to the PNS after entering the CNS.

    d. Both the **peripheral** and **central** processes of unipolar neurons are classified as **axons** because they are long and slender and have few branches (see Figure 2-2).

        (1) The **peripheral** process of a unipolar neuron is **axonal** in structure but **dendritic** in function because it conveys nerve impulses **toward** the perikaryon.

        (2) The **central** process is **axonal** both in structure and function because it conveys nerve impulses **away** from the perikaryon.

D. **Characteristics of interneurons**

    1. With a few exceptions, interneurons are **multipolar.**

    2. Their dendrites and axons remain in the CNS; no interneurons send axons into the PNS.

    3. The **perikarya** and **dendrites** of interneurons, along with **primary motoneurons,** form the **gray matter** of the brain and spinal cord. The number of interneurons greatly exceeds the number of primary sensory neurons and motoneurons combined.

    4. The **axons** of interneurons with their myelin sheaths form most of the **white matter** of the CNS.

E. **Characteristics of primary motoneurons** (efferent neurons)

    1. Primary motoneurons are **multipolar.** Their **perikarya** are located in the **gray matter** of the brain stem or spinal cord (see Chapter 1 III D 2).

    2. Their **axons** exit from the CNS through a ventral root of a spinal nerve or corresponding part of a cranial nerve.

    3. Motoneuron **impulses** reach their effectors **directly** or **indirectly.**

        a. The axons from motoneurons for **skeletal muscle** run uninterruptedly to the muscle cells, forming a **direct, one-neuron pathway.**

        b. The axons from motoneurons for **smooth** and **cardiac muscle** and **glands** synapse first on motor ganglia in the PNS. These **secondary** motoneurons in turn send axons to the effector cells, forming an **indirect, two-neuron pathway** (see Figures 5-1 and 5-5).

F. **Human behavior as expressed through motoneurons to the effectors**

    1. Behavioral psychologists may choose to disregard the mental activity produced by the interneuronal pool of the brain. By ignoring thought processes and emotions, which are private and unobservable, they analyze behavior. **Behavior** per se means any **observable change** produced by neural activation of an effector.

2. Nerve impulses can produce behavior in only two ways:
   a. By causing a **gland** to **secrete** something
   b. By causing **muscle fibers** to **shorten**
      (1) Shortening of muscle fibers may change the diameter of an orifice or internal organ or activate a skeletomuscular lever to change the angle of a joint.
      (2) By stopping the flow of nerve impulses, the nervous system can stop the shortening of muscle fibers, but it cannot actively lengthen them. Lengthening occurs passively, as when the heart refills with blood or when an antagonistic muscle contracts. Thus, after contracting your biceps, you have to straighten the elbow with the triceps or by the action of gravity for the biceps fibers to lengthen again.

3. Thus, all of our behavior consists of secreting substances and shortening muscle fibers.

G. **Reflex arcs**

1. A **reflex** is a reproducible, nearly automatic, neurally mediated response to a stimulus.

2. In **monosynaptic reflexes,** afferent axons of sensory neurons synapse directly on a motoneuron. Excitation of the motoneuron causes a twitch of a muscle fiber or activates a gland (see Figure 2-7).

3. In **polysynaptic reflexes,** one or more interneurons, excitatory or inhibitory, intervene between the afferent impulses and the motoneuron (Figure 2-8). Polysynaptic reflexes may involve a single muscle or the whole body (e.g., when postural reflexes adjust the body to changes in position).

H. **Axonal transport.** The organelles in the perikarya produce most of the energy and conduct most of the metabolism of the neuron. Because the axons lack most of the organelles necessary for cell metabolism, transport mechanisms move critical **metabolic substances** and **neurotransmitters** down the axon.

1. The axonal volume may exceed the perikaryal volume by a ratio of as much as 2000:1 in Golgi type I neurons.

2. Slow and rapid axonal transport mechanisms provide for the flow of materials down the axon from the perikaryon and back up to the perikaryon; dendritic flow also occurs.

3. If metabolic and toxic disorders interfere with the axonal transport mechanisms, metabolites cannot reach the entire axon. The distal tips of the longest axons then suffer, causing a **"dying back" neuropathy.**

FIGURE 2-8. Polysynaptic reflex arc consisting of a primary sensory neuron, a number of interneuronal synapses (N), and a motoneuron to an effector.

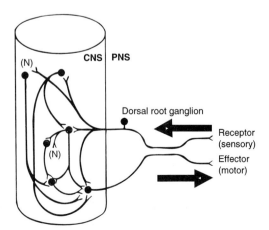

IV. PATHOLOGIC REACTIONS OF NEURONS

A. Doctrine of **selective vulnerability** of neurons

1. Metabolic diversity of neurons

    a. Nerve cells have a greater **diversity** of structure, function, and metabolic characteristics than all of the other cells of the body together.

    b. Each type of neuron is **genetically programmed** in terms of its particular structure and critical metabolic pathways.

        (1) Some neurons produce large quantities of **pigment,** others produce virtually none.

        (2) Some neurons respond to **chemical stimuli,** others respond to **physical stimuli.**

        (3) Some neurons produce **excitatory transmitters,** others produce **inhibitory transmitters.**

2. Selective vulnerability of neurons

    a. Because of metabolic differences, various types of neurons exhibit **differential susceptibility** to **pathogens.**

        (1) Some neurons succumb more quickly to **hypoxia,** others succumb more quickly to **hyperbilirubinemia.**

        (2) Certain **viruses** attack specific groups of neurons (e.g., the poliomyelitis virus prefers motoneurons over all other CNS neurons; herpes zoster prefers dorsal root ganglion neurons).

        (3) Genetic defects may produce types of neurons that lack an enzyme critical for their function. These disorders are called **inborn errors of metabolism.**

    b. Related neurons may undergo **systematized degeneration.**

        (1) If a pathogen selectively affects **retinal neurons,** it causes **blindness;** if it affects **auditory neurons,** it causes **deafness;** if it selects **motoneurons,** it causes **paralysis.**

        (2) In theory, and it is almost proved in reality, a toxic, viral, or genetic disease could exist for each anatomically and metabolically different group of neurons. (This text mentions some of these diseases when various parts of the nervous system are described.)

B. **Neuronal reactions to injury**

1. Wallerian degeneration is the **dissolution** of the **distal** part of an **axon** and its **myelin sheath** that follows transection and separation of the axon from its perikaryon. In fact, any bit of living neuron that is separated from the metabolic machinery in the perikaryon will die (Figure 2-9).

    a. After axonal injury, the axon may also degenerate for varying distances back toward the perikaryon.

    b. Wallerian degeneration of the distal segment of the axon always occurs, but the centripetal degeneration varies. Usually, it extends backward to the first collateral above the transection.

    c. If the axon has no collateral or is severed close to the perikaryon, the whole neuron may die.

    d. Neuroanatomists use Wallerian degeneration to determine the course of axonal pathways. After destroying neuronal perikarya or transecting nerve fibers, the observer can selectively stain degenerating myelin or axoplasm to trace the course of nerve fibers through serial sections to their termination (see VIII D).

2. Chromatolysis. After axonal injury, the neuronal perikaryon shows **cytoplasmic swelling, pallor** of Nissl bodies (endoplasmic reticulum), and **nuclear eccentricity** (Figure 2-10).

    a. The **Nissl bodies** stain less intensely than in the normal neuron, but their endoplasmic reticulum is merely diluted by cytoplasmic swelling, not destroyed.

    b. The **cytoplasmic swelling** also displaces the nucleus to the side of the neuron opposite the axon hillock (**nuclear eccentricity**).

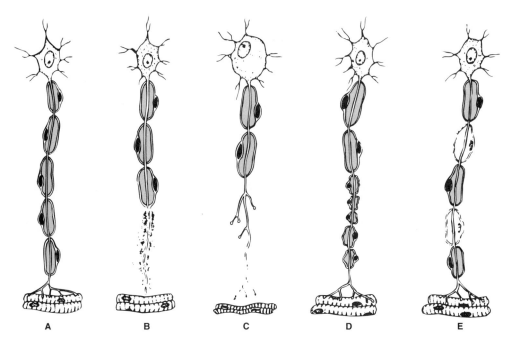

FIGURE 2-9. Wallerian degeneration. (A) Normal neuron with myelinated axon. (B) Degeneration of the axon and myelin sheath distal to its point of transection. (C) Regeneration of the axon after removal of axonal and myelin debris. (D) Irregular remyelination of regenerated axon. (E) Segmental demyelination.

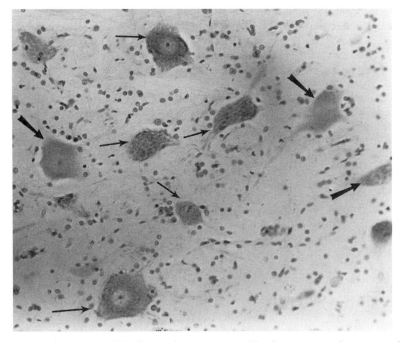

FIGURE 2-10. Microphotograph of Nissl-stained motoneurons. The thin arrows indicate normal motoneuronal perikarya, showing Nissl bodies. The thick arrows indicate motoneuron perikarya undergoing chromatolysis, showing dissolution of Nissl bodies.

3. Regeneration of neurons
   a. Whole, mature neurons, representing the most specialized cells of the body, do not multiply, but do have a limited capacity to regenerate axons after axonal death.
   b. Although the severed distal part of an axon always undergoes Wallerian degeneration, the proximal stump, which still retains contact with the perikaryon, may grow out again from the perikaryon to reestablish synaptic connection with an effector.
       (1) In the PNS, both motor and sensory neurons may regenerate axons and reestablish synaptic connections.
       (2) Although in theory any neuron could regenerate its axon, axons in the human CNS do not regenerate effectively.

4. Transplantation of embryonic neurons. After part of the brain is destroyed, transplanting embryonic tissue of the same type may allow functional regeneration to occur. The moral justification in terms of obtaining tissue from human fetuses, however, remains a troubling issue.

5. Direct neuronal death
   a. Interruption of the metabolic machinery in the perikaryon may cause the neuron to die.
   b. The entire neuron—dendrites, perikaryon, and axon with all its collaterals—dies, but neighboring neurons, including the next neuron in line, generally survive unless the disease also affects them directly.

6. Transsynaptic neuronal death
   a. If one neuron dies, the next neuron in line may undergo **transsynaptic degeneration** if it has no or few other sources of afferent fibers. For example, the retina supplies most of the axons that synapse on the neurons of a nucleus called the **lateral geniculate body.** Transection of the optic nerve, which conveys retinal axons to the geniculate body, results in degeneration of the optic nerve fibers. Denuded of all synapses, the geniculate body neurons undergo transsynaptic degeneration.
   b. Because most CNS neurons have multiple sources of synapses, they do not die after one source is destroyed.
   c. When an axon to a muscle cell dies, the muscle cell will atrophy and die because it has no other source of stimulation, thus illustrating transsynaptic degeneration in the PNS.
   d. Denervated glands may also undergo transsynaptic atrophy and death.

V. NEURON DOCTRINE

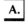
The neuron doctrine of Santiago Ramón y Cajal summarizes neuron structure and function and recapitulates this chapter to this point. The neuron doctrine is a special case of the general theory that the cell is the basic unit of living organisms. The neuron doctrine consists of **six tenets:**

1. Each neuron is an anatomical unit.
   a. A neuron is a cell consisting of a **nucleus,** a **perikaryon,** and **axonal** and **dendritic processes** (see Figure 2-1).
   b. The **perikaryon** and its processes are enclosed by a **continuous membrane** that keeps the neuron anatomically distinct from all other cells and from the extracellular fluid.

2. Each neuron is a genetic unit.
   a. Each neuron develops from an independent embryonic cell called a **neuroblast.**
   b. Each neuron contains a **genetic code,** which specifies its **structure, metabolism,** and **connections.**
   c. Although some variability of connections may result from learning, initially, genetic programming determines the connections of the nervous system.

3. **Each neuron is a functional unit.**
   a. A neuron is the smallest unit capable of receiving a **stimulus** and generating and transmitting a **nerve impulse.**
   b. Each neuron forms a unit in a **communication circuit.** A neuron in isolation, such as one growing in tissue culture, is functionally useless.
   c. **Intercellular communication** between neurons or effectors occurs after a stimulus generates a nerve impulse. The nerve impulse affects the next cell in line through a **synapse.**
      (1) Neurons synapse on other neurons or effectors.
      (2) A **neurotransmitter** released at the synapse transmits the effect of the nerve impulse to the next cell in line (see II C 2).
      (3) The neurotransmitter may **inhibit** (hyperpolarize) or **excite** (depolarize) the next cell in line. Whether any given neuron generates a nerve impulse depends on the algebraic summation of inhibitory and excitatory effects (see II C 3, 4).
   d. A neuron generates a nerve impulse according to an **all or none law;** it either produces an impulse or it does not. The impulse, considered as a depolarization wave, is always the same.

4. **Each neuron is a polarized unit.**
   a. A neuron, when stimulated under normal conditions, conducts nerve impulses in one direction; from dendrite, to perikaryon, to axon, and to the synaptic endings at the axonal tips.
   b. If a stimulus excites a neuronal membrane at a site other than its normal afferent source, the membrane conducts the nerve impulse in both directions from the site of stimulation, but it will transmit impulses to other neurons only at the synapse, which acts as a one-way valve.
   c. The discovery of dendrodendritic synapses and amacrine neurons indicates that the classical, strict dendritic-axonal polarity doctrine does not apply to all neurons.

5. **Each neuron is a pathologic unit.**
   a. Each neuron reacts to injury as a unit. If severely injured, the whole neuron—dendrites, perikaryon, and axon—will die as a cellular unit.
   b. Although each neuron reacts individually to injury, populations of **similar neurons** are **selectively vulnerable** to various toxins, metabolic derangements, viral infections, or genetic defects. This leads to **systematized degeneration** of structurally and metabolically similar neurons in response to specific pathogens or genetic defects.
   c. Any bit of cytoplasm, dendritic or axoplasmic, that is separated from its perikaryon will die, although the remainder of the cell itself may survive. The process of degeneration of an axon and its myelin sheath distal to a site of transection is called **Wallerian degeneration** (see IV B 1).

6. **Each neuron is a regenerative unit.**
   a. Mature neurons generally do not divide, but the perikarya of PNS axons may effectively regenerate motor and sensory axons.
   b. In humans, in general, **severed CNS axons do not effectively regenerate.** Axons may regenerate in the PNS if their perikaryon remains intact.

B. **Summary of the neuron doctrine.** The neuron is the **anatomical, genetic, functional, polarized, pathologic,** and **regenerative** unit of the nervous system.

VI. SUPPORTING TISSUES OF THE NERVOUS SYSTEM

A. **Functions.** Because of their specialization and unique role in intercellular communication, neurons cannot also support and maintain the structural integrity of the nervous system. Therefore, supporting tissues are needed to:

1. **Provide a scaffolding** to keep the neurons in place and hold them in synaptic contact

2. **Produce protective coverings,** such as the skull and meninges, which absorb and distribute blows

3. **Produce fluids,** such as **intercellular** and **cerebrospinal fluid (CSF)** that coat, support, protect, and nourish neurons

4. **Form a blood-neuronal (blood-brain) barrier**

5. **Proliferate to form scars** to heal the nervous tissue after injury

6. **Produce myelin sheaths**

B. **Classification.** The body contains two main types of supporting tissue: **fibrous connective tissue** and **glia.**

1. The **PNS** contains only **fibrous connective tissue.**

2. Within the **CNS** proper, all of the connective tissue consists of **glia.** However, fibrous connective tissue forms coverings around the CNS called **meninges** and accompanies the larger blood vessels that penetrate the CNS.

3. **Fibrous connective tissue consists of:**
   a. Fibrocytes
   b. Collagen and elastic fibrils
   c. Intercellular fluid
   d. Miscellaneous types of cells, including Schwann cells, in peripheral nerves

4. **Glial connective tissue** consists only of cells and intercellular fluid. It contains no extracellular fibrils and relatively little extracellular fluid.
   a. Glial cells. **Glia** consist of **astrocytes, oligodendrocytes, microglia,** and **ependyma.** The glia differ in location, size, shape, and function (Table 2-1).
      (1) **Ependymal cells** form simple columnar epithelium, which lines the ventricular cavities and central canal of the spinal cord. Ependymal cells have the simplest contours of any of the glia.

TABLE 2-1. Types of Glial Cells, Their Locations and Normal Functions

Cell Type	Location	Normal Function
Astroglia (astrocytes)		
Protoplasmic	Gray matter (perineuronal satellites)	Provide supportive scaffolding for the CNS, barrier end feet on vessels and
Fibrous	White matter	meninges; function as extracellular space of the CNS and control ionic balances; scavenge and bind to neurotransmitter molecules; modulate neuronal metabolism and polarization
Oligodendroglia	Gray matter (perineuronal satellites) White matter (interfascicular oligodendroglia)	Modulate neuronal function by influencing their metabolism or polarization Membranes surround the axons to form myelin sheaths in the CNS; Schwann cells form myelin sheaths in the PNS
Microglia	Perineuronal satellites Diffuse in white matter but concentrated around blood vessels	Modulate neuronal function by influencing their metabolism or polarization; form macrophages (also from blood monocytes); act as antigen presenters for the CNS immune system
Ependyma	Line cavities of the CNS	Serve as an epithelial barrier between CNS tissue and the CSF within the CNS cavities; act to control volume, secretion, and composition of the CSF

CNS = Central nervous system; CSF = cerebrospinal fluid.

> **(2) Astrocytes, oligodendroglia,** and **microglia** have complicated, branched contours (Figure 2-11).
> **b. Perineuronal satellite cells**
> **(1)** Three types of glial cells, **astrocytes, oligodendroglia,** and **microglia,** send processes that contact the membrane of neuronal perikarya in the CNS (Figure 2-12).
> **(2)** Although these contacts are not known to function as actual synapses, they may influence neurons by transferring metabolites.

C. **Blood-brain barrier and extracellular space in the CNS**

1. Aniline dyes, when injected into the blood stream, stain almost all organs and tissues except the CNS. Apart from a few tiny regions, the CNS remains uncolored (i.e., the dye does not penetrate the CNS from the blood).

2. We now know that some substances—oxygen, carbon dioxide, glucose, and certain amino acids—enter the CNS readily from the blood, whereas barrier mechanisms exclude other substances, particularly large molecules like proteins.

3. This **blood-brain barrier** may provide for active transport of some molecules and passive diffusion or active rejection of other molecules.

4. The **anatomical structures** that collectively form a barrier between the blood and brain include the following:
  a. Capillary endothelium (The endothelial cells of CNS capillaries have very tight junctions that oppose the passage of some substances.)
  b. Vessel walls

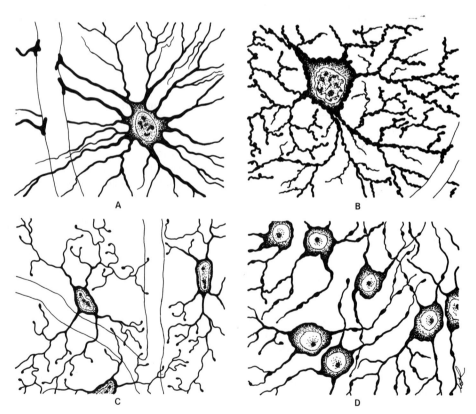

FIGURE 2-11. Branched glial cells. (A) Fibrous astrocyte. (B) Protoplasmic astrocyte. (C) Microgliocyte. (D) Oligodendrocyte.

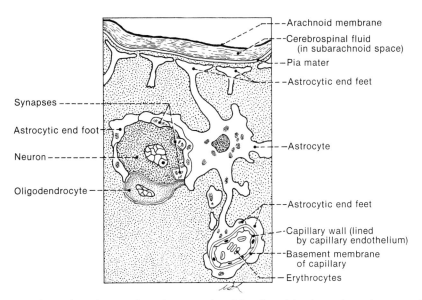

FIGURE 2-12. Relationship of astrocytic processes to the pial surface, blood vessels, and neurons. (Adapted with permission from De Robertis E, Gershenfeld HM: Submicroscopic morphology and function of glial cells. In *International Review of Neurobiology,* vol 3. Edited by Pfeiffer CC, Smythies JR. New York, Academic Press, 1961, p 20.)

   c. **Astrocytic end feet** (see Figure 2-12)

     (1) End feet of astrocytes form a **continuous covering** on the **external capillary wall.** Electron microphotographs of fixed (dead) tissue show that only very narrow extracellular spaces exist between the surface membranes of the astrocytes, other glia, and neurons and contiguous connective tissue. Just how much extracellular space exists during life and whether the astrocyte cytoplasm forms a functional "extracellular" space for the CNS remains unsettled.

     (2) Because the **astrocytic end feet** form a continuous covering on the blood vessels, they form part of the **blood-brain barrier.**

   d. **Perineuronal satellite cells** consist of oligodendroglia, microglia, and astrocytes. All glia contacting the neuronal surface may act to transmit or exclude specific substances from the neuronal surface membrane. How the satellite cells modulate neuronal activity remains unclear.

   e. **Glycoprotein and sialic acid** form the **surface covering** of the **neuronal membrane** and are the final possible components of the blood-brain barrier. Thus, the physical and chemical properties of the neuronal membrane may constitute the final censor of what will affect the firing of a neuron. In this sense, the barrier would best be called a **blood-neuronal barrier,** but blood-brain is the conventional term.

  5. The **blood-brain barrier functions** to make the **neuronal surface** a privileged site. It excludes extraneous substances, ensuring that only the appropriately released neurotransmitters and appropriate modulating substances will attach to receptors to control the polarization of neuronal membranes.

  6. Under **pathologic conditions,** the blood-brain barrier breaks down and substances normally excluded, such as fluid or metabolites from the CSF or blood, can leak into the CNS.

   a. The ensuing state of neuronal intoxication may inhibit or excite neuronal discharges.

   b. The accumulation of fluid in the cells, a state called **edema,** may impair cellular function or rupture cells and cause cell death.

VII. HISTOLOGIC METHODS FOR IDENTIFYING CELLS OF THE NERVOUS SYSTEM

A. Visualization techniques for microscopy

1. **Overview.** Neuroanatomists use numerous methods to selectively visualize particular tissue elements and their alterations induced by natural diseases, surgical lesions, or chemical reactions. Many visualization methods use true dyes, while other methods do not, although all are generically referred to as **staining.**

2. Various methods of fixation, embedding, and mordanting alter the affinity of the tissue components for the dyes or other agents used. By altering the processing and staining technique, the investigator can select one cell type or one tissue element (e.g., axons or myelin sheaths) for visualization, causing it to stand out against the background (see Figure 4-2). Alternately, the investigator can apply an all-purpose stain that colors most of the tissue components.

B. Types of stains using true dyes

1. **Nissl cellular stains.** Basic aniline dyes, such as **hematoxylin,** have a selective affinity for the nuclei of cells and for Nissl substance in the cytoplasm [deoxyribonucleic acid (DNA) and ribonucleic acid (RNA)]. These dyes demonstrate the location and arrangement of neuronal and glial perikarya but do not show dendrites, axons, or myelin sheaths (see Figures 2-10 and 3-9).

2. **All purpose stain.** The addition of a second dye, eosin, with hematoxylin—the **Ehrlich hematoxylin and eosin (H&E) stain**—results in hematoxylin staining the nuclei and Nissl bodies and eosin staining the remaining tissue. It is used extensively by pathologists for surveying slides for diagnostic purposes, but does not differentiate the individual tissue elements.

3. **Myelin sheath staining**
   a. **Iron-hematoxylin method.** Mordanting tissue with iron salts reduces the affinity of hematoxylin for nucleic acid and enhances its affinity for myelin sheaths, which then stand out against an unstained background (Figure 4-2D).
   b. **Luxol fast blue** also selectively stains myelin.

C. Other methods for visualizing neural elements. These include metallic impregnation, enzyme histochemistry, immunohistochemistry, radioactive tracers, and autoradiography.

1. **Metallic impregnation.** Several heavy metals, notably silver, gold, and osmium, enhance tissue components because of their property of precipitating on membranes; they precipitate on the surface membranes of cells or fibers or on the membranous organelles inside the cell.
   a. **Osmium** is deposited on cell membranes for **electron microscopy.**
   b. **Silver** is deposited on cell membranes for **light microscopy.**
      (1) Silver readily undergoes reduction when exposed to oxidizing agents or light, causing it to precipitate on membranes or other surfaces. For these reasons silver is used in photographic and radiographic film and to make mirrors by precipitation on a glass surface.
      (2) Varying the fixatives, reducing agent, or conditions of exposure of the tissue to silver salts will cause the silver ion to precipitate on specific tissue elements. By varying these factors, the examiner can cause the silver to selectively impregnate the various glial cells, neurons and axons, degenerating axoplasm, or fibrous connective tissue (Table 2-2).

2. **Histochemical reactions**
   a. **Enzyme histochemistry** involves exposing the tissue to an enzymatic substrate. The end product then can be stained to visualize the location of the enzyme. This method can display perikarya and certain neurotransmitters.
   b. **Autoradiography** of tissue slices will disclose the location of cells that metabolize or take up specific radioactive substrates.

TABLE 2-2. Metallic Impregnation Methods for Demonstrating Neural Elements by Light Microscopy

Element to be Demonstrated	Originator and Method
Normal axons	Bodian protagarol method
	Ramón y Cajal neurofibrillary impregnation
	Hortega neurofibrillary impregnation
	Glees neurofibrillary impregnation
	Bielschowsky neurofibrillary impregnation
Degenerating axons	Nauta-Gygax silver impregnation method
Astrocytes	Ramón y Cajal gold chloride sublimate
	Hortega silver impregnation method (I)
Micorglia/oligodendroglia	Hortega silver impregnation method (II)
Entire individual neurons	Golgi silver impregnation method
Reticulin	Laidlaw silver impregnation for reticulin

3. **Immunologic methods.** Specific antibodies attach to and allow differentiation of the various glial cells and of specific types of neurons and receptors. Antibodies also differentiate various neoplasms of neural tissue.

4. **Fluorescent microscopy.** Fluorescent methods identify a large population of catecholaminergic neurons and their axons, which other methods of visualization fail to show.

VIII. METHODS FOR TRACING NERVE TRACTS

A. **Gross dissection.** Many of the larger tracts can be followed by gross dissection along the fiber pathways (see Figure 12-5).

B. **Phylogenetic comparison.** Certain tracts stand out very clearly in some animals and may show an increase or decrease in size depending on the phylogenetic rank of the animal.

C. **Embryologic methods**

1. **Silver impregnation for axons (neurofibrillary impregnation).** The outgrowth and ultimate connections of axons may be directly observed in embryos of successive ages subjected to silver impregnation for axons. The method works best for tracts that appear early, before other pathways grow out and cause confusion when axons from many sources intermingle.

2. **Myelination.** Tracts that myelinate early can be visualized with myelin stains before adjacent tracts myelinate (see Figure 3-23).

3. **The Golgi method.** A special silver impregnation recipe causes entire cells—perikarya, dendrites, and axonal processes—to stand out against an unstained background (see Figure 13-32B). Although best applied to an immature CNS, it also works with the mature CNS.

D. **Wallerian (anterograde) degeneration.** Some methods use Wallerian degeneration to trace nerve tracts that have been selectively transected experimentally in animals or by natural disease in humans (see IV B 1).

1. **Axonal degeneration methods**
   a. The **silver method** of Nauta-Gygax selectively impregnates degenerating axoplasm without staining normal axons, giving a **positive trail** of the degenerating tract.

   b. Silver impregnation of degenerative synaptic end feet shows the sites of synaptic termination of a severed tract.

2. Myelin degeneration methods
   a. The Marchi method. Osmic acid reacts with degenerating myelinated fibers so that they show up against an unstained background, giving a **positive trail** of the degenerating tract.
   b. Iron-hematoxylin method. After a myelinated tract has degenerated, iron-hematoxylin staining shows the surrounding intact myelinated fibers, while the tract in question stands out as an unstained void, giving a **negative trail** of the tract.

E. Nuclear reaction methods

   1. Nissl chromatolysis method. After transection of a tract, the perikarya of origin of the axons can be identified by chromatolysis (see IV B 2; see Figure 2-10).

   2. Gudden method. After transection of a tract of axons, the nuclear group of origin may undergo complete (retrograde) degeneration. Nissl staining then shows a void of neurons at the site of the perikarya that originate the tract. The method works best in immature animals.

F. Injection-tracer methods. Neuronal perikarya will take up some substances injected nearby or directly into them. Intracellular transport mechanisms then distribute the substance through the neuronal perikarya, dendrites, and axons. The substance can be seen by microscopy either directly, after the tissue is subjected to a chemical reaction, or by radioactivity.

   1. Horseradish peroxidase, when injected around the perikarya or axonal terminals, is picked up by the neuron and distributed to all of its processes. An enzymatic reaction then permits visualization of the peroxidase in the axons and dendrites of individual perikarya.

   2. Fluorescence microscopy demonstrates a dye, **procion yellow,** absorbed by neurons and distributed into their processes.

   3. Autoradiography of tissue slices demonstrates radioactive substances introduced into neuronal perikarya and distributed into their processes.

G. Electrophysiologic methods for tracing pathways

   1. Evoked action potentials induced by stimulating neurons can be detected by placing recording electrodes along the course of a tract.

   2. Alternatively, stimulating a tract enables retrograde (antidromic) evoked potentials to be recorded at the site of the perikarya of origin.

   3. Clinicians can stimulate visual, auditory, or somatosensory afferents and record the evoked potentials from surface electrodes placed along the course of the pathway or on the scalp, over the relevant sensorimotor cortex (see Figure 8-3). The clinician can then objectively judge whether the sensory pathway is intact or interrupted in an unconscious patient or malingerer.

STUDY QUESTIONS

DIRECTIONS: Each of the numbered items or incomplete statements in this section is followed by answers or by completions of the statement. Select the ONE lettered answer or completion that is BEST in each case.

1. Which tenet of the classic neuron doctrine has been questioned most by new evidence?

(A) The neuron is a genetic unit
(B) The neuron is a pathologic unit in reacting to disease
(C) The neuron is a regenerative unit in regard to regrowth of axons
(D) The neuron is a polarized unit
(E) The neuron is an anatomical unit

2. Which of the following statements about synapses is true?

(A) Synapses are more common on axons than dendrites
(B) Synapses usually act by transmitting electrical messages across the gap
(C) Synapses typically permit the two-way transmission of nerve impulses
(D) Synapses may excite or inhibit the next cell in line
(E) Synapses characteristically consist of a pre- and postsynaptic membrane, one of which is derived from a glial cell

3. The ultimate function of the blood-brain barrier is to

(A) exclude small molecules such as O_2 and CO_2
(B) actively transport large protein molecules
(C) exclude white blood cells
(D) control the ingress of cholesterol into myelin
(E) protect the polarization of the neuronal membrane

4. The term Wallerian degeneration describes

(A) dissolution of a severed axon and its myelin sheath
(B) nuclear eccentricity
(C) pallor of Nissl substance
(D) systematized degeneration of related groups of neurons
(E) transsynaptic degeneration of neurons or muscle fibers

DIRECTIONS: Each of the numbered items or incomplete statements in this section is negatively phrased, as indicated by a capitalized word such as NOT, LEAST, or EXCEPT. Select the ONE lettered answer or completion that is BEST in each case.

5. All of the following statements about glia are true EXCEPT

(A) astrocytes provide a structural scaffolding for neurons
(B) oligodendrocytes produce myelin sheaths
(C) microglia are one type of perineuronal satellite cell
(D) ependymal cells are highly branched
(E) glia serve in place of the fibrous connective tissue of other organs

6. All of the following constitute effector cells that produce behavior directly when activated EXCEPT for

(A) skeletal muscle cells
(B) cardiac muscle cells
(C) glial cells
(D) gland cells
(E) smooth muscle cells

DIRECTIONS: Each set of matching questions in this section consists of a list of four to twenty-six lettered options followed by several numbered items. For each numbered item, select the appropriate lettered option(s). Each lettered option may be selected once, more than once, or not at all. EACH ITEM WILL STATE THE NUMBER OF OPTIONS TO SELECT. CHOOSE EXACTLY THIS NUMBER.

Questions 7–10

For each description, choose the corresponding cell.

(A) Amacrine neuron
(B) Astrocyte
(C) Oligodendroglia
(D) Ependymal cell
(E) Golgi type I neuron
(F) Golgi type II neuron
(G) Bipolar neuron
(H) Schwann cell
(I) Multipolar neuron
(J) Chromatolytic neuron
(K) Microglia

7. Cell in which the axonal volume may greatly exceed the volume of the perikaryon (SELECT 1 CELL)

8. Perineuronal satellite cells that nourish neurons and protect their surfaces (SELECT 3 CELLS) B C, K

9. Neurons classified by axonal length (SELECT 3 CELLS) A E F

10. Glial cells that have multiple branches (SELECT 3 CELLS) B, C, F

ANSWERS AND EXPLANATIONS

1. The answer is D [V A 4 c]. Neuroscientists generally accept the original neuron doctrine advocated by Ramón y Cajal, but newer information has modified some of the tenets. The demonstration of a number of dendrodendritic contacts in the nervous system, which appear to be synapses, has modified the law of strict polarity of neurons, which requires that impulses flow only from dendrites to axons. Some neurons (e.g., amacrine neurons) have only dendritic processes without axons. Nevertheless, for the majority of neurons, the original tenets of the neuron doctrine are generally true.

2. The answer is D [II C 1, 2, 3]. Synapses typically consist of a presynaptic membrane from an axonal terminal, a postsynaptic membrane from a dendrite or perikaryon, and an intervening synaptic cleft. Synapses typically transmit nerve impulses by releasing a chemical substance into the synaptic cleft between the two membranes. The released neurotransmitter may excite or inhibit the next cell in line when it attaches to a receptor on the postsynaptic membrane.

3. The answer is E [VI C 5]. The blood-brain barrier allows selective permeability of substances from the blood. Although it excludes red blood cells, under pathological conditions, white blood cells can penetrate the barrier. The ultimate function of the blood-brain barrier is to protect the surface membrane of the neuron. Many substances might enter the central nervous system (CNS) from the blood that could alter the electrical potential of the neuronal membrane, causing the neuron to function inappropriately. The neuron should discharge only in response to the orderly and appropriate release of neurotransmitters at its synaptic contacts. Otherwise, communication between neurons would be chaotic.

4. The answer is A [IV B 1; Figure 2-9]. Whenever a bit of cytoplasm is separated from the metabolic machinery of the perikaryon, that cytoplasm dies. The axon, a long extrusion of the neuronal membrane, is especially vulnerable because of its length. After transection of an axon, the entire distal part of the axon degenerates and its myelin sheath dissolves (Wallerian degeneration). The proximal stump of the axon, still attached to its perikaryon, may regenerate under some circumstances.

Regeneration is most successful in the peripheral nervous system (PNS). Neuroanatomists can selectively stain degenerating axoplasm or myelin to trace axonal pathways through the central nervous system (CNS) and PNS. Much of what we know about neuronal circuitry comes from the study of Wallerian degeneration.

5. The answer is D [VI B; Table 2-1]. Glial cells replace the fibrous connective tissue of other organs. They serve numerous functions. Ependymal cells are simple columnar or cuboidal epithelium that line the cavities of the central nervous system (CNS), rather than exhibiting numerous branches. The astrocytes produce a scaffolding and contribute end feet to the blood-brain barrier and brain-cerebrospinal fluid (CSF) barrier. In the CNS, oligodendrocytes produce myelin sheaths, which act like insulators for axons. In the peripheral nervous system (PNS), Schwann cells produce myelin. The perineuronal satellite glia may act to provide nourishment or metabolites or to influence neurotransmission or membrane polarity.

6. The answer is C [III F 1, 2]. Effector cells are the cells that ultimately respond to nerve impulses to produce behavior. The effectors are either gland cells or one of the three types of muscle cells—smooth, cardiac, or skeletal. The only behaviors that the nervous system can produce are to shorten muscle fibers and to cause glands to secrete. The basis of the clinical neurologic examination is an orderly set of rules for observing spontaneous and elicited behavior. The clinician uses commands and many reflexes to elicit behavior and "thinks through" the neuronal pathways to analyze whether the neural circuits work or not. The end point of each designated test or observation involves a defined response of an effector. For example, the clinician tests for pupillary reaction to light. The light is the stimulus and the constriction of the pupil is the designated and observed behavioral end point.

7. The answer is: E [I C 3 a; III H 1]. The Golgi type I neurons all have long axons that may exceed the perikaryal volume by a ratio of 2000:1. The longest Golgi type I axons in the central nervous system (CNS) extend from the pyramidal neurons of the motor cortex to the caudal end of the spinal cord. The longest axons of the peripheral nervous system (PNS) extend from the motoneurons of the spinal cord gray matter of the caudal end of the spinal cord to the muscles of the feet. In whales and giraffes, axonal lengths are measured in meters. The organelles of the perikaryon manufacture nutrients and neurotransmitters that are conveyed to the distal tip of the axon by active transport systems.

8. The answers are: B, C, K [VI B 4 b]. Neurons require special nutrients and carefully regulated ionic concentrations inside and outside their membranes to function. Perineuronal satellite cells in the central nervous system (CNS) cover, nourish, and protect the surface membrane of each neuron, making it a privileged site that is protected by the blood-neuronal barrier system. Whatever reaches the surface of the neuronal membrane may affect membrane polarity and, thus, neuronal function. The satellite cells ensure that only properly regulated substances, liberated appropriately by nerve impulses, affect neuronal activity.

9. The answers are: A, E, F [I C 3]. Neurons can be classified anatomically by many different characteristics, including size, shape, degree of branching, and length of processes. Axonal length is one important criterion because axons are the communication branch of most neurons. However, neurons vary greatly in respect to axon length. Amacrine neurons, which are an unusual neuronal type, have no axons and presumably communicate by dendrodendritic contacts. Golgi type I neurons produce lengthy axons. The named tracts of the central nervous system (CNS) consist of Golgi type I axons. Golgi type II neurons, with short axons, comprise most of the internuncial neurons of the CNS.

10. The answers are: B, C, K [VI B 4 a]. Almost all cells of the nervous system, neurons and glia, have multiple branches. Neurons have dendrites and axons, whereas glial cells send processes that cover the surfaces of the pia, blood vessels, and neurons. The ependymal cells, which are the cuboidal or columnar epithelial glia that line the ventricles and central canal of the spinal cord, have only a single tail that extends from the base of the cell into the neural tissue.

Chapter 3

Embryology of the Nervous System

I. BASIC MECHANISMS OF MORPHOGENESIS

A. **Stages of morphogenesis.** For convenience, morphogenesis can be divided into three stages: **cytogenesis, histogenesis,** and **organogenesis** (Table 3-1).

B. **Configurations adopted by developing cells.** Developing cells assume only a few configurations that may then vary greatly in detail:

1. Solid or hollow balls

2. Sheets or layers on or beneath surfaces

3. Nodular masses or protrusions

4. Rod-like masses, which may remain solid or canalize

5. Tubes, which may then evaginate or fold over on themselves

C. **Embryonic development.** The human embryonic disk and the embryo that develops from it show the sequence of cytogenesis, histogenesis, and organogenesis and display the basic cell configurations.

1. **Origin of the embryonic disk** (cytogenesis to histogenesis) [Figure 3-1]
   a. The fertilized ovum multiplies to form a solid, berry-like ball called a **morula.**
   b. The morula forms a fluid-filled ball called a **blastocyst.**
   c. Cells at one pole of the blastocyst multiply to form a **polar mass,** or **inner cell mass.**
   d. The polar mass secretes additional fluid, which separates it from the surface cells, forming a partition called the **embryonic disk.** This disk becomes the embryo proper.

2. **Origin of the three basic embryonic layers in the embryonic disk** (histogenesis)
   a. By proliferation, differentiation, and orientation of its cells, the embryonic disk forms into three layers: the **ectoderm, mesoderm,** and **entoderm** (see Figure 3-1). The ectoderm and entoderm are sheets of cells on the dorsal and ventral surfaces of the mesoderm, respectively. The mesoderm is sandwiched in the middle.
   b. The **ectodermal layer** becomes the epidermis and the neural tube.
   c. The **mesodermal layer** produces bone, muscle, fibrous connective tissue, the circulatory system, and much of the genitourinary tract.
   d. The **entodermal layer** becomes the gastrointestinal tube and its appendages and the lungs.

II. DEVELOPMENT OF THE EXTERNAL CONTOUR OF THE NEURAXIS (ORGANOGENESIS)

A. **Major organogenetic events of the neuraxis [central nervous system (CNS)]**

1. The **fundamental event** in organogenesis of the neuraxis is that the monolayer of ectodermal cells rolls up to form the **neural tube.** Thus, the neuraxis commences as a tube and remains a tube, although subsequent events expand some of its regions and cause it to fold into its final form.

2. The organogenetic events consist of:
   a. **Closure** of the neural tube (neurulation)
   b. **Transverse segmentation** of the neural tube
   c. **Evagination** of the neural tube walls

TABLE 3-1. Three Stages of Morphogenesis

Cytogenesis
Formation of gametes by mitosis and meiosis, followed by fertilization
Cell multiplication at proper time and site
Cell differentiation into various parenchymal and supporting cells
Programmed death of certain cell populations (apoptosis)
Histogenesis
Orientation of cells to each other and their supporting tissues
Establishment of intercellular contacts (synapses)
Migration of cell populations
Blending of migrating, multiplying, and differentiating parenchymal and connective tissue cells, and blood vessels, into tissues
Organogenesis
Blending of tissues into organs
Shaping of the external contour of organs
Shaping of the internal contour of organs
Growth to complete the somatotype of the individual

FIGURE 3-1. Development of an ovum into a morula, blastocyst, and embryonic disk, with lamination of the latter into ectoderm, mesoderm, and entoderm.

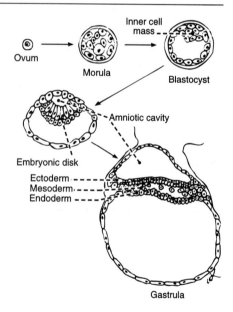

d. **Flexion** of the neural tube
e. **Protrusion** of masses (e.g., cerebellum, olivary eminences, quadrigeminal bodies)
f. **Fissuring** and **sulcation** of the cerebrum and cerebellum
g. **Growth** to adult size

B. **Neurulation or closure: formation of the neural tube.** Although neurulation and the other organogenetic events proceed simultaneously, this text, for conceptual simplicity, describes these events as if they occurred separately.

1. Neural organogenesis begins when the **primitive streak** and **primitive node** appear in the sagittal plane along the dorsal aspect of the embryonic disk (Figure 3-2A).

2. Next, a median **neural groove** flanked by **neural folds** appears in the sagittal plane of the embryonic disk (Figure 3-3).

3. Then, the dorsal margins of the neural folds **close** or **fuse** (see Figures 3-2 and 3-3).
   a. The fusion of the neural folds allows the neural tube to separate from the remainder of the surface ectoderm.
   b. The neural folds first close in the lower cervical and upper thoracic regions. From that site, the closure of the neural folds proceeds rostrally and caudally (see Figures 3-2C and 3-2D).
   c. Figures 3-2C and 3-2D show the incompletely closed ends of the neural tube. These ends, called the **anterior** and **posterior neuropores**, finally fuse so that the neural tube resembles an elongated balloon.

4. **Neurulation** completes the transformation from a single cell, to a ball of cells, to a sheet of cells, to a tube of cells. The neuraxis now is a simple, fluid-filled, elongated tube sealed at the ends. Neurulation can be easily simulated by rolling up a piece of paper into a tube and squeezing the ends together.

5. Failure of the tube to close properly at any site from the anterior to the posterior neuropore is called **dysraphism,** which is a relatively common type of congenital

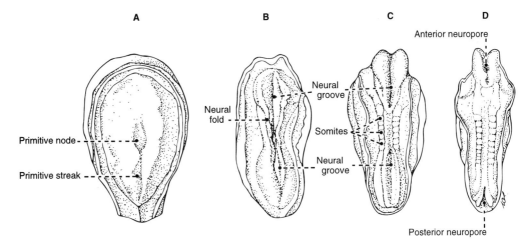

FIGURE 3-2. Dorsal view of the embryonic disk showing elevation and fusion of the neural folds to form the neural tube. (Adapted with permission from Streeter GL: Factors involved in the formation of the filum terminalis. *Am J Anat* 25:1–11, 1919.)

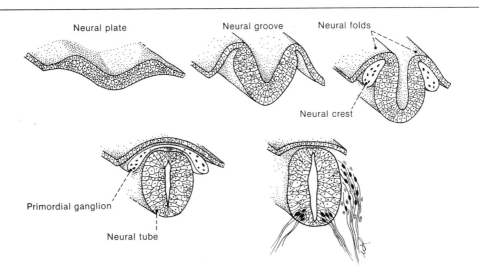

FIGURE 3-3. Formation of the neural tube by closure or fusion of its dorsal lips and sequestration from the surface ectoderm.

malformation. Various degrees and sites of dysraphism are called **myelomeningo-cele, encephalocele,** and **anencephaly.**

C. **Transverse subdivisions of the neural tube** proceed as the neuropores close (Figure 3-4).

1. Transverse segmentation first creates three transverse subdivisions of the brain: the forebrain, midbrain, and hindbrain.

2. The first and third units then segment into two each, making five final brain units.

3. The midbrain and spinal cord do not undergo further transverse subdivision.

4. The original fluid-filled lumen of the neural tube remains throughout its length.

D. **Evagination of the neural tube walls**

1. **Evagination** begins as **closure** and **transverse segmentation** proceed.
   a. Evagination involves the outpouching of a local part of the neural tube wall.
   b. The lumen of the neural tube extends out into the evaginations. See the development of the telencephalon in Figures 3-4 and 3-5.

2. Evagination produces the **pineal body, hypophysis, optic stalks,** and the **cerebral hemispheres** themselves and their evaginations, the **temporal lobes** and **olfactory stalks** (see Figure 3-5).
   a. Figure 3-5, a **lateral** view of the neuraxis, shows that the evaginations come only from the forebrain (the forebrain or prosencephalon comprises the diencephalon and telencephalon).
   b. Although Figure 3-5 depicts **evagination** as occurring after **closure** and **segmentation,** it actually begins before these events are complete.

3. **The pineal body** evaginates dorsally in the median plane at the diencephalic-midbrain junction (see Figure 3-5, 1).

4. **The hypophysis (pituitary gland)**
   a. The **neurohypophysis (posterior pituitary)** evaginates **ventrally** in the median plane near the junction of the diencephalon with the midbrain (see Figure 3-5, 2).
   b. The neurohypophysis meets another evagination, **Rathke's pouch,** which comes from the roof of the mouth. Rathke's pouch becomes the **adenohypophysis (anterior pituitary)** [see Figure 3-5, 3].
   c. The stalk of the neurohypophysis remains continuous with the neuraxis. The adenohypophyseal stalk atrophies. Thus, the adenohypophysis loses its connection with its origin.

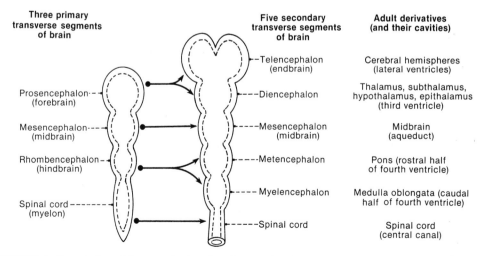

Three primary transverse segments of brain	Five secondary transverse segments of brain	Adult derivatives (and their cavities)
	Telencephalon (endbrain)	Cerebral hemispheres (lateral ventricles)
Prosencephalon (forebrain)	Diencephalon	Thalamus, subthalamus, hypothalamus, epithalamus (third ventricle)
Mesencephalon (midbrain)	Mesencephalon (midbrain)	Midbrain (aqueduct)
Rhombencephalon (hindbrain)	Metencephalon	Pons (rostral half of fourth ventricle)
	Myelencephalon	Medulla oblongata (caudal half of fourth ventricle)
Spinal cord (myelon)	Spinal cord	Spinal cord (central canal)

FIGURE 3-4. Dorsal view of the neural tube after closure, showing transverse segmentation into three and then five gross divisions.

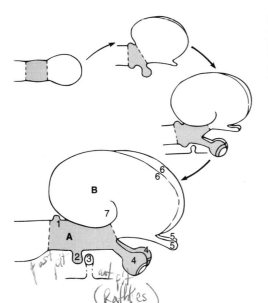

FIGURE 3-5. Lateral view of the forebrain. (*A*) The diencephalon and (*B*) telencephalon with the evaginations numbered. (*1*) Pineal body. (*2*) Neurohypophysis. (*3*) Adenohypophysis. (*4*) Optic bulb. (*5*) Olfactory stalks and bulbs. (*6*) Cerebral hemispheres. (*7*) Temporal lobe.

5. The optic evaginations

    a. The **optic stalks** evaginate from the diencephalon **ventrally** in the median plane and bifurcate (see Figure 3-5, 4). The pineal body and neurohypophysis, which also evaginate in the median plane, do not bifurcate.

    b. The optic stalks produce the **retinas** at their distal ends and conduct the retinal axons into the diencephalon, thus forming the **optic nerves** (see Figure 9-11).

        (1) Like the neurohypophysis, the optic stalks remain in continuity with the CNS. Thus, the olfactory, optic, and neurohypophyseal stalks originate from the neuraxis and remain continuous with it.

        (2) Being evaginations of the brain wall, the **optic nerves** have glial supporting cells. The myelin of the optic nerves comes from oligodendroglia. Hence, the demyelinating diseases that affect the CNS, such as multiple sclerosis, may affect the optic nerves. Conversely, the diseases that affect the true peripheral nerves spare the optic nerve.

        (3) The term **optic nerve** is thus a misnomer embryologically, histologically, and pathologically.

    c. The original neural tube lumen that extended into the pineal, neurohypophyseal, optic, and olfactory evaginations obliterates during maturation.

6. Cerebral hemispheres

    a. Two evaginations, the **cerebral hemispheres**, extend laterally from the telencephalon (see Figures 3-4 and 3-5, 6).

    b. The fissure between the cerebral hemispheres is the **interhemispheric fissure**.

    c. The two olfactory bulbs (see Figure 3-5, 5) and the temporal lobes (see Figure 3-5, 7) can be regarded as secondary evaginations from the original hemispheric evaginations. However, if the cerebrum is interpreted phylogenetically, the cerebral hemispheres can be regarded as evaginating from the olfactory bulbs, not the reverse (see Figure 13-10).

    d. The cerebral hemispheres and temporal lobes retain the original lumen of the neural tube as the **lateral ventricles**. The original lumen that extended into the olfactory bulbs obliterates.

E. Flexions

    1. As the neural tube elongates, the brain undergoes **flexions** that fit it more compactly into the intracranial space (Figure 3-6).

    2. These flexions as well as the evaginations and protuberances explain why the final form of the brain differs from a simple linear tube. The spinal cord, which does not undergo such pertubations, remains as a simple linear tube.

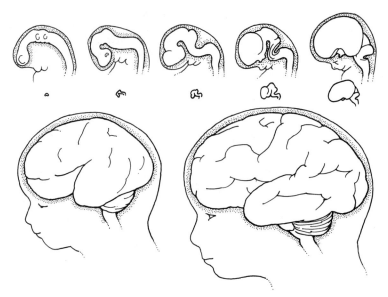

FIGURE 3-6. The flexions of the neural tube that fit the brain into the skull. (Adapted with permission from Cowan WM: The development of the brain. *Sci Am* 241:113–133, 1979.)

F. **Protuberances**

1. Proliferation of cells into masses at particular sites in the wall of the neural tube produces thickenings or actual protuberances.

2. The difference between protuberances in the wall and evaginations is that the ventricular lumen does not extend out into the protuberances, which are solid masses.

3. The **largest** protuberance, the **cerebellum,** grows from the dorsal aspect of the metencephalon (pons) [see Figure 10-5].

4. Additional protuberances include the:
   a. Inferior olivary eminences of the medulla
   b. Nuclei of the basis pontis
   c. Four elevations of the quadrigeminal plate of the midbrain
   d. Mamillary bodies of the diencephalon

G. **Formation of sulci and gyri** (see Chapter 13 I D)

III. CYTOGENESIS AND HISTOGENESIS IN THE WALL OF THE NEURAL TUBE

A. **Cytogenesis of neurons and glia** (Figure 3-7)

1. As the neural tube closes, blast cells multiply in the periventricular zone, producing **neuroblasts** and **glioblasts**.
   a. Theoretically, glioblasts and neuroblasts derive from a common precursor cell, which is pluripotential until a certain number of cell divisions have occurred.
   b. The blast cell then becomes "determined." It "breeds true" and produces only one type of mature glial cell or neuron.

2. Although most neurons and glia arise from the periventricular zone, some cells migrate into the CNS from the neural crest (see IV D).

3. After the fetal period, the periventricular cells lose their capacity to produce new neuroblasts and glioblasts; however, some glial cells, notably astrocytes, retain the

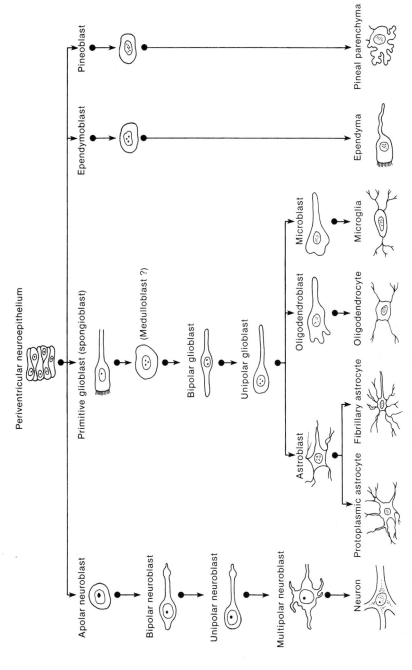

FIGURE 3-7. Cytogenesis of neurons and glia of the central nervous system (CNS).

ability to proliferate. The ependymal cells, which line the ventricles, are mature cell forms with little ability to proliferate.

B. **Cytogenesis and neoplasia.** The theory of neural cytogenesis shown in Figure 3-7 serves as a basis for the classification of CNS neoplasms.

1. CNS neoplasms consist of cell types that resemble the cell lineages seen during normal embryogenesis.

2. One theory of CNS neoplasia assumes that certain cells, perhaps nests of primitive embryonic cells, later undergo mitosis unrestrained by the normal influences that govern cell division during embryogenesis.

3. An alternative theory holds that neural cells, after differentiating into mature forms, can "dedifferentiate" to resemble their embryonic precursors.

C. **Cytogenesis of neurons**

1. The differentiating neuroblast initially produces protoplasmic expansions at opposite poles. Most neuroblasts pass through this **bipolar state** (Figure 3-8).

2. One of the bipolar processes continues to grow out, producing an **axon**, which seeks out its genetically determined synaptic contacts.

3. The other bipolar process undergoes atrophy, is replaced by a **dendritic tree**, and forms a **multipolar neuron** (see Figure 3-8).

D. **Histogenesis of CNS gray matter**

1. **Disposition of neuronal perikarya in gray matter**
   a. In the **CNS**, the perikarya of neuroblasts arrange themselves into one of three forms of gray matter: **nuclei**, **reticular formation** (RF), or **cortex** (Figure 3-9A–C).
   b. In the **peripheral nervous system** (PNS), the neuronal perikarya of differentiating neuroblasts arrange themselves into nodules called **ganglia** or into **plexuses** in the walls of the viscera (see Figure 3-9D).

2. **Migration of neuroblasts.** In the CNS, the neuroblasts undergo mitosis in the periventricular matrix zone, after which many migrate outward.
   a. The neuroblasts that remain in the periventricular matrix zone of the spinal cord, brain stem, cerebellum, or cerebrum, or those that migrate only a short distance away, form **nuclei**. In the brain stem, they also form **RF** (see Figure 3-9B).
   b. In the cerebrum and cerebellum, many neuroblasts separate from the periventricular nucleated zone. They migrate further outward to the surface, where they form cerebral or cerebellar **cortex** (Figure 3-10).

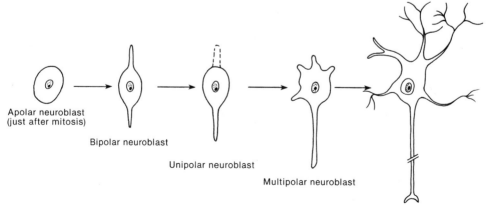

Apolar neuroblast
(just after mitosis)

Bipolar neuroblast

Unipolar neuroblast

Multipolar neuroblast

Mature multipolar neuron

FIGURE 3-8. Typical developmental stages in the cytogenesis of a multipolar neuron.

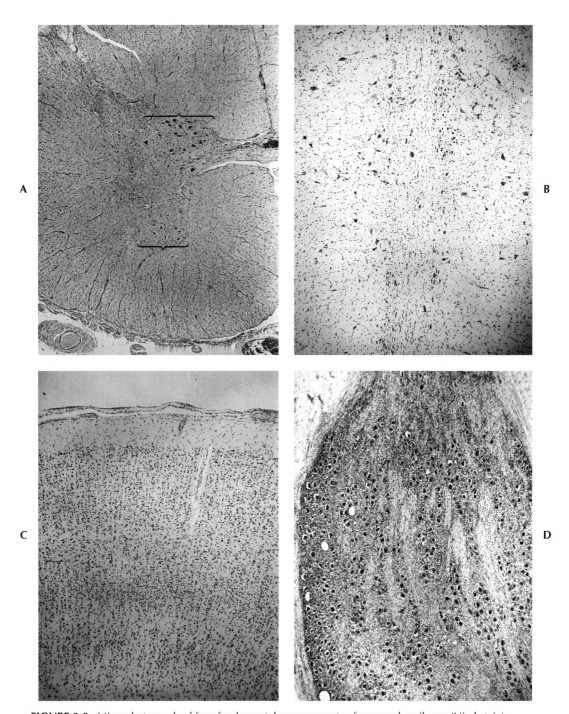

FIGURE 3-9. Microphotograph of four fundamental arrangements of neuronal perikarya (Nissl stain). (A) Nuclei in the ventral horn of the spinal cord (25×). (B) Reticular formation (RF) [40×]; section of the rostral medullary raphe and paramedian RF. (C) Cerebral cortex (40×). (D) Dorsal root ganglion (25×). A–C occur only in the central nervous system; D occurs only in the peripheral nervous system.

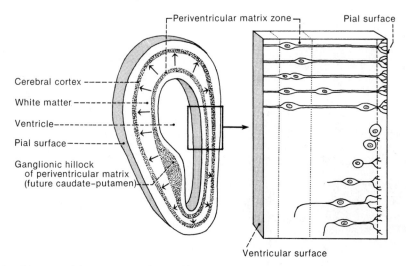

FIGURE 3-10. Diagram of the migration of neuroblasts from the periventricular matrix zone to the subpial zone to form cerebral cortex. After the nuclei migrate to the pial surface, the elongated cytoplasmic connection separates to form two individual cells from the preceding binucleate phase. The neuroblasts that remain along the ventricular lumen form the future caudate-putamen of the basal ganglia.

3. Disposition of nuclei
  a. Nuclei and cortex are the gray matter of the CNS. The nucleate arrangement in the CNS extends from the caudal tip of the spinal cord up through the brain stem, diencephalon, basal nuclei, and basal forebrain.
  b. The nuclei of the diencephalon (mainly the thalamus) are lined medially by ependyma and form the walls of the third ventricle (see Figure 11-2).
  c. The **caudate** nuclei in the telencephalon, which are also covered medially by ependyma, form the lateral wall of the anterior horn and the body of the lateral ventricle (see Figure 11-2).

4. Disposition of RF
  a. The RF is the next step up from nuclei in the complexity of neuronal disposition. It consists of loosely arranged neuronal groupings surrounding the denser nuclei proper, intermingled with numerous axonal connections and dendrites (see Figure 3-9B).
  b. The RF proper commences in the rostral end of the cervical cord and extends rostrally through the midbrain.
  c. The RF provides integrative, polysynaptic interneuronal circuits for behavior more complex than simple monosynaptic reflexes. It mediates activities such as breathing, swallowing, hiccoughing, pulse rate, blood pressure, and even consciousness itself.

5. Disposition of cortex and its relationship to underlying nuclei
  a. Cortex consists of layers of neuronal perikarya alternating with layers of dendrites and axons (see Figures 3-9C and 13-32).
    (1) Neuroblasts form the cerebral and cerebellar cortices by migrating to the surface.
    (2) By contrast, neuroblasts that remain close to the ventricular lumina form the basal nuclei and diencephalic nuclei.
    (3) The cerebellar and cerebral cortices then establish extensive axonal connections with their respective deep nuclei.
  b. The cerebellum and cerebrum contain the only true cortex. Although a stratified arrangement of neurons occurs in a few other sites, namely the retina, olfactory bulbs, and quadrigeminal plate of the midbrain, these are not true cortices.
  c. Cortex provides the ultimate in plasticity and variety of interneuronal circuits, allowing for more complex neural activity than either nuclei or RF.

IV. CYTOGENESIS AND HISTOGENESIS OF THE SPINAL CORD

A. **Three concentric layers of the spinal cord.** After the neural tube closes, the spinal cord develops as three concentric layers, which are, from the inside out, the **ependymal layer**, **mantle layer**, and **marginal layer** (Figure 3-11A).

1. The inner layer, the **ependymal layer**, surrounds the central canal.

2. The middle layer, the **mantle zone**, becomes nucleated gray matter as the neuroblasts within it differentiate.

3. The outer layer, the **marginal zone**, becomes the white matter as axons invade it from the dorsal root ganglia, spinal cord nuclei, brain stem, and cerebral cortex.

B. **Glial framework of the spinal cord.** Ependyma and astrocytes extend their processes from the deepest layer of the cord to the pial surface (Figure 3-12).

C. **Configuration of spinal cord gray matter** (see Figure 3-11B–D)

1. The neuroblasts invade and thicken the mantle zone to form paired **alar plates** dorsally and paired **basal plates** ventrally. The plane of the **sulcus limitans** separates the alar and basal plates (see Figure 3-11B and C).

2. Neuroblast proliferation thickens the gray matter of the alar and basal plates in the shape of an **H** (see Figure 3-11D), but the roof and floor plates remain thin.
   a. The **crossbar** of the H-shaped gray matter surrounds the central canal.
   b. The four limbs of the H become **dorsal** and **ventral** horns of gray matter.
   c. Just ventral to the plane of the sulcus limitans, an **intermediate** (intermediolateral) **horn** appears as neuroblasts thicken the region (see Figure 3-11D).

D. **Neural crest.** The neural crest consists of two longitudinal rows of cells that develop along the dorsolateral aspect of the neural tube, where surface ectoderm and neural ectoderm join (Figure 3-13; see Figure 3-3).

1. The neural crest consists of **rostral** and **caudal** parts.
   a. The **rostral (cranial)** neural crest is adjacent to the brain.
   b. The **caudal (spinal)** neural crest is adjacent to the spinal cord.

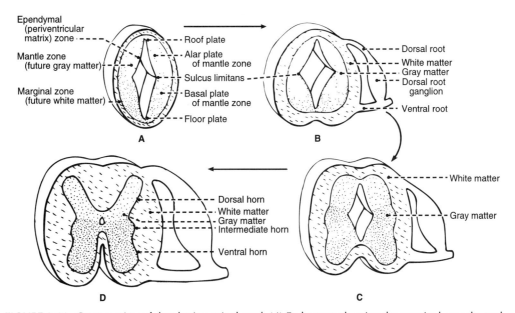

FIGURE 3-11. Cross section of developing spinal cord. (*A*) Early stage showing the marginal, mantle, and ependymal (periventricular matrix) zones. (*B*) and (*C*) Intermediate stages showing the fate of the sulcus limitans and the roof, floor, alar, and basal plates. (*D*) Final contour of the spinal cord.

FIGURE 3-12. Cross section of the embryonic spinal cord showing the ependymal and astrocytic framework. (*A*) Ependyma of the floor plate. (*B*) Central canal. (*C*) Ependyma of the dorsal part of the central canal and roof plate. (*D*) Astroblasts. (*E*) Ependyma of the midpart of the central canal. (Adapted with permission from Chambers W, Liu C: Anatomy of the spinal cord. In: *The Spinal Cord*, 2nd ed. Edited by Austin G. Springfield, IL, Thomas Publishing, 1971, p 12.)

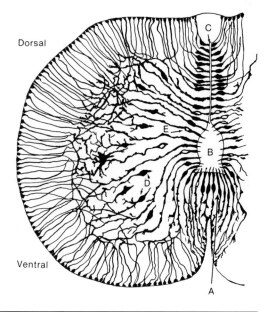

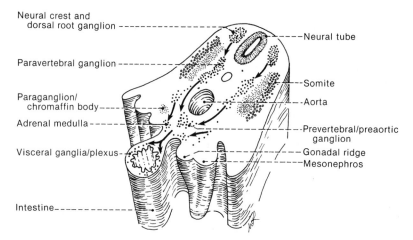

FIGURE 3-13. Cross section of the trunk of an embryo showing the migratory pathway of autonomic neuroblasts from the neural crest.

   2. Some neural crest cells remain near their site of origin, dorsolateral to the neural tube. Others migrate varying distances away (see Figure 3-13).
   a. The cells that remain dorsolateral to the neural tube, thus close to the vertebral column, become **dorsal root** ganglia, **paravertebral** ganglia, or **prevertebral** ganglia.
   b. The cells that migrate away from the paravertebral region become the more peripheral autonomic ganglia or plexuses in the walls of the viscera.
   c. Table 3-2 lists the neural derivatives of the spinal and cranial neural crest. Figure 3-14 depicts the cytogenesis of the neural and non-neural derivatives of the neural crest.

E. **Origin of neurons**

   1. As a rule, those neurons whose perikarya lie **outside** of the CNS originate from the neural crest, and those neurons whose perikarya lie **inside** of the CNS originate from the neural tube (ectoderm).

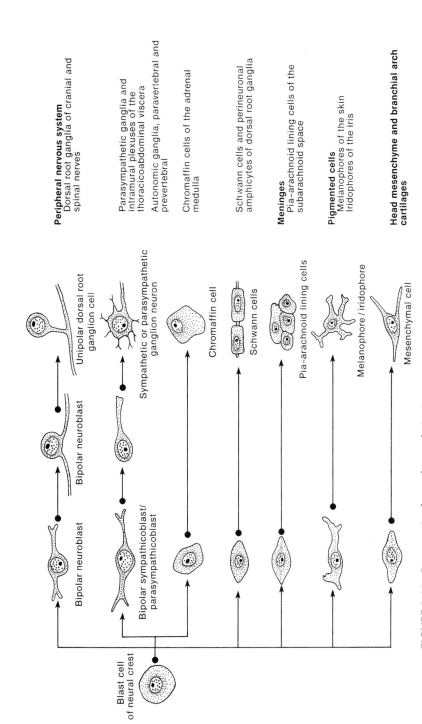

FIGURE 3-14. Cytogenesis of neural crest derivatives.

TABLE 3-2. Neural Derivatives of the Neural Crest

Derivative Structure	Cranial Neural Crest Derivatives	Spinal Neural Crest Derivatives
Sensory ganglia	Trigeminal (CN V) Geniculate (CN VII) Superior and inferior (CN IX) Superior and inferior (CN X)	All spinal dorsal root ganglia
Autonomic ganglia		
Parasympathetic ganglia	Ciliary Pterygopalatine Submandibular Otic	Pelvic plexus Enteric plexus
Sympathetic ganglia	None	Cervical Prevertebral Paravertebral Remak's sinoatrial ganglion Adrenal medulla
Supporting cells	Schwann cells Some meningeal cells Possibly some glial cells	Schwann cells Some meningeal cells Possibly some glial cells

CN = cranial nerve.

2. Neural crest cells produce the neurons of the dorsal root afferent system and the ganglionic neurons of the autonomic ganglia and plexuses.

3. While these rules are true in general, various studies suggest greater intermingling by migration of peripheral and central precursor cells than previously appreciated.

V. DEVELOPMENT OF THE SPINAL NERVES. The spinal cord has 31 pairs of spinal nerves. They attach at regular intervals corresponding to the paired somites (see VII) and to the paired nodules of the neural crest (see Figure 6-1). Each spinal nerve derives from **dorsal** and **ventral roots**, which unite to form a **nerve trunk** (Figure 3-15; see Figure 3-17).

A. Formation of the dorsal (posterior) roots. Each paired nodule of the neural crest produces neuroblasts for a dorsal root ganglion. Each neuroblast in the dorsal root ganglion produces a process that bifurcates into a **peripheral** and a **central** branch (see Figure 3-15).

1. The **central branch** pierces the dorsolateral aspect of the spinal cord, forming the **dorsal** root (see Figure 3-15). Upon entering the spinal cord, the dorsal root axon characteristically branches.
   a. One branch synapses on a spinal neuron, an interneuron or motoneuron, that is at or close to the level of entry (see Figure 6-7).
   b. The other branches then may run up or down the cord before synapsing.

2. The **peripheral** branch extends from the dorsal root ganglion to a receptor in the skin or viscera.

B. Formation of the ventral (anterior) roots

1. Neuroblasts in the ventral horn gray matter differentiate and produce axons that exit from the ventrolateral aspect of the spinal cord (see Figure 3-15).

2. Two types of axons enter the ventral roots: axons destined for **skeletal muscles** and axons destined for **autonomic ganglia** (Figure 3-16).

  a. The somatomotor axons destined for **skeletal muscles** issue from motoneurons in the **ventral** horns. They travel directly to the muscle without further synapses.

  b. The autonomic axons destined for autonomic ganglia issue from neurons in the **intermediate** horn.

   (1) These autonomic axons do not synapse directly on glands or smooth muscles. Instead, they synapse on a peripheral neuron in a ganglion or on a

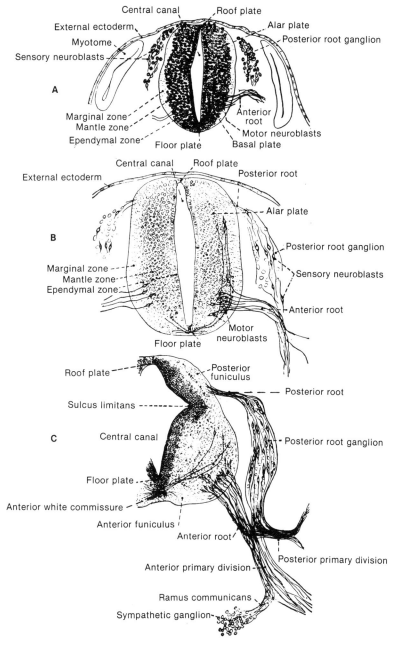

FIGURE 3-15. Cross section of the embryonic spinal cord and dorsal root to show neuronogenesis in the ventral horns and dorsal root ganglia. (Adapted with permission from Larsell O: *Anatomy of the Nervous System*, 2nd ed. New York, Appleton-Century-Crofts, 1951, p 56.)

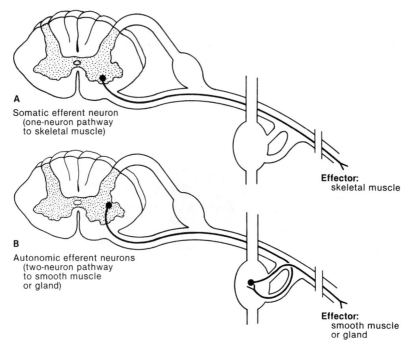

FIGURE 3-16. Spinal cord with an attached spinal nerve to contrast (*A*) the one-neuron pathway to skeletal muscles and (*B*) the two-neuron pathway to the autonomic effectors.

TABLE 3-3. Histologic Components of the Peripheral Nervous System and Their Embryologic Origin

Histologic Components	Function	Embryologic Origin
Axons of ventral roots	Purely motor	Neural ectoderm
Ganglia		
Dorsal root ganglia	Purely sensory	
Autonomic ganglia	Purely motor	Neural crest
Plexuses (located in sheets in the walls of viscera)	Smooth muscle contraction and glandular secretion	
Schwann cells	Produce myelin sheaths	
Fibrous connective tissue	Supports and strengthens the peripheral nervous system	Mesoderm
Blood vessels and lymphatic channels	Circulation of fluids	

    plexus neuron in the wall of a viscus. The peripheral neuron then innervates the effector.

(2) Thus, the autonomic pathway of the PNS involves two neurons; the skeletal muscle pathway involves only one neuron (see Figure 3-16).

(3) The preganglionic autonomic axon runs to the ganglion by a small ramus from the peripheral nerve trunk. The postganglionic axons rejoin the trunk by another ramus (see Figure 3-16).

(4) After traveling varying distances in the nerve trunk, the postganglionic axon departs from the spinal nerve to synapse on its effector.

C. Table 3-3 summarizes the histologic elements of the PNS and their embryologic origin from one of three sources: **neural ectoderm**, **neural crest**, and **mesoderm**.

VI. FUNCTIONAL CLASSIFICATION OF PERIPHERAL NERVE FIBERS

A. Division into sensory and motor axons

1. Because **dorsal** roots conduct sensory impulses **to** the CNS and **ventral** roots conduct motor impulses **away from** the CNS, a functional classification begins by recognizing two categories of nerve fiber: **afferent** and **efferent**.

2. The fact that the **dorsal roots** are **afferent**, or **sensory**, while the **ventral roots** are **efferent**, or **motor**, is called the **law of Bell and Magendie**.

3. The spinal cord gray matter reflects the division of function between dorsal and ventral roots.
   a. The **alar plates**, or **dorsal horns**, are primarily **sensory** in function.
   b. The **basal plates**, or **ventral horns**, are primarily **motor** in function.

B. Division into somatic and visceral axons

1. The **sensory axons** of neurons in the dorsal root ganglia conduct afferent impulses from either a **somatic** or a **visceral** structure. Although the perikarya of visceral and somatic neurons apparently intermingle in the dorsal root ganglia, the two types of axons separate upon entering the spinal cord and to reach their somatic or visceral end stations.

2. Separate **motor axons** also innervate either somatic or visceral effectors. Their perikarya of origin occupy different nuclear sites in the efferent plate of the spinal cord. Hence, somatic and visceral efferent axons commence separately in the spinal cord, exit together in the ventral root, pass through the main nerve trunk, and then separate again distal to the main trunk.

C. Theory of nerve components

1. The theory of nerve components combines the motor/sensory and somatic/visceral dichotomies to recognize **four functional types of axons** in spinal nerves (Figure 3-17).
   a. All axons destined for skeletal muscle of somite origin are classified as **general somatic efferent (GSE)** axons.
   b. All axons destined for autonomic ganglia or plexuses that then reach smooth muscle or glands are classified as **general visceral efferent (GVE)** axons.
   c. Afferent axons from the viscera are classified as **general visceral afferent (GVA)**.
   d. Afferent axons from the somatic or musculoskeletal system are classified as **general somatic afferent (GSA)**.

2. Special sensory and motor axons serve the special senses and special motor functions at the brain stem level (see Figures 7-8 and 7-25).

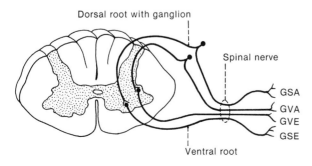

Dorsal root with ganglion

Spinal nerve

GSA
GVA
GVE
GSE

Ventral root

FIGURE 3-17. Four functional components of the typical spinal nerve. *GSA* = general somatic afferent; *GSE* = general somatic efferent; *GVA* = general visceral afferent; *GVE* = general visceral efferent.

3. Although functionally different, the individual motor and sensory axons in the peripheral nerves look exactly alike and are indistinguishable when viewed microscopically. However, in general, autonomic axons and nerves are smaller than somatic axons and nerves and are less well myelinated.

VII.   THE DEVELOPMENT AND INNERVATION OF SOMITES

A.   Composition and arrangement of somites

1. **Somites** develop as a series of regular, paired masses or corrugations of mesoderm on each side of the neural tube (see Figures 3-2C and 3-2D).

2. Somites produce the parietes, or somatic structures of the body, because their mesoderm differentiates into **dermatomes, myotomes,** and **sclerotomes** (Figure 3-18).
   a. The **dermatome** produces the dermis, which is the deep layer of skin beneath the epidermis. The epidermis derives from surface ectoderm.
   b. The **myotome** differentiates into skeletal muscle.
   c. The **sclerotome** differentiates into the skeleton and related connective tissues.

B.   Extent of the somite plan and the segmental part of the nervous system

1. The somites extend from the midbrain to the caudal end of the spinal cord.

2. At the spinal level, the somites form a continuous series.

3. At the brain stem level, the somites are discontinuous because some retrogress and disappear during the complicated development of the face.
   a. The **rostral**-most somite is opposite the midbrain and forms eye muscles. The rostral-most somite nerve, also the rostral-most motor nerve, CN III, issues from the midbrain to innervate eye muscles.
   b. Reflecting the extent of the somites, the **spinal cord** and **brain stem** (up to the midbrain level) constitute the **segmental part** of the nervous system. The **diencephalon** and **cerebrum** are the **suprasegmental part**.
      (1) Just like the spinal cord, the brain stem has alar and basal plates (see Figure 3-11). Thus, the brain stem can be interpreted simply as an expansion of the spinal cord.
      (2) The development of the diencephalon and cerebrum differs from the basic developmental plan of the segmental nervous system. If the basal or efferent plate stops at the midbrain, as most authorities advocate, then the cerebrum proper develops from expanded alar plates, as an elaborate interneuronal pool.

C.   Innervation of the somites

1. Each pair of somites receives a corresponding pair of somite nerves from the spinal cord or brain stem. The somite pairs also receive paired arteries from the aorta. Hence, each somite pair has one pair of primary nerves and one pair of primary arteries.

FIGURE 3-18. Cross section of the embryonic neural tube (spinal cord) and adjacent body wall showing the three derivatives of a somite: the dermatome, myotome, and sclerotome. The arrows show pathways of migration of the cells from the myotomes and sclerotomes to form muscles, bones, and connective tissue.

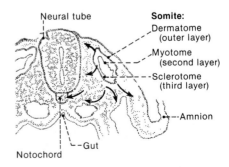

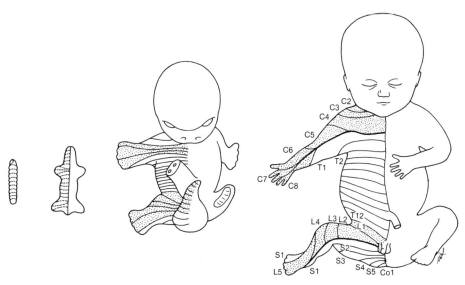

FIGURE 3-19. Translocation of dermatomes during the outgrowth of the limb buds. *C* = cervical; *L* = lumbar; *S* = sacral; *T* = thoracic.

    2. Each **somite nerve** consists of dorsal and ventral roots and innervates all of the tissues derived from its original somite and only those tissues.
      a. The somite nerve innervates the dermis derived from the particular somite's dermatome, the muscles derived from the somite's myotome, and the bone derived from its sclerotome (see Figure 4-12).
      b. This rule holds even when the somite derivatives migrate and undergo extensive transformations in the arm, leg, and face regions.
      c. Figure 3-19 shows the transformation of the dermatomes. Only the thoracic region retains the original somite simplicity because it is unaltered by face, arm, or leg growth.
    3. Paired paravertebral **autonomic ganglia**, corresponding to the pairs of somites, develop from the neural crest. Some ganglia coalesce in the cervical region, but the ganglia remain separate in the thoracic region (see Figure 5-1).

D. Formation of somatic nerve plexuses

    1. Axons of the PNS run through **plexuses** that distribute them to their end stations. Figure 3-20A shows that a spinal nerve trunk entering a plexus contains axons from only one spinal nerve serving only one spinal segment. Although axons of the individual nerve trunks intermingle in the plexus, each axon retains its own identity and does not anastomose with axons of another segment.

    2. Figure 3-20B shows that the peripheral nerves issuing from a somatic plexus may contain axons from more than one nerve trunk or spinal segment.

    3. Plexuses occur in the cervical, arm, and leg regions of the cord. No plexuses occur in the thoracic region, where the somites retain their original serial simplicity.

VIII. **MYELINATION IN THE PERIPHERAL NERVOUS SYSTEM AND CENTRAL NERVOUS SYSTEM**

A. Jelly-roll hypothesis of myelin formation

    1. The axons of the CNS and PNS initially grow out as naked cytoplasmic extensions. Many axons then receive a myelin sheath, while others remain unmyelinated.

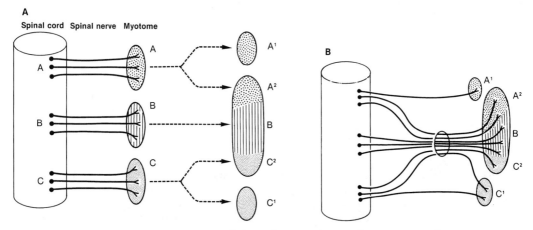

FIGURE 3-20. Diagrammatic representation of plexus formation by spinal nerves. (*A*) Each myotome receives one spinal nerve, but the myotome may split to contribute to a composite muscle. See *A¹* and *A²* and *C¹* and *C²*. (*B*) The axons that innervate a composite muscle still reach their original myotome but first run through a plexus (*circled*) to form a common nerve or nerves.

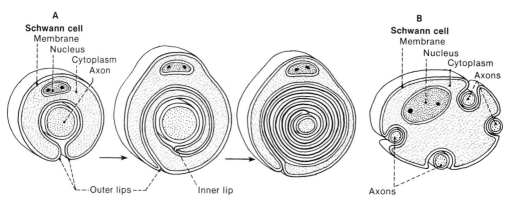

FIGURE 3-21. Cross section of a myelinating axon in the peripheral nervous system (PNS). (*A*) Three stages in the encircling of the axon by a lip of Schwann cell to form a "jelly roll" of myelin sheath. (*B*) The nonmyelinated axons indent the surface membrane of the Schwann cell but do not receive a jelly roll wrapping.

2. In the **PNS**, Schwann cells, which originate from the neural crest, form the myelin sheaths. In the **CNS**, oligodendroglial cells, which originate from the neural ectoderm, form the myelin sheaths.

3. In the **PNS**, the Schwann cells myelinate the axons by a lip of cytoplasm that slips under the other lip to encircle the axon in a "jelly roll" manner topologically (Figure 3-21A). The myelin sheath thus consists of layers of Schwann cell membrane.
    a. The axons that remain unmyelinated are imbedded in Schwann cell cytoplasm, but the lips of the Schwann cell do not encircle the fiber (see Figure 3-21B).
    b. Any given Schwann cell may accommodate both myelinated and unmyelinated fibers.
    c. In the PNS, the structure of the peripheral nerve is completed by the formation of blood vessels and fibrous connective tissue sheaths from the mesoderm.

4. In the **CNS**, **oligodendroglial** membranes form the myelin laminae, but the topology of the investment is more complicated than it is in the PNS. One oligodendroglia

cell myelinates many axons by means of cytoplasmic extensions that produce a "jelly roll."

B. **Junction of the CNS and PNS**

1. The Schwann cells and fibrous connective tissue of the PNS stop abruptly within a few millimeters of the site where a dorsal or ventral nerve root attaches to the CNS (see Figure 1-2).

2. **Central** to this junction, glial connective tissue comprised of oligodendrocytes and astrocytes replaces the Schwann cells and fibrous connective tissue of the PNS.

3. The junction of the two different types of connective tissues is called the **Obersteiner-Redlich zone** (Figure 3-22).

C. **Timetable of myelination in the CNS**

1. The various tracts or regions of the CNS myelinate in an orderly, regular sequence (Figure 3-23). In general, spinal and brain stem axons myelinate before cerebral axons.

2. Myelination slightly precedes assumption of function in the nerve fibers. Hence, the degree of myelination in the developing nervous system is one measure of its functional maturation.

D. **Demyelination**

1. Some diseases attack the myelin sheath but tend to spare the axons. Because most of the axons remain, the disease is called a **demyelinating disease**. In multiple sclerosis, the most common demyelinating disease of the CNS in young adults, patches of demyelination are scattered at various sites in the CNS white matter. The patient has a variety of signs and symptoms, depending on the site of the white matter lesions. Commonly, the demyelinating patches affect the optic nerves as well as the white matter of the cerebrum, brain stem, cerebellum, and spinal cord. Magnetic resonance imaging (MRI) scans of the CNS show the advance of myelination during normal development or its destruction under pathologic conditions.

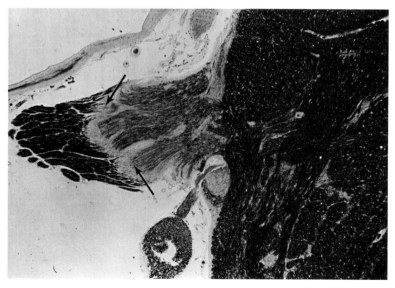

FIGURE 3-22. Microphotograph of myelin-stained section of nerve root attaching to the medulla. The central myelin meets the peripheral myelin at the Obersteiner-Redlich zone (*arrows*).

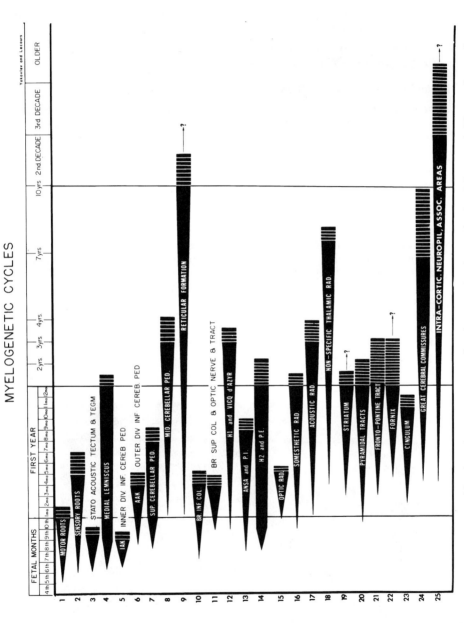

MYELOGENETIC CYCLES

FIGURE 3-23. Timetable of myelination. (Reprinted with permission from Yakovlev P, Lecours A: The myelogenetic cycles of regional maturation of the brain. In *Regional Development of the Brain in Early Life*. Edited by Minkowski A. Oxford, Blackwell Scientific, 1967, pp 3–70.)

2. Diseases that affect individual Schwann cells in the PNS may result in **segmental demyelination** (see Figure 2-9E), impairing the sensory or motor function of the peripheral nerves.

3. Remyelination may occur in the PNS (see Figure 2-9D) and possibly to some extent in the CNS. The Schwann cells or oligodendroglia then repeat the "jelly roll" sequence.

STUDY QUESTIONS

DIRECTIONS: Each of the numbered items or incomplete statements in this section is followed by answers or by completions of the statement. Select the ONE lettered answer or completion that is BEST in each case.

1. Demyelination is defined as

(A) loss of pre-existing axons and myelin sheaths in equal degree
(B) loss of pre-existing myelin sheaths with relative preservation of axons
(C) loss of pre-existing axons with relative preservation of myelin sheaths
(D) loss of pre-existing myelin sheaths uniformly throughout only the central nervous system (CNS)
(E) none of the above

2. The junction between the central and peripheral myelin occurs at the level of the

(A) nerve trunk
(B) dorsal root ganglion
(C) intervertebral foramina
(D) junction of dorsal and ventral roots
(E) none of the above

3. Select the statement that best describes the relationship of nerve roots to somite derivatives.

(A) All somite derivatives retain their original nerve root wherever they migrate
(B) Myotomes retain their original nerve roots when they migrate but dermatomes do not
(C) The dermatomes retain their original nerve roots but myotomes do not
(D) Nerve roots usually exchange somites when the somites migrate
(E) None of the above

4. The process of neurulation or neural tube closure requires

(A) migration of neuroblasts from the periventricular region
(B) segmentation of the encephalon
(C) fusion of the dorsal margins of the neural folds
(D) evagination
(E) none of the above

5. Destruction of the neural crest in an embryo would result in absence of which of the following?

(A) Afferent nerve fibers in the peripheral nerves
(B) Efferent nerve fibers in the peripheral nerves
(C) Collagen fibrils in the peripheral nerves
(D) Blood vessels in peripheral nerves
(E) None of the above

DIRECTIONS: Each of the numbered items or incomplete statements in this section is negatively phrased, as indicated by a capitalized word such as NOT, LEAST, or EXCEPT. Select the ONE lettered answer or completion that is BEST in each case.

6. The following structures develop by evagination, EXCEPT for the

(A) optic nerve
(B) olfactory bulb
(C) neurohypophysis
(D) cerebral hemispheres
(E) cerebellum

7. All of the following structures have glial supporting tissue EXCEPT for the

(A) optic nerve
(B) neurohypophysis
(C) olfactory tract
(D) dorsal root ganglia
(E) pineal body

8. Which of the following statements about the basal plates is INCORRECT?

(A) They are known to extend throughout the entire length of the neuraxis

(B) They contrast with the alar plates in being mainly motor in function

(C) They correspond to the segmental or somite level of the central nervous system (CNS)

(D) They contain neurons that provide axons for the ventral roots

(E) They are ventral to the plane of the sulcus limitans

[handwritten: alar = sens, basal = motor]

DIRECTIONS: Each set of matching questions in this section consists of a list of four to twenty-six lettered options (some of which may be in figures) followed by several numbered items. For each numbered item, select the ONE lettered option that is most closely associated with it. To avoid spending too much time on matching sets with large numbers of options, it is generally advisable to begin each set by reading the list of options. Then, for each item in the set, try to generate the correct answer and locate it in the option list, rather than evaluating each option individually. Each lettered option may be selected once, more than once, or not at all.

Questions 9–13

Match the adult derivative as specifically as possible with the embryologic units that are produced by transverse segmentation of the neuraxis.

(A) Telencephalon of the forebrain
(B) Rhombencephalon (hindbrain)
(C) Diencephalon
(D) Mesencephalon
(E) None of the above

9. Thalamus *C*

10. Pons *B*

11. Medulla *B*

12. Midbrain *D*

13. Cerebrum *A*

DIRECTIONS: Each set of matching questions in this section consists of a list of four to twenty- six lettered options followed by several numbered items. For each numbered item, select the appropriate lettered option(s). Each lettered option may be selected once, more than once, or not at all. EACH ITEM WILL STATE THE NUMBER OF OPTIONS TO SELECT. CHOOSE EXACTLY THIS NUMBER.

Questions 14–18

(A) Schwann cells
(B) Adenohypophysis (Rathke's pouch)
(C) Lining of the lung
(D) Epidermis
(E) Melanophores
(F) Thyroid gland
(G) Skeletal and smooth muscle fibers
(H) Blood vessels
(I) Dorsal horns of the spinal cord
(J) Heart
(K) Adrenal medulla
(L) Ventral motoneurons
(M) Preganglionic neurons of the autonomic nervous system
(N) Neural tube

Each adult cell type or structure has a specific, immediate embryologic precursor and arises in a definite, preprogrammed developmental sequence. For each numbered item, select the anatomic entity or entities that directly or immediately derive from or in the precursor.

14. Neural crest (SELECT 3 ENTITIES)
[handwritten: Schwann, Melanophores, adrenal]

15. Basal plate (SELECT 2 ENTITIES)
[handwritten: Ventral motor neurons pregang]

16. Alar plate (SELECT 1 ENTITY)
[handwritten: Dorsal horn]

17. Mesoderm (SELECT 3 ENTITIES)
[handwritten: muscle, blood vessels, heart]

18. Surface or oral ectoderm (SELECT 3 ENTITIES)
[handwritten: adeno (Rathke's), epidermis, neural tube]

ANSWERS AND EXPLANATIONS

1. The answer is B [VIII D]. Demyelination refers to the selective loss of myelin sheaths, with the relative preservation of axons. In these diseases, such as multiple sclerosis, demyelination is the primary event. Other diseases may affect the axon, with degeneration of the myelin sheath as a secondary event. Some diseases cause patchy demyelination in the central nervous system (CNS) or peripheral nervous system (PNS); other diseases cause diffuse demyelination. The lesions that destroy all of the tissue, glia, axons, and myelin sheaths, such as infarcts, are not classified as demyelinating diseases. Remyelination may restore the axons to normal function and occurs more readily in the PNS than in the CNS.

2. The answer is E [VIII B 1–3; Figure 3-22]. Two different cell types produce myelin: oligodendroglia in the central nervous system (CNS) and Schwann cells in the peripheral nervous system (PNS). The CNS and the PNS meet at a sharp junction near the site of attachment of the nerve roots to the surface of the brain stem and spinal cord, where the roots pierce the pia. The demyelinating diseases of the CNS that involve oligodendroglia generally spare Schwann cell myelin, and the demyelinating diseases of peripheral nerves that involve Schwann cells generally spare oligodendroglial myelin.

3. The answer is A [VII C 2 a, b]. When they migrate to different locations, somite derivatives retain axons from their original spinal cord levels. The axons, which originally would run from the spinal cord directly laterally to their somites, rearrange their course in the plexuses to reach the migrated somites. For example, the myotomes of the diaphragm originate opposite the 3rd, 4th, and 5th cervical levels, but migrate to the lower thoracic level. The diaphragm drags its original nerve supply from C3–5, named the phrenic nerve, along with it.

4. The answer is C [II B 1–5; Figures 3-2 and 3-3]. Neurulation, or neural tube closure, comes about after the neural folds elevate on either side of the neural groove. The dorsal margins of the neural folds then fuse, and a tube composed of surface ectoderm splits away from the surface. The open ends of the tube, the anterior and posterior neuropores, then fuse, giving the primitive neuraxis the

configuration of an elongated balloon. Neurulation may fail altogether, which is a condition incompatible with survival. Incomplete closure results in an individual born with a defect along the dorsal midline, from the forehead to the coccyx, along the expected line of neural tube closure.

5. The answer is A [IV D 1–2; Table 3-2; Figure 3-13]. The neural crest develops on each side of the neural tube as it closes and splits away from the surface ectoderm. Cells of the neural crest produce the dorsal root ganglia, which provide afferent nerve fibers for the spinal nerves, and the peripheral ganglia of the autonomic and parasympathetic systems. Because the adrenal medulla corresponds to a sympathetic ganglion, destruction of the neural crest would also result in its absence, as well as all other crest-derived peripheral structures.

6. The answer is E [II D, F 3; Figure 3-5]. Evagination, one of the fundamental events in organogenesis, drastically alters the configuration of the forebrain, producing the pineal body, neurohypophysis, optic and olfactory bulbs, cerebral hemispheres, and temporal lobes. In contrast, some structures, such as the cerebellum and basis pontis, develop as solid masses that thicken local sites in the wall of the neural tube and protrude from the tube.

7. The answer is D [II D 5 b (2); Table 3-3]. All structures that develop as evaginations from the wall of the forebrain tube have glial supporting tissue because they are basically extensions of the wall of the neural tube. None of the structures of the peripheral nervous system (PNS), such as the dorsal root and autonomic ganglia, contain glia per se, but they do have supporting tissue and cells derived from mesoderm or the neural crest. Initially during development, the afferent and efferent axons of the central nervous system (CNS) grow along pre-existing glial cells. PNS axons invade the body tissues as naked protoplasmic extensions and then acquire their collagenous supporting tissue, blood vessels, and Schwann cells secondarily.

8. The answer is A [IV C 1, 2; Figures 3-11 and 3-15]. The basal plates and the alar plates form the major plates of the segmental part of the nervous system. The sulcus limitans divides the two plates, with the basal plate being ventral. Many authors contend that the basal plates stop at the rostral end of the midbrain. No motor axons issue from the central nervous system (CNS) rostral to the midbrain. Ventral roots come from the basal plates; the cerebellum, diencephalon, and cerebrum originate from the alar plates. A roof plate connects the alar plates dorsally, and a floor plate connects the basal plates ventrally. If the neural tube fails to close, the alar plates will have a widely separated or absent roof plate, whereas the floor plate will still hold the basal plates together along their ventromedial margins.

9–13. The answers are 9-C, 10-B, 11-B, 12-D, 13-A [II C; Figure 3-4]. Transverse segmentation of the neural tube produces five final segments that become the definitive parts of the brain. Transverse segmentation has already begun before the neural tube closes completely. The forebrain, or prosencephalon, divides into the telencephalon and diencephalon, which produce the cerebrum and thalamus, respectively. In addition, the diencephalon produces the epithalamus, subthalamus, and hypothalamus. One transverse segment of the central nervous system (CNS), the mesencephalon, does not undergo further segmentation but remains as the definitive midbrain of the adult CNS. The hindbrain, or rhombencephalon, becomes the pons and medulla. From the level of the medulla to the tip of the spinal cord no further transverse segmentation occurs, although the spinal nerve roots attach at orderly intervals corresponding to the somites. The pons, in turn, gives rise to two major protuberances: a large bulging belly, which protrudes **ventrally**, and the cerebellum, which protrudes **dorsally**.

The original cavity of the neural tube, which extends from the rostral end of the forebrain to the tip of the spinal cord, continues through the various transverse segments and their adult derivatives. The original cavity includes the lateral ventricles in the cerebrum, the third ventricle in the diencephalon, the aqueduct in the midbrain, the fourth ventricle in the pons and medulla, and the central canal of the spinal cord.

14. The answers are: A, E, K [IV D; Figure 3-13]. The neural crest consists of columns of cells that develop just dorsolateral to the neural tube as neurulation procedes. These precursor cells develop into seemingly diverse derivatives, including the postganglionic neurons

of the autonomic nervous system, adrenal medulla, dorsal root ganglia, and melanophores. Disorders of development of the neural crest include the neurocristopathies, characterized by multiple pigmented spots and tumors of the peripheral and central nervous system, and the commonest tumor of early childhood, neuroblastoma, often found in association with the adrenal gland or at any site along the sympathetic chain.

[handwritten: Neural crest]

15. The answers are: L, M [IV C 1, 2, E; V B 2 a, b]. The basal plate of the neuraxis is the efferent plate in which the visceral and somatic motoneurons develop. Their axons leave the central nervous system (CNS) to form the ventral roots. The preganglionic visceromotor neurons arise in the intermediolateral horn of the basal plate and the motoneurons for skeletal muscle arise in the ventral horn per se. The visceromotoneurons commence the two-neuron pathway from the CNS to the periphery that characterizes the autonomic nervous system.

16. The answer is I [VI A 3 a]. The alar plates, which are dorsal to the basal plates, produce the neurons of the dorsal horn that receive the incoming afferents from the dorsal roots and initiate sensory pathways to the rest of the nervous system. Taken together, the basal plates and alar plates reflect the law of Bell and Magendie, which states that the dorsal roots are sensory and the ventral roots are motor.

17. The answers are: G, H, J [I C 2 c]. Mesoderm provides the skeletomuscular system, which includes the connective tissue outside of the central nervous system (CNS); smooth, skeletal, and cardiac muscle; and bone. The neural crest contributes to the facial skeleton. The heart is the only muscle of the body that contains its own intrinsic pacemaker, which causes it to contract. In the process of removing a heart for transplantation, the surgeon must sever the autonomic nerves that supply it. Under normal conditions, these autonomic connections alter its rate of contraction but do not initiate contractions. All other muscle, smooth and skeletal, must have an intact nerve supply to function. These muscles, when deprived of their nerve supply, degenerate and fail to function.

18. The answers are: B, D, N [I C 2 b; II D]. The surface ectoderm that initially covers the inner cell mass or embryonic disk becomes the epidermis and, by the process of neurulation, the neural tube. The dermis derives from the mesoderm. The oral ectoderm of the roof of the mouth produces an evagination called Rathke's pouch, which becomes the adenohypophysis. Failure of this evagination to develop results in aplasia of the adenohypophysis. The neurohypophysis, derived from the neural tube, may still develop.

Chapter 4

Nerve Roots, Plexuses, and Peripheral Nerves

I. MICROSCOPIC ANATOMY OF PERIPHERAL NERVES

A. Cross sections of peripheral nerves

1. Cross sections of a peripheral nerve disclose round fascicles of nerve fibers separated by connective tissue sheaths. Blood vessels penetrate the sheaths to nourish the nerve fibers (Figure 4-1).

2. The fascicles contain (Figure 4-2):
   a. Schwann cells and fibrocytes
   b. Axons
   c. Myelin sheaths
   d. Collagen fibrils of the endoneurium
   e. Blood vessels (see Figure 4-1)

B. Relation of Schwann cells to axons

1. Axons in a peripheral nerve vary in diameter from less than 1 μ to 15 μ. The smaller axons merely indent the surface membrane of Schwann cells, forming **un-myelinated** axons (Figure 4-3; see Figure 3-21).

2. Other axons receive circular wrappings by the surface membrane of Schwann cells, forming **myelinated axons** (see Figures 4-3 and 3-21).

3. One Schwann cell may accommodate myelinated and unmyelinated fibers.

4. **Nodes of Ranvier** and the **internodal segment of Schwann cells**
   a. A **node of Ranvier** is the site where one Schwann cell membrane stops and the next begins (Figure 4-4).
   b. **The internodal segment**
      (1) The internodal segment is the space between two nodes of Ranvier, occupied by one Schwann cell (see Figure 4-4).
      (2) One Schwann cell nucleus is present for each internodal segment.
      (3) In some neuropathies, such as in lead poisoning, individual Schwann cells along peripheral nerves will die, while other Schwann cells remain. The lesion is called **segmental demyelination** of Gombault and Stransky (see Figure 2-9E).

C. The three connective tissue sheaths in peripheral nerves are, from inside out, the endoneurium, perineurium, and epineurium.

1. The **endoneurium** consists of scattered fibrocytes and numerous collagen fibrils, which run longitudinal to the nerve fibers (see Figures 4-2C and 4-3).
   a. The collagen fibrils of the endoneurium run in the space between the surface membranes of the individual Schwann cells, which embed the axons.
   b. Those endoneurial collagenous fibrils close to the Schwann cell contact a carbohydrate matrix that covers the cell surface, thus forming a **basal lamina**.
   c. The outer surface of the Schwann cell, the basal lamina, and the immediately adjacent endoneurial fibrils form the **neurilemmal sheath** of classic light microscopy.
   d. The term **nerve fiber** designates the axon and, when present, its myelin and neurilemmal sheaths.
   e. The term **axon** refers only to the actual axoplasmic extension of the neuron and excludes the sheaths.

2. The **perineurium** divides the nerve into fascicles (see Figure 4-1).
   a. The perineurial sleeve around each fascicle consists of:
      (1) Concentric lamellae of fibrocytes, flattened and oriented circumferentially (see Figure 4-2A–C)
      (2) Collagen fibers oriented circumferentially and obliquely

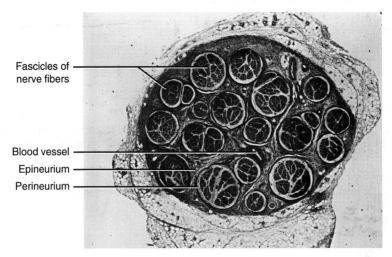

Fascicles of nerve fibers

Blood vessel

Epineurium

Perineurium

FIGURE 4-1. Low-power microphotographs (25 ×) of silver-impregnated cross section of peripheral nerve, showing round fascicles of nerve fibers separated by connective tissue, consisting of the ring-like perineurium and the looser epineurium, containing blood vessels.

  b. Electron microscopy shows that the perineurial cells have a basal lamina on their inside and outside surfaces and that the cell membranes form **tight junctions** where they contact each other.

 3. The **epineurium** is the outermost sheath of peripheral nerves (see Figure 4-1).
  a. It consists of fibrocytes and collagen fibers, and it conveys blood vessels and lymphatic vessels.
  b. The epineurium binds together the fascicles demarcated by the perineurium and conveys blood vessels destined for the interior of the nerve.

D. Functions of the connective tissue sheaths in peripheral nerves

 1. The connective tissue sheaths with their interwoven fibers provide **strength with flexibility** (compare a cable woven of many strands to a solid metal rod of equal diameter).
  a. The interweaving of the collagen strands and the undulating course of the fascicles allow for stretch when the extremities move.
  b. Although peripheral nerves have great tensile strength, they lack resistance to compression. Hence, the nerves may suffer **compression neuropathies** where they pass by bones or the edges of ligaments.

 2. The **perineurium** provides a **blood-nerve fiber barrier**.
  a. The tight junctions where the membranes of the perineurial cells contact each other provide a selective barrier to chemical substances. They may also block the access of viruses into the fascicles, and hence, into the axons.
  b. The perineurium and the amphicytes (satellite cells) around neurons of the ganglia provide a continuous protective barrier along the entire surface of neuronal membranes in the peripheral nervous system (PNS), in analogy with the blood-brain barrier and the brain-cerebrospinal fluid (CSF) barrier of the central nervous system (CNS) [see Chapter 2 VI C]. These anatomic constructions ensure that the surface of the neuronal membrane, with its rich and seductive array of receptors, remains a "privileged site" that is accessible only to the appropriate neurotransmitters.

E. Blending of the three meninges with the three connective tissue sheaths of peripheral nerves

 1. After the dorsal and ventral roots unite to exit from the vertebral canal at the **intervertebral foramina,** the three meningeal sheaths of the CNS merge with the three connective tissue sheaths of the PNS.
  a. The **dura mater** continues distally as the **epineurium**.
  b. The **pia-arachnoid,** or **leptomeninges,** continues distally as the **perineurium** and **endoneurium**.

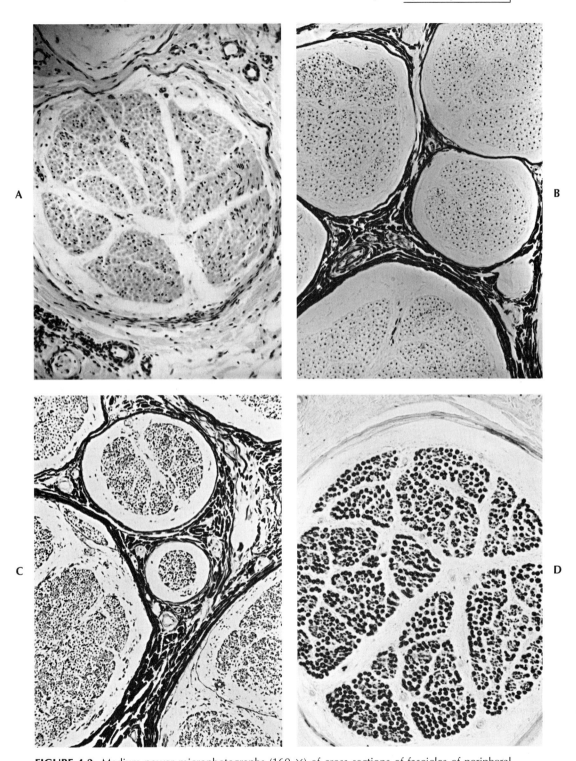

FIGURE 4-2. Medium-power microphotographs (160 ×) of cross sections of fascicles of peripheral nerve with surrounding perineurial sheaths. (*A*) Nissl stain, showing nuclei of Schwann cells and fibrocytes. Perineurial fibrocytes encircle the entire fascicle. Note blood vessels in the epineurium. (*B*) Selective silver impregnation showing axons. The surrounding myelin sheaths and endoneurium are unstained, but the perineurium and epineurium are well shown. (*C*) Less selective silver impregnation showing axons and endoneurium. (*D*) Selective iron-hematoxylin stain for myelin sheaths, which appear as small, dark rings around each axon. The axons, endoneurium, perineurium, and nuclei are unstained.

2. The nerve roots themselves, as they cross the subarachnoid space, lack an epineurium and a perineurial fascicular arrangement (Figure 4-5).
    a. Lacking the tensile strength provided by the two outer sheaths, nerve roots will avulse from the cord or suffer a stretch injury if a peripheral nerve is pulled too hard.
    b. Blunt trauma that stretches an extremity or traction on a baby's arm or shoulder during a difficult delivery may cause permanent paralysis.

II. CLASSIFICATION OF NERVE FIBERS

A. Anatomic versus functional classification

1. **Anatomically,** nerve fibers can be classified by:
    a. Diameter
    b. Length
    c. Presence or absence of a myelin sheath

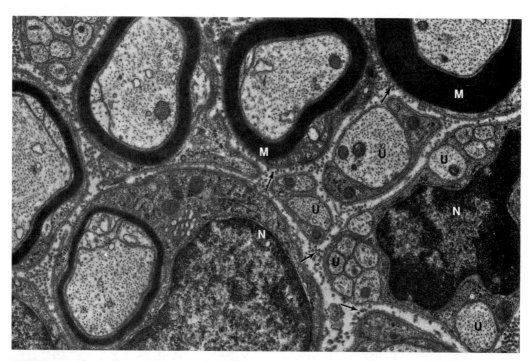

FIGURE 4-3. Electron microphotograph (22,500 ×) of a normal peripheral nerve in cross section. *Arrows* = endoneurial collagen fibrils cut in cross section (they are located in the extracellular space, between surface membranes of the Schwann cells); *M* = the myelin sheath enclosing a fairly large axon (notice the myelin lamination) [compare with Figure 3-21]; *N* = the nucleus of a Schwann cell; *U* = unmyelinated axons of various sizes indenting the cytoplasm of Schwann cells (some unmyelinated axons are in groups).

FIGURE 4-4. Longitudinal diagram of a myelinated axon showing the nodes of Ranvier and the internodal segment presided over by one Schwann cell and its nucleus.

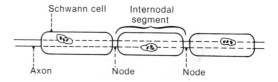

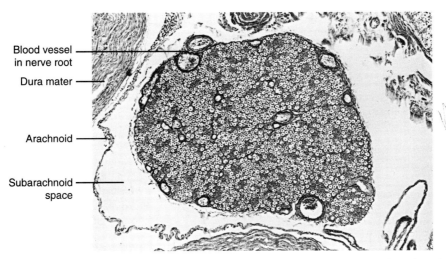

Blood vessel
in nerve root

Dura mater

Arachnoid

Subarachnoid
space

FIGURE 4-5. Medium-power microphotograph (160 ×) of cross section of nerve root in the subarachnoid space, silver impregnated for axons and collagen fibrils. Axons are small dots within clear spaces, which are the unstained myelin sheaths. Notice the scattered groups of small, unmyelinated axons. Compare with Figures 4-1 and 4-2B and C, and note the absence of fascicular structure and the absence of distinct epi- and perineurial sheaths.

     d. Cells of origin
     e. Distribution peripherally and centrally

  2. Functionally, nerve fibers can be classified by:
     a. Conduction velocity
     b. Conduction direction; afferent or efferent (sensory or motor)
     c. Type of sensory modality served
     d. Type of structure innervated; visceral or somatic
     e. Type of neurotransmitter

B. **Relation of nerve fiber diameter to conduction velocity**

  1. Human peripheral nerves contain fibers ranging in size from approximately 1–20 μ in diameter (myelin sheath included) and conducting at rates from approximately 1–120 m/sec.

  2. In general, the larger the axon, the thicker the myelin sheath, and the longer the internodal distance, the faster the conduction velocity. All fibers conducting faster than 3 m/sec are myelinated.

C. **Classification of nerve fibers by size and conduction velocity**

  1. Physiologists classify nerve fibers by a confusing mixture of the English and Greek alphabet and Roman numerals.

  2. The **A-B-C** system of Gasser and Erlanger classifies nerve fibers into three groups.
     a. Group A contains all small, medium, and large **myelinated** afferent and efferent somatic fibers (1–20 μ in diameter).
     b. Group B consists only of small preganglionic **myelinated** axons of the autonomic nervous system (ANS) [1–3 μ in diameter].
     c. Group C consists only of small, **unmyelinated** fibers: visceral afferents, pain and temperature afferents, and postganglionic autonomic efferents (less than 2 μ in diameter).

  3. The **Roman numeral system**, as defined originally by Lloyd, included **all** afferents, but now is frequently restricted to muscle afferents (Table 4-1). Authors usually designate the large cutaneous afferent fibers as A fibers, with Greek alphabet subscripts.

TABLE 4-1. Classification of Nerve Fibers by Diameter and Conduction Velocity

Type		Diameter (μ)*	Conduction Velocity (m/sec)	Terminal Field
Somatic and visceral efferents				
A	Alpha motoneurons	12–20	70–120	To extrafusal skeletal muscle fibers from alpha motoneurons
	Gamma motoneurons	2–8	10–50	To intrafusal muscle fibers from gamma motoneurons
B		< 3	3–15	To autonomic ganglia (preganglionic axons)
C		0.2–1.2	0.7–2.3	To smooth muscle and glands (postganglionic axons)
Cutaneous afferents				
A_α		12–20	70–120	From joint receptors
A_β		6–12	30–70	From pacinian corpuscle and touch receptors
A_δ		2–6	4–30	From touch, temperature, and pain endings
C		< 2	0.5–2	From pain, temperature, and some mechanoreceptor endings
Visceral afferents				
A		2–12	4–70	From visceral receptors
C		< 2	0.2–2	From visceral receptors
Muscle afferents				
I_α		12–20	70–120	From muscle spindles (annulospiral endings)
I_β		12–20	70–120	From Golgi tendon organs
II		6–12	30–70	From muscle spindles (flower-spray endings)
III		2–6	4–30	From pressure-pain endings
IV		< 2	0.5–2	From pain endings

*Myelin sheath included if present.

III. GROSS BRANCHES AND FIBER COMPONENTS OF THE PROTOTYPICAL SPINAL NERVE

A. **Gross branches.** Figure 4-6 shows the gross features of an **intercostal** nerve, which is a prototype for all spinal nerves.

1. Figure 4-6 shows the union of dorsal and ventral roots to form the **nerve trunk**, which branches into a **recurrent nerve, communicating rami**, and **dorsal** and **ventral primary rami**.

2. Figure 4-6 also shows the terminal **sensory** and **motor branches** of the dorsal and ventral primary rami.

B. **Fiber components.** The prototypical spinal nerve has all of the four standard nerve fiber components: general somatic afferent (GSA) axons; general visceral afferent (GVA) axons; general visceral efferent (GVE) axons; and general somatic efferent (GSE) axons (Figure 4-7).

IV. GROSS ANATOMY OF THE VERTEBRAE AND VERTEBRAL COLUMN

A. **The vertebral column** consists of:

1. Twenty-two more or less typical vertebrae (Figure 4-8)

2. Two atypical vertebrae, the **atlas** and **axis,** at its rostral end

3. Nine fused vertebrae, the **sacrum** and **coccyx,** at its caudal end

B. **Intervertebral disks**

1. **Location and function.** An **intervertebral disk** separates each vertebral body from its neighbor. The disks act as shock absorbers for the vertebral column.

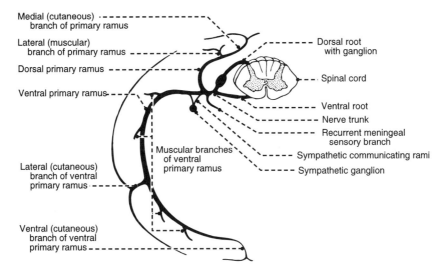

FIGURE 4-6. Gross components of a prototypical peripheral nerve (thoracic level). The dorsal primary ramus, ventral primary ramus, recurrent meningeal sensory branch, and sympathetic communicating rami are the basic branches of the nerve trunk.

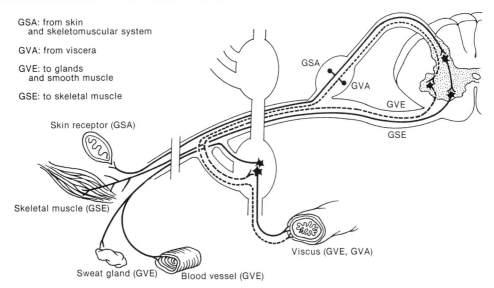

FIGURE 4-7. Four functional types of axons in prototypical peripheral nerve. *GSA* = general somatic afferent; *GSE* = general somatic efferent; *GVA* = general visceral afferent; *GVE* = general visceral efferent.

2. Structure. A disk consists of an **annulus fibrosus** surrounding a **nucleus pulposus** (Figure 4-9A).
   a. The **annulus fibrosis** is dense fibrous connective tissue.
   b. The **nucleus pulposus** is soft, pulpy material.

3. Rupture of disks
   a. Longitudinal ligaments, which run between the vertebral bodies, hold the disk in place.
   b. If the ligaments and the annulus fibrosus rupture, the nucleus pulposus herniates into the vertebral canal.
   c. The herniated disk may compress the spinal cord or a nerve root (see Figure 4-9B). In either case, it may cause loss of sensation or paralysis, depending on the root or part of the spinal cord involved.

C. **Innervation of the vertebra**

1. The vertebrae, joints, and ligaments receive sensory nerves from three sources:
   a. Direct branches from both the **dorsal and ventral primary rami** of the spinal nerves (see Figure 4-6)
   b. The recurrent sinu-vertebral nerve of Luschka (Figure 4-10; see Figure 4-6)

2. These nerves mediate pain (backache) and proprioception from the vertebral column.

FIGURE 4-8. Typical vertebra. (*A*) Superior (top) view. (*B*) Lateral view.

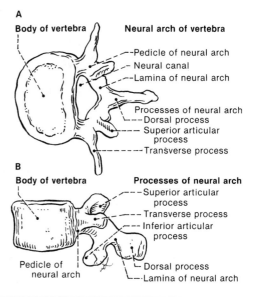

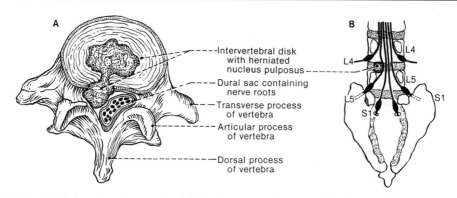

FIGURE 4-9. Herniation of an intervertebral disk. (*A*) Horizontal section of lumbar vertebra and cauda equina. (*B*) Dorsal view of the cauda equina with the arches removed from the pedicles, showing lateral herniation of an intervertebral disk impinging on root L5. (Only roots L4–L5 of the cauda are shown.)

A   B

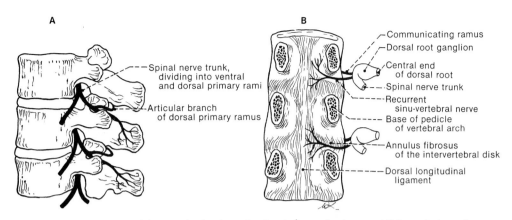

FIGURE 4-10. Innervation of the vertebral column by the sinu-vertebral nerve. (A) Lateral view of vertebrae showing the spinal nerves branching into dorsal and ventral rami as the nerve trunks clear the intervertebral foramina just distal to the dorsal root ganglia. (B) Dorsal view of the vertebrae with their neural
arches removed down to the base of their pedicles, exposing the dorsal root ganglia on the right. The ganglia were pulled laterally to emphasize the origins of the sinu-vertebral nerve of Luschka before the spinal
nerve trunk exits from the intervertebral foramina. [Adapted with permission from Pedersen HE, Blunk CFJ,
Gardner E, et al: The anatomy of lumbosacral posterior rami and branches of spinal nerves (sinu-vertebral
nerves). *J Bone Joint Surg* 38:377, 1956.]

D.   **Relationship of nerve roots, spinal nerves, and the spinal cord to vertebral levels**

1. Numbering of spinal nerves
   a. Humans have 31–32 pairs of spinal nerves, each pair corresponding to a pair of
       embryonic somites.
   b. The spinal nerves are numbered in relation to the vertebrae. There are 8 pairs of cer-
       vical nerves, 12 thoracic, 5 lumbar, 5 sacral, and 1 or 2 coccygeal (Figure 4-11).
   c. There are only **7 cervical vertebrae** but **8 cervical nerves** because cervical
       nerve 1 (C1) comes out **rostral** to the first cervical vertebra and cervical nerve 8
       (C8) comes out **caudal** to the seventh cervical vertebra.
   d. Caudal to the cervical level, the numbers assigned to the vertebrae and spinal
       nerves correspond (see Figure 4-11).

2. Effect of ascensus of the spinal cord on the length and angulation of nerve roots
   a. Because the vertebral column elongates faster during gestation than the spinal
       cord, the caudal tip of the cord, which originally lies opposite the coccyx, comes
       to lie opposite the first lumbar vertebra (L1).
   b. Because of this relative elevation (ascensus), the more **caudal** a nerve root, the
       further it must run to reach its intervertebral foramen and the greater its down-
       ward angulation (see Figure 4-11).
   c. Because the tip of the cord lies at L1, a physician can insert a needle into the
       subarachnoid space at L4–L5 or L5–S1 to obtain CSF for diagnostic analysis with-
       out fear of puncturing the cord. The nerve roots move aside and generally are
       undamaged by the needle.

V.   **THE SEGMENTAL (SOMITE) PATTERN OF SOMATIC SENSORY
       AND MOTOR INNERVATION**

A.   **Innervation of somite derivatives** (see Chapter 3 VII).

   1. One spinal nerve innervates the dermatome, myotome, and sclerotome derived
       from one somite.

   2. Wherever the somite derivative migrates during embryogenesis, it retains its original
       somite nerve.

FIGURE 4-11. Topographic relationship between nerve roots and spinal cord segments (Arabic numbers), and the bodies and spinous processes of the vertebrae (Roman numerals). (Adapted with permission from Haymaker W, Woodhall B: *Peripheral Nerve Injuries*, 2nd ed. Philadelphia, WB Saunders, 1953, p 32.)

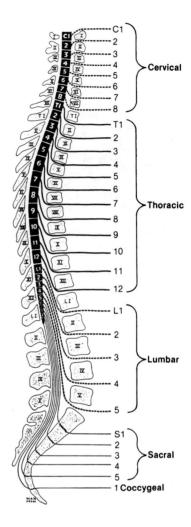

3. The somites rearrange most extensively in the head, arm, and leg regions. The thorax retains the simple serial somite plan, undisturbed by somite rearrangements (Figure 4-12).

4. The somatic nerve plexuses redistribute the axons from the spinal nerve trunks into convenient pathways to the migrated somite derivatives of the head, arms, and legs.

B. **Final distribution of somite derivatives**

1. Figure 4-13 shows the final arrangements in the leg of the **dermatomes**, **sclerotomes**, and **myotomes** with their segmental innervation.

2. Contrast the dermatomal distributions in Figure 4-12 with the peripheral nerve distributions in Figure 4-14.

C. **Important dermatomal distributions to remember**

1. No useful purpose is served by memorizing Figures 4-12 and 4-14. However, some knowledge of dermatomal levels is important because of the frequency of nerve root compression syndromes in everyday clinical practice.

2. Spinal dermatomes begin with **C2,** which abuts on the sensory area of cranial nerve (CN) V (see Figure 4-12). Spinal nerve C1 often departs from the prototype by lacking a dorsal root.

3. C3 and C4 innervate the cape area, which is where a graduation cape would rest on the neck and shoulders.

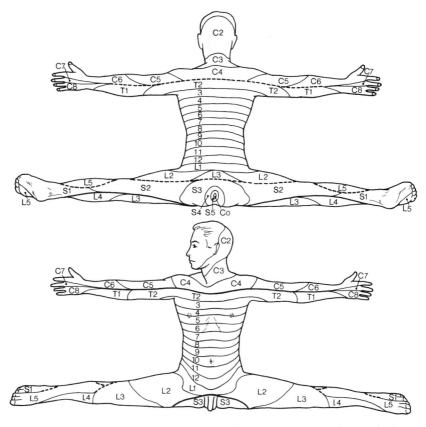

FIGURE 4-12. Distribution in the leg of the dermatomes (skin), myotomes (muscles), and sclerotomes (bones) by spinal segments L1 to S3. (Reprinted with permission from Bateman JE: *Trauma to Nerves in Limbs.* Philadelphia, WB Saunders, 1962, p 79.)

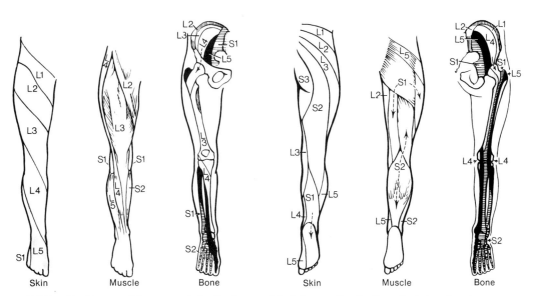

FIGURE 4-13. Pattern of dermatomal distributions and their innervation by the spinal dorsal roots. (Reprinted with permission from Haymaker W, Woodhall B: *Peripheral Nerve Injuries,* 2nd ed. Philadelphia, WB Saunders, 1953, p 19.)

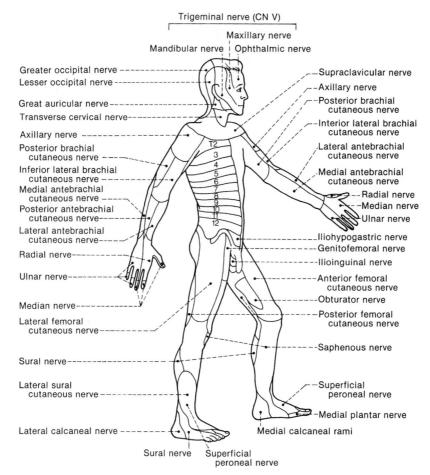

Trigeminal nerve (CN V)

Maxillary nerve
Mandibular nerve | Ophthalmic nerve

Greater occipital nerve --------------
Lesser occipital nerve --------------

Great auricular nerve--------------
Transverse cervical nerve--------------

Axillary nerve --------------
Posterior brachial
  cutaneous nerve ----
Inferior lateral brachial
  cutaneous nerve --------------
Medial antebrachial
  cutaneous nerve ----
Posterior antebrachial
  cutaneous nerve--------
Lateral antebrachial
  cutaneous nerve----

Radial nerve----------

Ulnar nerve--------

Median nerve--------------
Lateral femoral
  cutaneous nerve----------

Sural nerve--------------

Lateral sural
  cutaneous nerve --------------

Lateral calcaneal nerve --------

Sural nerve   Superficial
                peroneal nerve

--Supraclavicular nerve
--Axillary nerve
--Posterior brachial
  cutaneous nerve
--Interior lateral brachial
  cutaneous nerve
Lateral antebrachial
  cutaneous nerve
Medial antebrachial
  cutaneous nerve
--Radial nerve
--Median nerve
--Ulnar nerve

Iliohypogastric nerve
Genitofemoral nerve
Ilioinguinal nerve
Anterior femoral
  cutaneous nerve
Obturator nerve
Posterior femoral
  cutaneous nerve

Saphenous nerve

--Superficial
  peroneal nerve
--Medial plantar nerve
Medial calcaneal rami

T2
3
4
5
6
7
8
9
10
12

FIGURE 4-14. Pattern of cutaneous innervation by the peripheral nerves. Note that spinal nerves T2–T12 receive numbers only, whereas the other nerves, which run through plexuses, receive names. (Adapted with permission from Poeck K: *Einguhrung in die klinische Neurologie.* New York, Springer-Verlag, 1966, p 23.)

4. C5 and C6 run down the **top surface** of the arm, **C7** innervates the middle finger, and T1 and T2 run up the **under surface** side of the arm. Hence, merely remember the distribution of C7; C4–T2 are arranged in an orderly way around it.

5. **T4** innervates the level of the nipple; **T10** innervates the level of the umbilicus.

6. L2, L3, and L4 creep down the front of the leg; **L5** innervates the big toe and **S1** innervates the little toe. **S2**, **S3**, **S4**, and **S5** converge toward the tip of the coccyx. Hence, remember L5 and S1 and the S2–S5 convergence.

7. We have now reduced the problem to remembering **C2**, **C7**, **T4**, and **T10**; **L5** and **S1**; and the convergence of **S2–S5** on the **coccygeal bull's eye**.

D. **Overlapping of dermatomal innervation.** The sharp lines on the dermatomal charts (see Figure 4-12) give a false impression of the sharpness of dermatomal boundaries as disclosed by clinical examination.

1. The sensory nerve terminals overlap considerably at the dermatomal margins (Figure 4-15).

2. Anatomic overlapping explains the fact that a patient may experience pain or numbness in a dermatomal distribution but the physician, upon sensory examination with a wisp of cotton or a pin, may not detect any sensory loss. Thus, the description of the area of sensory loss by a reliable patient may prove a better guide to the involved dermatome and its sensory root than the examination.

3. Touch fibers overlap more at the dermatomal margins than do pain and temperature fibers. Hence, testing the distribution of loss of pain and temperature may delineate a dermatomal loss in a single root better than the testing of touch.

4. Peripheral nerve boundaries are generally sharper than dermatomal boundaries. Hence, peripheral nerve lesions produce a sharper sensory border than root lesions.

E. **The segmental innervation of myotomes** is given in Table 4-2 and that of spinal reflexes is given in Table 4-3.

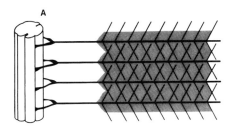
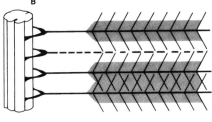
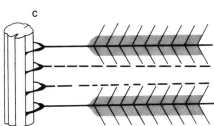

FIGURE 4-15. (*A*) The herringbone pattern represents the width of the band for touch innervation by each spinal nerve, which overlaps its neighbors. The shaded areas represent the narrower band of pain innervation for each spinal nerve, which does not overlap. (*B*) After one spinal nerve is destroyed, testing for touch may not disclose a loss because of overlapping bands of innervation, whereas a band of pain loss can be found because the pain bands do not overlap. (*C*) With two adjacent spinal nerves destroyed, the patient has a band of anesthesia for touch and pain, but the band of loss of pain is wider than the band of loss of touch.

TABLE 4-2. Segmental Innervation of Myotomes

Segment	Structures Innervated
C1–C4	Neck muscles
C3–C5	Diaphragm
C5–C6	Biceps, deltoid
C7–C8	Triceps; long muscles of the forearm
C8–T1	Some long muscles for finger and wrist movements; the small intrinsic muscles of the hand
T2–T12	Axial musculature; intervertebral muscles; intercostal muscles; abdominal muscles
L1–L2	Flexors of the thigh
L2–L4	Quadriceps of the thigh
L4–S1	Extensors of the foot and great toe
L5–S1	Gluteal muscles
S1–S2	Plantar flexors of the foot (calf muscles); intrinsic foot muscles
S3–S5	Muscles of the pelvic floor, bladder, sphincters, and external genitalia

TABLE 4-3. Segmental Innervation of Spinal Reflexes

Deep Muscle Reflexes	Superficial Reflexes	Methods of Elicitation	Normal Results	Segment Traversed
Biceps		Tap biceps tendon	Flexion of the forearm at the elbow	C5–C6
Triceps		Tap triceps tendon	Extension of the forearm at the elbow	C6–C7
Brachioradial		Tap styloid process of the radius, with forearm held in semipronation	Flexion of the forearm at the elbow	C7–C8
Finger flexion		Flick palmar surface of the tip of the finger	Flexion of the fingers	C7–T1
Abdominal muscle		Tap lowermost portion of the thorax or abdominal wall; or tap symphysis pubis	Contraction of the abdominal wall or, when the symphysis is tapped, adduction of the leg	T8–T12
	Abdominal skin and muscle	Stroke skin of the upper abdominal quadrants	Contraction of the abdominal muscle and retraction of the umbilicus to the stimulated side	T8–T12
	Cremaster	Stroke skin of the upper and inner thigh	Upward movement of the testicle	L1–L2
Adductor		Tap medial condyle of the tibia	Adduction of the leg	L2–L4
Quadriceps		Tap tendon of the quadriceps femoris	Extension of the lower leg	L2–L4
Triceps surae		Tap tendon Achillis	Plantar flexion of the foot	L5–S2
	Plantar	Stroke sole of the foot	Plantar flexion of the toes	S1–S2
	Anal	Prick skin of the perianal region	Contraction of the anal sphincter—"anal wink"	S4–Co1
	Bulbo-cavernous	Prick skin of the glans penis	Contraction of the bulbocavernosus muscle and constrictor urethrae	S3–S4

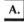

VI. PLEXUSES AND PERIPHERAL NERVE DISTRIBUTIONS

A. Distribution of nerve trunks

1. After the dorsal and ventral roots unite to form a single spinal nerve trunk, the trunk reaches its terminal distributions by one of two routes.
    a. The nerve trunk may extend directly to its end stations without interchanging fascicles with a neighboring nerve, as shown by the typical intercostal nerve in Figure 4-6.
    b. The nerve trunk may interchange fascicles with neighboring trunks. The interchange of fascicles from adjacent nerves produces a **plexus** (see Figure 3-20).

2. The distribution of the peripheral nerves that issue from the plexus differs considerably from the dermatomal distributions, except in the thoracic region, where no plexuses exist (compare Figure 4-12 to Figure 4-14).

B. Summary of the segmental relations among roots, plexuses, and their peripheral nerves

1. **Dorsal roots** convey **sensory** axons and **ventral roots** convey **motor** axons of only **one** somite (one segment).

2. **Intercostal nerves** (T2–T12) convey both **sensory and motor** axons of **only one** somite.

3. The **peripheral nerves** that issue from a **plexus** convey **sensory** and **motor axons** from **more than one** somite.

4. The intercostal nerves (T2–T12) and their nerve roots have no special name, only a number corresponding to their spinal cord level.

5. The peripheral nerves that issue from a plexus **always** receive a name.

6. The **histologic structure** of intercostal and plexus nerves is the same, although many plexus nerves are much larger than intercostal nerves.

C. The cervical plexus. The cervical is the first of the three plexuses: the **cervical, brachial,** and **lumbosacral.**

1. **Anatomical pattern** (Figure 4-16)

2. **Segmental origin: C1–C4**

3. **Motor distribution**
   a. The cervical plexus innervates muscles that turn, flex, and extend the head and open the jaw.
   b. It shares innervation of the trapezius muscles with CN XI.
   c. The cervical plexus **originates the phrenic nerve,** which is the most important spinal nerve in the body because it innervates the diaphragm, the most important muscle for breathing.
      (1) The phrenic nerve arises from roots C3–C5 but mainly from C4 (see Figure 4-16).
      (2) The nerve runs behind the anterior thoracic wall to reach the diaphragm.

4. **Sensory distribution**
   a. The cervical plexus innervates the skin on the back of the head (C2) via the **greater** and **lesser occipital nerves** (see Figure 4-14) and the cape area of the neck and shoulders by the supraclavicular nerves (C3 and C4).
   b. It conveys afferents from neck muscles and adjacent vertebrae.

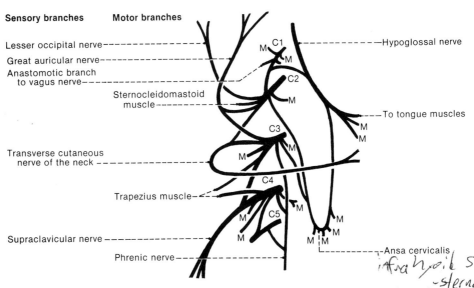

FIGURE 4-16. Frontal view of the right cervical plexus. *M* = motor to striated muscle.

D. **Brachial plexus**

1. **Anatomic pattern** (Figure 4-17)

2. **Segmental origin: C5–T1**

3. **Motor distribution.** The brachial plexus innervates the muscles of the shoulder girdle, upper chest wall, arms, and hands (Figure 4-18).

4. **Sensory distribution.** The brachial plexus innervates skin, bones, and muscles of the shoulders, arms, and hands (see Figures 4-14 and 4-17).

5. **Plan of the brachial plexus** (Table 4-4; see Figure 4-18)
   a. The brachial plexus derives from **five nerve roots** (C5–T1), which form **three nerve trunks** and **three cords**, and issues **five major terminal nerves** (see Figure 4-17, 1–5).
   b. The brachial plexus also issues a number of smaller nerves, most of which branch off at acute angles to the longitudinal axis of the plexus (see Figure 4-17, a–f). These nerves innervate muscles of the shoulder girdle and chest wall and the skin of the arm.
   c. The **five major terminal nerves** extend distally in the long axis of the plexus into the shoulder and arm (see Table 4-4; see Figures 4-17 and 4-18). These nerves comprise:
      (1) One for the **shoulder**—the **axillary or circumflex nerve**
      (2) Four for the **arm**—the **musculocutaneous, radial, median,** and **ulnar nerves**

6. **Mnemonic based on C7 to remember the plan of the brachial plexus**
   a. Notice that root **C7** forms an **axis of symmetry** (Figure 4-19).
   b. Of the five spinal nerve trunks that form the plexus, two (C5 and C6) are **rostral** to C7 and two (C8 and T1) are **caudal** to C7.
   c. C7 runs directly into its cord (although spoiling the purity of its symmetry by branching to the upper cord), whereas C5 and C6 unite and C8 and T1 unite (see Figure 4-19).

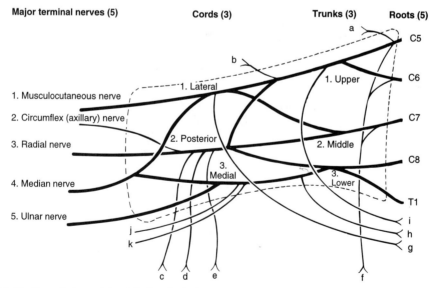

FIGURE 4-17. Frontal view of the right brachial plexus. The dashed line encloses the major roots and the largest branches. After the dorsal and ventral **roots** converge to form nerve **trunks**, the **cords** redistribute them to the major **terminal nerves**. a = Dorsal scapular nerve to rhomboid muscle; b = suprascapular nerve to supra- and infraspinatus muscles; c = inferior subscapular nerve to teres major muscle; d = thoracodorsal nerve to latissimus dorsi muscle; e = superior subscapular nerve to subscapular muscle; f = long thoracic nerve to serratus anterior muscle; g = lateral pectoral nerve to pectoralis muscle; h = medial pectoral nerve to pectoralis muscle; i = subclavian nerve to subclavius muscle; j = medial cutaneous nerve of the forearm; k = medial cutaneous nerve of the arm.

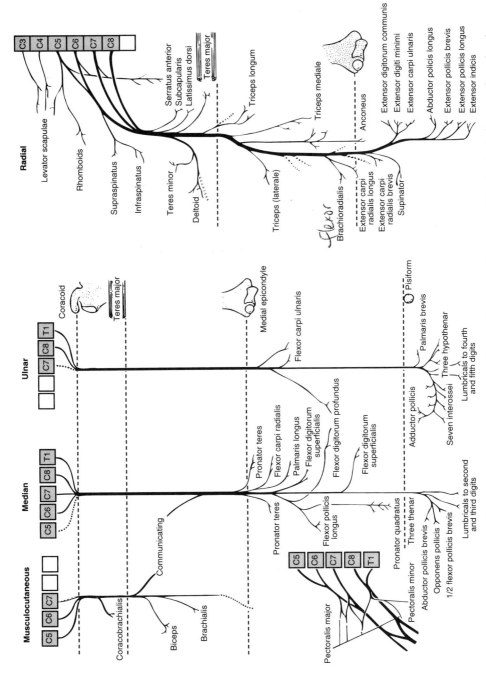

FIGURE 4-18. Innervation of the muscles in the upper extremities by the terminal branches of the brachial plexus. (Adapted with permission from Grant JCB: *An Atlas of Anatomy*, 5th ed. Baltimore, Williams & Wilkins, 1962.)

d. After receiving communications from the united trunks of C5 and C6 and C8 and T1, C7 forms the **posterior** cord on the **back** of the plexus.

  (1) The posterior cord **radiates** in a straight course **down the back of the arm** as the **radial nerve.**

  (2) Its only major proximal branch is the **axillary (circumflex) nerve.**

TABLE 4-4. Summary of the Motor Distributions of the Major Nerves of the Cervical, Brachial, and Lumbosacral Plexuses

Major Terminal Nerves	Segment of Origin	Distribution and Function
Cervical plexus	C1–C4	Supplies neck muscles that turn the head and open the jaw; shares trapezius muscle with CN XI
Phrenic nerve	C3–C5	Innervates diaphragm
Brachial plexus	C5–T1	
Axillary (circumflex) nerve	C5–C6	Elevates the arm (deltoid action); aids in sweeping arm forward and backward
Musculocutaneous nerve	C5–C7	Flexes arm at the shoulder and forearm at the elbow (except for brachioradialis muscle)
Radial nerve	C5–C8	Extensor nerve of the elbow, wrist, and fingers; supplies the brachioradialis muscle, a forearm flexor; extends the digits, except for the distal phalanges, which are extended by the intrinsic hand muscles
Median nerve	C6–C8, T1	Flexor nerve of the wrist (aided by the ulnar nerve) and of the distal phalanges of the fingers, innervates five hand muscles: the three thenar muscles (the flexor brevis, abductor, and opponens) and the two lumbricals (to the second and third digits)
Ulnar nerve	C7–C8, T1	Main mover of the fingers; innervates the flexo carpi ulnaris of the forearm and all interossei, the lumbricals to the fourth and fifth digits, the adductor pollicis, and ½ of the flexor pollicis brevis. (Lumbricals, supplied by the median and ulnar nerves, flex the proximal phalanges and extend the distal phalanges; the interossei waggle the finger laterally and flex the proximal phalanges and extend the distal. The actions of the thumb test three of the long nerves of the brachial plexus: extension, **radial;** opposition to the little finger and abduction, **median;** and adduction, **ulnar.**)
Lumbosacral plexus	T12–S5	
Obturator nerve	L2–L4	Adductor nerve of the thigh
Femoral nerve	L2–L4	Extensor nerve of the knee
Sciatic nerve	L4–L5, S1–S3	Flexor nerve of the knee; flexor and extensor nerve of the foot and toes; in the popliteal space, it divides into the tibial and peroneal nerves
Tibial nerve	L4–L5, S1–S2	Plantar flexor of the foot and toes and invertor of the foot; innervates all intrinsic foot muscles except the extensors
Peroneal nerve	L4–L5, S1–S2	Dorsiflexor (extensor) of the foot and toes and evertor of the foot; innervates long and intrinsic extensors of the toes
Pudendal nerve	S2–S4	Innervates the urogenital diaphragm and voluntary bowel and bladder sphincters; is afferent from the external genitalia
Pelvic splanchnic nerve	S2–S4	Afferent from and efferent to the bladder wall and involuntary sphincters; vasomotor for erection

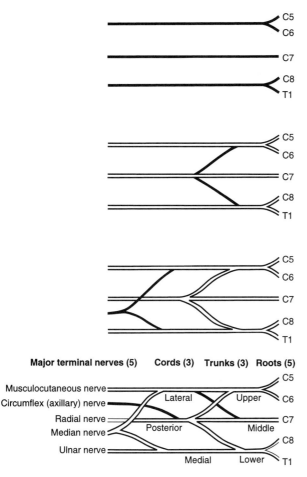

FIGURE 4-19. Progressogram to learn the plan of the brachial plexus. The black lines on each successive drawing show what has been added to the preceding drawing.

e. Ultimately, the C7 dermatomal fibers reach the **digit of symmetry** (the third digit), which has the same relation to the other digits (two on one side and two on the other) as root C7 does to roots C5 and C6 and C8 and T1.

f. To remember both the dermatomal pattern of the arm and the plan of the brachial plexus, learn the course and distribution of root C7.

E. **Lumbosacral plexus**

1. **Anatomic pattern** (Figure 4-20)

2. **Segmental origin: L1–S4**

3. **Plan of distribution** (see Table 4-4)
   a. Like the brachial plexus, the lumbosacral plexus gives off a number of short proximal nerves, in this case, to paravertebral and pelvic girdle muscles, before originating the major terminal branches to the lower extremity.
   b. As a mnemonic, consider the lumbosacral plexus as **two plexuses**: a purely **lumbar** (L1–L4) and a mainly **sacral** (L4–S5) plexus. One major anastomosis from L4–L5, the lumbosacral **anastomotic trunk of Furcle**, connects lumbar roots with the mainly sacral part of the two plexuses (see Figure 4-20).

4. **The lumbar plexus** provides two major **sensorimotor nerves**, the **femoral** and **obturator nerves**, and one purely **sensory nerve**, the **lateral femoral cutaneous nerve**.
   a. The **femoral** and **obturator nerves** innervate the **extensor** muscles of the knee and the **adductor** muscles of the thigh, respectively (Figure 4-21).
   b. **Innervation of the skin of the thigh** (see Figure 4-14)
      (1) The **lateral femoral cutaneous nerve** innervates the anterolateral aspect of the thigh. This nerve may become entrapped where it passes under the in-

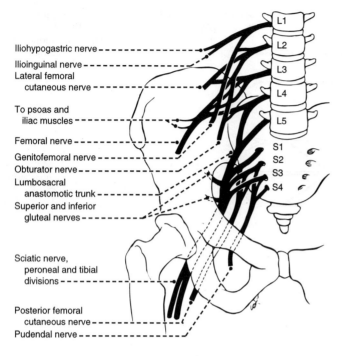

FIGURE 4-20. Frontal view of the right lumbosacral plexus, showing its origin in relation to vertebral levels and to the pelvis. The intermediate (anterior) and medial cutaneous nerves (see Figure 4-14) from the femoral nerve are omitted.

guinal ligament. The patient complains of pain and dysesthesia on the anterolateral aspect of the thigh.

(2) The **anterior femoral cutaneous nerve** from the femoral nerve innervates the anterior part of the thigh and the **posterior femoral cutaneous nerve** from the sacral plexus innervates the posterior part of the thigh.

(3) The **medial femoral cutaneous branch** of the obturator nerve innervates a small area of skin of the thigh medially.

5. The **sacral plexus** provides the **sciatic, pudendal,** and **pelvic splanchnic nerves** (see Figures 4-20, 4-21, and 6-22).

   a. The **sciatic nerve** is the **largest** and **longest** peripheral nerve of the body. It innervates the hamstring muscles of the thigh and all of the leg and foot muscles by its **tibial and peroneal branches**. Thus, consider the proximal part of the sciatic nerve as three nerves—the **hamstring, tibial,** and **peroneal**—bound by one epineurium.

   b. The **pudendal** nerve (see Figures 4-20 and 6-22) is **sensorimotor** to the anogenital region.

      (1) It is **motor** to the external anal and urethral sphincters and related pelvic and perineal muscles.

      (2) It is **sensory** to the glans penis, clitoris, and urethra.

   c. The **pelvic splanchnic nerve** (nervus erigens), a visceral nerve, is **motor** and **sensory** to the bladder and is **vasomotor** for erection (see Figure 6-22).

VII. CLINICAL MANIFESTATIONS OF ROOT, PLEXUS, AND PERIPHERAL NERVE LESIONS

A. **The clinical manifestations of a PNS lesion depend on:**

1. The **anatomic site** of the lesion along the pathway from nerve root to terminal distribution

2. The **functional type of axon** affected (i.e., **motor** or **sensory/somatic**, or **visceral**) [see Chapter 3 VI C]

3. Whether the lesion causes **deficit phenomena**, **irritative phenomena**, **or both**

B. **Definition of deficit phenomena**

    1. **Deficit phenomena** are **negative** signs or **symptoms**, indicating the reduction or loss of a function such as strength or sensation. Deficit phenomena result from interruption of the flow of nerve impulses.

    2. **Deficit phenomena** from interruption of **somatomotor** axons to skeletal muscle are:

        a. Weakness or paralysis of skeletal muscles depending on the number of axons affected

        b. Atrophy and ultimately death of permanently denervated muscle fibers

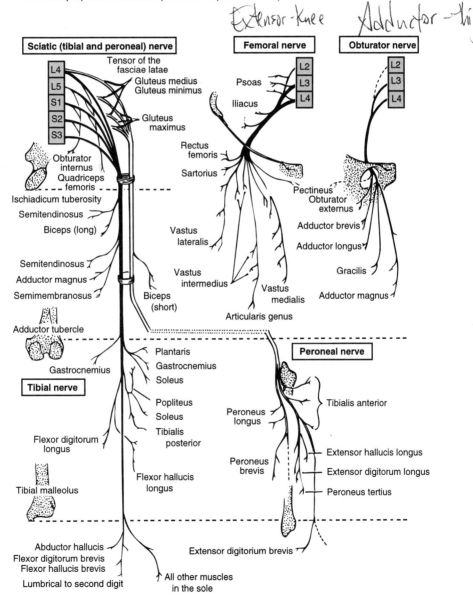

FIGURE 4-21. Innervation of the muscles in the lower extremities by the terminal nerves of the lumbosacral plexus. (Adapted with permission from Grant JCB: *An Atlas of Anatomy,* 5th ed. Baltimore, Williams & Wilkins, 1962).

3. **Deficit phenomena** from interruption of **visceromotor** axons to smooth muscle or glands are:
   a. Atony of visceral walls with lack of peristalsis and failure of propulsion or emptying
   b. Vasomotor paralysis with vasodilation
   c. Anhidrosis
   d. Trophic changes with loss of hair, thinning of the skin, and dystrophy of the nails

4. **Deficit phenomena** from interruption of **sensory axons** consist of numbness or anesthesia.

C. **Definition of irritative phenomena**

1. **Irritative phenomena are positive signs or symptoms**, indicating excessive sensation or the overactivity of a muscle or gland. Irritative phenomena result from either:
   a. Destabilization of the axonal membrane, causing excessive impulse flow
   b. An imbalance in afferent input, which enhances motor activity or a certain sensation

2. Irritative phenomena in the **somatic motor nerves** consist of twitches of muscle, which can be either myoclonic **jerks** or **fasciculations**.
   a. A **myoclonic jerk** is a twitch of all or most of a muscle, as if an electric current had stimulated its nerve.
   b. A **fasciculation** is a much smaller twitch of all of the muscle fibers innervated by one ventral horn cell axon (a **motor unit**) [see Chapter 6 IV C 3 c].

3. Irritative phenomena of the **autonomic axons** include **hyperhidrosis** and **vasoconstriction**.

4. Irritative phenomena in the **sensory system** include **pain, tingling (paresthesias or dysesthesias)**, and **hyperesthesia**.

5. Sometimes **mixtures of irritative and deficit phenomena** occur, as in a dysautonomia called **causalgia**, which may cause trophic changes, hyperhidrosis, and varying degrees of vasomotor paralysis, accompanied by severe pain.

D. **Methods of clinical examination for lesions of the PNS** (see Appendix, page 417)

1. **Motor system**
   a. Inspect the muscles for atrophy or abnormal twitches, and test the skin for excessive or absent sweating.
   b. Formally test the strength of neck, shoulder, and extremity movements by manual opposition, using movements designed to test individual muscles wherever possible.
   c. Formally list any weak muscles.

2. **Sensory system**
   a. Ask the patient to delineate the distribution of the sensory symptoms as carefully as possible.
   b. Formally test for deficits in the sensation of touch, pain, and temperature discrimination (see the Appendix).
      (1) Review of the dermatomal map (see Figure 4-12) will show why in testing for the level of sensory deficit in a dermatomal distribution the physician **circles the extremities** with the wisp of cotton or a pin but goes **up and down the chest**.
      (2) This pattern of testing gives the patient the best chance to compare the stimulus in the affected dermatomes with that in the adjacent intact dermatomes.

3. **Analysis of the findings from the clinical examination**
   a. Outline in ink on the patient's skin or on a drawing the borders of any sensory deficit discovered.
   b. Write down a list of the weak muscles.
   c. Consult charts of segmental innervation (dermatomes, myotomes, and sclerotomes) [see Figure 4-12] and peripheral nerve distributions (see Figure 4-14) to determine whether the deficits match dermatomal or peripheral nerve distributions.

E. How to "think circuitry:" the process of "thinking through" the circuitry of the nervous system

1. Knowledge of neuroanatomy enables the clinician to think systematically through the circuits of the nervous system. The clinician can then identify the sites where a lesion might explain the constellation of signs and symptoms presented by the patient.

2. To analyze a **motor deficit** in the PNS, such as weakness, think through the motor pathway.
   a. Follow along the course of impulse flow according to the neuron doctrine:
     (1) Neuronal perikaryon in the ventral horn
     (2) Central segment of the root (intra-axial course)
     (3) Ventral root (beginning of extra-axial course)
     (4) Nerve trunk
     (5) Plexus (roots, trunks, cords)
     (6) Peripheral nerve (main trunk and branches)
     (7) Neuromyal junction. Include the neuromyal junction in the analysis of weakness because diseases such as myasthenia gravis, a defect in cholinergic transmission, may cause weakness by affecting that site in the circuit.
     (8) Muscle. Include the muscle itself because of the many primary diseases of muscle that can cause weakness.
   b. Thus, in thinking through a motor nerve, travel from nerve cell to synapse to the effector itself.

3. To analyze a **sensory deficit** caused by a PNS lesion, commence with the area of the deficit drawn on the skin of the patient or on a sketch.
   a. Initially, assume that the lesion could be at any site along the sensory pathway. Start with the skin itself because some diseases, such as leprosy, characteristically involve the nerves of the skin. Including the skin is analogous to including the muscles in thinking through the motor system.
   b. In thinking through the sensory pathway consider:
     (1) Skin and receptor endings
     (2) Peripheral nerve (main trunk and branches)
     (3) Plexus (cords, trunks)
     (4) Roots
     (5) Central termination (dorsal horn or, via a spinal cord pathway, up to and including the sensory receptive area of the cerebral cortex). Irritation anywhere along a sensory pathway causes an experience of discomfort at the normal site of origin of stimuli of the pathway, not at the lesion site.

VIII. CLINICAL EXAMPLES OF USING SEGMENTAL AND PERIPHERAL NERVE CHARTS AND OF "THINKING CIRCUITRY"

A. Patient #1

1. **Clinical history.** A patient complains of pain and numbness down the leg and into the lateral side and bottom of the foot and pain in the lower back and hip.

2. **Examination** discloses mild weakness in foot movements and a mild decrease in pinprick perception on the lateral side of the foot.

3. **Analysis** requires **detecting the nerve or nerve root involved**.
   a. The sensory loss involving the lateral side of the foot suggests an S1 dermatomal distribution and thus an S1 nerve root lesion (see Figure 4-12).
   b. Because the S1 sclerotome contributes to the shaft and the proximal end of the femur, the hip pain might also come from irritation of the S1 dorsal root (see Figure 4-13).
   c. The pain in the back might come from rupture of the longitudinal ligament and the compressive effects of the herniated disk on intervertebral joints and adjacent tissue. The sinu-vertebral nerve of Luschka and the direct branches from the primary dorsal and ventral rami of the spinal nerves mediate the back pain.

d. The myotomes of S1 contribute to several of the muscles that move the foot. Weakness of the foot is consistent with involvement of the S1 motor root (see Table 4-2). The clinical findings thus suggest a segmental distribution of sensory and motor loss affecting the dorsal and ventral roots of S1.

4. Hypothesizing the cause for the nerve root syndrome. Statistically, the most common cause of such a syndrome would be herniation of the L5–S1 intervertebral disk, impinging on the dorsal and ventral S1 nerve roots as they join to exit from the vertebral canal.

B. **Patient #2**

1. Clinical history. A woman who sits long hours at a desk complains of persistent numbness over the top of her right foot, worsened by prolonged sitting with one knee crossed over the other. She has no backache.

2. Examination. The patient has decreased light touch and pain sensation over the dorsum of her foot. Sensation of the toes is normal. She also has mild weakness of dorsiflexion of the foot and large toe and of eversion, but strong plantar flexion.

3. Analysis
   a. Either an L5 root or a peroneal nerve lesion could cause the sensory abnormalities.
      (1) The lack of symptoms in the great toe and the lack of a sensory deficit there argues against a radicular lesion.
      (2) The distribution of sensory loss best matches that of the superficial peroneal nerve (see Figure 4-14).
      (3) The weakness of the anterior tibial muscle that dorsiflexes the foot might implicate an L4 or L5 motor root lesion, but that would not explain the sensory loss.
      (4) Interruption of the motor branches of the common peroneal nerve explains the weakness of eversion (peroneal muscles) and foot dorsiflexion (tibialis anterior).
      (5) Compression of the common peroneal nerve at the fibular head (see Figure 4-21) would explain the sensory and motor deficits.
   b. The history of sitting long hours, often with one knee crossed over the other, suggests compression of one common peroneal nerve by the opposite knee, hence producing an entrapment or compression neuropathy.
      (1) The treatment is merely to advise the patient not to sit with crossed legs.
      (2) Complete interruption of the common peroneal nerve at the fibular crossing results in complete footdrop and anesthesia in a triangular patch on the dorsum of the foot, extending somewhat up the leg. In this patient, the interruption is partial, and the chance of regeneration with restoration of function is excellent.

STUDY QUESTIONS

DIRECTIONS: Each of the numbered items or incomplete statements in this section is followed by answers or by completions of the statement. Select the ONE lettered answer or completion that is BEST in each case.

---

1. After fetal growth, the caudal tip of the spinal cord normally is at the level of the

(A) caudal thoracic vertebrae
(B) rostral lumbar vertebrae $- L1 - L2$
(C) caudal lumbar vertebrae
(D) rostral sacral vertebrae
(E) caudal sacral vertebrae

2. A patient complaining of tingling and pain down a leg into the little toe would most likely have a lesion of which sensory nerve root?

(A) L2
(B) L3
(C) L4
(D) L5
(E) S1

3. A patient has weakness of plantar flexion of his left foot. Your examination shows no muscle stretch reflex at the ankle; severe atrophy of the calf muscles (triceps surae); and loss of sensation over the back of the calf, sole, and lateral aspect of the foot. Most likely he has a

(A) femoral nerve lesion
(B) sciatic nerve lesion
(C) peroneal nerve lesion
(D) tibial nerve lesion
(E) primary disease of muscle

4. The dorsal root frequently missing in normal individuals is

(A) C1
(B) C3
(C) T1
(D) L5
(E) S1

5. The phrenic nerve typically originates from

(A) C1–C3
(B) C2–C3
(C) C3–C5
(D) C5–C8
(E) C6–T1

6. The "axis of symmetry" for the brachial plexus is

(A) C3
(B) C4
(C) C5
(D) C6
(E) C7

7. The spinal cord region that has one more nerve than the number of vertebrae is the

(A) sacral
(B) thoracic
(C) lumbar
(D) cervical
(E) none of the above

8. A patient with a stab wound in the shoulder is unable to elevate his arm at the shoulder but can flex and extend his elbow, wrist, and fingers with normal strength. The lesion most likely affects the

(A) circumflex (axillary) nerve
(B) lateral cord of the brachial plexus
(C) radial nerve
(D) C8–T1 nerve roots
(E) medial cord of the brachial plexus

9. The reason that a patient with a herniated lumbar disk that compresses a nerve root may feel severe pain in the hip or upper thigh, rather than or in addition to pain in the foot, is that

(A) the hip is often injured when the disk ruptures
(B) immobility of the leg causes a "frozen" hip joint, similar to the shoulder–hand syndrome
(C) the back spasm associated with disk pain alters the gait
(D) the piriform muscle goes into spasm, compressing the sciatic nerve
(E) the somite of the compressed dorsal root contributes dermatomes to the feet and sclerotomes to the femur

10. In "thinking through" to localize the site

of a lesion along the course of the motor pathway to the periphery, the clinician should commence at the

(A) neuromuscular synapse
(B) effector
(C) plexus
(D) ventral root
(E) motoneurons

11. Which of the following statements about Schwann cells is correct?

(A) Autonomic nerves contain no Schwann cells
(B) Degeneration of one Schwann cell causes degeneration of the neighboring Schwann cells
(C) The Schwann cells arise from glioblasts
(D) Each internode has one Schwann cell nucleus
(E) The Schwann cells are unable to regenerate a myelin sheath

12. Which of the following statements about the anatomy of nerve roots during their entire course through the subarachnoid space is true?

(A) They are strengthened by an astrocytic framework
(B) They have a strong fascicular arrangement and prominent perineurium
(C) They lose their Schwann cells at the intervertebral foramen
(D) They lack an epineurium
(E) They interchange axons freely with ventral roots

13. Select the one true statement about the innervation of the longitudinal ligament of the vertebrae and annulus fibrosus.

(A) Direct branches run from each ventral root to the ligaments
(B) Recurrent branches run from the spinal nerve trunks
(C) Special rami run from parasympathetic ganglia to the nucleus pulposus
(D) Direct branches run from the dorsal roots before they cross the subarachnoid space
(E) The longitudinal ligament and annulus receive no nerve supply

DIRECTIONS: Each of the numbered items or incomplete statements in this section is negatively phrased, as indicated by a capitalized word such as NOT, LEAST, or EXCEPT. Select the ONE lettered answer or completion that is BEST in each case.

14. Histologically, peripheral nerves contain all of the following structures EXCEPT

(A) fibrous connective tissue
(B) blood vessels
(C) myelinated axons
(D) astrocytes
(E) cells with basal laminae

15. The following are true statements about nerve sheaths EXCEPT

(A) the nerve sheaths strongly resist compression
(B) perineural fibers mainly orient circumferentially
(C) the perineurial sheaths divide the nerve into fascicles
(D) endoneurial fibers run in the space between Schwann cells
(E) the epineurium is continuous with the dura mater

16. Which of the following statements about intercostal nerves is INCORRECT?

(A) They contain general somatic efferent (GSE), general somatic afferent (GSA), general visceral efferent (GVE), and general visceral afferent (GVA) fibers
(B) They angulate sharply downward in running through the subarachnoid space
(C) They have simpler distributions than plexus nerves
(D) They receive numbers instead of names
(E) They communicate with the sympathetic ganglia

17. The nerve that does NOT have a cutaneous innervation is the

(A) femoral nerve
(B) common peroneal nerve
(C) pelvic splanchnic nerve
(D) obturator nerve
(E) genitofemoral nerve

18. Deficit phenomena after peripheral nerve lesions as contrasted to irritative phenomena include all of the following EXCEPT

(A) muscle atrophy
(B) vasodilation
(C) anhidrosis
(D) fasciculations
(E) hypesthesia

DIRECTIONS: Each set of matching questions in this section consists of a list of four to twenty-six lettered options followed by several numbered items. For each numbered item, select the appropriate lettered option(s). Each lettered option may be selected once, more than once, or not at all. EACH ITEM WILL STATE THE NUMBER OF OPTIONS TO SELECT. CHOOSE EXACTLY THIS NUMBER.

Questions 19–22

(A) Lesion of the C7 dorsal and ventral nerve roots
(B) Lesion of the C8 dorsal nerve root
(C) Lesion of the C5–C7 ventral nerve roots
(D) Lesion of the C8–T1 ventral nerve roots
(E) Lesion of the lateral (upper) trunk of the brachial plexus
(F) Lesion of the medial (lower) cord of the brachial plexus
(G) Lesion of the lateral (upper) trunk of the brachial plexus
(H) Radial neuropathy
(I) Ulnar neuropathy
(J) Combined radial and ulnar neuropathy
(K) Median neuropathy (carpal tunnel syndrome)
(L) Combined median and radial neuropathy

For each clinical problem, match the appropriate lesion. (Use Tables 4-2, 4-3, and 4-4 and Figures 4-12, 4-14, 4-17, and 4-18 to gain familiarity with how dermatomal, myotomal, and peripheral nerve distributions are used in analyzing neurologic deficits.)

19. A patient complains of intermittent pain and tingling in the little finger and, to some extent, in the adjacent finger. (SELECT 3 LESIONS)

20. During an auto accident, a patient fractures the left humerus and suffers a whiplash injury of the neck. The patient complains of pain and tingling along the top side of his left forearm and into the back of the index finger and thumb. The patient cannot dorsiflex his left wrist. (SELECT 1 LESION)

21. A newborn baby, after a prolonged and difficult delivery, cannot elevate the right arm or flex the right elbow. The muscle stretch reflex (MSR) of the right biceps is absent. (SELECT 2 LESIONS)

22. A computer programmer noticed the gradual development of numbness and a burning discomfort in the palm of her hand, extending mainly into the palmar aspect of the thumb and index finger. Examination discloses mild loss of sensation in that area and weakness of thumb movements, particularly abduction. (SELECT 1 LESION)

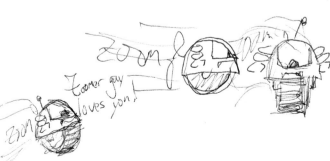

ANSWERS AND EXPLANATIONS

1. The answer is B [IV D 2 a; Figure 4-11]. Early in embryogenesis, the tip of the spinal cord lies opposite the sacral vertebrae, but the vertebral column elongates during fetal growth more than the spinal cord itself. The greater elongation of the vertebral column causes the tip of the cord to rise relative to the vertebral level. Because the cord ends at about L1–L2, the physician can insert a needle into the lower lumbar region to sample spinal fluid for diagnostic analysis without injuring the cord.

2. The answer is E [V C; Figure 4-13]. The patient who complains of tingling and pain radiating down into the little toe would most likely have a lesion of the S1 nerve root. The L5 nerve root typically innervates the big toe. The most common cause would be compression of the nerve root by a herniated intervertebral disk. Thus, the clinical localization of the sensory abnormality implicates the nerve root that is involved by the lesion.

3. The answer is D [VI E 5 a; VII D 3; Figure 4-21]. Loss of sensation over a restricted region of skin associated with severe atrophy of adjacent muscles generally suggests a lesion of a peripheral sensorimotor nerve. A primary lesion or disease of muscle would not cause a sensory loss. The nerve with the distribution most closely matching the sensorimotor findings is the tibial nerve. A lesion of the sciatic nerve would cause deficits in both the peroneal and tibial nerve functions.

4. The answer is A [V C 2; Figure 4-12]. Because of rearrangement of somites at the base of the skull at the transition point from the first cervical vertebra to the occipital bone, the first cervical dorsal root may undergo regression and disappear. Because the front half of the head is innervated by cranial nerve (CN) V, the back half of the head is then innervated by C2.

5. The answer is C [VI C 3 c (1); Table 4-4]. The most important spinal nerve of the body, the phrenic nerve, which causes the diaphragm to contract in breathing, originates typically from C3–C5. The nerve may originate a segment or two higher or lower; thus, from C2–C5 or from C4–C6. Interruption of the spinal cord caudal to the phrenic origin causes paralysis of the intercostal muscles, but the patient can maintain breathing by diaphragmatic action alone.

6. The answer is E [VI D 6 a; Figure 4-19]. To remember the plan of the brachial plexus, think of it as having an axis of symmetry around C7. The brachial plexus arises from two segments above C7 (C5 and C6) and from two segments below C7 (C8 and T1). The two nerve segments rostral to C7 (C5 and C6) unite into a trunk, as do those caudal to C7 (C8 and T1). C7 is located symmetrically between the two unions.

7. The answer is D [IV D 1; Figure 4-11]. The cervical region has seven vertebrae but eight spinal nerves. The reason for the discrepancy is that the first cervical nerve runs rostral to the first vertebra and the eighth cervical nerve runs caudal to the seventh cervical vertebra. The nerve root immediately caudal to cervical vertebra 7 is numbered C8. The number given to thoracic, lumbar, and sacral roots corresponds to the vertebral number.

8. The answer is A [VI D 5 c (1); Tables 4-2 and 4-4; Figure 4-18]. A patient who is unable to abduct his arm but has normal strength otherwise would have paralysis of the deltoid muscle, which is innervated by the circumflex (axillary) nerve. This muscle receives its innervation from the C5 and C6 nerve roots, which run through the posterior cord of the brachial plexus and then enter the circumflex nerve. If the lesion affected the lateral cord, the patient would have had weakness of the biceps muscle and weakness of flexion at the elbow.

9. The answer is E [V B 1; VIII A 3; Figure 4-13]. A patient with a herniated lumbar disk compressing a nerve root may feel discomfort in all of the structures derived from the somite innervated by that nerve root. Because each somite produces a sclerotome and a dermatome, the patient feels discomfort in either one or both of the somite derivatives innervated by that particular root. L5, for example, contributes a sclerotome to the femur and a dermatome to the foot. Root compression may cause pain referred to either site. Some patients will feel pain mostly in the hip, femur, or thigh and relatively little in the dermatomal distribution in the foot. This suggests a primary disease of the hip, such as arthritis, rather than the correct diagnosis of a disk herniation.

10. The answer is E [VII E 2]. In "thinking through" to localize a motor lesion in the peripheral nervous system (PNS), commence at the motoneurons and visualize the axon's course through the ventral root, nerve trunk, plexus if it is a plexus nerve, course of the peripheral nerve along bone and through muscle and fascial compartments, and its terminal distribution and neuromuscular synapse, and the muscle itself. In this way, the clinician will systematically consider the alternative sites for the lesion and can identify the site that best fits the clinical findings.

11. The answer is D [I B 4; Figure 4-4]. Each internode has one Schwann cell nucleus, which is longitudinally oriented. Degeneration of one Schwann cell does not by itself cause degeneration of neighboring Schwann cells because the membranes of the cells are completely independent and separated at the nodal points. Schwann cells can regenerate myelin sheaths after Wallerian degeneration or segmental degeneration. Although Schwann cells are much less numerous in autonomic nerves, they still provide the myelin sheaths for those autonomic fibers that are myelinated.

12. The answer is D [I E 2; Figure 4-5]. As the axons cross the subarachnoid space in the nerve roots, they still retain endoneurial supporting tissue and Schwann cells, but they lack the distinct connective tissue sheaths that divide the peripheral nerve into fascicles. The fascicular pattern, perineurium, and epineurium commence when the roots unite at the intervertebral foramina to form the nerve trunks.

13. The answer is B [IV B, C; Figure 4-10]. The vertebrae and their longitudinal ligaments receive their major innervation from recurrent branches of the spinal nerve trunks and from the dorsal and ventral primary rami. They do not receive any direct branches from the dorsal roots because the dorsal roots themselves enter the cord from the dorsal root ganglia. Because the sinu-vertebral nerves depart from the nerve trunks and curve back in through the intervertebral foramen to reach their terminations, they are called recurrent sinu-vertebral nerves (of Luschka).

14. The answer is D [I A, C; Figures 4-1 and 4-2C]. The peripheral nerves contain the peripheral type of connective tissue, which is fibrous, rather than the central type of connective tissue consisting of astrocytes and other glia.

15. The answer is A [I C 1, E 1 a]. The sheaths of the peripheral nerves have different orientations of their fibers and different reactions to disease. The sheaths allow flexibility and some stretch, but little resistance to compression. The endoneurium consists of connective tissue fibers, which have essentially a longitudinal orientation and run in the space between Schwann cells. The endoneurium undergoes proliferation after loss of nerve fibers, which is a feature readily disclosed by histologic examination of injured peripheral nerve.

16. The answer is B [III A, B; VI B 2, 4; Figures 4-6 and 4-14]. The intercostal nerves are the simplest of the nerves because their somites remain at their level of origin and the intercostal nerves extend directly laterally into them without going through a plexus. They are the prototype of the single spinal nerve–single somite relationship. The lowermost intercostal spinal nerves (T12) extend down onto the lower part of the abdomen, where they border on the lumbar nerves, but they do not angulate downward sharply in the subarachnoid space, as do the lumbosacral nerve roots.

17. The answer is C [VI E 4]. The major sensorimotor somatic nerves of the lumbar plexus include the femoral nerve and the obturator nerve. These nerves both convey a considerable number of sensory and motor fibers to somatic structures. The lateral femoral cutaneous nerve is purely sensory; therefore, lesions of the former two nerves cause both loss of sensation and motor function, whereas damage to the lateral femoral cutaneous nerve causes only sensory disturbances. The pelvic splanchnic nerve, while sensorimotor, innervates the bladder; thus it is visceral, not somatic. The pudendal nerve innervates the voluntary skeletal muscle sphincters of the bladder and anus and also sexual sensations from the glans and clitoris.

18. The answer is D [VII B, C]. Nerve lesions cause both deficit phenomena and irritative phenomena. Deficit phenomena include muscle atrophy, anesthesia, anhidrosis, and vasodilation. Vasodilation is the result of interruption of sympathetic vasoconstrictor fibers. Irritative phenomena include hyperesthesia or paresthesias, pain, and fasciculations. Some lesions cause a severe, burning type of pain called causalgia, with mixtures of deficit and irritative phenomena.

19. The answers are: B, F, I [Figures 4-12 and 4-17]. When a patient reports sensory complaints localized to one or two digits, the clinician starts the analysis by visualizing the relevant dorsal root and dermatome and "thinking through" the course of the sensory axons from their dorsal roots to their end stations. Irritation of a root causes the patient to experience sensation in the whole peripheral distribution of the root. The root that innervates the fifth and part of the fourth digits, C8, travels through the medial (lower) cord of the brachial plexus and down the arm in the ulnar nerve. Hence, a lesion at the C8 root level, lower cord of the plexus, or anywhere along the course of the ulnar nerve could cause the sensory complaint. The definitive localization of the site depends on disclosing any associated motor findings, recording nerve conduction velocities (which documents slowing across the site of the lesion), and sometimes radiography.

20. The answer is H [Figures 4-14 and 4-17]. After leaving the brachial plexus, the radial nerve passes obliquely downward, behind the humerus in the spinal groove of that bone. Thus, fractures of the humerus may cause a radial neuropathy. The patient experiences pain in the radial nerve sensory distribution and weakness or paralysis of the extensor muscles of the forearm. Inability to extend (dorsiflex) the wrist is called a "wrist drop." Similarly, a lesion of the common peroneal nerve, which innervates the extensors (dorsiflexors) of the foot, causes a "foot drop." Had the whiplash injury of the cervical spine affected the C6 dorsal root, the patient might have had a rather similar sensory complaint, but would not have had the "wrist drop."

21. The answers are: C, E [Figure 4-17]. Prolonged labor and difficult delivery, particularly with a large baby, may cause undue traction or stretch on the brachial plexus. The stretch commonly involves the C5–C6 sensory and motor root distributions. The clavicle, or less commonly the humerus, may also be fractured. After combining into the lateral (upper) trunk of the brachial plexus and running through the lateral cord, the C5 and C6 motor roots innervate the deltoid, biceps, and other arm flexors via the circumflex and musculocutaneous nerves. The lesion may consist of an actual avulsion of nerve roots from the spinal cord or only a mild stretch injury affecting the roots or the lateral trunk or cord of the plexus. Avulsions have a poor prognosis for recovery, whereas stretch injuries without physical separation of the nerves may allow complete recovery.

22. The answer is K [Table 4-4; Figures 4-12, 4-14, and 4-18]. The median nerve conveys the motor axons from C8 to the abductor pollicis brevis and the cutaneous innervation from C6 for the palmar aspect of the thumb and forefinger. The C6 dorsal root overlaps the median and radial nerve distributions. The transverse carpal ligament may compress the median nerve as it runs through the carpal tunnel at the wrist. This carpal tunnel syndrome is one of the most common entrapment neuropathies, particularly in persons who hold their hands in specific positions for prolonged periods of time (e.g., working at a computer keyboard). The syndrome may be severe enough to require surgical section of the transverse carpal ligament for relief.

Chapter 5

Peripheral Autonomic (Visceral) Nervous System

I. **RATIONALE FOR RECOGNIZING SOMATIC AND VISCERAL SUBDIVISIONS OF THE NERVOUS SYSTEM.** We will separate the **function** of the **somatic and visceral nervous systems** in the simplest possible way, which is by the **action** of the effectors, not by results or epiphenomena.

A. Somatic system and its effectors (skeletal muscles)

1. The function of the **somatic** or **skeletal** muscle fibers is to **contract** (shorten) or **relax**. In so doing, they activate a skeletomuscular lever or change the diameter of an external orifice (i.e., sphincter action); however, these changes are epiphenomena to the contraction or relaxation of the muscle fibers.

2. Skeletal muscles, being fast acting, tend to respond quickly to stimuli that impinge on the skin surface, eyes, or ears and that generally command conscious appreciation. The skeletal muscles act primarily under the direction of the voluntary motor system of the brain.

B. Visceral system and its effectors (smooth and cardiac muscles and glands)

1. The function of **smooth** and **cardiac muscle fibers** is to **contract** or **relax**.
   a. Because of their radial or circumferential orientation, the visceral muscles change the diameter of an internal organ or internal orifice.
   b. The change in diameter usually moves something along, as in peristalsis or pumping blood (the pupils being an exception).
   c. An organ like the heart functions solely to change its diameter. Blood in the chambers of the heart is moved along, but that is an epiphenomenon to the basic action of a change in the heart's diameter when its muscle fibers contract or relax.

2. The function of **glands** is **secretion**, either to lubricate, digest, control temperature, or change the internal chemistry of the body. If food happens to occupy the gastrointestinal (GI) tract, the process of changing diameter and secreting will move the food along and digest it, but these again are epiphenomena to the basic actions of the effectors.

3. The **somatic system**, with its fast-acting muscles, responds to **external** stimuli and external contingencies that register in consciousness.

4. The **visceral system**, with its slow-acting smooth muscles and glands, tends to respond slowly to **internal** stimuli and internal contingencies, which generally do not command conscious appreciation, except for distension and pain. The viscera are controlled mainly by an automatic or **autonomic system.**

II. **DEFINITIONS AND NOMENCLATURE OF THE AUTONOMIC NERVOUS SYSTEM (ANS)**

A. Definition of the ANS

1. The term **autonomic** comes from **auto** (meaning self) and **nomos** (meaning law); it is the **self-lawed nervous system** because it runs on by itself, largely unconsciously, and according to its own internal laws.

2. We can eliminate all ambiguities by defining the ANS operationally, by its effectors, as **the system that innervates smooth and cardiac muscle and glands**. In so doing, we may then properly include visceral afferent fibers as part of the autonomic sys-

tem because they return impulses from the territories of the effectors. Some authors limit the ANS to purely motor axons.

B. The ANS has two main subdivisions: the **sympathetic** and **parasympathetic** nervous systems.

1. The term **sympathetic** comes from the ancient intuition that the body contains some internal mechanism that mediates the obvious sympathy between the body parts—the swelling of the breasts in sympathy with the gravid uterus or the speeding up of the heart and breathing in sympathy with exercise.

2. Ancient physicians speculated that the pre- and paravertebral ganglia and their interconnections mediated this sympathy between the parts; today, we still classify these ganglia with the sympathetic nervous system.

3. Some authors recognize yet a third subdivision, the **enteric nervous system**, comprised of those neurons that form plexuses in the wall of the hollow viscera, such as the plexuses of Auerbach and Meissner in the gut. The latter are the most autonomic of all because they receive relatively little input from the central nervous system (CNS).

C. **Levels of origin of the parasympathetic and sympathetic nervous systems**

1. The levels of origin of their efferent axons distinguish these two parts of the ANS.

2. The **parasympathetic**, or **craniosacral**, **ANS** arises from the **brain stem** and **sacral** levels of the spinal cord.

3. The **thoracolumbar**, or **sympathetic**, **ANS** arises from the **thoracic** and **lumbar** levels of the spinal cord (Figure 5-1).

D. **The principle of a two-neuron motor pathway of the ANS**

1. A two-neuron pathway conveys motor impulses to the autonomic effectors (see Figure 5-1).
   a. The **perikaryon** of the **first** visceral efferent neuron is located **inside** the CNS, similar to the lower motoneurons to skeletal muscle. Its axon, called a **preganglionic** axon, synapses on a **ganglion** or **plexus** of neurons.
   b. The **perikaryon** of the **second** visceral efferent motoneuron is located **outside** of the CNS, in a **ganglion** or **plexus of neurons**. Its axon, called a **postganglionic** axon, synapses on an autonomic effector.

2. The **perikarya** of **visceral afferent axons** are located in a dorsal root ganglion.

E. **Location of the effectors of the ANS**

1. **Locate the effectors by tracing around the periphery of Figure 5-1.**

2. **Location of smooth muscle**
   a. Iris
   b. All blood vessels
   c. Pulmonary tree
   d. Walls of the GI tract from the lower portion of the esophagus to the internal anal sphincter
   e. Walls and tubes of the genitourinary tract
   f. Piloerector muscles
   g. Splenic capsule

3. **Location and types of glands**
   a. **Mucosal surfaces**
      (1) Salivary glands
      (2) Tear glands
      (3) Mucous glands
   b. **Skin**
      (1) Sweat glands
      (2) Sebaceous glands

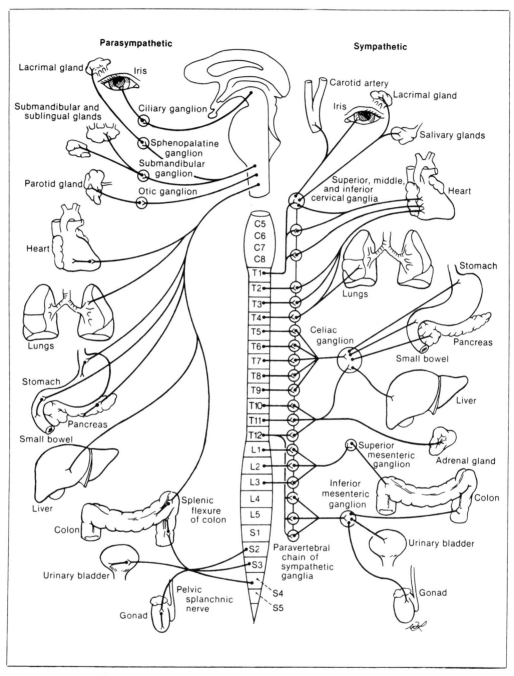

FIGURE 5-1. Diagram of the autonomic nervous system (ANS). The parasympathetic division (*left*) arises from cranial nerve (CN) III, CN VII, CN IX, and CN X and from spinal cord segments S2–S4. The sympathetic division (*right*) arises from spinal cord segments T1–T12.

   c. **Body cavities**
   (1) Adrenal glands
   (2) Pancreas
   (3) Thymus and lymphoid glands and spleen
   (4) Liver
   (5) Pineal gland

4. **Location of cardiac muscle:** heart

III. PARASYMPATHETIC (CRANIOSACRAL) AUTONOMIC NERVOUS SYSTEM (ANS)

A. **Cranial division: level of origin and distribution of preganglionic axons.** Of the twelve pairs of **cranial nerves** (CN), four nerves—CN III, CN VII, CN IX, and CN X—convey preganglionic parasympathetic efferent axons (Table 5-1; see Figure 5-1).

B. **Sacral division: level of origin and distribution**

1. The sacral parasympathetic preganglionic axons arise from the sacral region of the spinal cord, segments S2–S4. They exit through the ventral roots, forming the **sacral plexus**, and then enter the **pelvic splanchnic nerves** (nervi erigentes) [see Figure 6-22].

2. The pelvic splanchnic nerves form a plexus with the pelvic sympathetic axons and run to postganglionic neurons located in the walls of the bladder, the genitalia, the descending colon (from the splenic fixture distally), and the rectum (Table 5-2; see Chapter 6 VI C and Figure 6-22).

TABLE 5-1. Parasympathetic Components of the Cranial Nerves

Cranial Nerve	Site of Nucleus	Preganglionic Nucleus	Postganglionic Nucleus	Effector/Function
III	Midbrain	Edinger-Westphal nucleus	Ciliary ganglion	Pupilloconstrictor muscle of iris
				Ciliary muscle
VII	Pons	Superior salivatory nucleus	Submandibular ganglion	Sublingual and submandibular salivary glands
			Pterygopalatine ganglion	Tear glands and glands of the nasal mucosa
IX	Medulla oblongata	Inferior salivatory nucleus	Otic ganglion	Parotid gland
X	Medulla oblongata	Dorsal motor nucleus of the vagus	Cardiac ganglion	S-A and A-V nodes
			Plexuses	Wall of pulmonary tree
				Smooth muscles and glands of gastrointestinal tract to the splenic flexure of the colon
				Kidney

TABLE 5-2. Parasympathetic Components of the Sacral Plexus

Organ	Preganglionic Neuron Level	Postganglionic Neuron Site	Effect of Stimulation
Distal colon	S2–S4	Intramural ganglion	Enhanced peristalsis
		Hypogastric plexus	Secretion
			Defecation
			Inhibition of anal sphincter
Urinary bladder	S2–S4	Intramural ganglion (vesical plexus)	Contraction of bladder wall
		Hypogastric plexus	Inhibition of urethral sphincter
Genitals	S2–S4	Hypogastric plexus (pelvic plexus)	Vasodilation, penile/clitoral erection

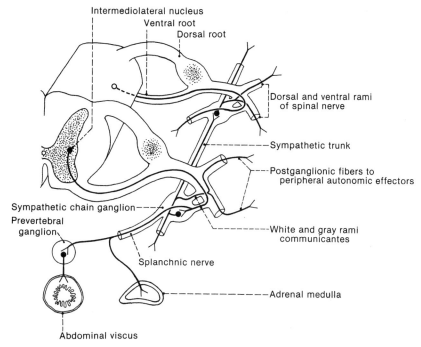

FIGURE 5-2. Formation of the sympathetic chain by ascending and descending axons between the sympathetic ganglia.

IV. SYMPATHETIC OR THORACICOLUMBAR AUTONOMIC NERVOUS SYSTEM (ANS)

A. Level of origin and preganglionic distribution

1. Preganglionic sympathetic axons arise in the intermediolateral cell column of the spinal cord and exit with the ventral roots of spinal nerves T1–L2 (Figure 5-2).

2. The axons enter the nerve trunk and take one of three courses.
   a. They may form a white ramus to synapse with a paravertebral postganglionic neuron at the level of the nerve trunk (see Figure 5-2). The ramus is white because preganglionic axons are myelinated.
   b. They may run rostrally or caudally to synapse on neighboring ganglia, forming a sympathetic chain (see Figure 5-2).
   c. They may bypass the **paravertebral chain** to synapse in a **prevertebral ganglion** (see the celiac, superior mesenteric, and inferior mesenteric ganglia in Figure 5-1).

B. Distribution of postganglionic axons from the para- and prevertebral ganglia

1. From a **paravertebral ganglion**, an axon rejoins an adjacent nerve trunk by way of a gray ramus or travels rostrally or caudally in the sympathetic chain to another nerve trunk. This ramus is gray because the axons are unmyelinated.

2. Typically, the axon then travels distally through a peripheral nerve or along the wall of a blood vessel to its effector (Figure 5-3).

3. In the cervical region, the one-to-one correspondence of paravertebral ganglia with somites is lost and the ganglia fuse.
   a. The rostral-most of these fused sympathetic ganglia, the **superior** cervical ganglion, contains the postganglionic neurons for the head (Figure 5-4).
   b. The **middle** and the **inferior** or **stellate** ganglia provide postganglionic axons to the sweat glands and blood vessels of the arms via the brachial plexus.

FIGURE 5-3. Sympathetic pathway from a preganglionic axon to the arm via the brachial plexus and the subclavian artery.

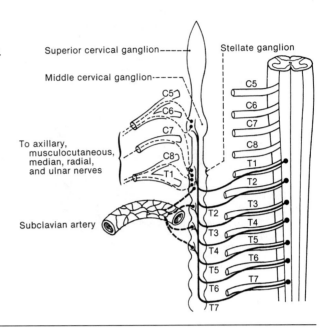

FIGURE 5-4. Sympathetic pathway to the pupillodilator and superior tarsal muscles, sweat glands of the face, and the smooth muscle of the carotid arteries.

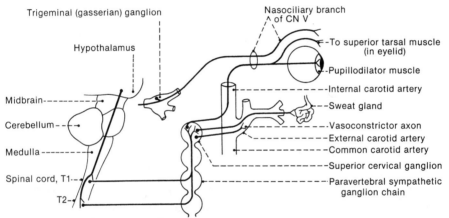

V. COMPARISON OF THE SYMPATHETIC AND PARASYMPATHETIC NERVOUS SYSTEMS

A. **Function.** Both components of the ANS act to maintain homeostasis with the body at rest or in action.

1. The **sympathetic nervous system** dominates during **action**. It prepares us for fight, flight, or fright. It is catabolic and energy expending because it:
   a. Increases heart rate and breathing
   b. Dilates blood vessels in skeletal and cardiac muscles and constricts them in the GI tract
   c. Dilates the bronchial passages
   d. Dilates the pupils
   e. Erects the hairs for protection and display
   f. Increases sweat secretion
   g. Mobilizes glucose

2. The **parasympathetic nervous system** dominates during rest. It prepares us to go to sleep and to digest. It is anabolic and energy conserving because it:
   a. Constricts the pupils
   b. Decreases the heart rate
   c. Increases GI peristalsis and secretion
   d. Expels waste via bladder and bowel function

B. **Location of sympathetic and parasympathetic ganglia.** The ganglia of the sympathetic and parasympathetic nervous systems typically differ in their locations (Figure 5-5).

1. **Sympathetic ganglia** are usually **proximally located** in the **paravertebral** chains or in **prevertebral** masses associated with the abdominal aorta and its branches.

2. **Parasympathetic ganglia** are generally more **distally located**, near or within the organ they innervate, and are isolated rather than in chains. The second neuron in the pathway to the smooth muscle of the hollow, tubular viscera is usually located in an intramural plexus of neurons (submucosal plexus of Meissner and myenteric plexus of Auerbach in the GI tract). Probably by means of interneuronal circuits, these plexuses regulate GI tract motility, mucosal secretion and absorption, and local blood flow.

C. **Neurotransmitters of the ANS**

1. **Cholinergic axons** include:
   a. All preganglionic axons of the ANS, both parasympathetic and sympathetic
   b. All postganglionic neurons of the parasympathetic nervous system
   c. The postganglionic axons of the sympathetic nervous system to the sweat glands and piloerector muscles

2. **Adrenergic axons** include the postganglionic sympathetic axons to most of the remaining smooth muscles and glands (see Figure 5-5).

3. **Additional neurotransmitters.** The discovery of additional neuropeptidergic and amino acid-related transmitters has altered the classical sharp dichotomy into sympathetic and parasympathetic neurons, but these two subdivisions still serve a useful purpose in predicting the effects of various mimetic drugs.

D. **Oppositional action of the sympathetic and parasympathetic nervous systems**

1. The actions of the sympathetic and parasympathetic nervous systems typically are directly antagonistic (Table 5-3), as in pupillodilation (sympathetic) and pupilloconstriction (parasympathetic).

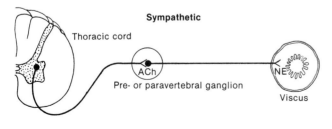

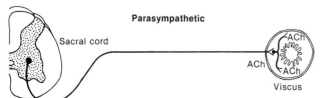

FIGURE 5-5. Comparison of the sympathetic and parasympathetic ganglia. Sympathetic ganglia are paravertebral or prevertebral in location, while parasympathetic ganglia are in or near the organs they innervate. The neurotransmitters of the postganglionic sympathetic neurons are adrenergic, except those for sweat glands and piloerector muscles, which are cholinergic. By contrast, all postganglionic parasympathetic neurons are cholinergic. *ACh* = acetylcholine; *NE* = norepinephrine.

TABLE 5-3. Oppositional Actions of the Sympathetic and Parasympathetic Nervous Systems

Functions Affected	Sympathetic	Parasympathetic
Pupillary size	↑	↓
Heart rate	↑	↓
Blood pressure	↑	↓
Bronchial size	↑	↓
Constriction of smooth muscle sphincters	↑	↓
Constriction of bladder wall	↓	↑
Gastrointestinal peristalsis	↓	↑

2. Some excitatory effects of the sympathetic nervous system lack parasympathetic opposition, including:
   a. Splenic capsule contraction
   b. Sweating and piloerection
   c. Elevation of the upper eyelid by the superior tarsal muscle

VI. GENERAL VISCERAL AFFERENT (GVA) FIBERS OF THE AUTONOMIC NERVOUS SYSTEM (ANS)

A. Functional considerations

1. The GVA fibers as a group do not mediate sensations such as touch, position, and vibration, which are adequate stimuli for skin afferents. The adequate stimuli for consciously appreciated visceral sensation are distension and pain.
   a. Distension, or stretch of a viscus—the bladder, bowel, rectum, or bile duct—produces intense discomfort and pain.
   b. Conversely, constriction of a portion of the wall of a viscus, which causes tension or stretch on the wall, produces cramping pain.

2. Similar or allied mechanisms may produce pain from blood vessel walls. The pain from some headaches, like migraine, has a throbbing character.

B. Anatomic routes for GVA fibers to the CNS. In general, afferent fibers that mediate visceral sensation travel to the CNS by three routes:

1. Parasympathetic nerves: CN IX, CN X, and the pelvic splanchnic nerve

2. Sympathetic nerves: thoracicoabdominal splanchnic nerves

3. Some somatic nerve trunks: phrenic, intercostal, and certain branches of the brachial and lumbosacral plexuses.

C. GVA fibers in parasympathetic nerves

1. GVA fibers travel to the CNS in CN IX, CN X, and the pelvic splanchnic nerves (see Figure 5-1).
   a. **CN IX** conveys GVA fibers from the carotid body and carotid sinus, which influence breathing and blood pressure, and from the pharyngeal mucosa.
   b. **CN X** conveys GVA fibers from the laryngeal mucosa and trachea and from thoracicoabdominal viscera as far distal as the splenic flexure of the colon.
   c. The **pelvic splanchnic nerves** convey GVA fibers from the colon distal to the splenic flexure, the rectum, and the bladder.

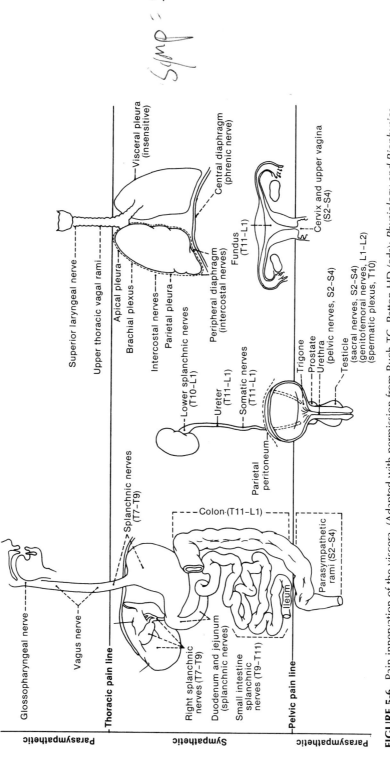

Symp = splanc

FIGURE 5-6. Pain innervation of the viscera. (Adapted with permission from Ruch TC, Patton HD (eds): *Physiology and Biophysics.* Philadelphia, WB Saunders, 1965, p 195.)

106 | CHAPTER 5 VI C

FIGURE 5-7. Sites of referral for some common sources of visceral pain.

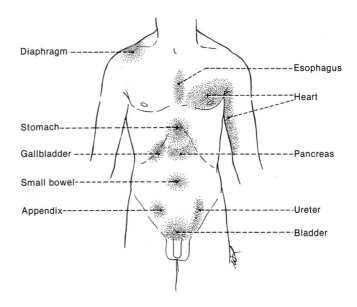

2. Thus, the afferent and efferent fibers of the cranial division of the parasympathetic nervous system, carried by CN X, reach the splenic flexure of the colon, whereupon fibers from the sacral division, carried by the pelvic splanchnic nerves, replace them to innervate the distal colon, rectum, and bladder.

D. **GVA fibers in sympathetic nerves**

1. The nerves that leave the sympathetic chains and pre- and paravertebral ganglia convey GVA fibers back from the viscera and blood vessel walls.

2. These fibers reach the dorsal roots via the communicating rami of the sympathetic ganglia.

E. **GVA fibers in somatic nerves.** Some GVA fibers go directly to the nerve trunk and dorsal root ganglia without passing through the sympathetic chain, and some may join branches of somatic nerves, such as the intercostal and phrenic nerves that innervate the pleura.

F. **Visceral pain and referred pain**

1. Most pain fibers from the viscera run in autonomic nerves (Figure 5-6).

2. Some visceral pain has a fairly accurate localization; for example, we feel a full bladder at the site of the bladder. In general, pain mediated through the parasympathetic nerves (see Figure 5-6) is better localized than pain traveling through the sympathetic fibers.

3. Pain of some visceral structures, notably those innervated by sympathetic nerves, tends to be experienced at a site distant from its site of origin (e.g., pain referred to the left arm from cardiac ischemia); a phenomenon called **referred pain** (Figure 5-7).

■ STUDY QUESTIONS

DIRECTIONS: Each of the numbered items or incomplete statements in this section is followed by answers or by completions of the statement. Select the ONE lettered answer or completion that is BEST in each case.

---

1. The parasympathetic innervation by CN X extends to the

(A) bladder neck
(B) splenic flexure of the colon
(C) ileocecal valve
(D) ileum
(E) ureter

2. Parasympathetic fibers to the bladder would be interrupted by a lesion of spinal cord segments

(A) C1–S5
(B) T1–L2
(C) L1–S5
(D) L2–L5
(E) S2–S4

3. Sweat glands are innervated by what kind of endings?

(A) Cholinergic
(B) Adrenergic
(C) Dopaminergic
(D) Histaminergic
(E) None of these

4. Which statement about the autonomic nervous system (ANS) is correct?

(A) It makes quick adjustments of the postural reflexes
(B) It innervates smooth muscles
(C) It acts through the largest myelinated axons
(D) It conveys the pain afferents from the skin
(E) It sends axons directly to end organs without synapsing in peripheral ganglia

---

DIRECTIONS: Each of the numbered items or incomplete statements in this section is negatively phrased, as indicated by a capitalized word such as NOT, LEAST, or EXCEPT. Select the ONE lettered answer or completion that is BEST in each case.

---

5. Which statement concerning transmitters in the autonomic nervous system (ANS) is IN-CORRECT?

(A) Preganglionic axons are cholinergic
(B) Postganglionic sympathetic axons are cholinergic and adrenergic
(C) Pre- and postganglionic parasympathetic neurons are cholinergic
(D) Autonomic axons of the cranial nerves are adrenergic
(E) Axons that stimulate epinephrine secretion by the adrenal cortex are cholinergic

6. The cranial nerve (CN) that does NOT convey parasympathetic axons from the central nervous system (CNS) to effectors is

(A) CN II
(B) CN III
(C) CN VII
(D) CN IX
(E) CN X

7. All of the following statements about visceral pain are true EXCEPT

(A) it is generally poorly localized
(B) it is frequently referred to a site distant from the lesion
(C) it is generally caused by distension of a viscus or traction on the viscus
(D) it has a more varied route through the peripheral nervous system (PNS) and the central nervous system (CNS)
(E) it does not arise from nerves to blood vessels

8. Fright or flight reactions, mediated by the sympathetic nervous system, include all of the following EXCEPT

(A) cardiac acceleration
(B) bronchodilation
(C) sweating
(D) pupillodilation
(E) salivary secretion

ANSWERS AND EXPLANATIONS

1. The answer is B [III A; VI C 2; Figure 5-1; Table 5-1]. Cranial nerve (CN) X, the vagus nerve, provides parasympathetic innervation to the gut from the pharynx down to the splenic flexure of the colon. This extensive field of innervation is by far the longest of any nerve in the body. The vagus nerve is the caudal-most cranial nerve to contain parasympathetic axons, and CN III is the rostral-most nerve of the cranial division of the parasympathetic nervous system.

2. The answer is E [III B; Figure 5-1; Table 5-2]. The parasympathetic axons for the distal colon and bladder arise from sacral segments S2–S4 and reach their terminal fields by the pelvic splanchnic nerve. A lesion of either the sacral cord or the pelvic splanchnic nerve would interrupt the parasympathetic innervation to the pelvic viscera.

3. The answer is A [V C 1]. The end organs of the autonomic nervous system (ANS) are generally innervated by cholinergic or catecholaminergic nerve fibers. The sweat glands receive their innervation from the cholinergic system. The salivary glands and lacrimal glands also receive cholinergic innervation. Thus, the exocrine gland system in general receives cholinergic, parasympathetic activation.

4. The answer is B [I B 4]. The autonomic nervous system (ANS) provides all of the innervation for the smooth muscles. These muscles and the autonomic reflexes in general react relatively slowly, in contrast to skeletal muscles and their reflexes, such as the postural reflexes, which typically react quickly.

5. The answer is D [V C]. The peripheral part of the autonomic nervous system (ANS) has well-defined neurotransmitters. All preganglionic axons are cholinergic. The autonomic axons in the cranial and sacral nerves are parasympathetic preganglionics. Postganglionic sympathetic axons are either cholinergic or adrenergic, with the cholinergic fibers innervating the sweat glands. The pre- and postganglionic parasympathetic neurons are cholinergic. Because the adrenal medulla corresponds to a sympathetic ganglion, its innervation corresponds to the preganglionic cholinergic fibers.

6. The answer is A [Table 5-1]. Parasympathetic axons travel from the brain stem through cranial nerve (CN) III, CN VII, CN IX, and CN X. CN II, the optic nerve, is an afferent nerve that conveys no axons to glands or muscle. CN III is the only somite cranial nerve to convey parasympathetic axons. Of the five branchial cranial nerves (CN V, CN VII, CN IX, CN X, and CN XI), two—CN V and CN XI—do not convey autonomic preganglionic axons, nor do any of the other cranial nerves (CN IV, CN VI, CN VIII, and CN XII).

7. The answer is E [VI A 2, F 2, 3]. Visceral pain, as compared with somatic pain, is poorly localized and often is referred to a distant site. Thus, gallbladder pain may be referred to the anterior chest region or cardiac pain to the left arm. Generally, the pain is caused by distension of a viscus or traction on it. Both in the peripheral nervous system and the central nervous system, the pathways are more diffuse for visceral than somatic pain. Two of the most painful headaches, migraine and temporal arteritis, may arise from pain receptors in the arterial walls, activated by dilation or inflammation.

8. The answer is E [V A 1]. A generalized discharge of impulses from the sympathetic nervous system prepares for the energy expenditure that occurs during fright or flight, when the individual faces an overwhelming stress. Fear or anxiety induces a dry mouth when an individual attempts to speak in front of an audience. Included in the reaction are tachycardia, bronchodilation, sweating ("sweaty palms"), and pupillodilation. The blood vessels to the muscles and heart will dilate, whereas those to the gut will constrict, thus shunting the blood to the muscles for action and reducing the digestive, anabolic processes of the body.

Chapter 6

The Spinal Cord

I. GROSS ANATOMY OF THE SPINAL CORD

A. Size and extent of the spinal cord

1. The spinal cord is a column of central nervous system (CNS) tissue approximately 43 cm long, with the diameter of your finger. It extends in the vertebral canal from the level of the foramen magnum to the level of vertebra L1 or L2 (Figure 6-1; see Figure 1-3).

2. **Rostral and caudal limits of the spinal cord**
   a. **Rostrally**, the spinal cord, or **medulla spinalis**, expands uninterruptedly into the bulb-like **medulla oblongata**. The dividing line, at the foramen magnum, is arbitrary (see Figure 1-3).
   b. **Caudally**, the spinal cord tapers as the **conus medullaris** to end at the level of vertebra L1 or L2 (see Figure 6-1).
   c. A thin strand, the **filum terminale**, composed of glial tissue covered by pia, extends from the tip of the **conus medullaris** to the sacrum (see Figure 6-1).
      (1) The filum stretches out during the ascensus of the cord in prenatal development.
      (2) After the ascensus, the dorsal and ventral spinal nerve roots angle **downward** on either side of the filum terminale. These roots extend from the lumbosacral cord to exit from the vertebral canal at their original lumbar and sacral vertebral levels. They are named the **cauda equina** because of a resemblance to a horse's tail (see Figure 6-1).

B. Levels of the spinal cord. The spinal cord has 5 levels, with a total of 31–32 pairs of spinal nerves (see Figures 6-1 and 4-11):

1. **Cervical** level, with 8 pairs of spinal nerves

2. **Thoracic** level, with 12 pairs of spinal nerves

3. **Lumbar** level, with 5 pairs of spinal nerves

4. **Sacral** level, with 5 pairs of spinal nerves

5. **Coccygeal** level, with 1–3 pairs of vestigial spinal nerves

C. External longitudinal grooves of the spinal cord (Figure 6-2)

1. A shallow **dorsal median sulcus** and a deep **ventral median fissure** mark the exact sagittal plane of the spinal cord.

2. Shallow **dorsolateral** and **ventrolateral sulci** mark the line of attachment of the dorsal and ventral nerve roots.

3. A shallow **dorsal intermediate sulcus** occurs in the cervical region.

D. Cross sectional anatomy of the spinal cord

1. The spinal cord levels vary in **shape** from round to oval and in **diameter** from 1–1.5 cm. The thoracic region is the narrowest and roundest (Figure 6-3).

2. Two **enlargements** of the spinal cord, the **cervical** and the **lumbosacral**, accommodate the extra neurons that innervate the limbs (see Figures 6-1 and 6-3).

3. **Gray and white matter.** Any cross section of the spinal cord reveals a core of gray matter **centrally** and white matter **peripherally**.
   a. **Gray matter**
      (1) **Composition.** The spinal gray matter consists of neuronal perikarya, dendrites with their synapses, glial supporting cells, and blood vessels.
      (2) **Shape.** The gray matter has an H-shape or, better stated, a **butterfly-**shape. The butterfly projects **dorsal horns, ventral horns,** and **lateral**

(or **intermediolateral**) **horns**. The **cross bar** contains a tiny **central canal** (see Figure 6-2).

b. White matter

(1) Composition. The white matter consists of nerve fibers, glia, and blood vessels. The nerve fibers run rostrally and caudally peripheral to the gray matter.

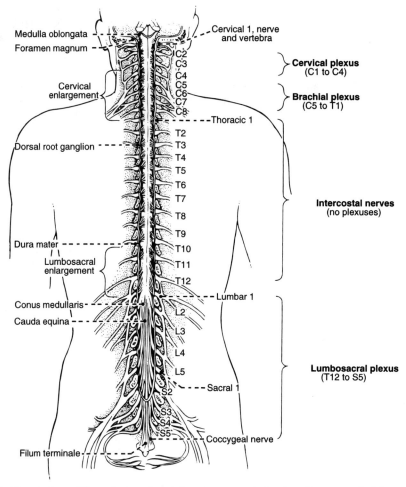

FIGURE 6-1. Dorsal view of the spinal cord and dorsal nerve roots in situ, after removal of the neural arches of the vertebrae.

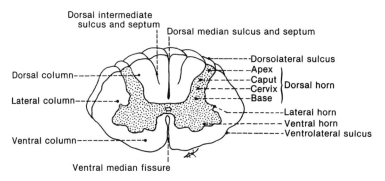

FIGURE 6-2. Cross section of the spinal cord with nomenclature for its crevices and regions.

C3   C7   T5

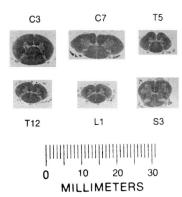

T12   L1   S3

|||||||||||||||||||||||||||||||
0   10   20   30
MILLIMETERS

FIGURE 6-3. Cross sections of myelin stained spinal cord, actual size. The central, lighter, unstained H- or butterfly-shaped area is gray matter. The ventral horns of the gray matter face up. The surrounding area consists of darkly stained myelinated nerve fibers.

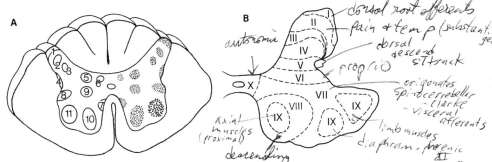

FIGURE 6-4. Nuclear and laminar subdivisions of the spinal cord gray matter. (*A*) Conventional nomenclature of the nuclei. *1* = dorsomarginal nucleus; *2* = substantia gelatinosa; *3* = nucleus proprius; *4* = reticular nucleus; *5* = nucleus dorsalis of Clarke; *6* = dorsal commissural nucleus; *7* = ventral commissural nucleus; *8* = intermediolateral nucleus; *9* = intermediomedial nucleus; *10* = medial motor nucleus; *11* = lateral motor nucleus. (*B*) Laminae of Rexed (Roman numerals I–X).

> **(2) Columns of white matter.** The gray H and the external longitudinal sulci demarcate three **columns** or **funiculi** of white matter, the **dorsal, lateral,** and **ventral** columns, which extend the length of the cord (see Figure 6-2). The exit track of the ventral roots marks the boundary between the ventral and lateral columns in the interior of the cord (see Figure 6-8).

II. THE NUCLEI AND LAMINAE OF THE SPINAL CORD GRAY MATTER

A. Spinal cord nuclei

1. Neuronal perikarya of similar size, shape, and function assemble into columns, called **nuclei** (Figure 6-4A).

2. The perikarya in the various nuclei may differ greatly in size, shape, and connections. Figure 6-5A shows typical neurons of selected nuclei.

3. The nuclear columns in the spinal cord vary in longitudinal extent (Figure 6-6).

B. Laminae of spinal cord gray matter

1. Rexed divided the perikaryal columns into regions or wafers called **laminae** (see Figure 6-4B).

2. The nuclear designations and laminae do not completely correspond (Table 6-1; see Figure 6-4).

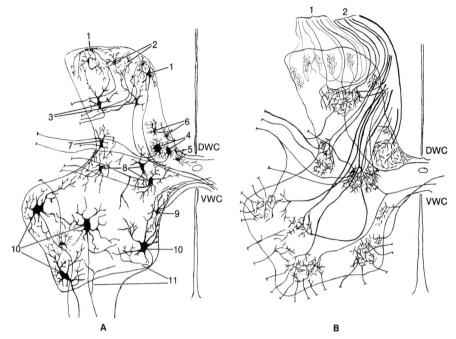

FIGURE 6-5. Cross sections of the right half of the spinal cord. (*A*) Typical neurons of some of the spinal cord nuclei (Golgi impregnation). *1* = dorsomarginal nucleus; *2* = substantia gelatinosa; *3* = nucleus proprius; *4* = nucleus dorsalis of Clarke; *5* = dorsal commissural nucleus; *6* = medial basal nucleus; *7* = lateral basal nucleus; *8* = intermediomedial and intermediolateral nuclei; *9* = ventral commissural nucleus; *10* = medial and lateral motoneuron nucleus; *11* = recurrent collaterals from axons of ventral motoneurons. *DWC* = dorsal white commissure; *VWC* = ventral white commissure. (*B*) Typical distribution of dorsal root afferent axons (silver impregnation). Compare the distribution of axonal terminals shown in Figure 6-5B with the nuclear groups upon which they end, as shown in Figure 6-5A. *1* = Lateral division of dorsal root (small unmyelinated axons, type C fibers); *2* = Medial division of dorsal root (large myelinated axons, type A or class I fibers).

III. FUNCTIONAL ORGANIZATION OF THE SPINAL CORD

A. Organization of the spinal cord gray matter

1. The function of the spinal cord nuclei reflects the division of the peripheral nervous system (PNS) into dorsal roots that are **sensory** and ventral roots that are **motor** (the law of Bell and Magendie), and into somatic and visceral nerve fibers (the theory of nerve components).

2. The **dorsal horns**, like the dorsal roots, mediate **sensation**. They receive general somatic afferent (GSA) and general visceral afferent (GVA) fibers and relay sensory impulses to the rest of the CNS. Dorsal root afferents also extend directly into the ventral horns to synapse on interneurons or motoneurons.

3. The **ventral** horns, like the **ventral** roots, mediate **motor** function. Their perikarya originate general somatic efferent (GSE) axons for the ventral roots.

4. The **intermediate** region receives GVA axons and originates general visceral efferent (GVE) axons.

B. Organization of afferents to spinal neurons

1. The nuclei of one level or segment of the cord receive afferent axons from:
   a. Dorsal roots of the same segment or of rostral or caudal segments
   b. Internuncial neurons (interneurons) of the same segment or of rostral or caudal segments
   c. Descending axons from the brain stem and cerebrum

2. Therefore, the nuclei of any one spinal cord segment receive:
   a. Intrasegmental afferents from the same segment
   b. Intersegmental afferents from caudal and rostral segments
   c. Suprasegmental afferents from the brain stem and cerebrum

3. Table 6-1 summarizes the spinal cord nuclei, their location in the spinal cord, and their connections or functions.

C. **Organization and dispersion of the dorsal roots**

1. Medial and lateral divisions of the dorsal roots
   a. As the dorsal root axons pierce the spinal cord at the dorsolateral sulcus, the **small** axons segregate into a **lateral** bundle and the **large** into a **medial** bundle (see Figure 6-5B).

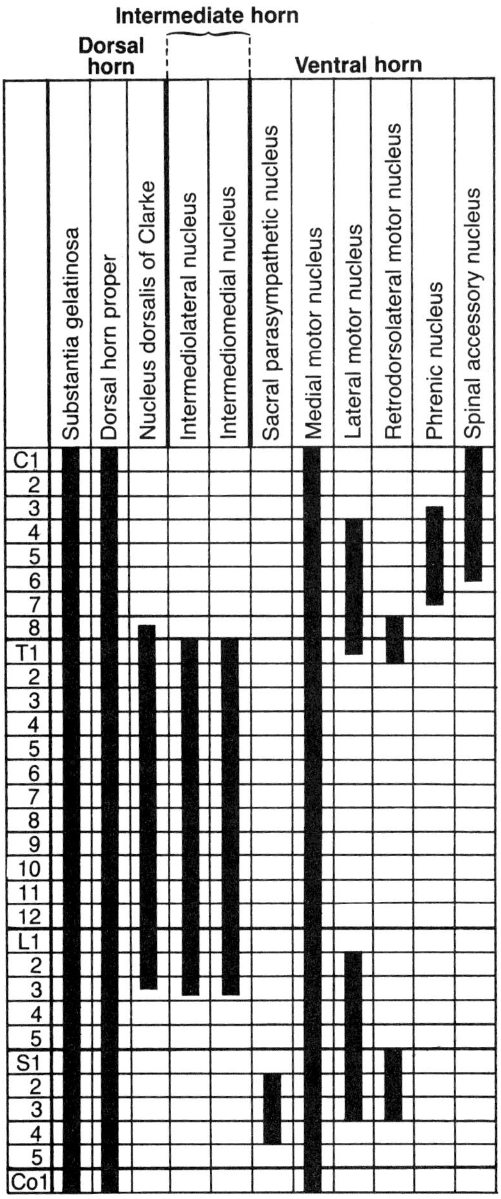

FIGURE 6-6. Longitudinal extent of the spinal cord nuclei.

Column headings (left to right), grouped as **Dorsal horn**, **Intermediate horn**, and **Ventral horn**:

- Substantia gelatinosa
- Dorsal horn proper
- Nucleus dorsalis of Clarke
- Intermediolateral nucleus
- Intermediomedial nucleus
- Sacral parasympathetic nucleus
- Medial motor nucleus
- Lateral motor nucleus
- Retrodorsolateral motor nucleus
- Phrenic nucleus
- Spinal accessory nucleus

Row labels (spinal cord segments): C1, 2, 3, 4, 5, 6, 7, 8, T1, 2, 3, 4, 5, 6, 7, 8, 9, 10, 11, 12, L1, 2, 3, 4, 5, S1, 2, 3, 4, 5, Co1

CHAPTER 6 III C

b. Each dorsal root axon in either the medial or lateral bundle typically trifurcates into **horizontal**, **ascending**, and **descending** branches (Figure 6-7).

c. Thus, the entering axon may synapse on nuclei at its level of entry or travel varying distances up and down the cord before synapsing.

TABLE 6-1. Spinal Cord Nuclei Collated with Laminae and Some Connections or Functions

Horn	Nuclear Column	Lamina	Extent in Cord	Some Connections or Functions
Dorsal	Dorsomarginal n.	I	Entire cord	Receives dorsal root afferents; sends some spinothalamic axons
	Substantia gelatinosa of Rolando	II	Entire cord	Relay nucleus for pain and temperature
	N. proprius of the dorsal horn	III, IV, V	Entire cord	Receives dorsal root afferents and descending brain pathways; originates spinothalamic tracts
	. . .	VI	Present in limb regions of cord (C4–T1; L2–S3)	Processes proprioceptive information from muscles
	N. dorsalis of Clarke	VII	C8–L3	Originates the dorsal spinocerebellar tract
Intermediate	Intermediomedial n.	VII	T1–L3	Receives visceral afferents
	Intermediolateral n.	VII	T1–L3	Originates preganglionic sympathic axons
	Periependymal (central) gray matter	X	Entire cord	Related to autonomic nervous system
Ventral	. . .	VIII	Entire cord, largest in limb regions	Receives descending axons from the brain
	Medial motoneuron n.	IX	Entire cord	Innervates axial (proximal) muscles
	Lateral motoneuron n.	IX	Present in limb regions of cord (C4–T1; L2–S3)	Innervates appendicular (limb) muscles
	Phrenic n.	IX	C3–C5	Innervates the diaphragm
	Spinal accessory n.	IX	C1–C6	Innervates sternocleidomastoid and trapezius muscles
	N. of Onufrowicz	IX	S1–S3	Innervates voluntary sphincters of the urethra and anus

N., n. = nucleus.

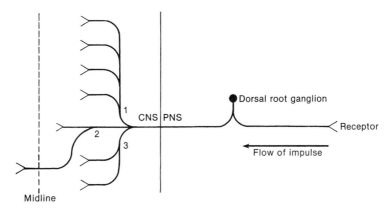

FIGURE 6-7. Typical branching of entering dorsal root axon. *1* = ascending branch; *2* = horizontal branch; *3* = descending branch.

      d. Most branches end in the **ipsilateral** spinal gray matter, but some cross to the **contralateral** gray matter.

  2. Dispersion of the lateral division of the dorsal roots
    a. Composition. The **lateral** bundle of primary sensory axons consists of small, mostly unmyelinated C fibers and lightly myelinated A-delta fibers (see Table 4-1.)
    b. Function. The lateral afferents mediate **pain** and **temperature** sensation.
    c. Termination of the lateral bundle of dorsal root axons. These axons terminate in nuclei of the dorsal horn. Section V B 4 details this pathway.

  3. Dispersion of the medial division of the dorsal roots
    a. Composition. The **medial** bundle of primary sensory afferents consists of the **larger, heavily myelinated A fibers** of peripheral nerve (see Table 4-1).
    b. Function. Such large fibers, in both the PNS and CNS, mediate discriminatory sensory modalities involving touch, texture, form, kinesthesia, and a modality termed **proprioception**.
    c. Termination of the medial bundle of root axons
      (1) The fibers branch into the typical **horizontal, ascending,** and **descending** branches (see Figure 6-7).
      (2) Many of the ascending branches travel up the dorsal columns of spinal white matter to terminate on the nuclei gracilis and cuneatus, at the cervicomedullary junction. Section V B 5 details this pathway.
      (3) The horizontal branches, at or near the level of entry, distribute to nuclei in the dorsal and ventral horns at intra- and intersegmental levels as follows.
        (a) Some branches go to the **substantia gelatinosa** (lamina II) and to the **nucleus propri** (laminae III and IV). These may in part mediate touch.
        (b) Some go to the **nucleus dorsalis** of Clarke and to other parts of laminae VII and VIII. These mediate proprioception.
        (c) Many synapse in lamina IX, upon the **GSE motoneurons** of the ventral horns, to mediate monosynaptic muscle stretch reflexes (MSRs).

IV. VENTRAL HORNS, MOTONEURONS, MOTOR UNITS, AND MUSCLE STRETCH REFLEXES (MSRs)

A.   **Nuclei and laminae of the ventral horn**

    1. Lamina VII. Rexed's lamina VII, or the **intermediate zone** located between the ventral and dorsal horns, contains the **intermediomedial** and **intermediolateral nuclei,** among other nuclei.

    a. The intermediomedial nucleus receives GVA fibers from the dorsal roots and relays fibers to the intermediolateral nucleus.

    b. The intermediolateral nucleus originates the sympathetic preganglionic GVE visceromotor axons for the ventral roots. It extends from T1–L3 (see Table 6-1).

2. Lamina VIII. Lamina VIII consists of a heterogeneous internuncial pool of the ventral horn. It receives suprasegmental and dorsal root fibers.

    a. It connects with ventral horn motor neurons.

    b. With several other laminae, it originates spinothalamic tracts that mediate pain and temperature.

3. Lamina IX

    a. Lamina IX contains **medial** and **lateral** columns of neurons that send GSE axons to the skeletal muscles (see Figure 6-4).

        (1) The **medial** motor cell column innervates the **axial** muscles.

        (2) The **lateral** motor cell column innervates the **appendicular** muscles (see Figure 6-4B for Rexed's division of the lateral motor cell column into two groups).

    b. In the cervical and lumbosacral regions, the most **dorsolateral** of these two lateral groups of neurons innervate the small, intrinsic muscles of the hands and feet.

B. **Somatomotoneurons of the ventral horn**

1. Lamina IX contains two types of motoneurons:

    a. Large, or **alpha**, motoneurons

    b. Small, or **gamma**, motoneurons

2. Characteristics of alpha motoneurons

    a. The alpha motoneurons of the medial and lateral cell columns exhibit very large, multipolar perikarya. By far the largest neurons in the spinal cord, they are among the largest in the nervous system (see Figure 6-5A, 10). In general, large perikarya have large dendritic trees and large, long axons, **alpha** axons, that conduct very rapidly (see Table 4-1). The name **alpha motoneurons** derives from their large alpha axons. Synonyms or near-synonyms for alpha motoneurons are:

        (1) Ventral motoneurons or ventral horn cells

        (2) Lamina IX of Rexed

        (3) Lower motoneurons (LMNs)

        (4) Final common pathway

    b. Similar large motoneurons occur in the GSE and special visceral efferent (SVE) nuclei of the brain stem.

    c. Alpha motoneurons innervate only striated muscle fibers. They do so in the form of **motor units**.

C. **Motor Units**

1. Definition. A **motor unit** is a motoneuron, its axon, and all of the muscle fibers it innervates (Figure 6-8).

    a. A motoneuron, in brain stem or spinal cord, may innervate only a few or hundreds of muscle fibers.

        (1) In the **smaller**, finer muscles, such as the extraocular muscles, the ratio may be nearly 1:1; that is, one neuron and its axon per muscle fiber.

        (2) In the **larger** muscles, such as the quadriceps femoris, one axon of a ventral motoneuron may branch to innervate hundreds of muscle fibers.

    b. Each muscle fiber receives only one axonal end foot.

    c. A motor unit is the smallest **unit of behavior** because the neuron responds on an all-or-none principle, the axon conducts on an all-or-none principle, and a muscle fiber responds all-or-none.

        (1) If an impulse starts down the main trunk of the axon, it will propagate to all of the axonal terminals.

        (2) Hence, to grade the strength of a contraction, the nervous system has to increase the number of motor units firing and the frequency with which they fire. The clinician can record the action potentials from the motor units as they fire by **electromyography**.

Muscle fiber

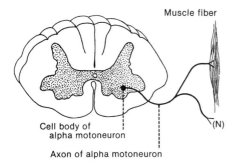

FIGURE 6-8. Motor unit consisting of an alpha motoneuron, its axon, and all of the muscle fibers it innervates. *N* = any number of additional fibers from one to several hundred.

Cell body of
alpha motoneuron
(N)

Axon of alpha motoneuron

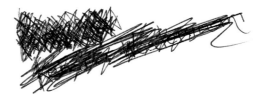

2. **Two types of motor units**
   a. Type I motor units predominate in red muscle, which is specialized for long, slow contractions, as in the leg muscles of birds with which the bird grasps a perch for hours at a time. The smaller motoneurons, with fibers that are approximately 10 micra meters in diameter, innervate the type I muscle fiber units.
   b. Type II motor units predominate in white muscle, which is called the "quick twitch" muscle and is specialized for quick, powerful contractions, such as the breast muscle of a bird. The larger motoneurons, with fibers up to 20 micra meters in diameter, innervate type II fibers.
   c. Diseases may affect type I and type II muscle fibers differently. For example, selective atrophy of type I muscle fibers may occur in some congenital myopathies.

3. **Pathophysiologic reactions of motor units**
   a. Death of a motoneuron or interruption of its axon results in paralysis of all of the muscle fibers of that motor unit.
   b. Unless the axon regenerates, the muscle fibers of the motor unit will ultimately die because they receive no stimulation.
      (1) If the axon regenerates, it reestablishes the motor unit.
      (2) If one axon dies but an adjacent one remains, the remaining axon may sprout new collaterals to innervate the denervated muscle fibers, as well as its original fibers. This enlarges the size of the motor unit. The electromyogram will then record **giant action potentials**.
   c. **Motor units and fasciculations**
      (1) Diseases of the alpha motoneuron or its axon may destabilize its membrane, causing impulses to arise spontaneously, rather than only in response to normal synaptic excitation of the perikaryon.
      (2) In this case, the muscle fibers innervated by the axon contract, producing a visible ripple or twitch of the activated muscle fibers. The twitch, evident on clinical inspection and recordable by electromyography, is called a **fasciculation**.
      (3) Thus, the motor unit is the anatomic, genetic, functional, pathologic, and regenerative unit of the neuromuscular system, in accordance with the Neuron Doctrine (see Chapter 2 V).

D. **Gamma motoneurons and muscle spindles**
   1. The smaller **gamma motoneurons** of the ventral horn send gamma-sized axons (see Table 4-1) into the peripheral nerves. The axons of gamma motoneurons end on specialized skeletal muscle fibers contained in **muscle spindles**.

   2. **Muscle spindles**
      a. Muscle spindles are specialized, spindle-shaped structures scattered throughout all skeletal muscles (Figure 6-9).
      b. Because **fusus** in Latin means **spindle**, the muscle fibers inside of a spindle, innervated by gamma motoneurons, are called **intrafusal muscle fibers**. The regular muscle fibers outside, innervated by alpha motoneurons, are **extrafusal fibers**.
      c. Muscle spindles are the receptors for the **muscle stretch reflexes (MSRs)** that clinicians routinely elicit in the neurologic examination (see Appendix VII F).

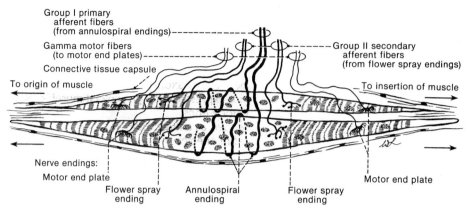

Group I primary
afferent fibers
(from annulospiral endings)
Gamma motor fibers
(to motor end plates)
Connective tissue capsule
To origin of muscle

Group II secondary
afferent fibers
(from flower spray endings)
To insertion of muscle

Nerve endings:
Motor end plate
Flower spray
ending
Annulospiral
ending
Flower spray
ending
Motor end plate

FIGURE 6-9. Muscle spindle and its innervation by gamma motoneuron efferents and type I afferents.

3. MSRs *muscle stretch reflexes*

a. A **monosynaptic reflex arc** (see Figure 2-7) links two neurons, an afferent (receptor) neuron with an efferent (motor) neuron, to activate an effector.

b. In the simplest reflex of skeletal muscles, the **MSR**, the muscle responds to a single stretch by exhibiting a single twitch.

(1) The **receptor** for the MSR is the **muscle spindle** (see Figure 6-9).

(2) Stretch of the muscle spindle from a pull on the muscle (usually via its tendon) activates receptor endings in the muscle spindle. A volley of **impulses** travels to the CNS through large, class I or alpha-myelinated afferents (see Table 4-1).

(3) The afferent axons traverse the **medial bundle** of the **dorsal root**. They proceed into the ventral horns to form **direct (monosynaptic) synapses** on **alpha motoneurons**.

(4) Firing of the alpha motoneurons contracts all of the **extrafusal fibers** that they innervate, with a resultant **twitch** of the muscle. The limb shows a jerk, such as extension of the knee, or the **knee jerk**.

c. Contraction of the intrafusal muscle fibers as governed by the activity of **gamma motoneurons** sets the tension in the muscle spindles and their sensitivity to stretch.

d. Various impulses from the brain and spinal cord play on the gamma system to govern postural reflexes and to maintain muscle tone as a foundation for voluntary movements.

E. **Excitation and inhibition of alpha motoneurons**

1. **Inhibition by Renshaw cells.** The alpha motoneurons send collateral axons to interneurons called **Renshaw cells**, which send an inhibitory synapse back to the alpha motoneuron.

2. **Excitation by alpha afferent and other axons.** The impulses from the muscle spindles excite the alpha motoneurons. The sum total of excitatory and inhibitory influences from all afferent sources, from the brain and spinal levels, determines whether motoneurons discharge impulses. Afferent sources include:

a. **Dorsal roots**, mainly the medial divisions of the segment where the motoneuron originates

b. **Intrasegmental interneurons** of the spinal cord, including Renshaw cells

c. **Intersegmental sensory afferent neurons and interneurons**

d. **Suprasegmental tracts** descending from the brain (Figure 6-10 and Table 6-2).

3. Interruption of various afferent pathways may **increase** or **decrease** the magnitude of the MSR depending on the ensuing balance between excitation and inhibition of alpha and gamma motoneurons and Renshaw cells. A lesion of the monosynaptic reflex arc itself, affecting either the afferent or efferent axons, reduces or abolishes the MSR, as

may disease of the muscle itself. The neurologic examination discloses the increase or decrease in the amplitude of the MSRs caused by disease of the CNS or PNS.

F. **Alpha motoneurons as the final common pathway from the CNS**

1. The alpha motoneuron is called the **final common pathway** out of the CNS.
   a. The alpha motoneurons provide the only axons to skeletal muscle.
   b. All reflex and voluntary behavior expressed through skeletal muscles must result from activation of the alpha motoneurons.
   c. The rest of the CNS can be regarded as a huge multi-circuited interneuronal pool that can ultimately express itself in effector activity (i.e., behavior).

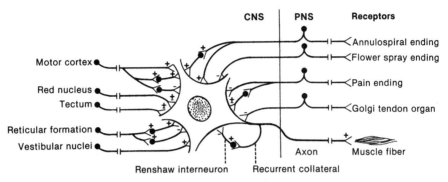

FIGURE 6-10. Summary of various excitatory and inhibitory afferents to an alpha motoneuron. Minus signs indicate an inhibitory influence on the alpha motoneuron; plus signs indicate an excitatory influence.

TABLE 6-2. Tracts of the Spinal Cord

Ascending tracts	Descending tracts (continued)
Primary (first-order) axons (from dorsal root ganglia)	Supraspinal in origin (brain stem)
Fasciculus gracilis (Goll's column)	Tectospinal tract
Fasciculus cuneatus (Burdach's column)	Rubrospinal tract
Secondary (second-order) axons (from internuncial neurons)	Reticulospinal tract
Ventral spinothalamic tract	Cerulospinal tract
Lateral spinothalamic tract	Vestibulospinal tract
Ventral spinocerebellar tract	Olivospinal tract
Dorsal spinocerebellar tract	Spinal in origin
Spino-olivary tract	In dorsal columns
Spinovestibular tract	Interfascicular fasciculus (Schultze's comma tract or semilunar tract)
Spinotectal tract	Septomarginal fasciculus
Spinoreticular tract	In ventral columns
Spinocervical tract (importance in humans is questionable)	Sulcomarginal fasciculus
Descending tracts (ultimately acting on the motoneurons)	**Mixed ascending and descending tracts**
Supraspinal in origin (cortical)*	Dorsolateral tract of Lissauer (primary axons from dorsal roots plus axons of intrinsic spinal neurons)
Ventral corticospinal tract	Fasciculi proprii (ground bundles) [secondary axons from internuncial neurons of gray matter] and branches from dorsal roots
Lateral corticospinal tract	

*Notice that no tracts of known clinical significance descend directly into the spinal cord from the cerebellum, basal ganglia, thalamus, or cerebral cortex, apart from the region around the central sulcus (sensorimotor cortex), which originates the pyramidal tract.

2. The large GSE motoneurons of the medial and lateral nuclei of the ventral horns and the corresponding brain stem neurons are also called **LMNs**. The **LMNs** contrast with the **upper motoneurons (UMNs)**, which descend from the brain (see V C 2 e).

V. PATHWAYS OF THE SPINAL CORD WHITE MATTER

A. Introduction

1. **Summary of ascending and descending spinal cord pathways.** Table 6-2 lists important spinal pathways that can be located in spinal cord cross sections in Figures 6-11, 6-12, 6-17, and 6-21.

2. **Spinal pathways arise from five sources**:
   a. Dorsal roots
   b. Internuncial neurons of the spinal cord gray matter
   c. Brain stem tegmentum [reticular formation (RF) and some nuclei]
   d. Cerebral cortex
   e. Hypothalamus

3. Some **morphologic laws** aid in remembering the **origin, course, location**, and **termination** of spinal pathways:
   a. **Law of the peripheral position of long fibers**
   b. **Law of lamination by phylogenesis**
   c. **Law of lamination by level of entry or body topography**
   d. **Law of separation of sensory pathways by sensory modalities**

4. **The concentric arrangement of the spinal pathways reflects the law of lamination by phylogenesis and the law of the peripheral position of the long fibers.**
   a. On cross section, the spinal cord exhibits three concentric zones (see Figure 6-12):
      (1) A **central** H-shaped core of gray matter
      (2) A **proximal** sleeve of short-running nerve fibers called **fasciculi proprii**, or **ground bundles**
      (3) A **peripheral sleeve** of long-running nerve fibers

FIGURE 6-11. Cross section of the spinal cord showing the ground bundles or fasciculi proprii of short fibers (*stippled*), immediately surrounding the gray matter.

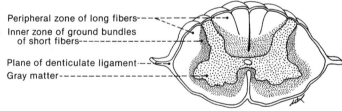

Peripheral zone of long fibers
Inner zone of ground bundles of short fibers
Plane of denticulate ligament
Gray matter

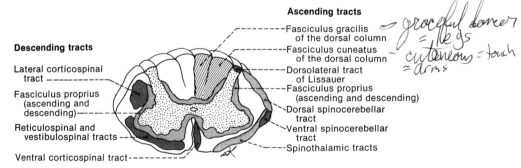

Descending tracts

Lateral corticospinal tract
Fasciculus proprius (ascending and descending)
Reticulospinal and vestibulospinal tracts
Ventral corticospinal tract

Ascending tracts

Fasciculus gracilis of the dorsal column
Fasciculus cuneatus of the dorsal column
Dorsolateral tract of Lissauer
Fasciculus proprius (ascending and descending)
Dorsal spinocerebellar tract
Ventral spinocerebellar tract
Spinothalamic tracts

FIGURE 6-12. Cross section of the spinal cord showing the location of the major ascending and descending tracts.

   b. The phylogenetically old, **short** fibers, the **ground bundles**, ascend and descend in a nearly concentric zone adjacent to the gray matter.
     (1) The ground bundles arise from:
       (a) Interneurons of the spinal cord gray matter
       (b) Dorsal root collaterals
     (2) The individual axons of the ground bundles extend only a few spinal cord segments at most. Thus, they mediate **intrasegmental** spinal reflexes (e.g., MSRs) and **intersegmental** reflexes between adjacent segments.
   c. The phylogenetically recent **long** fibers surround the ground bundles. They ascend and descend in the concentric zone of white matter between the ground bundles and the pial surface of the cord (see Figure 6-11).
     (1) The **ascending long fibers** arise from:
       (a) Interneurons of the spinal cord gray matter, which send axons to rostral levels of the spinal gray matter and to the brain
       (b) Dorsal root branches
     (2) Most **descending long fibers** come from the brain. Some dorsal root fibers descend in the dorsal columns (see Figure 6-7).

5. Anatomic demonstration of the ground bundles
   a. A transecting cut **rostral** and **caudal** to one spinal cord segment will isolate that segment from the rest of the cord (Figure 6-13A).
     (1) The **rostral cut** interrupts all long axons that arise **rostral** to the isolated segment and **descend** through it.
     (2) The **caudal cut** interrupts all long axons that arise **caudal** to the isolated segment and **ascend** through it.
     (3) After some weeks, all interrupted ascending and descending axons and myelin sheaths disappear because of Wallerian degeneration. Then, only the short-running axons whose perikarya lie in dorsal root ganglia or spinal cord gray matter of the isolated segment remain between the two cuts (see Figure 6-13B).
   b. The transections **impair** the individual's ability to **function**.
     (1) Interruption of all **ascending** sensory axons causes anesthesia caudal to the rostral cut.
     (2) Interruption of all **descending** motor axons from the brain causes paraplegia. Intrasegmental reflexes (e.g., MSRs) of the isolated segment of the distal cord remain, as do the spinal reflexes of the intact spinal cord, caudal to the cuts.

B.   **Ascending pathways of the spinal cord**

1. Features of the ascending pathways
   a. Pathways ascend in all three **columns** of white matter: the **dorsal**, **lateral**, and **ventral** columns.
   b. Ascending long pathways transmit impulses that originate from sensory receptors and are destined to:
     (1) Produce conscious sensation, somatic or visceral
     (2) Mediate reflexes, somatic or visceral
     (3) Guide the motor centers in the cerebellum, brain stem, diencephalon, basal ganglia, and cortex
   c. Ascending **afferent** pathways mediate both **conscious** and **unconscious** sensory functions.
     (1) Pathways that mediate **conscious** sensations are:
       (a) **Ventrolateral spinothalamic pathways** mediate touch, pain, and temperature.
       (b) **Dorsal column pathways** (fasciculus gracilis and fasciculus cuneatus) mediate **discriminative modalities**, such as touch, form, texture, movement, and position sense.
     (2) Common plan of the somatosensory pathways for conscious sensation
       (a) Each somatosensory pathway for conscious sensation extends from a peripheral receptor to the cerebral cortex.

FIGURE 6-13. (*A*) Surgical isolation of a thoracic segment of cat spinal cord by transverse cuts rostral and caudal to that segment. (*B*) Myelin-stained transverse histologic section of the isolated segment of the spinal cord (ventral horns facing down). No myelinated fibers remain in zone 1, the periphery that transmits the long tracts. Zone 2 shows the preserved ground bundles adjacent to zone 3, the gray matter from which the ground bundles arise. (Adapted with permission from Anderson FD: The structure of a chronically isolated segment of the cat spinal cord. *J Comp Neur* 120:297–316, 1963.)

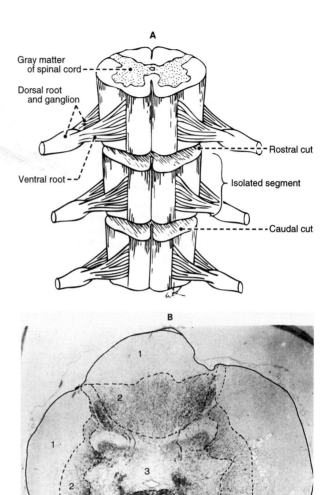

(i) The pathway begins in a **receptor** in the **skin** (Figure 6-14) or the **skeletomuscular** and **proprioceptive systems**.

(ii) Some sensory modalities arise in specific sensory receptors and have discrete central pathways, while other modalities appear to share peripheral receptors and central pathways.

(b) The perikaryon of the **primary** or **first-order neuron** in the pathway is in a dorsal root ganglion (Figure 6-15).

(c) The perikaryon of the **secondary** or **second-order neuron** is in the spinal cord gray matter. Its axon decussates and ascends to the brain stem, where these pathways join in the **medial lemniscus** to synapse on tertiary neurons in the contralateral thalamus.

(d) The perikaryon of the **tertiary** or **third-order neuron** is in the thalamus. It sends its axon to the ipsilateral sensorimotor cortex of the postcentral gyrus.

(3) Pathways that mediate **unconscious** sensory functions

(a) **Spinocerebellar pathways** relay information for coordinating volitional movements and posture.

(b) **Spinoreticular pathways** relay information to the brain stem tegmentum and RF that mediates somatic and visceral reflexes.

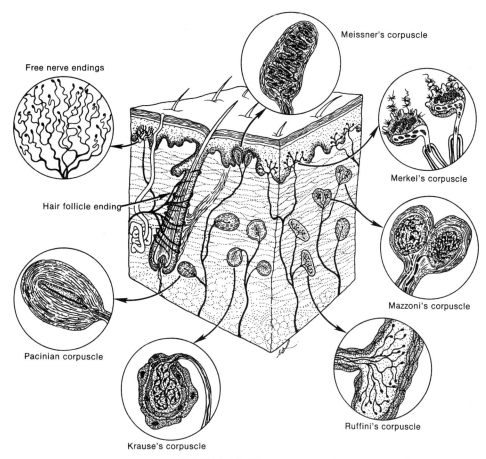

FIGURE 6-14. Skin receptors.

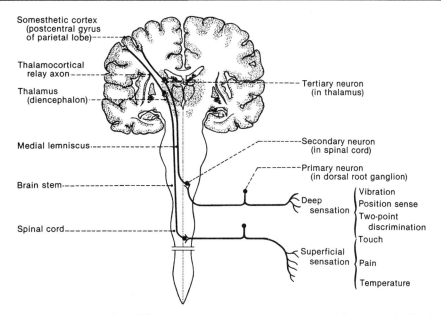

FIGURE 6-15. Three-neuron plan of the somatic sensory system. Notice the difference in the level of decussation of the pathways for superficial and deep sensation and the dual pathways for touch. (Reprinted with permission from DeMyer W: *Technique of the Neurologic Examination: A Programmed Text,* 4th ed. New York, McGraw-Hill, 1994.)

2. **Thinking through the circuitry.** In localizing the cause for sensory disorders, the clinician must "think through" this entire circuitry, which requires knowledge of the:
   a. Receptor location
   b. Route through the PNS (nerve branch, plexus, and dorsal root)
   c. Location of primary, secondary, and tertiary perikarya
   d. Level of decussation of second-order neuron, which occurs at the level of the perikaryon of the second-order neuron
   e. Column of the cord—dorsal, lateral, or ventral—by which the pathway ascends
   f. Brain stem course via the medial lemniscus
   g. Location of the thalamic relay nucleus and the pathway of its axon through the white matter to the cerebral cortex (see Chapter 12 II E)
   h. Cortical receptive area

3. **Dorsal column pathways and their sensory modalities**
   a. Function
      (1) The dorsal columns convey axons that mediate touch localization, form, texture, position sense, pressure, vibration, and kinesthesia. Because these sensations are very specific as to stimulus, location, and spatial and temporal discrimination, they are called **discriminative modalities**.
      (2) Interruption of the dorsal columns in patients causes:
         (a) Loss of position sense
         (b) Loss of vibration sense
         (c) Inability to recognize numbers written on the skin (graphanesthesia)
         (d) Loss of recognition of the form of objects handled (stereoanesthesia)
         (e) Sensory ataxia
         (f) Inability to detect movement, such as the direction of a scratch (kinanesthesia)
      (3) Because of the ventrolateral column pathways, touch, pain, and temperature sensations are retained when the dorsal columns are interrupted.
   b. Peripheral course of the dorsal column pathways
      (1) Dorsal column pathways begin in **encapsulated receptors** in the skin and the skeletomuscular system.
         (a) **Skin** receptors include **Meissner's** and **Pacinian corpuscles**, which are innervated by medium to large **A** fibers (see Figure 6-14 and Table 4-1).
         (b) **Skeletomuscular receptors** include **muscle spindles** and **Golgi tendon organs**, which are innervated by medium to large **Ia** and **Ib** fibers (see Figure 6-9 and Table 4-1.)
      (2) The **peripheral axons** arise from dorsal root ganglia and enter the spinal cord through the **medial** division of the dorsal roots (see Figure 6-5B).
   c. Central course of the dorsal column pathways
      (1) After the axon enters the spinal cord through the medial division of the root and divides, its **ascending branch** runs up the **ipsilateral** dorsal column (Figure 6-16). Hence, the dorsal columns of the cord contain:
         (a) Primary sensory axons whose cell body is located **outside** of the CNS, in the dorsal root ganglia of the PNS
         (b) Primary axons that also form the dorsolateral **fasciculus of Lissauer**, but via the lateral division of the dorsal root
      (2) **Descending** branches of the dorsal root **fibers** form the **fasciculus interfascicularis** and the **sulcomarginal fasciculus** in the dorsal columns, but their function is unknown.
      (3) Both **ascending and descending axonal branches** send numerous collaterals into the spinal gray matter (see Figure 6-7).
   d. The **ascending** dorsal column fibers illustrate the **law of lamination** by level of entry, or body topography (Figure 6-17).
      (1) The **sacral** fibers serving the anogenital region and legs form the **medial**-most wafers of axons, the **fasciculus gracilis** (of Goll) [see Figure 6-12].
      (2) The **cervical** fibers serving the arms form the **lateral**-most wafers of axons, the **fasciculus cuneatus** (of Burdach) [see Figure 6-12].

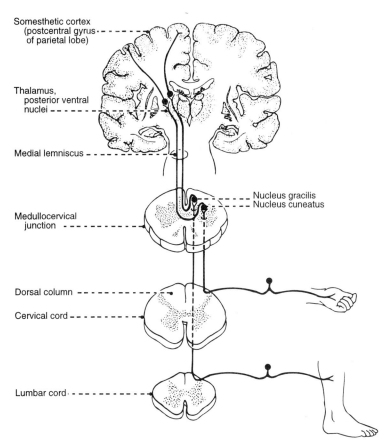

FIGURE 6-16. Somatosensory pathway for dorsal column modalities. (Adapted with permission from DeMyer W: *Technique of the Neurologic Examination: A Programmed Text*, 4th ed. New York, McGraw-Hill, 1994.)

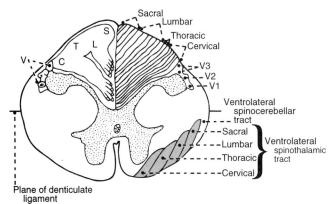

FIGURE 6-17. Cross section diagram of the spinal cord at C1. It shows the lamination of ascending sensory axons by level of entry in the dorsal columns (discriminative modalities) and ventrolateral columns (pain and temperature). V1, V2, and V3 refer to the first, second, and third sensory divisions of CN V.

e. **Course of the ascending dorsal column axons in the brain**
   (1) The ascending dorsal column axons synapse on the **nuclei gracilis** and **cuneatus**, which straddle the cervico-medullary junction and contain **second-order** neurons.
   (2) From these dorsal column nuclei the axons decussate, forming the **medial lemniscus**, which ascends to the **thalamus** of the diencephalon (see Figure 6-16).
   (3) After a synapse on the **third-order sensory neurons** in the thalamus, the pathway ascends to the **somesthetic cortex** located in the postcentral gyrus.

4. Pain and temperature pathways and the ventrolateral spinothalamic tracts (Figure 6-18).
  a. Peripheral course of the pain and temperature pathways
    (1) The pathway begins in terminal ramifications of unmyelinated C fibers and lightly myelinated A fibers that pervade the skin, skeletomuscular apparatus, and certain parts of the viscera.
    (2) The axons travel centrally via the somatic and visceral nerves to enter the CNS via the lateral divisions of the dorsal roots (see Figure 6-5B).
  b. Central course of the pain and temperature pathways
    (1) As the lateral bundle of root fibers divide into horizontal, ascending, and descending fibers at the apex of the dorsal horn, they form the **dorsolateral tract (of Lissauer)** [see Figure 6-12]. Most of these axons synapse at the segment of entry or after traveling up or down only a segment or two.
    (2) These primary axons of the dorsolateral tract synapse on secondary neurons of the adjacent **dorsomarginal nucleus** (lamina I), the **substantia gelatinosa** (lamina II), the **nucleus proprius** (lamina III–V), and some extend to lamina X.
    (3) By means of complicated interconnections that remain in some doubt, the secondary axons from these sensory nuclei may synapse on interneurons in laminae VI, VII, and VIII.
    (4) The axons of various neurons of laminae I–VIII decussate just ventral to the central canal, in the **ventral white commissure**. They then **ascend** in the con-

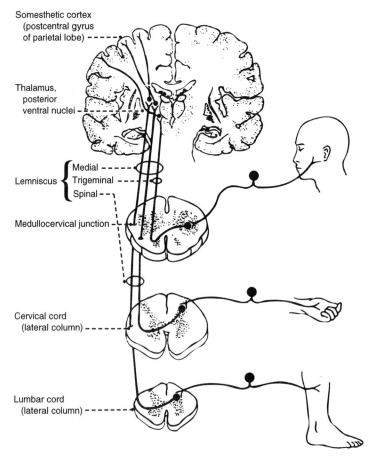

FIGURE 6-18. Somatosensory pathway for pain and temperature. Notice that the second-order axon crosses at the level of entry of the primary axon from the dorsal root. Compare with Figure 6-16. (Reprinted with permission from DeMyer W: *Technique of the Neurologic Examination: A Programmed Text,* 4th ed. New York, McGraw-Hill, 1994.)

tralateral white matter as the **ventrolateral spinothalamic tract** [see V B 5 a (2) and Figure 6-12].

  (5) The ventrolateral spinothalamic tract, being on the periphery of the cord, illustrates the **law of the peripheral position of long fibers**. It also illustrates the **law of lamination by level of entry** (see Figure 6-17).

c. **Termination of the spinothalamic pathway**
  (1) At brain stem levels, the axons send collaterals into the RF of the brain and join the medial lemniscus to synapse in the somatosensory nucleus of thalamus, which relays to the somatosensory area of the cerebral cortex (see Figure 6-18).
  (2) Additional terminals synapse on the intralaminar nuclei of the thalamus.
  (3) Interneurons of various laminae in the cord appear to originate ascending somatosensory pathways in the ventrolateral columns with at least three terminations:
    (a) The classical ventrolateral spinothalamic pathway just described
    (b) A spinoreticular pathway
    (c) A spinomesencephalic pathway

d. **Additional pain pathways**
  (1) Because we experience several types pf pain—**immediate pain; sharp, pricking pain; long-lasting, dull pain**—and **hyperalgesia** with an exaggerated feeling of pain, no single, simplistic diagram of one pathway explains all of the phenomena. Much remains unknown about pain pathways.
  (2) Some observations suggest alternate pathways for the ascent of pain sensations to consciousness.
    (a) Interruption of the ventrolateral spinothalamic tract, the classic pain and temperature pathway, causes at least temporary loss of pain and temperature sensation on the contralateral side of the body. Visceral pain is less affected and may have a more diffuse pathway than somatic pain.
    (b) After surgical interruption of the tract to relieve pain, called **tractotomy** or **cordotomy**, the level of pain will drop several segments over a period of time. If the level of pain and temperature loss is C2, the final level may drop to C5. Some pain and temperature sensation may return.
  (3) Alternate pain pathways, particularly polysynaptic pathways for visceral pain, may ascend in the spinal cord. Some may form a **spinocervical tract** to reach a nucleus in the cervical cord, which would relay impulses to the brain. A role of touch fibers in pain is also suggested.
  (4) Descending tracts from the brain stem RF inhibit the transmission of pain impulses from the dorsal roots to the spinal neurons (see Chapter 14).

5. **Summary of touch pathways**
  a. Two pathways apparently convey touch impulses to consciousness (see Figure 6-15):
    (1) The **dorsal column pathway** (see Figure 6-16)
    (2) The **ventrolateral spinothalamic tract**, which resembles the ventrolateral spinothalamic tract for pain and temperature (see Figure 6-18)
  b. Interruption of the ventral pathway causes little or no clinical deficit in touch sensation, but interruption of both the ventral and dorsal column pathways impairs touch sensation. Certainly, spinal cord transection abolishes all touch sensation caudal to the level of the lesion.

6. **The dorsal and ventral spinocerebellar tracts** (Figure 6-19)
  a. **Function**
    (1) The spinocerebellar pathways convey proprioceptive impulses to the cerebellum, which coordinates the contractions of skeletal muscles. The tracts do not convey any impulses known to reach consciousness.
    (2) The tracts serve mainly the lower extremities.
  b. **Peripheral course.** From pressure receptors in the skin and from the **Golgi tendon organs** and **muscle spindles**, Ib afferents course centrally in somatic nerves. They enter the CNS through the medial division of the dorsal roots.

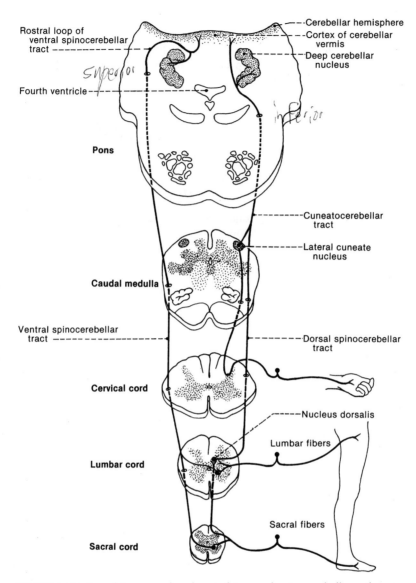

FIGURE 6-19. Dorsal (*uncrossed*) and ventral (*crossed*) spinocerebellar pathways.

c. **Central course.** Spinocerebellar impulses travel by **dorsal** and **ventral** spinocerebellar tracts (see Figures 6-12 and 6-19).
  (1) **The dorsal, uncrossed spinocerebellar tract**
     (a) The entering fibers traverse the medial division of the dorsal roots from
         C1–S5 and synapse on the **nucleus dorsalis of Clarke** (see Figure 6-4A).
         (i) The neurons of the nucleus dorsalis send their axons laterally to the
             periphery of the **ipsilateral** lateral column, where they ascend as the
             dorsal spinocerebellar tract.
         (ii) Because the nucleus dorsalis extends only to the L2–L3 level of the
             cord, the fibers from the sacral and lumbar roots have to ascend in
             the dorsal columns to reach their synapse.
     (b) A similar arrangement exists for the arm.
         (i) Some spinocerebellar fibers from the arms ascend into the brain stem
             where they synapse on the homolog of nucleus dorsalis, the **lateral or
             accessory cuneate nucleus**.

(ii) The lateral cuneate nucleus transmits axons **ipsilaterally** to the cerebellum.

(2) Ventral, crossed spinocerebellar tract

(a) The ventral spinocerebellar tract conveys axons originating in the caudal segments of the cord.

(b) This tract resembles the dorsal tract in its origin in peripheral receptors and its course to the spinal cord gray matter.

(3) Differences in the dorsal and ventral spinocerebellar tracts

(a) The dorsal tract arises from a discrete nucleus in lamina VII, the nucleus dorsalis, but the ventral tract arises more diffusely from lamina VII.

(b) The **dorsal** spinocerebellar tracts from secondary neurons ascend **ipsilaterally**, but the secondary axons of the ventral tract decussate in the white commissure of the spinal cord and ascend **contralaterally** (see Figure 6-19).

(c) In the pons, where the two tracts turn dorsally into the cerebellum, the **dorsal tract** enters through the **inferior (caudal) cerebellar peduncle** and the **ventral tract** enters through the **superior (rostral) peduncle**.

d. Cuneocerebellar tract from the arm

(1) Fibers from receptors in the arm ascend in the ipsilateral fasciculus cuneatus to synapse on the **lateral** or **external cuneate nucleus** in the caudal medulla (see Figure 7-13).

(2) The lateral cuneate nucleus relays impulses to the cerebellum. It corresponds to the nucleus dorsalis of Clarke.

7. Miscellaneous ascending spinal tracts. The **spino-olivary**, **spinovestibular**, and **spinotectal tracts** cannot be tested at the bedside and are not further described here.

C. Descending pathways in the spinal cord

1. Descending pathways in the spinal cord originate from either **supraspinal** or **spinal** sources.

a. Spinal sources of descending pathways include:

(1) Short intra- and intersegmental pathways in the ground bundles, arising in internuncial neurons of the spinal gray matter

(2) Descending collaterals of dorsal root axons in the dorsal columns and in the dorsolateral tract of Lissauer

b. Supraspinal sources include the **cerebral cortex** and **brain stem** (see Table 6-2).

(1) From the **cerebrum**, only the **sensorimotor cortex** around the central sulcus sends axons into the spinal cord. The basal ganglia, thalamus, and cerebellum send no axons of known clinical importance directly to the spinal cord.

(2) From the **brain stem tectum** and **tegmentum**, many tracts descend into the spinal cord (see Table 6-2). Some autonomic axons descend from the hypothalamus.

2. The pyramidal tract (the corticospinal and corticobulbar tracts)

a. Origin and function

(1) The **pyramidal tract** arises from the cerebral motor cortex. The **motor cortex** occupies the region around the central sulcus, mainly the **precentral gyrus** (see Figure 1-4).

(2) The pyramidal tract has two components:

(a) A **corticobulbar tract** to the brain stem

(b) A **corticospinal** tract to the spinal cord

(3) The pyramidal tract mediates voluntary contractions of skeletal muscles. Interruption of this tract causes weakness or paralysis of volitional movements.

b. Course through the brain

(1) Both components of the pyramidal tract travel ipsilaterally from the motor cortex, through the deep white matter of the cerebrum (internal capsule), and onto the ventral surface of the midbrain.

    (2) Corticobulbar fibers depart **ipsilaterally** and **contralaterally** into the brain stem at various levels (Figure 6-20), as detailed in the discussion of cranial nerves (see Chapter 7 VIII).

    (3) Corticospinal fibers continue **ipsilaterally** through the brain stem, passing through the **medullary pyramids** to the cervicomedullary junction, where most decussate (see Figure 7-11).

  c. Distribution of pyramidal fibers in the spinal cord. At the cervicomedullary junction, each pyramidal tract divides into two bundles, one descending in the **lateral** white column and the other in the **ventral** white column.

    (1) The lateral corticospinal tract

      (a) The **lateral** corticospinal tract consists mostly of decussated fibers, but some undecussated fibers descend in the lateral bundle. Thus, the lateral corticospinal tract consists of a **majority** of **crossed** fibers and a **minority** of **uncrossed** fibers.

      (b) The lateral corticospinal tract occupies a zone dorsal to the transverse plane of the denticulate ligament (Figure 6-21).

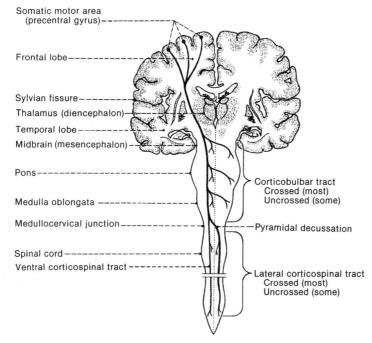

FIGURE 6-20. Course of the corticobulbar and corticospinal tracts. (Reprinted with permission from DeMyer W: *Technique of the Neurologic Examination: A Programmed Text*, 4th ed. New York, McGraw-Hill, 1994.)

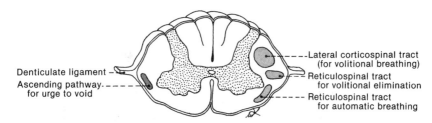

FIGURE 6-21. Transverse section of the spinal cord showing the location of the pathways for the control of breathing and elimination by the bladder and bowel.

(2) The ventral corticospinal tract. A minority of fibers from each medullary pyramid continue **ipsilaterally** into the ventral column as the **ventral** corticospinal tract (see Figure 6-12).

d. Termination of corticospinal axons

(1) The **lateral corticospinal tract** descends the length of the cord, synapsing along its length. Extending from cortex to conus medullaris, it is thus the longest continuous tract in the CNS.

(a) It sends axons into the gray matter at all levels. Hence, it gradually diminishes in size as it descends.

(b) The **lateral** corticospinal axons veer into the intermediate region of the spinal gray matter to synapse on:

(i) Neurons of laminae IV–VII (majority of terminals)

(ii) Alpha motoneurons of lamina IX (minority of terminals, estimated at 10% in humans)

(c) The **uncrossed lateral** corticospinal axons terminate at synapses in the base of the dorsal horn, intermediate zone, and central parts of the ventral horn.

(2) The **ventral corticospinal tract** crosses in the ventral white commissure to synapse mainly in lamina VII.

e. The concept of UMNs. Although the term LMN applies only to the alpha motoneurons, the term **UMN** has two meanings, one general and the other restricted. Thus, depending on the context, UMNs may mean either:

(1) All descending tracts from the brain that ultimately play on the LMNs

(2) Only the descending pathway from the cortex, that is, the **pyramidal tract**

f. Clinical importance of the corticospinal tract decussation

(1) Interruption of one pyramidal tract will paralyze voluntary movement on one side of the body, a condition called **hemiplegia.**

(2) The **side** of the paralysis depends on whether the lesion interrupts the pyramidal tract **rostral** or **caudal** to the decussation of its fibers.

(a) A lesion **rostral** to the decussation causes **contralateral** weakness. Certain corticobulbar movements will also be paralyzed, most notably voluntary movements of the lower part of the face (see Chapter 7 XIV B 1).

(b) A lesion in the rostral part of the spinal cord, **caudal** to the decussation, causes **ipsilateral** weakness; the face is spared. ↑ pyramidal

(3) Bilateral interruption of the corticospinal tracts rostral to the decussation causes bilateral paralysis.

(a) Because of some variability in the number of decussating fibers in the corticospinal tracts, particularly the size of the ventral tract, unilateral interruption of one lateral corticospinal tract may not cause complete paralysis in some individuals.

(b) The ipsilateral fibers may account for some degree of recovery after a corticospinal tract lesion.

g. Clinical signs of corticospinal tract (UMN) lesions and LMN lesions

(1) Both UMN and LMN lesions cause paresis or paralysis, but the lesions differ in location, cause, and clinical features (Table 6-3).

(2) Acute, severe UMN lesions

(a) Acute complete or nearly complete interruption of UMNs may result in a transient stage called **spinal shock** or **cerebral shock.** During this stage, in addition to total paralysis, the affected side of the body exhibits:

(i) Hypotonia

(ii) Absence of MSRs

(iii) Absence of abdominal and cremasteric reflexes

(iv) Absence of plantar responses

(b) If the lesion transects the cord, the patient also shows:

(i) Hypotonic paralysis of bowel and bladder

(ii) Hypotension and anhidrosis

(c) Within hours, days, or weeks, the hypotonia changes to spasticity, the MSRs become hyperactive, and the large toe extends in response to a

TABLE 6-3. Clinical Features of UMN and LMN Lesions (Chronic Stage of Lesion)

UMN lesions (pyramidal syndrome)
Paralyze movements in hemiplegic, quadriplegic, or paraplegic distribution, not individual muscles
Atrophy of disuse only (late and slight)
Hyperactive MSRs and spasticity
Clonus
Absent abdominal and cremasteric reflexes
Extensor toe sign (Babinski sign)

LMN Lesions
Paralyze individual muscles or sets of muscles in root or peripheral nerve distribution
Atrophy of denervation (early and severe)
Fasciculations and fibrillations
Hypoactive or absent MSRs
Hypotonia

LMN = lower motoneuron; MSRs = muscle stretch reflexes; UMN = upper motoneuron.

plantar stimulus (Babinski sign), the classical signs of UMN lesions (see Table 6-3).

(d) The exact pathophysiologic mechanisms of the changes in reflexes and plantar responses in acute or chronic UMN lesions is not known.

3. **Descending tracts from the brain stem**
   a. **Tectospinal, rubrospinal, coerulospinal,** and **olivospinal tracts** are not testable clinically.
   b. **Vestibulospinal tracts** participate in controlling postural reflexes (see Chapter 8 II F 3 b).
   c. **Reticulospinal tracts** affect both somatic and visceral motor functions.
      (1) Lesions rarely interrupt these pathways exclusively and do not result in specific clinical syndromes.
      (2) Section VI discusses the control of visceral functions by reticulospinal and pyramidal pathways.

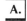

VI. ASCENDING AND DESCENDING SPINAL PATHWAYS FOR VISCERAL FUNCTIONS

A. Volitional and reflex control of visceromotor actions

1. Ascending and descending pathways in the brain and spinal cord control the following visceral motor functions:
   a. Breathing
   b. Digestion and elimination
   c. Blood pressure and pulse
   d. Sweating and other glandular secretions
   e. Piloerection
   f. Penile/clitoral erection

2. Volitional and autonomic pathways both collaborate in the control of many visceral functions, notably breathing and the bladder and bowel sphincters. Volition may result in activation or inhibition, as with the detrusor muscle of the bladder. Involuntary autonomic reflexes control the remaining visceral functions.

3. The viscerosensory and autonomic visceromotor tracts occupy the ventrolateral quadrant of the spinal cord. They intermingle considerably with each other and with the ventral and lateral spinothalamic tracts.

B. **Role of the spinal cord in breathing**

1. **UMN control.** Breathing is controlled by volitional and automatic UMN pathways. Both ultimately activate the same LMNs to the diaphragm and intercostal muscles.
   a. The **lateral corticospinal tract** controls **volitional** breathing. It occupies the plane dorsal to the denticulate ligament (see Figure 6-21).
   b. The **medullary (lateral) reticulospinal tract (bulboreticulospinal tract)** controls **automatic** breathing.
      (1) The reticulospinal respiratory pathway arises in the respiratory center in the medullary RF (see Chapter 7 XII F 1 and Figure 7-40).
      (2) This tract runs **ventral** to the plane of the denticulate ligament, in the ventrolateral white matter just off of the tip of the ventral horn (see Figure 6-21).
      (3) Reticulospinal tracts also coordinate the action of breathing with swallowing and with defecation and urination.

2. **LMN innervation for breathing**
   a. Ventral motoneurons of spinal segments C3–C5 innervate the diaphragm through the phrenic nerve.
   b. Spinal segments T2–T12 innervate the intercostal and abdominal muscles through the intercostal nerves.

3. **Afferent pathways for the control of breathing**
   a. Afferent pathways run in CN IX and CN X (see Figure 7-40).
   b. An ascending pathway of unknown origin also runs to the medullary respiratory center via the ventrolateral quadrant of the cord.

4. **Effect of spinal cord lesions on breathing** (see also Chapter 7 XII D)
   a. **Transection of the cord at or rostral to C2** paralyzes all volitional and automatic breathing. The patient dies unless given artificial respiration because **the spinal cord contains no centers that can initiate or maintain breathing**.
   b. **Hemisection of the cord at or rostral to C2** paralyzes both volitional and automatic breathing by the ipsilateral diaphragm and intercostal muscles.
   c. **Ventrolateral quadrant section** interrupts both the descending autonomic pathways for breathing and the ascending pathways, which provide part of the drive to breathe.
      (1) **Interruption of the ascending pathway in the ventrolateral quadrant** reduces the ventilatory response to carbon dioxide.
      (2) **Bilateral section of the ventrolateral quadrants of the cord at C2** paralyzes automatic breathing, which condemns the patient to stay awake to breathe by using pyramidal pathways **(Ondine's curse)** [see Chapter 7 XII H 2].
   d. **Transection of the cord at C6** paralyzes intercostal breathing, but with the phrenic nerve intact the diaphragm can maintain adequate ventilation, at least with the patient at rest.
   e. **Transection of the dorsal roots of all intercostal nerves** reduces breathing; the reason is uncertain.

C. **Role of the spinal cord in micturition**

Para = pelvic
splanch

1. **LMN or segmental innervation of the bladder** (Figure 6-22)
   a. Efferents run to the bladder and its sphincters from the three motor systems:
      (1) **Sympathetic (T6–L3)** via the hypogastric nerve and plexus
      (2) **Parasympathetic (S2–S4)** via the pelvic splanchnic nerves
      (3) **Somatomotor (S2–S4)** via the pudendal nerve (Motor axons for the voluntary sphincters of bladder and bowel arise in the nucleus of Onufrowicz in the ventral horn.)
   b. **Afferents** return to the spinal cord from all three nerves (see Figure 6-22).

2. **Reflex emptying of the bladder**
   a. Unlike breathing, micturition and ejaculation can occur reflexly after spinal cord transection. Reflex defecation is less successful.
   b. The sacral segments of the cord contain a center for reflex micturition, but brain stem and cerebral centers superimpose UMN control. During maturation, young children learn to use these UMN pathways to control the excretory reflexes.

FIGURE 6-22. Innervation of the bladder by the hypogastric plexus (sympathetic), pelvic splanchnic nerve (parasympathetic and visceral sensory), and pudendal nerve (somatosensorimotor).

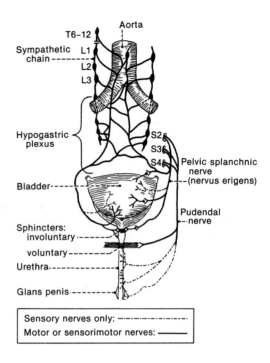

3. UMN innervation of the bladder
   a. The UMN pathway for volitional micturition arises in the posterior, medial part of the frontal lobe, which represents the genitalia (see Figure 13-37).
   b. The frontal cortex projects to a micturition center in the pontine RF and also directly to the sacral level of the spinal cord. The pontine micturition center also receives and sends pathways to and from the sacral level of the cord.
   c. In the spinal cord, the pathway for volitional micturition descends in the white matter midway between the intermediolateral horn and the periphery of the cord (see Figure 6-21). Hence, it lies at or just ventral to the plane of the denticulate ligaments.
   d. The volitional pathway apparently is not part of the pyramidal tract per se. It runs somewhat ventral to the lateral corticospinal tract, and in amyotrophic lateral sclerosis, even after severe pyramidal tract degeneration paralyzes the legs, the patient tends to retain sphincter control.
   e. Spinal cord transection or interruption of the ventrolateral quadrants of the cord causes an immediate flaccid paralysis of the bladder, which will later begin to empty reflexly.

4. Ascending pathways for bladder sensation
   a. The major ascending pathway for the urge to void apparently travels in the periphery of the cord (see Figure 6-21). It corresponds more or less with the sacral fibers in the lateral spinothalamic tract (see Figure 6-17).
   b. The dorsal columns may convey urethral sensation in the sacral wafers (see Figure 6-17).

D. **Role of the spinal cord in defecation**
   1. The **descending** pathways for volitional control of defecation appear to overlap those for micturition but may be a little more lateral.
   2. The **ascending** pathway is presumably similar to that for micturition.
   3. Reflex bowel emptying can occur after spinal cord transection, but less effectively than reflex bladder emptying.

E. **Vasomotor, sudomotor, and pupillomotor pathways**
   1. Vasomotor and sudomotor autonomic UMN pathways from the hypothalamus and RF descend in the ventrolateral columns of white matter, intermingled with and medial to the lateral spinothalamic tract. The LMNs of the autonomic system, located in the **intermediolateral** nucleus, provide preganglionic efferent axons.

2. Interruption of descending UMN autonomic pathways results in loss of sweating caudal to the level of the lesion and vasodilation with hypotension.
   a. The hypotension is **orthostatic** and may be severe enough to cause fainting. When the patient is elevated from a horizontal to a vertical position, the brain cannot produce reflex vasoconstriction through the interrupted descending autonomic pathway. The pull of gravity causes pooling of blood in the dilated vessels.
   b. Because of insufficient return of blood, the heart cannot maintain the intracranial circulation and the patient faints.
   c. In **Shy-Drager syndrome**, the patient has orthostatic hypotension and fainting because the neurons in the autonomic ganglia selectively degenerate, blocking the central activation of vasomotor tone.

3. A pupillodilator/sudomotor/vasomotor pathway runs from the hypothalamus to the intermediolateral nucleus of the lower cervical–upper thoracic region of the cord. Its interruption causes Horner's syndrome (see Figure 5-4).

VII. CLINICO-ANATOMIC SYNDROMES OF THE SPINAL CORD (FIGURE 6-23)

A. Motoneuron diseases

1. **Diseases of LMNs** (see Figure 6-23A). Two diseases may relatively selectively destroy alpha motoneurons.
   a. **Progressive muscular atrophy** is a heredofamilial degenerative disease, which in pure form causes death of the ventral motoneurons. The patient gradually becomes weaker and dies. It is the somatomotor concomitant of Shy-Drager syndrome, which causes death of visceromotor neurons.
   b. **Poliomyelitis** is an acute inflammatory viral infection.
      (1) The virus has a predilection for the LMNs, although it may also involve other neurons to lesser degrees.
      (2) It may affect only a segment or part of a segment of the cord or brain stem and cause only a selective atrophy of the relevant muscles or part of one muscle.

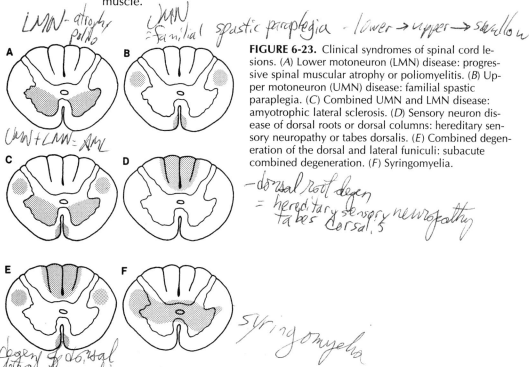

FIGURE 6-23. Clinical syndromes of spinal cord lesions. (*A*) Lower motoneuron (LMN) disease: progressive spinal muscular atrophy or poliomyelitis. (*B*) Upper motoneuron (UMN) disease: familial spastic paraplegia. (*C*) Combined UMN and LMN disease: amyotrophic lateral sclerosis. (*D*) Sensory neuron disease of dorsal roots or dorsal columns: hereditary sensory neuropathy or tabes dorsalis. (*E*) Combined degeneration of the dorsal and lateral funiculi: subacute combined degeneration. (*F*) Syringomyelia.

2. **Diseases of UMNs** (see Figure 6-23B). In **familial spastic paraplegia**, the pyramidal tracts undergo a dying back process in a **distal to proximal sequence**. The patient first has lower extremity paralysis, then upper extremity, and finally corticobulbar paralysis, with difficulty speaking and swallowing.

3. **Combined UMN and LMN diseases** (see Figure 6-23C). **Amyotrophic lateral sclerosis** (Lou Gehrig disease) is the prototypic disease involving both UMNs and LMNs.
   a. The **amyotrophy** refers to the muscular atrophy from degeneration of the LMNs.
   b. The **lateral sclerosis** refers to the pyramidal tract degeneration, which results in astrocytic proliferation, and therefore scar formation or sclerosis in the lateral columns (see Chapter 3 VIII D 1).
   c. The neurological examination shows a combination of UMN and LMN signs.

B. **Sensory neuron diseases of dorsal roots and dorsal columns**

1. In **hereditary sensory neuropathy**, the dorsal roots selectively degenerate, causing loss of sensation.

2. In **tabes dorsalis**, a form of **syphilis**, the dorsal columns degenerate. The patient loses dorsal column modalities, but retains pain sensation and often has lancinating pains in the extremities. The lower extremities are more affected than the upper, and leg fibers of the dorsal column degenerate more severely than arm fibers (see Figure 6-23D).

C. **Diseases with combined degeneration of dorsal and lateral columns**

1. **Subacute combined degeneration of the dorsal and lateral funiculi**, or **posterolateral sclerosis**, is caused by a deficiency of vitamin B_{12}. The patient has a combination of UMN signs and dorsal column sensory loss (see Figure 6-23E).

2. **Spinocerebellar degenerative diseases** involve the dorsal columns and spinocerebellar tracts and, to varying degrees, the pyramidal tracts.

3. **Clinical effects of combined dorsal and lateral column lesions**
   a. Patients with dorsal and lateral column diseases may show hyperreflexia or hyporeflexia, depending on which column shows the most advanced lesion.
   b. With severe dorsal column involvement, the MSRs ultimately disappear because of interruption of the afferent arc, in spite of the corticospinal tract lesions, which should result in hyperactive MSRs.

D. **Syringomyelia syndrome** (see Figure 6-23F). In syringomyelia, a cavitating process causes destruction of tissue around the central canal and extending out from it. It most commonly occurs in the cervical cord or medulla.

1. The first fibers affected are the pain and temperature fibers, which decussate in the ventral white commissure to turn rostrally into the lateral spinothalamic tract.

2. The patient loses pain and temperature sensation and may suffer burns of the fingers because of loss of the protective sensory modalities.

3. The lesion may expand out to involve one or both corticospinal tracts, or the alpha motoneurons, causing UMN and LMN signs in addition to the sensory loss.

E. **Syndromes of partial or complete transection of the spinal cord**. Trauma, neoplasms, vascular occlusion, and multiple sclerosis commonly affect all or part of the spinal cord.

1. **Complete transection** (Figure 6-24A) causes **quadriplegia** if **rostral** to the arm level and **paraplegia** if **caudal** to the arm level. Caudal to the level of the lesion, the patient shows:
   a. Paralysis of all voluntary movements, with UMN signs
   b. Anesthesia
   c. Loss of volitional bladder and bowel control (although reflex emptying may occur)
   d. Anhidrosis and loss of vasomotor tone
   e. Paralysis of all volitional and automatic breathing if the transection is rostral to C3

2. **Ventrolateral quadrant transection** (see Figure 6-24B)

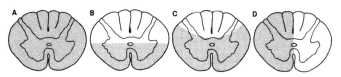

FIGURE 6-24. Syndromes of partial or complete interruption of the spinal cord at the cervical level. (*A*) Complete transection of the spinal cord. (*B*) Transection of the ventrolateral quadrants of the spinal cord. (*C*) Transection of the ventral two thirds of the spinal cord. (*D*) Lateral hemitransection (hemisection) of the spinal cord.

TABLE 6-4. Clinical Features of Brown-Séquard Syndrome (Spinal Cord Hemisection)

Clinical Findings	Anatomic Basis
Contralateral effects	
Loss of pain and temperature sensation caudal to the level of the lesion	Interruption of the spinothalamic tract
Ipsilateral effects	
Paralysis of voluntary movements caudal to the level of the lesion; hyperreflexia, spasticity, and extensor toe sign	Interruption of the lateral corticospinal tract
Loss of vibration, position sense, form perception, and two-point discrimination	Interruption of the dorsal columns
Segmental weakness and atrophy	Destruction of the ventral motoneurons at the level of the lesion
Segmental anesthesia	Destruction of the dorsal rootlets at the level of the lesion
Loss of sweating caudal to the level of the lesion, and, if the lesion is cervical, ipsilateral Horner's syndrome (pupilloconstriction, ptosis, and hemifacial anhidrosis)	Interruption of the descending autonomic fibers in the ventral funiculus
Hemidiaphragmatic paralysis (high cervical lesion)	Interruption of UMN pathways for breathing

UMN = upper motoneuron.

      a. Transection of the ventrolateral quadrants in the **cervical region** results in:
         (1) Paralysis of automatic breathing and decreased sensitivity to carbon dioxide, if rostral to C3
         (2) Loss of voluntary bladder and bowel control, with preservation of reflex emptying
         (3) Loss of the urge to urinate
         (4) Loss of pain and temperature sensation
         (5) Anhidrosis caudal to the lesion level
         (6) Hypotension
      b. The patient retains voluntary movement of the skeletal muscles and retains dorsal column modalities.

   3. Transection of the ventral two thirds of the cord (see Figure 6-24C)
      a. Occlusion of the ventral spinal artery (see Chapter 15 II A) results in infarction of the ventral two thirds of the spinal cord.
      b. The patient shows paralysis of voluntary movements in addition to the signs of ventrolateral quadrant transection listed in section VII E 2 a.

   4. Hemisection of the spinal cord (Brown-Séquard's syndrome) [Table 6-4; see Figure 6-24D]. This classic syndrome is the testing ground for knowledge of clinical spinal cord anatomy.

STUDY QUESTIONS

DIRECTIONS: Each of the numbered items or incomplete statements in this section is followed by answers or by completions of the statement. Select the ONE lettered answer or completion that is BEST in each case.

---

1. In doing a cordotomy to relieve pain in a patient with inoperable pelvic carcinoma, the neurosurgeon would insert the knife

(A) in the fasciculus gracilis of Goll
(B) deep in the dorsal median sulcus
(C) deep in the ventral median fissure
(D) just ventral to the plane of the denticulate ligament
(E) just dorsal to the plane of the denticulate ligament

2. The axons that innervate the distal muscles of the limbs derive from

(A) the intermediolateral cell column
(B) the intermediomedial cell column
(C) the medial cell column of the ventral horn
(D) the lateral cell column of the ventral horn
(E) the nucleus dorsalis of Clarke

3. Which of the following statements about the diameter of the spinal cord is true?

(A) The thoracic cord has the greatest diameter
(B) The transverse diameter at C8–T1 exceeds the anteroposterior diameter
(C) The diameter of the pyramidal tract area is smaller in the cervical than in the thoracic region
(D) The diameter of the fasciculus cuneatus is largest in the thoracic region
(E) The diameter of the substantia gelatinosa is smallest in the lumbosacral and cervical enlargements

4. Which of the following statements about the ventral corticospinal tract is true?

(A) It is located along the ventral median fissure
(B) It is larger than the lateral corticospinal tract
(C) It is composed of decussated axons
(D) It is composed of fibers known to regulate elimination
(E) None of the above

5. A neurosurgeon wishing to eliminate pain in a particular dermatome without causing loss of the sense of touch or a motor deficit would best make a cut at which one of the following sites?

(A) In the nerve trunk approximately 1 cm distal to the ganglion
(B) Just at the distal edge of the dorsal root ganglion
(C) Just after the dorsal root enters the subarachnoid space from the intervertebral foramen
(D) In the midportion of the root as it crosses the subarachnoid space
(E) Where the fibers of the lateral division of the dorsal root attach to the cord

6. To demonstrate only the crossed axons of both lateral corticospinal tracts by staining the products of Wallerian degeneration, an experimenter should

(A) cut one medullary pyramid transversely
(B) transect the sacral region of the spinal cord
(C) make a midsagittal cut at the cervico-medullary junction
(D) make a transverse cut in the ventral columns of the cord in the lower cervical region
(E) transect the dorsal columns high in the cervical region

7. The afferent axons for the muscle stretch reflexes (MSRs) synapse on the

(A) substantia gelatinosa
(B) lamina I of Rexed
(C) ventral motoneurons
(D) lamina VII of Rexed
(E) dorsal root ganglion

monosynaptic

8. A patient shows weakness of all arm and hand movements, slight atrophy of the arm muscles, hyperreflexia, and slight clasp-knife spasticity. The most likely cause is

(A) an upper motoneuron (UMN) lesion
(B) a cerebellar lesion
(C) a primary lesion of muscle
(D) a peripheral nerve lesion
(E) a nerve root lesion

9. A patient who failed to recognize a coin placed in his hand when his eyes were shut would most likely have a lesion of the

(A) spinoreticular tracts
(B) spinocerebellar tracts
(C) dorsal column pathways
(D) ground bundles of the spinal cord
(E) none of the above

10. Which of the following is the correct source of axons for the dorsal columns?

(A) Substantia gelatinosa
(B) Dorsal root ganglia
(C) Intermediolateral cell column
(D) Nucleus dorsalis of Clarke
(E) None of the above

11. Which general statement about the long tracts of the spinal cord is true?

(A) Most arise in the cerebrum
(B) Few are sensory pathways
(C) The long descending motor pathways stop short of the sacral cord
(D) The long tracts tend to run on the periphery of the spinal cord
(E) None of the above

12. Which of the following statements about the denticulate ligaments is true?

(A) A line drawn between the two ligaments bisects the spinal cord into right and left halves
(B) They consist of glia rather than collagen
(C) They attach directly to the vertebral bodies
(D) They travel along the dorsal roots
(E) None of the above

DIRECTIONS: Each of the numbered items or incomplete statements in this section is negatively phrased, as indicated by a capitalized word such as NOT, LEAST, or EXCEPT. Select the ONE lettered answer or completion that is BEST in each case.

---

13. The following nuclei or cell columns extend along the entire spinal cord EXCEPT for the

(A) medial motor cell column of the ventral horn
(B) intermediolateral cell column
(C) substantia gelatinosa (lamina II of Rexed)
(D) nucleus proprius (lamina III, IV, and V of Rexed)
(E) dorsomarginal nucleus (lamina I of Rexed)

14. The large fibers entering from the dorsal roots synapse on all of these nuclei EXCEPT for the

(A) ventral motoneurons
(B) nucleus dorsalis of Clarke
(C) nucleus gracilis
(D) intermediolateral nucleus = LMN of autonomic system
(E) nucleus cuneatus

15. Clinical effects seen immediately after complete transection of the spinal cord at T6 are likely to include all of the following EXCEPT for

(A) loss of voluntary control of the bladder and bowel
(B) paralysis of volitional leg movements
(C) loss of vasomotor reflexes in the legs
(D) hypotonia
(E) hyperactive muscle stretch reflexes (MSRs)

16. After complete spinal cord transection at C2, which one of the following functions CANNOT take place automatically through local spinal reflexes?

(A) Micturition and defecation
(B) Ejaculation
(C) Intestinal peristalsis
(D) Breathing
(E) Piloerection and sweating

17. After spinal cord hemisection at C2 (i.e., section of the dorsal, lateral, and ventral columns on one side), the patient shows the following clinical deficits caudal to the lesion EXCEPT for

(A) nearly complete ipsilateral loss of touch
(B) contralateral loss of pain and temperature sensation
(C) ipsilateral loss of dorsal column modalities
(D) ipsilateral paralysis of the arm and leg
(E) ipsilateral Horner's syndrome of ptosis and miosis

DIRECTIONS: Each set of matching questions in this section consists of a list of four to twenty-six lettered options (some of which may be in figures) followed by several numbered items. For each numbered item, select the ONE lettered option that is most closely associated with it. To avoid spending too much time on matching sets with large numbers of options, it is generally advisable to begin each set by reading the list of options. Then, for each item in the set, try to generate the correct answer and locate it in the option list, rather than evaluating each option individually. Each lettered option may be selected once, more than once, or not at all.

Questions 18–22

Match each name listed below with its characteristic or definition.

(A) Alpha motoneuron
(B) Motor unit
(C) Muscle spindle
(D) Fasciculation
(E) Renshaw neuron
(F) Interneuron

18. Largest neurons in the spinal cord

19. A motoneuron and all of the muscle fibers it innervates

20. A twitch caused by the contraction of all muscle fibers innervated by one axon

21. A neuron that provides an inhibitory synapse to motoneurons

22. A structure innervated by gamma motoneurons and Ia fibers

---

DIRECTIONS: Each set of matching questions in this section consists of a list of four to twenty-six lettered options followed by several numbered items. For each numbered item, select the appropriate lettered option(s). Each lettered option may be selected once, more than once, or not at all. EACH ITEM WILL STATE THE NUMBER OF OPTIONS TO SELECT. CHOOSE EXACTLY THIS NUMBER.

Questions 23–26

(A) Volitional movements of the extremities
(B) Volitional control of the bladder and bowel
(C) Ground bundles for intra- and intersegmental reflexes
(D) Automatic breathing pathway
(E) Touch
(F) Position sense and vibration
(G) Pain and temperature
(H) Direction of an object moving on the skin (directional scratch test)
(I) Awareness of bladder fullness
(J) Proprioception to the cerebellum

For the columns of the spinal cord, select the sensory or motor function(s) conveyed, in whole or in part, by that column.

23. Dorsal columns (SELECT 4 FUNCTIONS)

24. Lateral columns (SELECT 8 FUNCTIONS)

25. Ventral columns (SELECT 5 FUNCTIONS)

26. Ventrolateral and dorsal columns (SELECT 1 FUNCTION)

ANSWERS AND EXPLANATIONS

1. The answer is D [V B 4 b (5); Figure 6-17]. The sacral fibers run in the spinothalamic tracts in a plane just ventral to the denticulate ligaments. This tract, which mediates pain and temperature, has a distinct somatotopic lamination. The lamination reflects the law of lamination by level of entry. The sacral fibers are most dorsolateral, with the leg, trunk, and arm fibers extending ventromedially in order. The topography extends through the brain stem and thalamic sensory nucleus to the postcentral gyrus.

2. The answer is D [IV A 3]. The motor cell columns of the ventral horn (lamina IX of Rexed) reflect the body topography. The medial motor cell column (the medial nuclear group of motoneurons) supplies the axial muscles and the lateral motor cell column (the lateral nuclear group) supplies the appendicular muscles. Axons for the most distal muscles, the intrinsic muscles of the hands, come from the most laterodorsal neurons of the lateral nuclear complex. In amyotrophic lateral sclerosis, the neurons of the lateral group usually degenerate first.

3. The answer is B [I D 1, 2; Figure 6-3]. The diameter and shape of the cord and its tracts and nuclei vary with the levels. At C8–T1, the transverse diameter exceeds the anteroposterior diameter because of the lateral expansion of the gray matter by the greater number of neurons needed to innervate the arms. The thoracic region has the smallest diameter. The motor tracts decrease in area or size as they descend and the sensory tracts increase in size as they ascend. Because the descending tracts end at all levels of the cord, only a few axons remain at the distal end of the descending tract. Sensory tracts, like the spinothalamic, increase in size as they go up the cord because they continue to receive additional fibers from all levels as they ascend to the brain stem or thalamus.

4. The answer is A [V C 2 c (2), d (2); Figure 6-12]. The ventral corticospinal tract borders on the ventral median fissure. While often rather sizeable, it is smaller than the lateral corticospinal tract. The ventral corticospinal tract consists of myelinated axons of various sizes. The axons run straight down into the cord before decussating. However, many of these axons are thought to decussate before terminating in the ventral horns. Their func-

tion, whether different from the lateral corticospinal tract, is unknown.

5. The answer is E [III C 2]. The dorsal roots divide into medial and lateral bundles. The lateral bundle, which consists of small, poorly myelinated fibers, mediates pain and temperature. Neurosurgeons have attempted to treat some types of chronic pain by selective section of these roots just where they attach to the cord, leaving the larger, heavily myelinated touch and proprioceptive fibers of the medial division of the root intact. Elsewhere in the nerve root and trunk, the fibers intermingle too much to permit selective sectioning of pain axons. Moreover, section of the nerve trunk after the ventral root joins the dorsal root would also cause a motor deficit.

6. The answer is C [V C 2 b, c (1)]. Demonstrating a tract by Wallerian degeneration requires transecting axons prior to their entering the region of interest. To demonstrate only the lateral corticospinal tracts by Wallerian degeneration, leaving the ventral corticospinal tracts and all other fiber systems intact, it is best to make a midsagittal cut through the pyramidal decussation near the cervicomedullary junction. The cut would sever only the crossing axons that form the lateral corticospinal tract. By applying the appropriate stains to sections of the spinal cord, it is possible to demonstrate the trail of degenerating axons and myelin sheaths.

7. The answer is C [IV D 3]. The muscle stretch reflexes (MSRs) are monosynaptic. The afferent axons that elicit the reflex synapse directly on the ventral motoneurons, which send their motor axons to the muscle fibers. The clinician elicits these reflexes as part of the routine neurologic examination.

8. The answer is A [V C 2 g (1); VII A 2; Table 6-3]. Lesions of each of the components of the motor system cause a different clinical syndrome. The classical upper motoneuron (UMN) syndrome consists of exaggeration of the muscle stretch reflexes (MSRs) [hyperreflexia], spasticity, weakness of all movements, and slight disuse atrophy of the muscles. Lesions of the other motor circuits in the brain, the basal motor nuclei, or cerebellum do not produce this characteristic syndrome. Lesions affecting the afferent or efferent arc of the MSRs or disease of the muscles will reduce or abolish the MSRs, thus causing hyporeflexia or areflexia rather than hyperreflexia.

9. The answer is C [V B 1 c (1) (b), 3 a]. Recognition of an object felt but not seen requires superficial and deep sensation. The superficial sensation gives information as to touch and temperature. Apparently, both spinothalamic and dorsal column pathways mediate touch. The deep sensation, which travels through dorsal column pathways, provides a sense of form or stereognosis and texture. The brain integrates these pieces of information to identify the form and nature of an object felt by the fingers. Vision is unnecessary for recognition of the form of the object. In the standard neurologic examination, the clinician routinely tests patients for stereognosis by placing coins or other objects in the patient's hand for recognition without allowing the patient to see the object.

10. The answer is B [V B 3 b (2)]. The dorsal column axons consist of the central process of perikarya in the dorsal root ganglia. They enter the cord with the medial division of the dorsal roots and ascend ipsilaterally to the nuclei gracilis and cuneatus at the cervicomedullary junction. The axons from these nuclei decussate, form the medial lemniscus, and terminate in the thalamus. The dorsal columns do contain some descending fibers that arise at spinal levels, but do not convey known descending motor tracts from the brain.

11. The answer is D [V A 4 c]. The long tracts of the spinal cord tend to run on the periphery. Thus, they surround the ground bundles, which are the short, inter- and intrasegmental connecting pathways. The long pathways consist of both motor and sensory fibers. The long motor pathways, such as the pyramidal pathways, extend the length of the cord. All of the primary sensory fibers from the spinal dorsal root ganglia synapse before the sensory pathway continues through the brain stem, except for dorsal root proprioceptive fibers from the arm and neck, which reach the lateral cuneate nucleus. This tract corresponds to the dorsal spinocerebellar tract of the remainder of the cord.

12. The answer is E [V C 2 c (1) (b); Figures 6-11 and 6-21]. The denticulate ligaments attach to the lateral aspect of the spinal cord midway between the dorsal and ventral roots.

They extend from the pia to the dura and are composed of fibrous connective tissue, not glia. A transverse line connecting the denticulate ligaments on each side separates the dorsal half of the lateral white column, which contains the bulk of the corticospinal axons, from the ventral half, which conveys axons for the control of automatic breathing, bladder, and bowel function.

13. The answer is B [Table 6-1; Figure 6-6]. The nuclear groups or cell columns of the spinal cord extend for varying lengths up and down the cord. Some nuclear groups have a restricted location; the intermediomedial and intermediolateral nuclei and the nucleus dorsalis extend from about C8 to L2 or L3. The intermediolateral nucleus contains preganglionic sympathetic neurons. Parasympathetic preganglionic neurons occur in the sacral part of the cord. Thus, only the cervical part of the cord rostral to C8 has no autonomic preganglionic neurons. Other nuclei extend throughout the length of the cord, such as the medial motor cell column, which innervates the axial muscles, and the substantia gelatinosa, which mediates pain and temperature sensations from the entire body.

14. The answer is D [III C 3 c]. The large fibers that enter along the medial division of the dorsal roots synapse on motoneurons of the ventral horns and on the nucleus dorsalis of Clarke, the nucleus gracilis, and the nucleus cuneatus. In addition, they synapse on many interneurons of the dorsal and ventral horns. They do not synapse on the intermediolateral column of preganglionic sympathetic neurons.

15. The answer is E [V C 2 g (2) (a); Table 6-3]. Immediately after transection of the cord, the patient undergoes a stage of spinal shock with hypotonia and absence of muscle stretch reflexes (MSRs). This immediate, acute stage differs from the usual upper motoneuron (UMN) syndrome seen in the chronic stage, in which the patient has spasticity and hyperreflexia. In both acute and chronic stages, the patient loses voluntary control of the bladder and bowel, has paralysis of the muscles caudal to the lesion, and has no abdominal or cremasteric skin-muscle reflexes.

16. The answer is D [VI B 4 a, C 2, 3 e, D 3]. After spinal cord transection, the patient loses all volitional movements distal to the lesion, but a number of visceral reflexes remain. The patient cannot breathe, however, because the spinal cord lacks its own intrinsic rhythm generator for breathing. This is a function of the brain stem reticular formation (RF). Retained reflex actions include micturition, defecation, intestinal peristalsis, and ejaculation. Thus, a quadriplegic male can still have a reflex erection and ejaculate in response to penile stimulation, although he may have no sensation of the sexual act.

17. The answer is A [VII E 4; Figure 6-24; Table 6-4]. Hemisection of the spinal cord would cause a Brown-Séquard syndrome. After hemisection at the C1 or C2 level, the patient loses pain and temperature sensation contralaterally because the lesion interrupts the crossed spinothalamic tract in the ventrolateral quadrant of the cord, which conveys these modalities to the thalamus. The ipsilateral arm and leg would be paralyzed because of interruption of the descending pyramidal tract fibers in the lateral columns, which crossed at the level of the medullary decussation. Touch sensation might be mildly impaired, but because the touch pathways ascend by crossed and uncrossed tracts through the cord, the sensation of touch is not greatly affected. The ipsilateral Horner's syndrome indicates loss of the descending sympathetic pathway from the hypothalamus to the intermediolateral cell column. The lesion would also affect the ipsilateral respiratory muscles.

18–22. The answers are 18-A, 19-B, 20-D, 21-E, 22-C [IV B–E]. The alpha motoneurons are among the largest in the spinal cord and in the entire central nervous system (CNS). Any of the huge motoneurons of the lumbosacral cord sends its axon to numerous muscle fibers, numbering in the hundreds, in the lower extremities. The large size of the neuron reflects the large diameter and extensive distribution of the axon. A motoneuron, its axon, and all of the muscle fibers it innervates is called a motor unit. When a motoneuron fires, it activates all and only its own muscle fibers. When a single motoneuron fires, the clinician can see the resultant twitch of the many hundreds of muscle fibers as a faint ripple under the skin, which is called a fasciculation, and can record it by electromyography. Afferent volleys from muscle spindles, which are bags of specialized muscle fibers located within the regular muscle fibers, also activate the motoneurons of the motor unit during a muscle stretch reflex (MSR). Gamma efferents innervate the specialized muscle fibers of the muscle spindles and alter the sensitivity of the

spindles to stretch. Numerous other inhibitory and excitatory pathways also influence the activity of the motor units. From a certain constellation of clinical findings, the clinician can recognize a lower motoneuron (LMN) syndrome. The LMN syndrome consists of weakness, reduced MSRs, atrophy, and fasciculations. Only disease of the LMNs, somewhere between the ventral horn and the neuromyal junction, produces this unique, diagnostic constellation of findings. Having localized the disease to a specific part of the nervous system, the clinician then knows the most likely disease processes to consider in the differential diagnosis.

23. The answers are: C, E, F, H [V B 3 a (1); Figures 6-12 and 6-17]. The dorsal columns, consisting of the fasciculi gracilis and cuneatus, convey the "discriminative modalities." These include stereognosis, position sense of the body parts, degree of pressure, weight, graphesthesia, and the direction of an object moving on the skin. Detection of movement serves as a sensitive screening test for dorsal column lesions. For the directional scratch test, the patient, with eyes closed, reports the direction of a light stroke on the skin. All three columns convey ground bundles that mediate intra- and intersegmental reflexes. These connections permit rather complex reflex behaviors (e.g., withdrawal of a leg from a stimulus) to persist in the segments of the spinal cord caudal to a transection.

24. The answers are: A, B, C, D, E, G, I, J [Figures 6-12, 6-17, and 6-21]. The lateral columns convey pathways for numerous functions: the lateral corticospinal tracts for voluntary movements, the spinocerebellar tracts for proprioception, the lumbosacral wafers of the spinothalamic tract for pain and temperature, and the ascending pathway for the urge to void. This latter pathway, signaling as it does discomfort, is closely allied to or nearly identical with the spinothalamic pain pathway from the sacral region. Touch pathways ascend in the ventral and lateral columns as part of the decussated spinothalamic system. Some controversy exists as to whether the dorsal parts of the lateral columns convey vibration and position sense in addition to, or instead of, the classical dorsal column route.

25. The answers are: A, C, D, E, G [Figures 6-12, 6-17, and 6-21]. The ventral columns convey the vestibulospinal and most of the reticulospinal and spinoreticular pathways.

Part of the spinothalamic pathway for touch occupies the ventral and lateral columns similar to the pain and temperature pathway. Most important, the reticulospinal tract for automatic breathing descends in the region ventrolateral to the rounded tip of the ventral horn, mostly in the ventral column. Without this tract, the patient fails to sustain breathing upon going to sleep and may die. This condition (Ondine's curse) condemns the patient to remain forever awake in order to breath. The ventral corticospinal tract, consisting of uncrossed axons, occupies the region adjacent to the ventral median sulcus. It varies considerably in size from person to person. Its fibers are presumed to cross before synapsing on the lower motoneurons (LMNs) or interneurons of the ventral horns.

26. The answer is E [V B 5 a, b]. Isolated lesions of neither the ventrolateral columns nor the dorsal columns abolish touch. Thus, pathways through both columns are presumed to mediate touch sensation. The touch pathways of the ventral columns travel in the vicinity of the lateral spinothalamic tract for pain and temperature, but a discrete and separate touch pathway has not been identified.

Chapter 7

The Brain Stem and Cranial Nerves

I. INTRODUCTION TO THE BRAIN STEM

A. **Definition**

1. The brain stem consists of three gross transverse subdivisions, the **midbrain, pons, and medulla oblongata,** in rostrocaudal order (Figures 7-1 to 7-3; see Figure 1-3).

2. Nine of the twelve pairs of cranial nerves attach to the brain stem (see Figures 7-1 to 7-3).

B. **New features of the brain stem.** Although the basic somite plan of the spinal cord continues through the brain stem, several major new features appear that are not present in the spinal cord.

1. Special motoneurons for a special set of cranial nerves that innervate the branchial arches

2. Special nuclei and pathways that mediate the special senses of taste, hearing, and equilibrium

3. Pathways that control eye movements

4. Reticular formation (RF)

5. Nuclei that supplement the motor and sensory systems

6. Quadrigeminal plate of the midbrain

7. The cerebellum, which protrudes from the dorsum of the pons

II. EMBRYOLOGY OF THE BRAIN STEM

A. **Early development of the brain stem.** Conceptually, the brain stem represents a bulbous, phylogenetic expansion of the basic structure of the spinal cord and it displays the same embryologic sequences.

1. The neural tube closes around a neural canal.

2. Roof and floor plates and paired basal and alar plates develop.

3. The wall of the neural tube develops the same ependymal, mantle, and marginal layers (see Figure 3-11A).

B. **Rhombencephalic roof plate and the rhomboid fossa**

1. The rhombencephalon becomes the pons and medulla (see Figure 3-4). The central canal of the rhombencephalon enlarges to become the fourth ventricle. The rhomboid-shaped floor of the fourth ventricle, the **rhomboid fossa,** explains the term **rhombencephalon** (Figure 7-4; see Figure 7-3).

2. The roof plate attaches along the margins of the rhomboid fossa. The margins, in fact the dorsal lips of the alar plate of the rhombencephalon, angle laterally, stretching out the roof plate (see Figure 7-4). It forms the superior and inferior medullary vela that roof the fourth ventricle.

3. The roof plates of both the hindbrain and forebrain develop initially as a two-layered membrane.
   a. **Pia mater,** derived from mesenchyme, forms the outer layer of the membrane.
   b. **Ependymal cells,** the neural element derived from neural ectoderm, forms a monolayer of cells as the inner layer of the membrane.

4. Perforations of the rhombencephalic roof plate
   a. On approximately the fiftieth day of gestation, the posterior medullary velum perforates in the midline to form the median **foramen of Magendie.**
   b. Similar perforations occur in the pia-ependymal roof plate membrane at the lateral angles of the rhomboid, forming lateral **foramina of Luschka.**

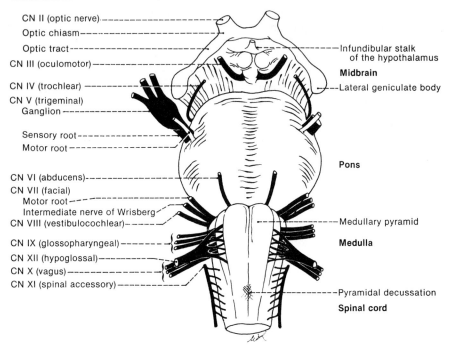

Cranial nerves

CN II (optic nerve)
Optic chiasm
Optic tract
CN III (oculomotor)
CN IV (trochlear)
CN V (trigeminal)
Ganglion
Sensory root
Motor root
CN VI (abducens)
CN VII (facial)
Motor root
Intermediate nerve of Wrisberg
CN VIII (vestibulocochlear)
CN IX (glossopharyngeal)
CN XII (hypoglossal)
CN X (vagus)
CN XI (spinal accessory)

Infundibular stalk of the hypothalamus
Midbrain
Lateral geniculate body
Pons
Medullary pyramid
Medulla
Pyramidal decussation
Spinal cord

FIGURE 7-1. Ventral view of the brain stem and cranial nerves.

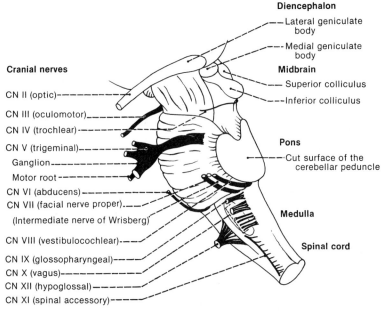

Diencephalon
Lateral geniculate body
Medial geniculate body
Midbrain
Superior colliculus
Inferior colliculus

Cranial nerves

CN II (optic)
CN III (oculomotor)
CN IV (trochlear)
CN V (trigeminal)
Ganglion
Motor root
CN VI (abducens)
CN VII (facial nerve proper)
(Intermediate nerve of Wrisberg)
CN VIII (vestibulocochlear)
CN IX (glossopharyngeal)
CN X (vagus)
CN XII (hypoglossal)
CN XI (spinal accessory)

Pons
Cut surface of the cerebellar peduncle
Medulla
Spinal cord

FIGURE 7-2. Lateral view of the brain stem and cranial nerves.

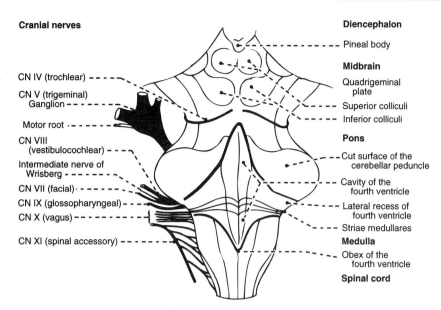

Cranial nerves

CN IV (trochlear)

CN V (trigeminal) Ganglion

Motor root

CN VIII (vestibulocochlear)

Intermediate nerve of Wrisberg

CN VII (facial)

CN IX (glossopharyngeal)

CN X (vagus)

CN XI (spinal accessory)

Diencephalon

Pineal body

Midbrain

Quadrigeminal plate

Superior colliculi

Inferior colliculi

Pons

Cut surface of the cerebellar peduncle

Cavity of the fourth ventricle

Lateral recess of fourth ventricle

Striae medullares

Medulla

Obex of the fourth ventricle

Spinal cord

FIGURE 7-3. Dorsal view of the brain stem and cranial nerves.

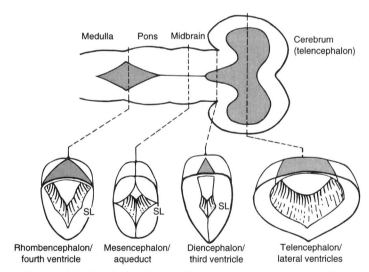

Medulla Pons Midbrain

Cerebrum (telencephalon)

Rhombencephalon/ fourth ventricle

Mesencephalon/ aqueduct

Diencephalon/ third ventricle

Telencephalon/ lateral ventricles

FIGURE 7-4. Dorsal view of the developing brain and representative cross sections. The membraneous portions of the roof plate are shaded. *SL* = sulcus limitans.

    c. These perforations allow cerebrospinal fluid (CSF) to escape from the neural canal into the subarachnoid space. If the roof plate fails to perforate, the CSF produced by the choroid plexuses of the roof plates dams up. The ventricular cavities and aqueduct balloon out, causing the wall of the cerebrum to thin and the head to enlarge. This condition, termed **hydrocephalus**, is treated by inserting a catheter into a ventricle to drain the fluid artificially.

5. Extent of the fourth ventricle
    a. Rostrally, the fourth ventricle narrows into the aqueduct of the midbrain (see Figure 1-7).

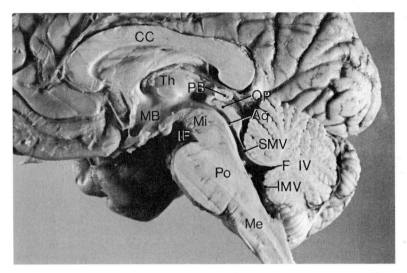

FIGURE 7-5. Midsagittal section of the brain. *Aq* = aqueduct; *CC* = corpus callosum; *F IV* = fastigium of the fourth ventricle; *IF* = interpeduncular fossa of the midbrain; *IMV* = inferior medullary velum; *MB* = mamillary body; *Me* = medulla; *Mi* = midbrain; *PB* = pineal body; *Po* = pons; *QP* = quadrigeminal plate; *SMV* = superior medullary velum; *Th* = thalamus.

       b. **Caudally,** the fourth ventricle narrows into the central canal of the spinal cord.

       c. **Laterally,** the fourth ventricle has its widest diameter at the **lateral recesses** of the rhomboid fossa (see Figures 7-3 and 7-4).

          (1) The plane across the lateral recesses marks the plane of the **pontomedullary sulcus,** which separates the pons from the medulla.

          (2) This plane also marks the peak of the fourth ventricle, the **fastigium,** where the anterior and posterior medullary vela meet (Figure 7-5).

C. **Derivatives of the rhombic lips of the alar plates**

    1. Neuroblasts proliferate prodigiously in the rhombic lips of the alar plates (see Figure 10-5). While some neuroblasts remain more or less in situ dorsally, others migrate ventrally into the expanding mantle zone and tegmentum:

       a. The neuroblasts that remain more or less in situ dorsally form the:

          (1) Cerebellum from the pontine rhombic lips

          (2) Auditory (cochlear) and vestibular nuclei, the special somatic afferent (SSA) nuclei

       b. The neuroblasts that migrate **peripherally** into the tegmentum form the:

          (1) **Inferior olivary nuclei** of the medullary tegmentum for the olivocerebellar motor pathways

          (2) **Superior olivary nuclei** of the pontine tegmentum for the auditory pathways

          (3) **Pontine nuclei** of the pontine basis for the corticopontocerebellar motor pathway

    2. **Surface protrusions from the brain stem**

       a. Three of these new rhombic lip derivatives form protrusions visible on the external surface of the brain stem:

          (1) Cerebellum (see Figure 7-5)

          (2) Inferior olivary complex (see Figure 7-9)

          (3) Bulk of the belly of the basis pontis (see Figure 7-9B)

       b. Massive circuitry links these three structures of common embryologic origin into a system that coordinates skeletal muscle contraction during voluntary movement, as described in Chapter 10 II B.

III. COMPOSITION OF THE BRAIN STEM

A. Composite cross section of the brain stem

1. Although in cross section the contour of the midbrain, pons, and medulla differs somewhat, a single, composite contour represents all three (Figure 7-6).

2. Any cross section of the brain stem (see Figure 7-10) exhibits three laminae: the **tectum**, **tegmentum**, and **basis**. Each laminae extends the entire length of the brain stem, through the midbrain, pons, and medulla, as does the original neural canal (Figure 7-7).

B. Composition of the tectum

1. **Definition.** The tectum is the lamina of brain stem tissue **dorsal** to the plane of the aqueduct (tectum means roof) [see Figure 7-7]. It develops from the roof plate of the brain stem.

2. **In rostrocaudal order the tectum consists of the:**
   a. Quadrigeminal plate over the midbrain
   b. Superior medullary velum over the pons
   c. Inferior medullary velum over the medulla (see Figure 7-5)

3. Notice in Figure 7-5 that:
   a. The **rostral** part of the tectum, the quadrigeminal plate of the midbrain, roofs the aqueductal part of the original neural canal.

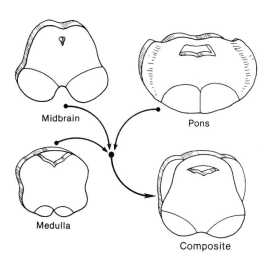

FIGURE 7-6. Composite of the cross-sectional contour of the midbrain, pons, and medulla.

Midbrain

Pons

Medulla

Composite

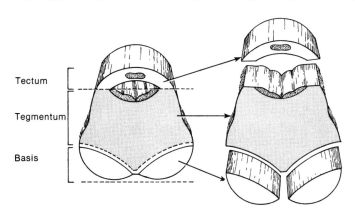

FIGURE 7-7. Exploded view of a composite cross section of the brain stem to show the three longitudinal subdivisions into the tectum, tegmentum, and basis.

Tectum

Tegmentum

Basis

    b. The **caudal** part of the tectum, the **superior** and **inferior medullary vela,** roof the fourth ventricular part of the original neural canal. The vela meet at the peak of the fourth ventricle, called the **fastigium.**

  4. The tectum contains no cranial nerve nuclei and no RF. No long motor or sensory pathways course longitudinally through it, as they do through the tegmentum and basis.

C. **Composition of the basis**

  1. The basis transmits descending cortical efferent motor tracts (see Figures 7-19 to 7-21), which consist of the:

    a. Corticopontine tracts

    b. Pyramidal tracts. The pyramidal tracts consist of:

      (1) Corticobulbar tracts to brain stem neurons

      (2) Corticospinal tracts to spinal neurons

  2. Differences in the basis of the midbrain, pons, and medulla

    a. The **midbrain** basis conveys corticobulbar, corticospinal, and corticopontine tracts, but contains no nuclei (see Figures 7-19 to 7-21).

    b. The **pontine** basis is the largest basis because it contains masses of nuclei upon which the corticopontine efferents synapse.

      (1) After receiving the corticopontine axons, the nuclei of the basis pontis project to the cerebellum, completing a cortico-ponto-cerebellar pathway.

      (2) All corticospinal fibers, and some remaining corticobulbar fibers, proceed longitudinally (caudally) past the pontine nuclei, through the pontine basis, and into the medullary basis, where the pyramidal tracts become visible on the ventral surface (see Figure 7-1)

    c. The **medullary basis** is the smallest (see Figure 7-6) because:

      (1) The corticopontine fibers terminated on the nuclei in the basis pontis.

      (2) Most corticobulbar fibers to tegmental neurons have already left the pyramidal tract to enter the tegmentum **rostral** to the medulla (see Figure 6-20). A few proceed into the medullary basis before entering the medullary tegmentum.

    d. Because the corticofugal tracts in the medullary basis have an oval or pyramidal shape on cross section, they are called the **medullary pyramids**, and, hence, the **pyramidal tracts.**

D. **Composition of the brain stem tegmentum** (tegmen means covering, the covering of the basis).

  1. Definition. The tegmentum is the plate of neurons and tracts sandwiched between the tectum and basis of the brain stem (see Figure 7-7). In contrast to the relative simplicity of the basis and tectum, the tegmentum consists of a complicated mixture of gray and white matter.

  2. Diagrammatic cross section of the tegmentum. Notice in Figure 7-8 that:

    a. The **general somatomotor and general sensory cranial nerve nuclei** cluster in the dorsal tier of the tegmentum. No cranial nerve nuclei occupy the tectum or basis.

    b. Special visceral efferent (SVE) nuclei migrate to a position ventrolateral to the general somatic efferent (GSE) motoneurons.

    c. Supplementary motor nuclei occupy the ventral tier of the tegmentum or basis pontis.

      (1) In the medulla, these are the inferior olivary nuclei.

      (2) In the pons, these are nuclei of the basis.

      (3) In the midbrain, these include the red nucleus and substantia nigra.

    d. Sensory tracts to the thalamus, called **lemnisci,** run in the ventral and lateral part of the tegmentum.

    e. RF fills in the space in the tegmentum unoccupied by cranial nerve nuclei, supplementary motor and special sensory nuclei, and long tracts.

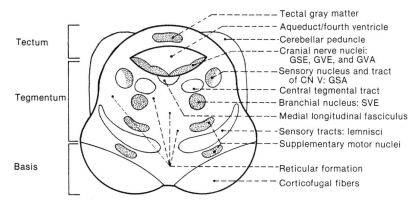

FIGURE 7-8. Diagrammatic cross section of the brain stem tegmentum. *GSA* = general somatic afferent; *GSE* = general somatic efferent; *GVA* = general visceral afferent; *GVE* = general visceral efferent; *SVE* = special visceral (branchial) efferent.

    3. **Neuronal arrangements in the tegmentum consist of:**
        a. **General and special motor and sensory nuclei** of CN III to CN XII, with the exception of CN XI
        b. **RF,** including certain chemically specified nuclei and tracts
        c. **Supplementary motor nuclei**
    4. **Pathways of the tegmentum consist of:**
        a. **All long sensory tracts** that ascend from the spinal cord to brain stem nuclei, RF, cerebellum, and diencephalon
        b. **Medial longitudinal fasciculus** (MLF), the ground bundle of the brain stem that belongs to the optomotor system
        c. **Cerebellar afferent and efferent pathways**
        d. **The central tegmental tract,** which interconnects the tegmentum, diencephalon, and basal forebrain gray matter
        e. **Hypothalamic pathways to the tegmentum,** particularly to the RF
        f. **Profuse, unnamed short and long ascending and descending pathways** within the RF

IV. **AN ATLAS OF THE INTERNAL ANATOMY OF THE BRAIN STEM.** Figures 7-9 through 7-21 present transverse brain stem levels in serial order, rather than scattering them throughout the text. Thus, it is possible to conveniently trace the changes in the nuclei and the course of the ascending and descending tracts from level to level, as the text describes them.

V. **DETAILED EXTERNAL AND INTERNAL ANATOMY OF THE MEDULLA OBLONGATA**

A. Gross external anatomy of the medulla (see Figure 7-9C)

B. Cross-sectional anatomy of the medulla
    1. **The medulla is an elaborated, bulbous expansion of the spinal cord.**
        a. The alar and basal plates angle outward (see Figure 7-4).
        b. The roof plate (tectum) stretches out thin.

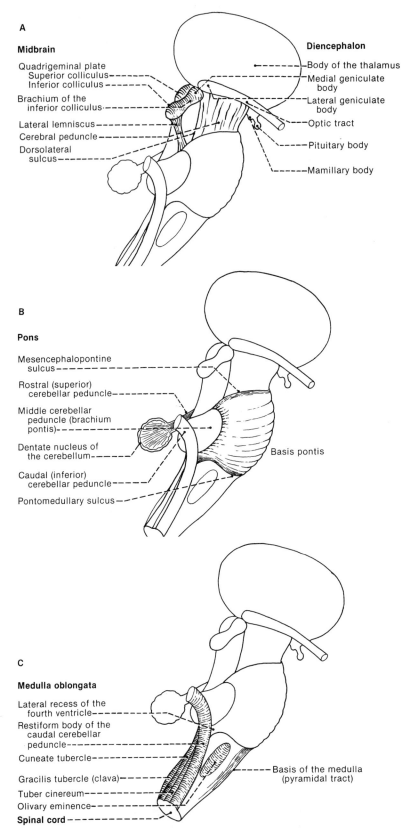

A

Midbrain

Quadrigeminal plate
  Superior colliculus
  Inferior colliculus
Brachium of the
  inferior colliculus
Lateral lemniscus
Cerebral peduncle
Dorsolateral
  sulcus

Diencephalon

Body of the thalamus
Medial geniculate
  body
Lateral geniculate
  body
Optic tract
Pituitary body
Mamillary body

B

Pons

Mesencephalopontine
  sulcus
Rostral (superior)
  cerebellar peduncle
Middle cerebellar
  peduncle (brachium
  pontis)
Dentate nucleus of
  the cerebellum
Caudal (inferior)
  cerebellar peduncle
Pontomedullary sulcus

Basis pontis

C

Medulla oblongata

Lateral recess of the
  fourth ventricle
Restiform body of the
  caudal cerebellar
  peduncle
Cuneate tubercle
Gracilis tubercle (clava)
Tuber cinereum
Olivary eminence
Spinal cord

Basis of the medulla
  (pyramidal tract)

FIGURE 7-9. Gross external anatomy of the brain stem.

c. The gray matter (tegmentum) thickens because of the RF and supplementary nuclei (see Figures 7-12 to 7-15).

d. The long tracts assemble, as a shell, around the periphery of the gray matter. Using Figures 7-12 and 7-13, start in the upper right and trace around the white matter shell, which consists of:

(1) The cerebellar peduncle (upper right)

(2) The descending root of CN V

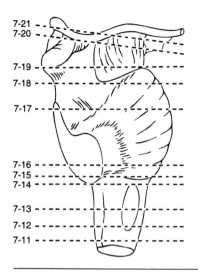

FIGURE 7-10. Key to the levels of the brain stem illustrated in Figures 7-11 through 7-21.

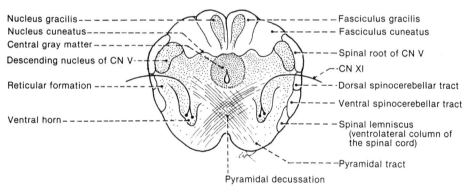

FIGURE 7-11. Transverse section of the cervicomedullary junction.

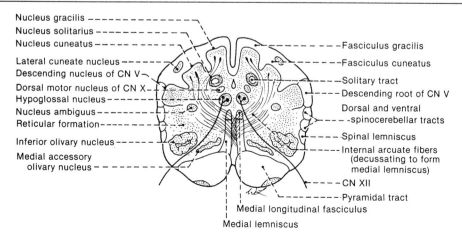

FIGURE 7-12. Caudal-most transverse section of the medulla oblongata.

(3) The dorsal and ventral spinocerebellar tracts

(4) The spinal lemniscus

(5) The pyramidal tract, and dorsal to it, the medial lemniscus and MLF

2. The area postrema

a. The area postrema, a specialized paraventricular organelle, occupies the caudal end of the fourth ventricle, in a region called the **obex** (see Figure 7-3).

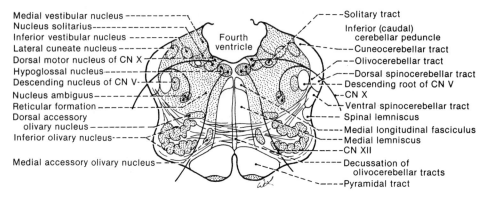

FIGURE 7-13. Caudal transverse section of the medulla oblongata.

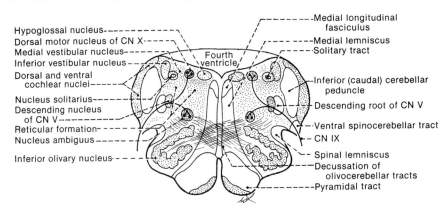

FIGURE 7-14. Midlevel transverse section of the medulla oblongata.

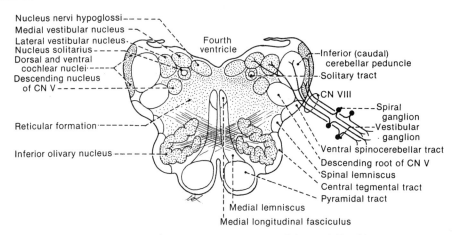

FIGURE 7-15. Rostral-most transverse section of the medulla oblongata.

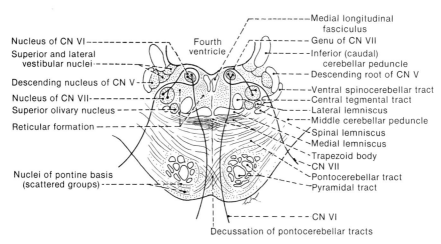

FIGURE 7-16. Caudal transverse section of the pons.

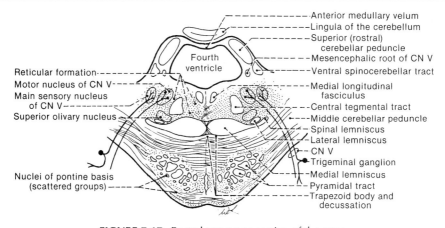

FIGURE 7-17. Rostral transverse section of the pons.

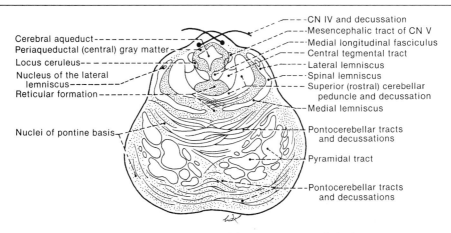

FIGURE 7-18. Transverse section of the pontomesencephalic junction.

b. The area postrema is an area of increased blood-brain barrier permeability, unlike the central nervous system (CNS) in general, containing highly specialized cells that act as chemoreceptors that trigger vomiting in response to bloodborne substances, such as apomorphine, digitalis, and other chemicals.

c. It mediates vomiting through its afferent connections with the nucleus solitarius, its efferent connections through the medullary RF, and the projections from the RF to motor nuclei of the brain stem and spinal cord.

C. **Corresponding structures of the spinal cord and medulla** (Table 7-1)

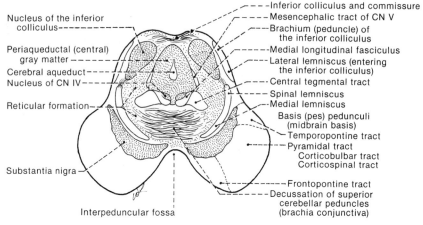

FIGURE 7-19. Caudal transverse section of the midbrain.

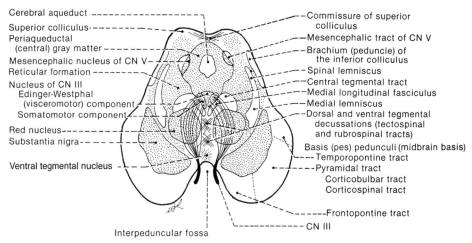

FIGURE 7-20. Rostral transverse section of the midbrain.

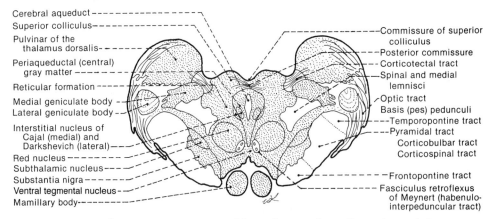

FIGURE 7-21. Rostral-most transverse section of the midbrain at the midbrain-diencephalic junction.

TABLE 7-1. Homologies and Analogies Between the Medulla and Spinal Cord

Spinal Cord Structure	Medullary Structure
Central canal	Fourth ventricle
Roof plate	Posterior medullary velum
Ventral motoneurons	Nucleus of CN XII
Motoneurons of CN XI	Nucleus ambiguus
Preganglionic parasympathetic neurons of the sacral cord	Dorsal motor nucleus of the vagus nerve
Reticular nucleus	Reticular formation
Substantia gelatinosa of Rolando and dorsolateral fasciculus of Lissauer	Spinal nucleus and tract of CN V
Nucleus dorsalis of Clarke	Lateral cuneate nucleus
Intersegmental ground bundles	Medial longitudinal fasciculus
Spinal lemniscus (lateral and ventral spinothalamic tracts)	Continues into the medial lemniscus, which is also joined by the trigeminal lemniscus
Dorsal column pathway	Continues into the medulla as the medial lemniscus after synapsing in the nuclei gracilis and cuneatus
Spinocerebellar tracts	Continues through the medulla into the pons and cerebellum
Pyramidal tract	Continues from the medulla through the length of the spinal cord

D. **Gray matter at the cervicomedullary transition zone.** Trace the following structures through Figures 7-11 to 7-15:

1. General somatic afferent (GSA) nuclei gracilis and cuneatus of the dorsal column pathway to the thalamus

2. GSA spinal nucleus and the tract of CN V (pain and temperature component), which merge with the substantia gelatinosa and the dorsolateral fasciculus of Lissauer

3. SVE nucleus of motoneurons for CN XI

4. SVE nucleus ambiguus of motoneurons for CN IX and CN X

5. GSE nucleus of motoneurons for CN XII

6. General visceral efferent (GVE) dorsal motor nucleus of CN X (the nucleus ambiguus is the ventral motor nucleus of CN X)

7. General visceral afferent (GVA) and special visceral afferent (SVA) nuclei of tractus solitarius for CN VII, CN IX, and CN X

8. SSA vestibular nuclei

9. Inferior olivary complex

E. **Decussations at or near the cervicomedullary junction.** Five clinically important decussations occur at the cervicomedullary transition zone:

1. **The reticulospinal respiratory pathways** for automatic breathing, just ventral to the obex of the fourth ventricle (see Figure 7-40)

2. **The pyramidal tract** decussation (see Figure 7-11)

3. **The three decussations that form internal arcuate fibers** consist of the:
   a. **Trigeminal lemniscus,** from the spinal nucleus of CN V (see Figure 7-30)
   b. **Medial lemniscus,** from the nuclei gracilis and cuneatus (see Figure 7-14)
   c. **Olivocerebellar tracts,** from the inferior olivary nuclei (see Figure 7-13) (Decussation extends throughout the length of the medulla.)

F. **The medial lemniscus**

1. **Origin.** The medial lemniscus originates from neurons of the nuclei gracilis and cuneatus at the cervicomedullary junction. These neurons are the secondary neurons that relay the dorsal column pathway from the spinal cord to the thalamus and somatosensory cortex.

    a. As these axons sweep ventromedially to decussate, they form the **caudal** part of the **internal arcuate decussation** (see Figure 7-12).

    b. The crossing of the olivocerebellar tracts forms the **rostral** part of the internal arcuate decussation (see Figure 7-13).

2. **Course of the medial lemniscus**

    a. At its origin and through the medulla, the medial lemniscus runs in the paramedian zone (see Figures 7-12 through 7-15).

    b. As the medial lemniscus ascends, two changes occur:

       (1) Its location shifts

       (2) Other fiber systems join it

    c. As it ascends into the pons, the medial lemniscus flattens out (see Figures 7-16 and 7-17). In the midbrain, it shifts dorsolaterally and contacts the lateral lemniscus (see Figure 7-18).

3. **Additional fiber systems in the medial lemniscus**

    a. As it **ascends** into the pons, two other ascending sensory pathways join the medial lemniscus:

       (1) The **trigeminal lemniscus**, which originates in the spinal nucleus of CN V and began its decussation at the medullocervical junction zone

       (2) The **spinal lemniscus**, consisting of the spinothalamic tracts, which have decussated in the spinal cord (see Figure 6-18)

    b. Some **corticobulbar fibers** depart from the corticobulbar tract in the midbrain to **descend** in the medial lemniscus.

    c. Thus, the composition and position of the medial lemniscus varies depending on the brain stem level.

4. **Termination of the medial lemniscus**

    a. By definition, all lemnisci end in a specific thalamic sensory relay nucleus. The medial lemniscus ends in the nucleus ventralis posterior, which relays to the somatosensory receptive area in the postcentral gyrus of the parietal lobe.

    b. The ascending pain and temperature fibers of the spinal lemniscus send collaterals into the RF along the way to the thalamus, but the medial lemniscal fibers, continuing the dorsal column pathway, apparently do not.

G. **Cranial nerve nuclei of the medulla.** The medulla contains the motor and sensory nuclei of CN IX and CN X and portions of the sensory nuclei of CN V and CN VIII (Figure 7-22).

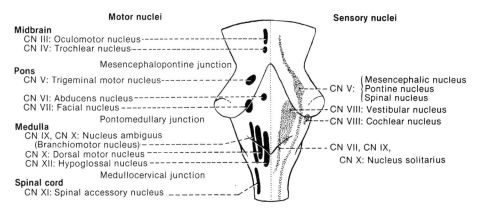

FIGURE 7-22. Dorsal view of the brain stem showing the location of the motor and sensory nuclei of the cranial nerves.

VI. DETAILED EXTERNAL AND INTERNAL ANATOMY OF THE PONS

A. **Gross external anatomy of the pons** (see Figure 7-9B)

B. **Triads of the pons.** The **five** triads of the pons include the **longitudinal** triad, **cerebellar peduncular** triad, **motor cranial nerve** triad, **sensory cranial nerve** triad, and **decussational** triad.

1. The **longitudinal triad of the pons** consists of the tectum, tegmentum, and basis.
   a. The pontine **tectum** consists of the superior medullary velum.
   b. The pontine **tegmentum** is a relatively thin plate of gray matter bounded by the ventral border of the medial lemniscus (see Figure 7-16).
   c. The bulging pontine **basis** consists of longitudinally coursing cortical efferent fibers and nuclear masses, which relay the corticopontocerebellar pathway.

2. **Pontine cerebellar peduncular triad.** Three paired peduncles, **caudal, middle,** and **rostral,** attach the cerebellum to the pons. They consist of afferent and efferent cerebellar tracts, but no gray matter (see Figure 7-9 and Figure 10-10).

3. The **pontine motor cranial nerve triad** consists of CN V, CN VI, and CN VII (see Figure 7-22).
   a. The three motor nuclei, CN V (SVE), CN VI (GSE), and CN VII (SVE), occupy the positions expected from the theory of nerve components (see Figure 7-16).
   b. One major peculiarity is the internal loop of CN VII over the nucleus of CN VI (see Figure 7-16).

4. **Pontine sensory cranial nerve triad**
   a. The pons contains parts of three different sensory nuclei: rostral continuations of the **cochlear and vestibular nuclei of CN VIII** and part of the **sensory nucleus of CN V.**
   b. The sensory nucleus of CN V has three divisions (see Figure 7-22), which are the:
      (1) Mesencephalic nucleus (GSA for proprioception)
      (2) Main sensory nucleus (GSA for touch)
      (3) Spinal nucleus of CN V, which is located in the medulla and rostral end of the cervical cord (GSA for pain and temperature) [see Figure 7-30]
   c. **The trigeminal ganglion divides into three main peripheral sensory branches** (see Figure 7-30), which are the:
      (1) Ophthalmic (V1)
      (2) Mandibular (V2)
      (3) Maxillary (V3)

5. **Decussational triad of the pons**
   a. The **auditory pathways** partially decussate through the trapezoid body and superior olivary nuclei.
   b. The **pontocerebellar pathways** from the nuclei of the basis pontis decussate to form the middle cerebellar peduncle (see Figures 7-16 and 10-12).
   c. The **cerebellovestibular pathway** partially decussates across the roof of the fourth ventricle (see Figure 10-11).

C. **Anatomic features of the pontomedullary junction.** Like the cervicomedullary junction, it is critical to learn the pontomedullary junction.

1. CN VI, CN VII, and CN VIII attach in ventrodorsal order to the pontomedullary sulcus (see Figure 7-1).
   a. The **somite** nerve (CN VI) attaches most ventrally, in the paramedian plane, as is typical of somite nerves.
   b. The **branchial** nerve (CN VII) attaches dorsolaterally, as is typical of branchial nerves.
   c. The purely **sensory** nerve (CN VIII) attaches most dorsolaterally, as is typical of sensory roots.

2. If CN VI, CN VII, and CN VIII attach in a transverse line at the pontomedullary sulcus, then as a mnemonic notice that CN I through CN V must attach **rostral** to that plane and CN IX through CN XII must attach **caudal** to it.

3. The nuclei of CN VI and CN VII, and the internal genu of CN VII lie just rostral to the plane of the pontomedullary junction.

4. CN V commences the transition from the pontine nucleus to the spinal nucleus, which mediates pain and temperature (see Figure 7-30).

5. Salivatory nuclei are located in the dorsal tegmentum at the pontomedullary junction.

6. The cochlear and vestibular nuclei straddle the plane of the pontomedullary junction.

7. The pontomedullary plane separates the superior olivary complex and trapezoid body of the pons (the auditory system) from the inferior olivary complex of the medulla (the olivocerebellar component of the somatomotor system).

8. The **tallest point of the fourth ventricle,** the **fastigium,** and the **widest point,** the **lateral recesses,** are in the plane of the pontomedullary junction.

9. The cerebellum, with its deep nuclei, lies over the fastigium.

10. The caudal cerebellar peduncle, conveying the dorsal spinocerebellar tract, turns dorsally into the cerebellum just rostral to the plane of the pontomedullary junction.

11. The medial lemniscus begins to migrate laterally from its paramedian location in the medulla. It flattens out into a fillet as the other ascending lemnisci join it.

12. Ventrally, the pyramidal tracts emerge from the basis pontis to form the medullary basis (see Figure 7-9C).

13. Ventrally, the vertebral arteries unite to form the basilar artery (see Figure 15-9).

D. **Anatomic features of the ponto-midbrain junction** (see Figure 7-9)

1. The bulging belly of the pons abruptly replaces the midbrain, which forms a narrow **isthmus** between it and the diencephalon and cerebral hemispheres.

2. The cerebral peduncle, with its pyramidal tract, disappears abruptly into the pontine belly.

3. The aqueduct becomes continuous with the rostral tip of the fourth ventricle.

4. CN IV emerges at the junction between the anterior medullary velum of the pons and the inferior colliculus of the quadrigeminal plate of the midbrain (see Figure 7-18).

5. The rostral tip of the cerebellum ends at the ponto-midbrain plane.

6. Ventrally, the basilar artery branches into the posterior cerebral arteries (see Figure 15-17).

VII. DETAILED EXTERNAL AND INTERNAL ANATOMY OF THE MIDBRAIN (MESENCEPHALON)

A. **Gross external anatomy of the midbrain** (see Figure 7-9A)

B. **Gray matter of the midbrain tegmentum consists of:**

1. **Two cranial nerve nuclei** (see Figure 7-22), which are the:
   a. Oculomotor nucleus of CN III with a GSE component and a GVE component (Edinger-Westphal nucleus)
   b. Trochlear nucleus of CN IV

2. **Two supplementary motor nuclei**
   a. The **red nucleus** receives the cerebellorubrothalamic tract after it decussates (see Figures 7-20 and 7-21).
   b. **Substantia nigra** projects to the forebrain (see Figures 7-19 through 7-21).

3. **RF,** including accessory optomotor nuclei around CM III.

C. **The quadrigeminal plate of the midbrain**

1. The midbrain **tectum**, or the **quadrigeminal plate,** consists of paired colliculi, two superior and two inferior, and closely related brachia (see Figures 7-5 and 7-9A).
   a. The **superior** colliculus consists of layers of fibers and neurons connected to the RF, and adjacent accessory nuclei of the optic system. It receives axons from the retina via the **superior** brachium and from the cerebral cortex and multiple sites in the brain stem.
   b. The **inferior** colliculus receives connections from the lateral lemniscus and relays to the medial geniculate body by the **inferior** brachium (see Figure 7-9A).
   c. Both the superior and inferior colliculi send a number of decussating and nondecussating pathways to RF, adjacent midbrain nuclei, and spinal cord (tectospinal tracts).

2. While the colliculi act as **integrating centers** for optic and auditory reflexes, we know of no specific syndromes of quadrigeminal plate lesions in humans.

D. **Composition of the midbrain basis.** The midbrain basis contains the corticopontine tracts and the pyramidal tract, which are shown topographically in Figure 7-21.

1. The two components of the **corticopontine tracts** are the:
   a. Frontopontine tracts
   b. Temporopontine tracts

2. The two components of the **pyramidal tract** are the:
   a. Corticobulbar tract
   b. Corticospinal tract

E. **Decussations of the midbrain**

1. The **dentatorubral** and **dentatothalamic tracts** of the rostral cerebellar peduncle (brachium conjunctivum) decussate in the caudal part of the pontine tegmentum (see Figures 7-19 and 10-12).

2. The corticobulbar pathway for volitional horizontal eye movements decussates caudally in the midbrain tegmentum and rostral pons (see Figure 9-20).

3. Other decussations include efferent pathways between the colliculi of the tectum, their tectospinal tracts, and the rubrospinal tract. Their functional roles in humans are unknown.

VIII. **THE NOMENCLATURE AND FUNCTIONAL CLASSIFICATION OF THE CRANIAL NERVES** (based on ontogeny-phylogeny and the theory of nerve components)

A. **Definition.** A cranial nerve is any one of the twelve paired nerves that pass through a major foramen in the base of the skull (Figure 7-23).

B. **The cranial nerves receive a number and a name.**

1. The **number** reflects:
   a. The rostrocaudal order in which the nerves exit from the foramina in the base of the skull (see Figure 7-23)
   b. The rostrocaudal order in which the nerves attach to the neuraxis, except for CN XI, which attaches to the rostral end of the spinal cord (see Figure 7-1)

2. The **name** reflects something about the course or function of the nerve, but derives from no specific rules (Table 7-2).

3. These nerves differ in embryologic origin, phylogeny, and functional type of axon.

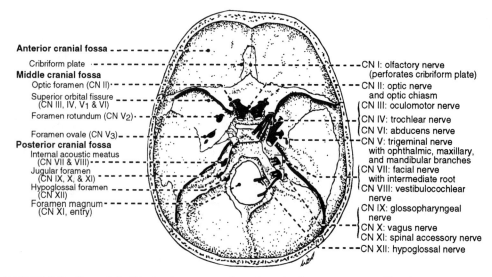

Anterior cranial fossa

Cribriform plate

Middle cranial fossa

Optic foramen (CN II)

Superior orbital fissure (CN III, IV, V₁ & VI)

Foramen rotundum (CN V₂)

Foramen ovale (CN V₃)

Posterior cranial fossa

Internal acoustic meatus (CN VII & VIII)

Jugular foramen (CN IX, X, & XI)

Hypoglossal foramen (CN XII)

Foramen magnum (CN XI, entry)

CN I: olfactory nerve (perforates cribriform plate)

CN II: optic nerve and optic chiasm

CN III: oculomotor nerve

CN IV: trochlear nerve

CN VI: abducens nerve

CN V: trigeminal nerve with ophthalmic, maxillary, and mandibular branches

CN VII: facial nerve with intermediate root

CN VIII: vestibulocochlear nerve

CN IX: glossopharyngeal nerve

CN X: vagus nerve

CN XI: spinal accessory nerve

CN XII: hypoglossal nerve

FIGURE 7-23. Base of skull (calvarium removed) to show the foramina traversed by the cranial nerves.

TABLE 7-2. The Twelve Cranial Nerves

Number/Name/Derivation of Name	Brief Summary of Function
I Olfactory	Smells
II Optic	Sees
III Oculomotor	Moves eyeball and constricts pupil
IV Trochlear [tendon runs through trochlea (pulley)]	Moves eyeball
V Trigeminal (three large sensory branches)	Feels front half of head and chews
VI Abducens (leads eyeball away from sagittal plane)	Moves eyeball
VII Facial	Moves face; tears, tastes, and salivates
VIII Vestibulocochlear (to vestibule and cochlea)	Equilibrates and hears
IX Glossopharyngeal (runs to tongue and pharynx)	Tastes, salivates, and swallows and monitors carotid body and sinus
X Vagus (vagrant, wandering from pharynx to splenic flexure of colon)	Tastes, swallows, lifts palate, and phonates; sensorimotor to thoracicoabdominal viscera
XI Spinal accessory (arises in spinal cord to convey asccessory fibers from medulla to CN X)	Turns head and shrugs shoulders
XII Hypoglossal (runs under tongue)	Moves tongue

C. **Brain stem somites and their cranial nerves: CN III, CN IV, CN VI, and CN XII.**

1. Somite plan and somite neuronal columns

a. The somite plan of the spinal cord continues to the rostral end of the midbrain, where the rostral-most motor cranial nerve, CN III, exits (see Figure 7-1).

b. Corresponding to the spinal cord, the brain stem develops **motor** nuclei in its basal plates and **sensory** nuclei in its alar plates, separated by a sulcus limitans (see Figures 7-4 and 7-25).

2. **Fate of the rostral, intermediate, and caudal groups of cranial somites**
   a. The **rostral** group of the cranial somites, opposite the midbrain, produces the **extraocular** muscles that rotate the eyeballs. CN III and CN IV innervate these muscles.
   b. The **caudal** group of cranial somites, opposite the medulla, produces the **tongue** muscles. The ventral roots of several adjacent caudal somites unite to form CN XII, which innervates the tongue muscles.
   c. The **intermediate** group of cranial somites, opposite the pons, mostly disappears, as do the tegmental nuclei, which would have formed their cranial nerves. Only the nucleus of CN VI, which innervates one extraocular muscle, the lateral rectus, remains in the GSE column in the pons. The GSE column, which is continuous through the entire spinal cord and caudal medulla, thus becomes discontinuous through the pontine tegmentum and midbrain. See the motor nuclei of CN III, CN IV, CN VI, and CN XII in Figure 7-22.

3. The dorsal roots of many of the somites remain and adapt to serve the general and special sensory functions of the brain stem.

D. **Branchial arches and their cranial nerves**

1. **Plan of the branchial arches**
   a. The branchial or gill arches of water-dwelling vertebrates are incorporated in land-dwellers into the:
      (1) Cheeks, jaws, and ears
      (2) Pharynx, larynx, and upper esophagus
   b. Branchial arches parallel somites in:
      (1) Having a serial order (Figure 7-24)
      (2) Receiving a single nerve
      (3) Receiving a single artery
      (4) Differentiating into skin, muscle, and bone
      (5) Retaining their original innervation as they undergo phylogenetic adaption

2. **Innervation of branchial arches**
   a. The five rostral-most branchial arches each receive and retain one nerve: CN V, CN VII, CN IX, CN X, or CN XI (see Figure 7-24).
   b. The five branchiomotor nuclei for these nerves arise from neuroblasts that migrate from the periventricular matrix zone of the basal plate to a ventrolateral site in the tegmentum (see Figure 7-8).

E. **Theory of nerve components as applied to the cranial nerves**

1. Because CN III, CN IV, CN VI, and CN XII are somite nerves, they contain one or more of the four types of axons found in the spinal nerves: GSE, GVA, GVE, and GSA axons (see Figure 4-7).

2. The remaining cranial nerves contain components that serve special functions.
   a. **SVA** axons serve the special senses of taste and smell.
   b. **SSA** axons serve the senses of hearing and equilibrium.
   c. **SVE** [branchial efferent (BE)] axons serve the striated muscles of the branchial arches. The motor nuclei of CN V, CN VII, CN IX, CN X, and CN XI, which innervate these muscles, consist of alpha motoneurons similar to GSE neurons (Figure 7-25). Nevertheless, the theory of nerve components designates them as SVE

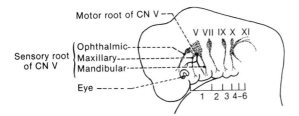

Motor root of CN V

Sensory root of CN V { Ophthalmic / Maxillary / Mandibular

Eye

V VII IX X XI

1 2 3 4-6

FIGURE 7-24. Lateral view of the head of an embryo showing the innervation of branchial arches (*Arabic numerals*) by branchial cranial nerves (*Roman numerals*).

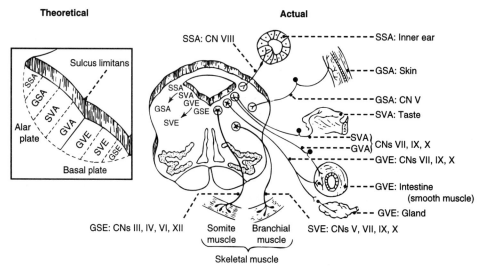

Theoretical

Sulcus limitans

Alar plate

Basal plate

SSA
GSA
SVA
GVA
GVE
SVE
GSE

Actual

SSA: CN VIII

SSA
SVA
GVE
GSA
GSE
SVE

GSE: CNs III, IV, VI, XII

Somite muscle

Branchial muscle

Skeletal muscle

SSA: Inner ear

GSA: Skin

GSA: CN V

SVA: Taste

SVA
GVA } CNs VII, IX, X

GVE: CNs VII, IX, X

GVE: Intestine (smooth muscle)

GVE: Gland

SVE: CNs V, VII, IX, X

FIGURE 7-25. Theory of nerve components as applied to the medulla. *GSA* = general somatic afferent; *GSE* = general somatic efferent; *GVA* = general visceral afferent; *GVE* = general visceral efferent; *SSA* = special somatic afferent; *SVA* = special visceral afferent; *SVE* = special visceral (branchial) efferent.

because the branchial arches or gills originally served a special visceral function, which was oxygenation of the blood.

3. These special motor and sensory functions require additional brain stem nuclei and pathways. Compare Figure 4-7 to Figure 7-25.

F. **A three-set classification of the cranial nerves.** Grouping the 12 pairs of cranial nerves into three sets, **special sensory, somatomotor** or **somitomotor**, and **branchial** (Table 7-3), based on the theory of nerve components, makes them much easier to learn.

1. **Solely special sensory set (SSSS): CN I, CN II, and CN VIII.** These three nerves contain no motor axons (see Table 7-3).
   a. **CN I**, the **olfactory nerve**, is not quite a nerve. It consists of axonal filaments, which perforate the cribriform plate to synapse on the olfactory bulb (Figure 7-26).
   b. **CN II**, the **optic nerve**, conveys axons from the retina, but it develops as an evagination from the diencephalon, not as an actual peripheral nerve (see Figure 3-5). All cranial nerves after CN I and CN II are true peripheral nerves ontogenetically and histologically.
   c. **CN VIII**, the **vestibulocochlear nerve**, consists of vestibular and cochlear (auditory) divisions. CN VIII develops as a homolog of dorsal root ganglia and has no ventral root.

2. **The somitic or somatomotor (GSE) set: CN III, CN IV, CN VI, and CN XII.**
   a. Setting aside CN I, CN II, and CN VIII leaves only nine cranial nerves to consider, four in the somatomotor (GSE) set and five in the SVE set. The somatomotor set contrasts directly with the SSSS because of the following.
      (1) The nerves are all somite nerves directly homologous with spinal nerves.
      (2) The nerves are essentially motor (GSE) in function.
      (3) The nerves convey only a small GSA sensory component, serving proprioception and no other special or general sensation. Although the nerves convey some proprioceptive afferents from the muscles, they lack individual dorsal root ganglia. The perikarya for their proprioceptive afferent axons may be:
         (a) Scattered along the course of the nerves
         (b) Derived from CN V, with the proprioceptive fibers entering the somite cranial nerves by peripheral anastomoses with the branches of CN V
   b. **Peripheral distributions of CN III, CN IV, and CN VI**
      (1) CN III, CN IV, and CN VI innervate only muscles of the eyes, thus forming an **optomotor** group (Figure 7-27).

TABLE 7-3. Functional Components of the Three Sets of Cranial Nerves

		GSE	SVE	GVE	GVA	SVA	GSA	SSA
Solely special sensory set	I					+		
	II							+
	VIII							+
Somatomotor set	III	+		+			+*	
	IV	+					+*	
	VI	+					+*	
	XII	+					+*	
Branchial set	V		+				+	
	VII		+	+	+	+	+	
	IX		+	+	+	+	+	
	X		+	+	+	+	+	
	XI		+				+*	

GSA = general somatic afferent; GSE = general somatic efferent; GVA = general visceral afferent; GVE = general visceral efferent; SSA = special somatic afferent; SVA = special visceral afferent; SVE = special visceral efferent.
*Proprioceptive GSA components only; no cutaneous or special senses.

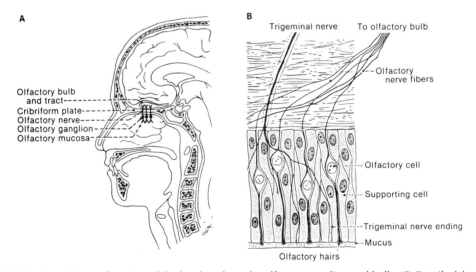

FIGURE 7-26. (*A*) Sagittal section of the head to show the olfactory ganglion and bulb. (*B*) Detail of the olfactory mucosa to show its dual innervation, the olfactory nerve for smell, and CN V for other sensations (Adapted with permission from Amoore JE, Johnston JW Jr, Rubin M: The stereochemical theory of odor. *Sci Am* 210:42, 1964).

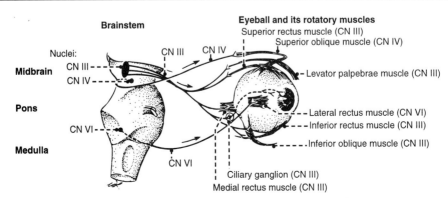

FIGURE 7-27. Peripheral distribution of CN III, CN IV, and CN VI.

(2) Only CN III of the somatomotor group conveys autonomic axons, consisting of parasympathetic axons to the ciliary and pupilloconstrictor muscles.

(3) CN XII innervates the tongue muscles. It conveys proprioceptive sensation but no taste, touch, or other sensations.

c. Setting aside the **three solely sensory** cranial nerves and the **four somite nerves** reduces the problem to the **five** cranial nerves of the branchial arch set.

3. **The branchial arch (SVE) set: CN V, CN VII, CN IX, CN X, and CN XI** (see Figure 7-24).

a. Each SVE nerve innervates striated muscles of branchial arch origin. Two of the nerves, CN V and CN XI, convey no other motor components, and neither convey special senses.

b. **First, set aside CN XI.**

(1) The simplest of the branchial set, CN XI is essentially a motor nerve innervating only striated muscles (mainly the trapezius and sternocleidomastoid muscles). It closely resembles the somatomotor set because it has only a proprioceptive sensory component.

(2) CN XI differs from all other cranial nerves because it arises in the gray matter of the cervical spinal cord and enters the skull through the foramen magnum (see Figure 7-23) before exiting through the jugular foramen.

(3) Now only four branchial cranial nerves remain, all sensorimotor.

c. **Next, set aside CN V.**

(1) The striated muscles innervated by the SVE motor root of CN V are the chewing muscles.

(2) CN V differs from CN XI and the remaining branchial nerves, CN VII, CN IX, and CN X, because it has a huge dorsal root ganglion and three huge (GSA) sensory divisions (see Figure 7-30).

(3) CN V does not convey any special sensory fibers or motor fibers to glands or smooth muscle.

d. Setting aside CN V and CN XI, the first and last of the branchial group, leaves only CN VII, CN IX, and CN X, which, while complex, share a common plan. They all contain axons of five functional types: SVE, GVE, GVA, SVA, and GSA (Table 7-4).

IX. ANATOMIC RELATIONSHIPS OF THE CRANIAL NERVES TO THE BRAIN STEM AND FORAMINA OF THE SKULL BASE

A. Location of the cranial nerve nuclei within the brain stem

1. The cranial nerve nuclei of the brain stem occupy distinct **motor** and **sensory** columns, which the theory of nerve components predicts (see Figures 7-8 and 7-22).

2. **Sensory nuclei are located dorsolaterally in the brain stem tegmentum,** in the part derived from the alar plate (see Figure 7-25).

a. The **trigeminal sensory nucleus of CN V** extends from the midbrain into the rostral end of the spinal cord (see Figure 7-22). It is the only sensory or motor nuclear column that extends throughout the entire length of the brain stem.

b. The **nucleus solitarius** is confined to the medulla. It mediates SVA (taste) and GVA sensation from CN VII, CN IX, and CN X.

c. The **cochlear** and **vestibular** nuclei of CN VIII start in the medulla and straddle the pontomedullary junction (see Figure 7-22).

3. **Motor nuclei.** Gaps exist in the columns of the various somatomotor and visceromotor nuclei of the brain stem. The gaps appear because various nuclei have disappeared during phylogenetic retrogression of their peripheral somite or branchial arch tissues.

a. The **somatomotor (GSE) nuclei,** CN III, CN IV, CN VI, and CN XII, all occupy the paramedian plane, just ventral to the floor of the fourth ventricle or aqueduct. To remember their paramedian location, draw a colored line through these nuclei in Figure 7-22.

TABLE 7-4. Nerve Components of CN VII, CN IX, and CN X and Their Peripheral Distribution

	Branchiomotor (SVE)	Visceromotor (GVE) (All Parasympathetic Nerves)	GVA	Taste (SVA)	GSA
CN VII	To all muscles of the face and facial orifices and to the stapedius muscles	To lacrimal, submandibular, and sublingual glands of the head, except the parotid gland; to the nasal mucosa	From the posterior nasopharynx and soft palate; from the salivary glands	From the anterior two thirds of the tongue (clinically significant)	Twig from the skin of the ear.
CN IX	To the pharyngeal muscles for swallowing	To the parotid gland and the pharyngeal mucosa	From the soft palate and upper pharynx; from the carotid body and sinus	From the posterior one third of the tongue (clinically insignificant)	Twig from the skin of the ear.
CN X	To the pharyngeal plexus and laryngeal muscles (via the accessory branch of CN XI)	To the glands of the pharyngeal and laryngeal mucosa and to the glands and smooth muscle of the thoracicoabdominal viscera; sends inhibitory axons to the heart	From the pharynx and larynx and the thoracicoabdominal viscera; from the aortic bodies	From the region of the epiglottis (clinically insignificant)	Twig from the skin of the ear.

GSA = general somatic afferent; GVA = general visceral afferent; GVE = general visceral efferent; SVA = special visceral afferent; SVE = special visceral efferent.

167

FIGURE 7-28. Segments of cranial nerves for "thinking through" the course of nerve impulses.

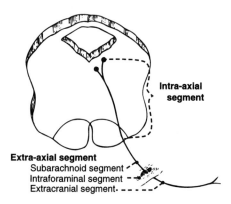

Intra-axial segment

Extra-axial segment
Subarachnoid segment
Intraforaminal segment
Extracranial segment

      b. The **branchiomotor (BE or SVE) nuclei,** CN V, CN VII, CN IX, and CN X, all migrate into the ventrolateral part of the brain stem tegmentum (see Figure 7-22).
          (1) One continuous branchiomotor or SVE nucleus in the medulla, the **nucleus ambiguus,** serves CN IX and CN X.
          (2) Draw a line of another color through the branchiomotor nuclei in Figure 7-22 to remember their location.
      c. The **visceromotor nuclei (GVE),** the preganglionic parasympathetic nuclei, occupy in general the location predicted from their site in the spinal gray matter (see Figures 7-22 and 7-25; see Table 4-1). Because of the scale, Figure 7-22 shows only the dorsal motor nucleus of CN X, the vagus nerve, not the more rostral GVE nuclei.

B. **Anatomic segments of the cranial nerves.** Clinicians divide the cranial nerves into segments to think through their course to localize lesions (Figure 7-28).

C. **Intra-axial segments of the motor divisions of the cranial nerves.** The intra-axial course and sites of exit of the motor cranial nerves are predictable.

  1. Somatomotor (GSE) group
      a. Somatomotor nerves III, VI, and XII drop fairly straight down (ventrally) in the paramedian plane (see CN XII in Figure 7-13) to exit in the paramedian plane on the ventral surface of the brain stem (see Figure 7-1).
      b. CN IV is an exception.
          (1) Its axons undergo a complete internal decussation before exiting (see Figure 7-18).
          (2) It **exits dorsally** through the tectum at the junction of the quadrigeminal plate with the anterior medullary velum. Again, however, being a somite nerve, it exits in the paramedian plane.

  2. Branchial arch (SVE) group. The branchial arch nerves tend to undergo an internal loop before exiting.
      a. CN VII makes the most distinctive loop, forming an actual **genu** around the nucleus of CN VI (see Figure 7-16).
      b. CN V of this group does not make such a distinct internal loop.

D. **Sites of attachment of the cranial nerves to the neuraxis**

  1. Three of the twelve cranial nerves do not attach to the brain stem.
      a. CN I, the **olfactory nerve,** attaches to the olfactory bulb, which develops as an evagination from the cerebrum (see Figure 3-5). No other nerve attaches directly to the cerebrum itself (see Figure 7-26A).
      b. CN II, the **optic nerve,** is the only cranial nerve to develop as an evagination from the diencephalon (see Figure 3-5). It is not a true peripheral nerve.
      c. CN XI attaches to the spinal cord, the only cranial nerve to do so.

  2. The remaining cranial nerves all attach to the brain stem proper.
      a. The **somatomotor (GSE) nerves** all attach in a line along the paramedian plane. CN III, CN VI, and CN XII attach ventrally, and CN IV attaches dorsally. Draw a colored line through them on Figure 7-1.

   b. The **branchial arch (SVE) nerves** all attach to the brain stem in a line **dorsolateral to the somatomotor nerves.** Identify these attachment sites in Figures 7-1 and 7-2.

   3. CN VI, CN VII, and CN VIII attach in numerical, **ventrodorsal order** at the pontomedullary sulcus (see Figures 7-1 and 7-2).

E. **Sites of exit of the cranial nerves from the skull.** The cranial nerves all cross the subarachnoid space to exit through foramina in the base of the skull (see Figure 7-23).

   1. CN III, CN IV, CN VI, and V1 (ophthalmic division) of CN V traverse the **superior orbital fissure**.

   2. V2 (maxillary division) of CN V traverses the **foramen rotundum**, and V3 (mandibular division) traverses the **foramen ovale.** The motor root exits through the foramen ovale.

   3. CN VII and CN VIII traverse the **internal auditory foramen**.

   4. CN IX, CN X, and CN XI traverse the **jugular foramen** (see Figure 7-35).

X. PERIPHERAL DISTRIBUTION OF THE BRANCHIAL CRANIAL NERVES (V, VII, IX, AND XI) AND CN XII

A. **Explanatory note.** This section groups these nerves because the features they share, when contrasted with their differences, makes them easier to remember. See Chapter 9 for descriptions of CN II, CN III, CN IV, and CN VI.

B. **CN V (trigeminal nerve)** [Figures 7-29 and 7-30]

   1. Functional components. CN V has an **SVE motor root** and a **GSA sensory root.**
     a. SVE axons innervate the chewing muscles, the temporalis, and the pterygoids, as well as the tensor tympani and tensor palatini.
     b. GSA axons
       (1) These axons mediate touch and pain sensation from the face; mucous membranes of the nose, sinuses, and tongue; and the dura mater. Notice in Figures 4-12 and 7-30 that the sensory territory of CN V abuts on C2 at about the interaural line. C1 usually lacks a sensory root.
       (2) The GSA axons also mediate proprioception from most of the head muscles, directly or by anastomosis with other cranial nerves.

   2. The motor nucleus (SVE) of CN V is in the rostral pontine tegmentum (see Figure 7-22). The motor axons exit laterally under the cover of the sensory root (see Figure 7-1).
     a. The motor root crosses the subarachnoid space to exit from the skull through the foramen ovale with V3 (see Figure 7-23).
     b. It innervates the chewing muscles, the temporalis, pterygoids, and masseters (see Figure 7-29), as well as the tensor tympani and tensor veli palatini.

   3. The peripheral ganglion of CN V is the trigeminal (semilunar, gasserian) ganglion (GSA).
     a. The trigeminal ganglion contains the primary unipolar neurons for CN V (see Figure 7-30). It is the largest sensory ganglion of the peripheral nervous system (PNS).
     b. Peripheral divisions of the trigeminal ganglion consist of:
       (1) V1: ophthalmic division
       (2) V2: maxillary division
       (3) V3: mandibular division
     c. The three divisions gather into one huge sensory root proximal to the ganglion to attach to the dorsolateral aspect of the basis pontis (see Figures 7-1 and 7-2). It is from these three huge sensory branches that the name **trigeminal** arises.

   4. The three trigeminal brain stem sensory nuclei: mesencephalic, main sensory, and spinal (see Figures 7-22 and 7-30)

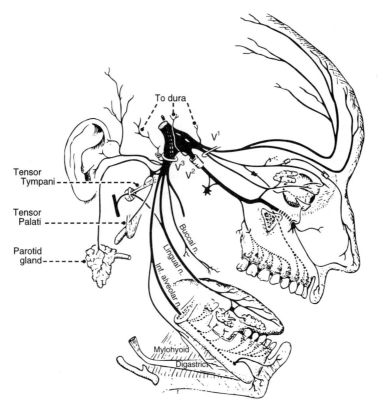

FIGURE 7-29. Peripheral distribution of CN V, the trigeminal nerve. V^1 = ophthalmic branch; V^2 = maxillary branch; V^3 = mandibular branch. (Adapted with permission from Grant JCB: *An Atlas of Anatomy,* 2nd ed. Baltimore, Williams and Wilkins, 1947, p 468.)

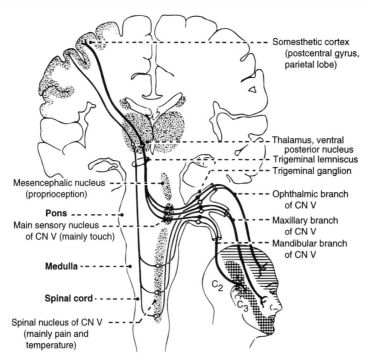

FIGURE 7-30. Sensory pathways of the trigeminal nerve (CN V). (Reprinted with permission from DeMyer W: *Technique of the Neurologic Examination: A Programmed Text,* 4th ed. New York, McGraw-Hill, 1994.)

a. The mesencephalic nucleus of CN V
(1) This unique nucleus is the only example of dorsal, root-type (unipolar) neurons located in the CNS.
(2) Peripheral axons of the mesencephalic nucleus follow the sensory root into the three major peripheral sensory divisions, and also enter the motor root.
(3) The axons are thought to serve as proprioceptive afferents from the ocular, facial, and bulbar muscles.
b. The principal sensory nucleus receives afferents from the trigeminal ganglion and subserves touch from the face, eyeball, and mucous membranes of the head.
c. The spinal nucleus subserves pain and temperature sensation for the facial skin; eyeball; mucous membranes of the sinuses, nose, and mouth; teeth; and meninges. As such, it mediates some of the most common and severe pain that we experience; for example, the pain of toothaches, earache, sinusitis, meningitis, photophobia, iritis, trigeminal neuralgia, temporal arteritis, and other forms of headache.

5. **Intra-axial course of primary trigeminal afferent axons**
   a. Upon entering the pons, the afferent trigeminal axons, like the spinal afferents, typically branch to end at various levels of the trigeminal nuclei and RF.
   b. The descending or spinal root of CN V conveys C fibers for pain and temperature sensation. It corresponds to and is continuous with the dorsolateral fasciculus of Lissauer.
   c. The spinal nucleus of CN V consists of substantia gelatinosa. It extends from the medulla into the spinal cord, where it is continuous with the substantia gelatinosa of the cervical level of the cord. Thus, the substantia gelatinosa is one continuous, topographic nuclear column, mediating pain and temperature for the entire body, from the face to the coccyx.

6. **Efferent pathways from the trigeminal sensory nuclei**
   a. The **trigeminal lemniscus** has two components.
   (1) The first component, from the spinal nucleus of CN V, decussates at the medullary level and joins the medial lemniscus at pontine levels to ascend to the thalamus (see Figure 7-30).
   (2) The second, uncrossed component arises from more rostral portions of CN V, and ascends as the ipsilateral trigeminal lemniscus.
   b. Other connections of the trigeminal sensory nuclei mediate clinically important reflexes by running directly to cranial nerve nuclei or indirectly through the RF. These reflexes include:
   (1) Jaw jerk, which is a muscle stretch reflex (MSR) [V–V reflex]
   (2) Corneal reflex (V–VII reflex)
   (3) Tearing (V–VII reflex)
   (4) Sneezing (V–RF reflex via respiratory center)
   (5) Many developmental reflexes (e.g., rooting, sucking, and chewing)

7. **Major clinical findings of CN V lesions**
   a. Pain or loss of sensation occurs in one or more of the three peripheral sensory divisions: V1, V2, and V3. In trigeminal neuralgia, the patient suffers unbearable lightening-like flashes of pain in one or more of the three sensory branches.
   b. Loss of the corneal reflex if V1 is affected.
   c. Ipsilateral chewing muscles and tensor tympani and tensor palatini are paralyzed.

C. **CN VII (facial nerve)** [Figure 7-31]

1. **CN VII as a prototype branchial nerve for CN IX and CN X.** CN VII serves as the prototype of the three complicated branchial nerves, CN VII, CN IX, and CN X, illustrating their common components and features.

2. **Functional components of CN VII**
   a. CN VII has five components: SVE, GVE, GVA, SVA, and GSA (see Table 7-3). By setting aside the relatively insignificant GSA twig to the ear and the minor GVA component to the palate and posterior nasal cavity (see Table 7-4), we can focus on the highly important **SVE, GVE,** and **SVA** components.
   b. The **SVE** axons innervate the facial muscles and stapedius.

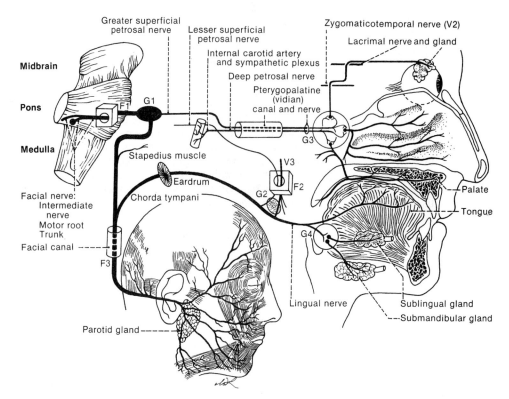

FIGURE 7-31. Peripheral distribution of CN VII, the facial nerve. *F1* = internal acoustic foramen (meatus); *F2* = foramen ovale; *F3* = stylomastoid foramen; *G1* = geniculate ganglion; *G2* = otic ganglion; *G3* = pterygopalatine (sphenopalatine) ganglion; *G4* = submandibular ganglion; *V2 and V3* = CN V branches.

    c. The **GVE** axons innervate the lacrimal and sublingual and submaxillary salivary glands.

    d. The **SVA** axons innervate taste.

3. Peripheral ganglia of CN VII

    a. The **sensory perikarya** are located in the geniculate ganglion (see Figures 7-31 and 7-32), where CN VII forms a **knee** or **genu** at the distal end of the internal auditory canal to enter the middle ear.

    b. The **parasympathetic ganglia** include sphenopalatine (pterygopalatine) and submandibular ganglia (see Figure 7-31; see Table 5-1).

4. The tegmental sensory nucleus of CN VII. The nucleus solitarius, which is located in the medulla, mediates the GSA and SVA (taste) functions of CN VII, CN IX, and CN X.

5. Motor nuclei of CN VII

    a. The **SVE** nucleus is the facial nucleus in the caudal pontine tegmentum (see Figures 7-16, 7-22, and 7-32).

    b. The **GVE** nuclei are the salivatory nuclei in the caudal pontine tegmentum.

6. Peripheral distribution of CN VII. To simplify the distribution of CN VII, consider first that two nerves combine to form its trunk. The two nerves are:

    a. The **facial nerve proper**, that is, the **SVE** motor root to the facial muscles, stapedius, and platysma

    b. The **intermediate nerve of Wrisburg** (glossopalatine nerve) [see Figure 7-31]

7. Course of the facial nerve proper (SVE motor root)

    a. After crossing the subarachnoid space and entering the internal acoustic meatus, CN VII runs through the **middle ear**, where it supplies the **stapedius muscle** and separates from the **chorda tympani**.

    b. It drops through the **facial canal** to emerge through the **stylomastoid foramen**.

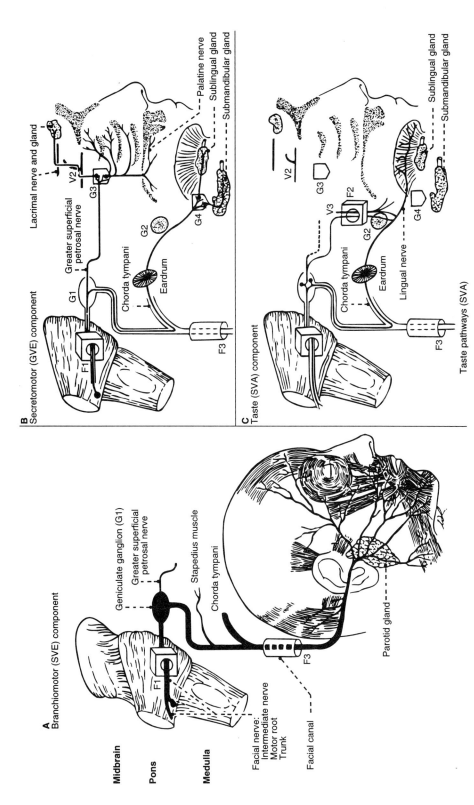

FIGURE 7-32. Peripheral distribution of CN VII, the facial nerve, considered as three different components. (A) Special visceral efferent (SVE) component to facial muscles. (B) General visceral efferent (GVE) secretomotor component of intermediate nerve to glands. (C) Special visceral afferent (SVA) component of intermediate nerve for taste on the anterior two thirds of the tongue. *F1* = internal acoustic foramen (meatus); *F2* = foramen ovale; *F3* = stylomastoid foramen; *G1* = geniculate ganglion; *G2* = otic ganglion; *G3* = pterygopalatine (sphenopalatine) ganglion; *G4* = submandibular ganglion; *V2 and V3* = CN V branches.

   c. It runs through, but not to, the **parotid gland** to disperse to the **facial muscles.** The SVE component of CN VII innervates all of the muscles of facial expression, including the sphincters of the eye and mouth, the orbicularis oculi and oris, the frontalis and buccinator, and the platysma. It also innervates the stapedius, the posterior belly of the digastric, and the stylohyoid.

   d. As a further aid to learning the course of CN VII, Figure 7-32 subdivides it into its three main functional components. Thus, CN VII consists of three nerves: SVE, GVE, and SVA.

8. The intermediate nerve of Wrisberg

   a. It is called **intermediate** because it attaches to the brain stem at the pontomedullary sulcus, between CN VII proper and CN VIII.

   b. As a sensorimotor nerve, it conveys **preganglionic parasympathetic (GVE)** axons for secretions and **taste (SVA)** axons for the tongue (see Figure 7-32).

   c. Notice that axons of the facial nerve proper and its intermediate root:

     (1) Separate where they attach to the pontomedullary sulcus (see Figure 7-2)

     (2) Unite to cross the subarachnoid space and run through the internal auditory meatus (see Figure 7-32)

     (3) Separate again at the geniculate ganglion and chorda tympani nerve to reach their terminations via the greater superficial petrosal nerve and chorda tympani (see Figure 7-32).

   d. The preganglionic parasympathetic axons of the intermediate nerve divide into two streams as they pass through, but do not synapse in, the geniculate ganglion (see Figure 7-32).

     (1) One stream, via the **greater superficial petrosal nerve,** synapses in the **sphenopalatine ganglion.** The axons from perikarya in the sphenopalatine ganglion then innervate the **lacrimal gland** and **glands of the nasal mucosa.**

     (2) The other stream, via the **chorda tympani,** synapses in the **submandibular ganglion.** Its axons innervate the **submandibular** and **sublingual salivary glands** and **glands of the oral mucosa.**

9. The pathway for taste

   a. Peripheral pathway. The SVA axons for taste traverse four named peripheral nerve segments. In distal proximal order, starting with the taste buds on the tongue, they are the (see Figures 7-31 and 7-32):

     (1) Lingual branch of the trigeminal nerve

     (2) Chorda tympani

     (3) Trunk of CN VII

     (4) Intermediate nerve of Wrisburg

   b. Central pathway for taste

     (1) The primary afferents for taste from CN VII, CN IX, and CN X (SVA) synapse in the nucleus solitarius, where a group of neurons form a "gustatory center."

     (2) The nucleus solitarius connects with the adjacent RF and dorsal motor nucleus (GVE) of CN X to mediate salivatory and lingual reflexes.

     (3) Neurons of the nucleus solitarius also form part of the medullary respiratory center and project to the phrenic nucleus and thoracic segments of the cord involved in reflexes such as coughing and vomiting.

     (4) The nucleus solitarius sends two pathways rostrally.

       (a) One taste pathway ascends through the central tegmental tract to nucleus ventralis posteromedialis of the thalamus (see Chapter 12 II F 1 b). This is a nonlemniscal pathway to the thalamus.

       (b) A second taste pathway relays to the **parabrachial nuclei** of the RF. The parabrachial nuclei are so called because they surround the medial and lateral part of the brachium conjunctivum of the superior cerebellar peduncle. The parabrachial nuclei then relay to the thalamus and hypothalamus of the diencephalon, and to the amygdala of the telencephalon.

     (5) Nucleus ventralis posteromedialis of the thalamus relays taste impulses to the cerebral cortex, in the caudal orbitofrontal region, and to the rostral insular and opercular cortices.

    c. The SVA axons from the taste buds and the GVE axons to the salivary glands may meander from nerve to nerve at the base of the skull, resulting in the following consequences.

      (1) The petrosal nerves and the otic and submandibular ganglia do not divide the innervation of the parotid and the submandibular and sublingual glands as neatly as Figures 7-31 and 7-32 suggest.

      (2) Some afferent axons for taste may detour through the greater superficial petrosal nerve rather than remaining in the chorda tympani. Nevertheless, the simplified diagrams given here suffice for clinical purposes.

10. The clinical signs of CN VII lesions. The signs depend on the site of the lesion along the course of the nerve and the fiber components affected. A proximal lesion affecting the main trunk of the nerve causes:

    a. Paralysis of all the ipsilateral facial muscles

    b. Hyperacusis due to stapedius muscle paralysis (the stapedius muscle dampens loud sounds)

    c. Dry eye (xerophthalmia) from absence of lacrimation

    d. Dry mouth (xerostomia) from absence of salivary secretion

    e. Ipsilateral loss of taste on the anterior two thirds of the tongue, but not loss of touch, which is a CN V function. If the lesion is **distal** to the chorda tympani, such as in the facial canal (see Figure 7-31), taste is preserved.

    f. In **Bell's palsy,** a common, presumably viral mononeuritis, the patient displays most or all of the deficits listed in a–e above.

D. **CN IX (glossopharyngeal nerve)** [Figure 7-33]

1. Functional components. CN IX contains the same five axonal components as CN VII and CN X (see Table 7-4).

    a. The **SVE** axons innervate the palate and pharyngeal constrictors.

    b. The **GVE** axons innervate the parotid gland.

    c. The **SVA** axons innervate taste on the posterior third of the tongue.

2. Peripheral ganglia of CN IX

    a. Sensory components of CN IX

      (1) GSA. The superior (jugular) ganglion provides afferents from the twig to the skin of the ear (see Table 7-4).

      (2) GVA and SVA. The inferior (petrosal) ganglion provides the visceral afferents from the carotid sinus, palate, and taste from the posterior third of the tongue (see Figure 7-33).

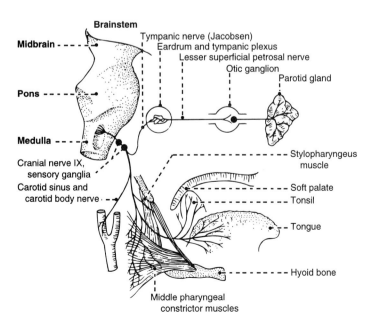

FIGURE 7-33. Peripheral distribution of CN IX, the glossopharyngeal nerve.

b. Parasympathetic ganglion of CN IX

(1) The otic ganglion provides secretory axons to the parotid gland, and corresponds to the sphenopalatine ganglion of CN VII (see Figure 7-31).

(2) Notice in Figures 7-32 and 7-33 that the **lesser** superficial petrosal nerve of CN IX corresponds to the **greater** superficial petrosal nerve of CN VII.

3. Central sensory nuclei of CN IX

a. GVA: nucleus tractus solitarius (see Figure 7-22)

b. SVA: nucleus tractus solitarius for taste, shared with CN VII and CN X

c. GSA: main trigeminal sensory nucleus for skin of the ear

4. Motor nuclei of CN IX (see Figure 7-22)

a. SVE: nucleus ambiguus in the medullary tegmentum

b. GVE: inferior salivatory nucleus in the rostral part of the medullary tegmentum

5. Proximity of central and peripheral distributions of CN IX and CN X

a. Isolated lesions of CN IX or CN X are rare because:

(1) CN IX and CN X share a common motor nucleus, the nucleus ambiguus, and a common GVA sensory nucleus, the nucleus solitarius.

(2) After exiting from the ventrolateral aspect of the medulla, they cross the subarachnoid space together and both exit through the jugular foramen (see Figure 7-23 and 7-35).

(3) CN IX follows the course of CN X in the neck as far as CN IX goes, and both go similarly to the palate and pharynx.

b. CN IX shares pharyngeal and, in some individuals, palatal muscles with CN X. The one muscle innervated exclusively by CN IX, the stylopharyngeus muscle, cannot be tested clinically.

c. Three cranial nerves innervate the palatal muscles.

(1) CN V innervates the tensor palatini, a clinically unimportant muscle.

(2) CN IX, but mainly CN X, innervates the levator palatini, the clinically most important muscle for palatal elevation. A lesion of CN X or, in some individuals, of CN IX causes paralysis of elevation of the ipsilateral half of the soft palate and eliminates the gag reflex.

d. CN IX innervates the carotid body and carotid sinus.

(1) The carotid and aortic bodies stimulate breathing in response to low oxygen tension in the arterial blood.

(2) The carotid sinus initiates reflexes that slow the heart in response to increased blood pressure.

(3) CN X innervates the aortic bodies and may overlap with CN IX in innervating the carotid body.

6. Clinical effects of CN IX lesions

a. Palatal palsy and loss of gag reflex caused by interruption of afferent or efferent palatal axons

b. Dysphagia caused by paralysis of the pharyngeal constrictor muscles

c. Loss of carotid sinus and carotid body reflexes

d. Loss of taste on the posterior third of the tongue, which the patient may not notice and which is difficult to test clinically (in contrast with the anterior two thirds of the tongue, the territory of CN VII)

E. **CN X (vagus nerve)** [Figure 7-34]

1. Functional components. CN X conveys the same five axonal components as CN VII and CN IX (see Table 7-3).

a. SVE axons innervate striated muscles of the palate, larynx, pharyngeal constrictors, and the upper two thirds of the esophagus (see Figure 7-34). CN X innervates all intrinsic laryngeal muscles through the **recurrent laryngeal nerve** (see Figure 7-34).

b. GVE axons innervate parasympathetic ganglia and plexuses of the thoracicoabdominal viscera.

c. SVA axons innervate epiglottal taste buds, but they are clinically insignificant.

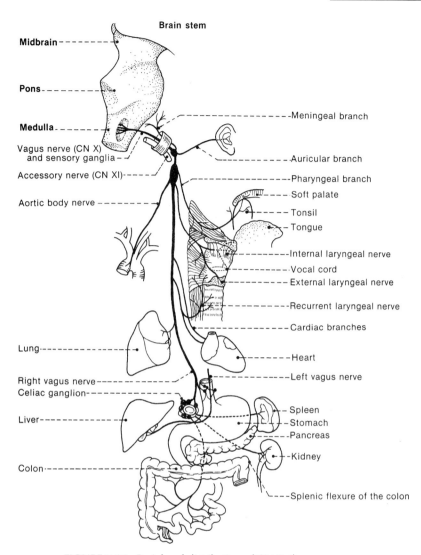

FIGURE 7-34. Peripheral distribution of CN X, the vagus nerve.

2. Peripheral ganglia of CN X
  a. Sensory: superior ganglion for GSA and inferior ganglion for GVA and SVA
  b. Parasympathetic (GVE): all parasympathetic ganglia and plexuses of the thoracicoabdominal viscera
    (1) CN X innervates no parasympathetic ganglia in the head.
    (2) CN X extends to the splenic flexure (see Figure 7-34), where the sacral parasympathetic system takes over. It innervates the **submucosal plexus** of Meissner and the **myenteric plexus** of Auerbach, which are intrinsic plexuses of the intestinal wall. To a large degree, these plexuses function autonomously, controlling peristalsis.

3. Central sensory nuclei of CN X
  a. SVA and GVA: nucleus solitarius
  b. GSA (ear twig): main trigeminal sensory nucleus

4. Motor nuclei of CN X
  a. SVE: nucleus ambiguus in medullary tegmentum (shared with CN IX)
  b. GVE: dorsal motor nucleus of the vagus nerve

5. **Functional effects of vagal stimulation**
   a. Cardiac inhibition with slowing of pulse
   b. Increased peristalsis that moves food through the esophagus, empties the stomach and gallbladder, and promotes passage of food products through the intestine
   c. Increased secretions in the tracheobronchial passages and stomach, and release of insulin and glucagon
   d. Constricted tracheobronchial passages
   e. Uncertain effect on coronary circulation and liver function

6. **Clinical effects of CN X lesions**
   a. Dysphagia caused by paralysis of pharyngeal constrictors and levator palatini
   b. Palatal palsy with nasal speech caused by paralysis of the levator palatini muscle
   c. Hoarseness because of vocal cord paralysis (bilateral paralysis of the vocal cord abductors may lead to death by asphyxia)
   d. Absence of vagus-mediated cardioinhibitory, respiratory, and gastrointestinal reflexes
   e. Loss of cardioinhibitory reflexes from carotid sinus
   f. Anorexia, vomiting, and progressive weight loss follow bilateral interruption of CN X

F. **CN XI (spinal accessory nerve)** [Figure 7-35]

1. **Functional components**
   a. **SVE**: to the sternocleidomastoid muscle and part of the trapezius muscle
   b. **GSA**: proprioception from the muscles innervated

2. **Peripheral ganglion**: presumably, the dorsal root of C2 serves proprioception

3. **Motor nuclei (SVE)** consist of:
   a. Caudal neurons of nucleus ambiguus
   b. Supraspinal nucleus, consisting of ventral horn neurons homologous to the nucleus ambiguus, but located in the rostral limit of the spinal cord

4. **Nomenclature of the spinal accessory nerve**
   a. The **spinal** part of the nerve arises in the spinal cord and innervates the sternocleidomastoid muscle and part of the trapezius muscle.

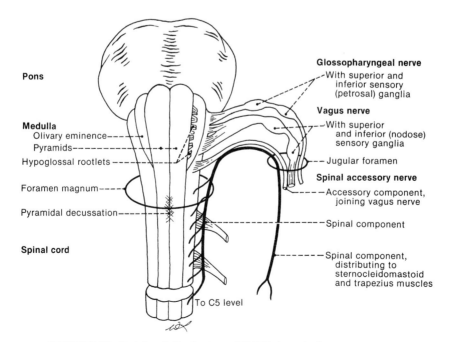

FIGURE 7-35. Peripheral distribution of CN XI, the spinal accessory nerve.

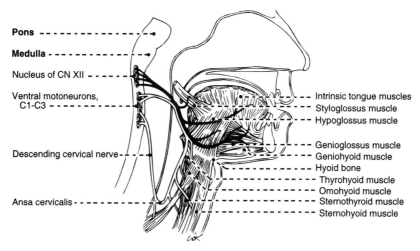

Pons
Medulla
Nucleus of CN XII
Ventral motoneurons, C1-C3
Descending cervical nerve
Ansa cervicalis

Intrinsic tongue muscles
Styloglossus muscle
Hypoglossus muscle
Genioglossus muscle
Geniohyoid muscle
Hyoid bone
Thyrohyoid muscle
Omohyoid muscle
Sternothyroid muscle
Sternohyoid muscle

FIGURE 7-36. Peripheral distribution of CN XII, the hypoglossal nerve. The hypoglossal nerve is in black; the cervical nerves are in white.

    b. The **accessory** part of the nerve merely conveys some vagal fibers, which accompany the spinal part of the nerve after it enters the posterior fossa via the foramen magnum. These accessory fibers to the vagus nerve arise in the nucleus ambiguus and innervate the larynx (vocal cords) through the inferior (recurrent) laryngeal nerve (see Figure 7-35).

5. Clinical signs of nerve interruption
    a. Weakness of head rotation because of sternocleidomastoid muscle paralysis
    b. Weakness of shoulder shrugging from paralysis of the upper part of the trapezius muscle
    c. Vocal cord paralysis and hoarseness if accessory fibers to CN X are involved

CN XII (hypoglossal nerve) [Figure 7-36]

1. Functional components of CN XII
    a. GSE: innervates intrinsic and extrinsic tongue muscles
    b. GSA: presumably comes from peripheral anastomoses with CN V (proprioception only)

2. Motor nucleus: the hypoglossal nucleus is in the caudal medullary tegmentum (see Figures 7-13 and 7-22)

3. Clinical effects of CN XII lesions
    a. Paralysis and atrophy of ipsilateral tongue muscles
    b. Dysarthria because of difficulty making lingual sounds
    c. Dysphagia from difficulty initiating the swallowing reflex because a paralyzed tongue cannot throw the food bolus into the back of the mouth

XI. RETICULAR FORMATION (RF)

Definition

1. RF consists of widely spaced neurons loosely arranged into nuclear groups throughout the entire brain stem tegmentum. Huge dendritic trees and the immense, highly collateralized afferent and efferent network of axons that separate the RF perikarya cause the "reticular" appearance in microscopic sections (see Figure 3-9B). This appearance contrasts with the dense packing of most other CNS nuclei and the lamination of cortex. As a type of neuronal organization, RF is a defining characteristic of the brain stem tegmentum.

2. The RF has the most heterogeneous connections of any other single part of the CNS. Stated epigrammatically, the RF receives impulses from and sends impulses to all of the CNS; thus, it influences all mental, motor, and sensory functions.

B. **Anatomic extent of the RF**

1. RF extends continuously throughout the entire length of the brain stem tegmentum. It fills all of the space not occupied by cranial nerve nuclei, supplementary sensory and motor nuclei, and named long and short tracts.

2. The **caudal** limit is generally regarded as the medullocervical junction, but lamina VII and the reticular nucleus of the spinal cord may forecast the RF proper of the brain stem level.

3. The **rostral** limit is less easily stated. Technically, the RF ends at the midbrain-diencephalic junction, but functionally, it represents a continuum between the spinal cord and diencephalic and cerebral connections.

C. **Morphology of RF neurons**

1. Although RF neurons differ greatly in size and shape, a characteristic, large type of RF neuron (gigantocellular neuron) is featured by:
   a. A large nucleus
   b. Long, smooth-surface dendrites that extend in bundles that are 0.5 mm or more from the perikaryon, and orient transversely to the long axis of the brain stem. The bundles of dendrites form dendrodendritic contacts. This cell type is called **isodendritic.**
   c. Long, highly branched axons (Golgi type I neurons) that collateralize locally and bifurcate into long ascending and descending branches. Branches of a given axon may reach targets ranging from the spinal cord to the cerebrum (Figure 7-37). The axons are unmyelinated or thinly myelinated.

2. The lateral and raphe nuclei of the RF consist of smaller neurons.

3. RF contains few, if any, Golgi type II neurons.

4. Physiologically, RF neurons are characterized by recruitment, divergence, and after-discharge. The RF is particularly sensitive to general anesthetics and certain psychoactive drugs (e.g., stimulants, tranquilizers), which have much less effect on the lemniscal and other specific afferent sensory systems.

D. **Disposition of perikarya in the RF**

1. In contrast to the densely packed perikarya of most other brain stem nuclei, the RF perikarya tend to form much looser nuclear groups, often with vague boundaries (see Figure 3-9B). Neuroanatomists, therefore, differ as to their identification.

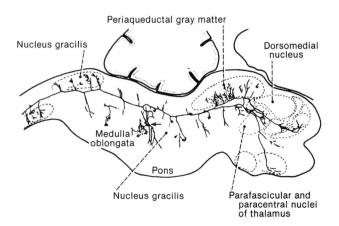

FIGURE 7-37. Golgi impregnation of single magnocellular neuron of the reticular formation (RF) in the brain stem of a 2-day old rat. The arrow points to the perikaryon. The axon branches profusely, distributing from the spinal cord to the diencephalon. (Adapted with permission from Scheibel ME, Scheibel AB: Structural substrates for integrative patterns in the brain stem reticular core. In *Reticular Formation of the Brain.* Edited by Jasper HH, et al, Boston, Little, Brown, 1958, p 46.)

Periaqueductal gray matter

Nucleus gracilis

Dorsomedial nucleus

Medulla oblongata

Pons

Nucleus gracilis

Parafascicular and paracentral nuclei of thalamus

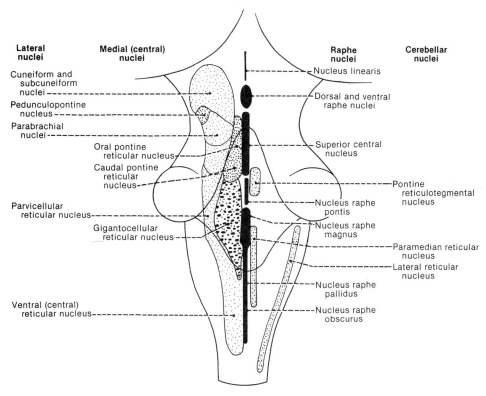

| Lateral nuclei | Medial (central) nuclei | | Raphe nuclei | Cerebellar nuclei |

Cuneiform and subcuneiform nuclei - - - - - - - - - - -
Pedunculopontine nucleus - - - - - - - - -
Parabrachial nuclei - - - - - - - - - - - -
Oral pontine reticular nucleus-
Caudal pontine reticular nucleus- -
Parvicellular reticular nucleus- - - - - - - - - - -
Gigantocellular reticular nucleus- -
Ventral (central) reticular nucleus- - - - - - - - - - - - - -

Nucleus linearis
Dorsal and ventral raphe nuclei
Superior central nucleus
Pontine reticulotegmental nucleus
Nucleus raphe pontis
Nucleus raphe magnus
Paramedian reticular nucleus
Lateral reticular nucleus
Nucleus raphe pallidus
Nucleus raphe obscurus

FIGURE 7-38. Dorsal view of the brain stem showing the location of the four groups of reticular formation (RF) nuclei.

2. The classification of many satellite nuclei clustered around the cranial nerve nuclei and scattered along tracts and of catecholaminergic nuclei (see Chapter 14) is controversial. For example, some authors classify the red nucleus with the RF, while others do not.

3. The nuclear groupings of the RF recognized by earlier neuroanatomists using Nissl (nucleic acid) stains do not clearly coincide with some of the centers demonstrated by physiologic evidence and may vary from groupings identified by the newer and more specific cytochemical and immunocytologic methods.

E. **Simplified classification of RF nuclei into four nuclear regions** (Figure 7-38)

1. Raphe nuclei extend the entire length of the median plane of the brain stem. The midline decussation of axons of brain stem pathways forms the raphe itself.

2. Medial (central) gigantocellular nuclei extend through the pontomedullary tegmentum, lateral to the raphe nuclei. They contain the conspicuous gigantocellular neurons seen in Figure 7-38.

3. Lateral parvicellular (small-celled) nuclei extend from the medullocervical region into the midbrain. In the medulla and pons, these nuclei are just lateral to the magnocellular group (see Figure 7-38). The midbrain also contains the interpeduncular nucleus (not shown in Figure 7-38).

4. Cerebellar RF nuclei mainly connect with the cerebellum (see Figure 7-38). Some authors exclude these three nuclei from the RF because of their strong cerebellar connections.

F. **Afferents to the RF**

1. Overview of afferent connections

    a. RF receives collaterals from most ascending or descending pathways through the brain stem, whatever the origin of the pathway in spinal cord or brain and whatever its function: visceral or somatic, motor or sensory. An exception is the medial lemniscus (**sensu strictorii**). Its fibers that relay discriminative sensations from the dorsal columns apparently do not collateralize to the RF, but the lateral spinothalamic and trigeminothalamic tracts, which join the medial lemniscus after its origin, do collateralize.

  b. Afferents to the RF arise in the **spinal cord, brain stem, cerebellum, diencephalon,** and **forebrain.** The RF receives the most varied, heterogeneous input of any neuronal groupings in the nervous system.

    (1) In principle, the afferents from sensory pathways reach the RF from collaterals of axons from secondary neurons, not by direct, primary afferents.

    (2) Afferents tend to synapse in the lateral, parvicellular nuclei, which then relay to the gigantocellular medial nuclei that disperse the RF efferents.

  c. The afferent fibers that bypass the RF are the discriminative or one-to-one systems designed to preserve the topographic order of the information transmitted and include the:

    (1) Dorsal column pathway through the medial lemniscus

    (2) Retino-geniculo-calcarine tract

    (3) Tonotopic fibers of the auditory system

  d. Auditory and optic pathways reach the RF, as inferred by the prompt startle response to loud sound or a sudden bright light, but the one-to-one component of these systems bypasses the RF.

2. **Spinal afferents to the RF**

  a. Spinoreticular tracts for RF nuclei arise at all levels of the cord.

  b. The spinothalamic tracts send collaterals to the RF.

3. **Brain stem afferents to the RF**

  a. **Collaterals of secondary/tertiary tracts from sensory nuclei of the cranial nerves:**

    (1) Trigeminal

    (2) Cochlear

    (3) Vestibular

    (4) Nucleus solitarius

  b. **Tectoreticular tracts** from the superior and inferior colliculi (midbrain tectum)

  c. **Reticuloreticular pathways.** RF neurons contact each other by means of innumerable axodendritic and dendrodendritic synapses.

4. **Cerebellar afferents to the RF.** Deep cerebellar nuclei, particularly from the nucleus fastigius, project to the RF. The cerebellar nuclei of the RF in turn project to the deep cerebellar nuclei and cerebellar cortex.

5. **Forebrain afferents to the RF**

  a. **Limbic system afferents arise from:**

    (1) **The basal forebrain and hypothalamus** via the medial forebrain bundle

    (2) **Mamillary bodies** of the hypothalamus via the mamillotegmental tract, and other hypothalamic nuclei via the longitudinal bundle of Schultze through the periaqueductal gray matter, which itself connects diffusely with the RF

    (3) **Habenular nuclei** of the diencephalon via the habenulointerpeduncular tract

  b. **Basal ganglia afferents to the RF.** The globus pallidus of the forebrain and substantia nigra of the midbrain send fibers to the pedunculopontine nucleus of the midbrain RF.

  c. **Cerebral cortex afferents to the RF.** Although direct corticobulbar pathways and collaterals reach most of the RF, they end most strongly in the:

    (1) **Gigantocellular nucleus** of the pons and medulla, which originate the reticulospinal tracts (this pathway would appear to provide the cortex with access to spinal neurons apart from the pyramidal tract)

    (2) **Cerebellar nuclei** of the RF

    (3) **Pedunculopontine nucleus**, which receives afferents from the motor cortex and connects with the basal motor nuclei. It acts as a locomotor center

G. **Efferents from the RF**

1. The RF integrates the great variety of afferent information it receives, runs it through multisynaptic circuits of appropriate complexity, and disperses its axons widely. RF efferents reach all parts of the CNS, from spinal cord through cerebral cortex. RF efferents generally run in the afferent pathways (see XI F), making them two-way fiber systems.

2. The **lateral**, or **parvicellular, nuclei** (see Figure 7-38) receive the majority of afferents to the RF. The lateral nuclei relay to the **medial gigantocellular nuclei** that originate the majority of efferents, but the dichotomy between afferent and efferent centers is incomplete.

3. **Specific efferent RF pathways**
   a. **Specific neurotransmitter pathways** travel to all parts of the CNS (see Chapter 14).
   b. **Reticulobulbar tracts** run to all cranial nerve nuclei.
   c. **Reticulospinal tracts** run in the ventrolateral columns of the spinal cord. The tracts arise from the medial RF nuclei.
      (1) Pontine reticulospinal tracts arise from the oral and caudal pontine reticular nuclei (see Figure 7-38). After descending in the medial longitudinal fasciculus (MLF), they end in laminae VII and VIII at all cord levels and overlap extensively with the termination fields of the vestibular nuclei. These pathways act on the axial muscles, particularly those of the neck, to mediate somatomotor functions, such as postural reflexes and muscle tone.
      (2) A medullary reticulospinal tract arises from nucleus reticularis gigantocellularis and synapses at all cord levels in laminae VII and IX. Their field of termination overlaps with the terminals of the corticospinal and rubrospinal tracts.
      (3) Although a minority of reticulospinal somatomotor axons end on ventral motoneurons, most end on internuncial neurons of laminae VII to IX.

H. **Overview of RF functions**

1. **Methods of discovering RF functions**
   a. **Transecting** the tegmentum or **destroying** tegmental regions
      (1) Natural lesions rarely affect discrete nuclear groups of the RF to allow clinicopathologic correlation of the lesion site with dysfunction.
      (2) The RF has a built-in redundancy or safety factor that requires bilateral lesions or complete transections of the tegmentum before abolishing the function of given regions.
   b. **Stimulating** various regions to determine the physiologic effects, which are usually the opposite of the effect of destructive lesions
   c. **Recording** the electrical activity of the RF during specific actions such as waking, sleeping, and breathing
   d. **Scanning by positron emission tomography (PET) scan,** which registers blood flow

2. **Range of functions mediated by the RF**
   a. **Mental state**. The RF mediates consciousness, attention span, alerting responses, and the sleep-wake cycle. The RF is tonically active during wake and sleep, but in different ways and through different nuclei.
   b. **Homeostasis and neurovegetative reflexes**. The RF mediates reflexes that control the activity of viscera and glands in the interest of homeostasis.
      (1) In concert with the forebrain, RF centers control breathing, pulse, blood pressure, gastrointestinal and genitourinary system motility, electrolyte balance, pupillary size, and ocular movements.
      (2) Reticulospinal tracts from noradrenergic neurons in the ventrolateral medulla that control blood pressure synapse on the intermediolateral cell column of the spinal cord.
      (3) RF circuitry mediates the reflexes of the upper gastrointestinal and respiratory tracts through afferents from CN V, CN IX, and CN X: coughing, sneezing, swallowing, vomiting, hiccuping, gagging, chewing, sucking, and feeding.

    (4) The **parabrachial nuclei** (so called because they surround the medial and lateral part of the brachium conjunctivum of the superior cerebellar peduncle) relay SVA (taste) and GVA afferents from the nucleus solitarius to the thalamus. The nuclei also relay taste impulses to the hypothalamus and amygdala.

    (5) The **Kolliker-Fuse nucleus,** ventral to the parabrachial nuclei, projects to the nucleus solitarius as part of the central regulatory system for respiration.

  c. Somatomotor and sensorimotor reflexes

    (1) RF mediates postural reflexes, extensor and flexor muscle tone, and vestibular reflexes affecting the eyes and somatic muscles.

    (2) Stimulation of the gigantocellular effector zone in the **medullary** RF tends to **inhibit** somatomotor activity by reducing MSRs, flexion reflexes, extensor tone, and cortically induced movements.

    (3) Stimulation of the gigantocellular effector zone in the **pontine** RF and in the mesencephalic reticular nuclei tends to **facilitate** somatomotor activity, including cortically induced movements.

    (4) Destructive lesions in these regions tend to cause an effect opposite to stimulation.

    (5) Although these effects occur in experimental animals, clinical use of this information is difficult because natural lesions are rarely limited to single, discrete nuclear regions of the RF.

3. Effects of stimulation of the raphe and periaqueductal gray matter

  a. Stimulation of the nucleus raphe magnus of the medulla or of the periaqueductal gray matter in experimental animals abolishes behavioral responses to pain.

  b. Reticulospinal pathways are presumed to reduce or gate the transmission of pain impulses by presynaptic inhibition at the level of the substantia gelatinosa (see Figure 14-2).

  c. The raphe nuclei of the medulla also belong to the sleep-inducing system of the brain stem.

I.   **Rostral-caudal dichotomy of RF function**

1. Transection of the tegmentum at the midpontine level divides the RF into **rostral** and **caudal** halves.

2. The **rostral** half of the RF is essential for arousal, consciousness, and an attentive, alert waking state.

3. The **caudal** half of the RF is essential for automatic breathing; vestibular reflexes; cardiovascular, pulmonary, and gastrointestinal reflexes, which are mediated through CN VII, CN IX, and CN X; and genitourinary and defecation reflexes. The caudal RF acts via reticulospinal tracts to the spinal centers corresponding to these functions.

J.   **Function of the rostral half of the RF and the ascending reticular activating system (ARAS)**

1. Destruction of the rostral pontine and midbrain RF

  a. Destruction or transection of the RF of the rostral pontine tegmentum causes transitory loss of consciousness.

  b. Destruction of the RF or transection of the midbrain permanently abolishes consciousness. In both instances, the unconscious individual maintains breathing, blood pressure, and other reflexes mediated through the caudal half of the RF.

  c. Transection of the brain stem rostral to the midpontine level deprives the forebrain of the entire afferent input from the huge sensory ganglion of CN V as well as all other ascending sensory influences that arise caudal to the level of the lesion. The optic and olfactory inputs, the only major ones remaining, do not seem sufficient by themselves to sustain consciousness. In a state of unconsciousness called the **persistent vegetative state**, which is caused by interruption of the ARAS, the patient's eyes are open, presumably allowing visual impulses to enter the brain, but the patient shows no evidence of conscious awareness or of any goal-directed, volitional movements.

2. Stimulation of the ARAS
   a. The rostral half of the RF projects to the forebrain by an **ARAS.**
   b. Stimulation of the ARAS by inserted electrodes causes the converse of destruction. It will cause a sleeping animal to arouse and maintains the cerebrum in a conscious, waking state. The RF controls the four As of the sleep-wake states:
      (1) Asleep
      (2) Awake (arousal)
      (3) Alert
      (4) Attentive (awareness or vigilance)
   c. The ARAS arises in neurons of the tegmentum and activates the cerebral cortex directly and, via thalamic connections, indirectly. Thus, the maintenance of the conscious waking state requires three neuronal pools and their interconnections, the:
      (1) Rostral RF
      (2) Thalamus
      (3) Cerebral cortex
   d. Bilateral destruction of any of these three neuronal groups results in unconsciousness, as does interruption of their connecting fiber pathways, which run through diencephalon and cerebral white matter.

K. **Functions of the caudal half of the RF**
Lesions of the caudal half of the pontine or the medullary tegmentum result in:

1. Respiratory dysrhythmia of a predictable type or apnea (see XII D)

2. Abolition of reflexes mediated through CN VII, CN IX, and CN X

3. Hypotension and Horner's syndrome because of loss of sympathetic pathways that descend from the hypothalamus through the RF or its reticulospinal pathways (see Figure 5-4)

L. **Relations of the RF to sleep**

1. Various regions of the RF of the brain stem, the hypothalamus, thalamus, and basal forebrain control the balance between wake and sleep. No single sleep center can be identified. The hypnagogic regions and the ARAS appear to be competitive; thus, increased activity in one system coincides with or leads to decreased activity in the other. The suprachiasmatic nucleus of the hypothalamus appears to act as a universal generator of circadian rhythms and, thus, participates in the control of the sleep-wake cycle.

2. Different sets of brain stem nuclei control the ARAS and rapid eye movement (REM) and non-REM sleep. Pontine tegmental lesions cause loss of REM sleep in humans, suggesting that REM sleep originates in this region.

3. The uncertainties and unresolved controversies about the neuroanatomy of sleep preclude a complete review (see Culebras A: Neuroanatomic and neurologic correlates of sleep disturbances. *Neurology* 42(supp16):19–27, 1992).

XII. **CENTRAL PATHWAYS FOR CONTROLLING BREATHING**

A. **Breathing serves three different functions: speech, emotional expression, and homeostasis.**

1. Speech and other volitional control of breathing is mediated through pyramidal pathways.

2. Emotional expression (laughing, crying, sighing, and the automatic utterance of expletives as in Tourette's syndrome) is mediated by limbic-extrapyramidal pathways.

3. Homeostasis (oxygen and carbon dioxide exchange and acid-base balance) is mediated through the medullary respiratory neurons and their reticulospinal pathways.

4. All pathways that affect breathing ultimately act through the same lower motoneurons (LMNs) of the cranial, phrenic, and intercostal nerves, and all centers are ultimately interconnected.

B. **Pyramidal pathways for the volitional control of breathing by the waking brain**

1. A center in the parasylvian area of the left cerebral hemisphere controls speech and, ultimately, the breathing patterns necessary for speech (see Chapter 13 VI G 3). The speech center and all centers for the volitional control of breathing act through pyramidal pathways.

2. The forebrain, when awake, also provides a general drive to breathe, mediated in part through pyramidal pathways to the LMNs of the respiratory muscles.

3. Sleep, coma, diffuse cerebral disease, or pyramidal tract interruption reduce the drive to breathe provided by the forebrain, but do not cause respiratory failure because the RF centers maintain breathing automatically.

C. **Limbic-extrapyramidal pathways for controlling breathing for emotional expression**

1. The neural drive for automatic crying, laughing, sighing, or expletive speech presumably arises in limbic circuits, or at least extrapyramidal circuits of the forebrain.

2. After loss of voluntary speech because of a left parasylvian lesion (aphasia) or because of bilateral corticobulbar tract lesions, the patient may still cry, laugh, sigh, or utter expletives automatically.

3. Bilateral corticobulbar tract lesions may even result in exaggerated crying or laughing (see **pseudobulbar palsy,** XIV C 3).

4. Emotional states in general may increase or decrease breathing.
   a. Patients with anxiety commonly **hyperventilate,** which may result in syncope or epileptic seizures.
   b. Young children may react to anger or frustration by **breathholding** spells that terminate in loss of consciousness.

D. **RF lesions and respiratory dysrhythmias** (to review the effects of spinal cord lesions on breathing, see Chapter 6 VI B 4)

1. Networks of neurons in the pontomedullary RF collaborate to produce an automatic, rhythmic drive to breathe to maintain appropriate oxygen and carbon dioxide levels in the blood.

2. The respiratory centers in the RF automatically maintain a level of breathing adequate for survival, even after hemispheric destruction or rostral brain stem transection; however, such lesions alter the respiratory rhythm and rate in characteristic ways (Figure 7-39).

3. The more caudal the lesion in the RF, the more disastrous the effects on breathing. Lesions of the caudal-most medullary RF or of the medullocervical junction may cause complete respiratory arrest (apnea).

E. **Location of medullary respiratory centers for automatic breathing.** Current evidence suggests two groups of respiratory neurons.

1. **Group I**, a **dorsal** respiratory group (DRG) of neurons, occupies the ventrolateral part of nucleus solitarius. It consists primarily of **inspiratory** neurons (Figure 7-40).

2. **Group II,** a **ventral** respiratory group (VRG) of neurons, occupies the ventrolateral part of the medulla, in association with the nucleus ambiguus and nucleus retroambigualis.
   a. Group II consists both of **inspiratory** and **expiratory** neurons.
   b. This assembly of neurons extends into the medullocervical junction, nearly to the level of C1.
   c. Also, the ventrolateral part of the medulla contains receptors, perhaps neurons themselves, sensitive to the carbon dioxide concentration, bicarbonate ion, and

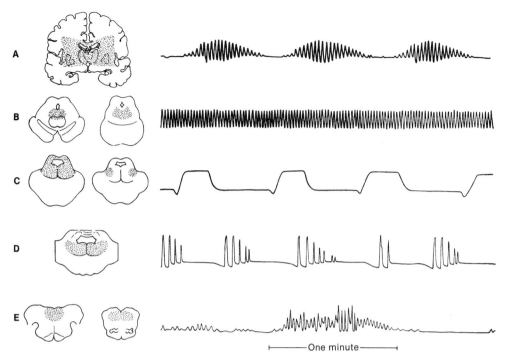

FIGURE 7-39. Correlation of intra-axial brain stem lesions (*shaded areas*) at successive levels, with the type of respiratory dysrhythmia produced. (*A*) Cheyne-Stokes respiration. (*B*) Central neurogenic hyperventilation. (*C*) Apneustic breathing. (*D*) Cluster breathing. (*E*) Ataxic breathing. (Redrawn with permission from Plum P, Posner J: *The Diagnosis of Stupor and Coma.* Philadelphia, F.A. Davis Company, 1966, p 16.)

acid-base balance. These receptors, acting through the neurons of the DRG or VRG, increase or decrease breathing to alter carbon dioxide levels as needed for acid-base balance.

F. **Reticulospinal tracts from the medullary respiratory centers**

1. The reticulospinal pathways from the medullary respiratory neurons decussate just ventral to the obex (caudal tip of the fourth ventricle) to descend to the LMNs that activate the diaphragm (C3–C5) and intercostal muscles (T2–T12) [see Figure 7-40].

2. Either a **transverse** or **sagittal** cut can interrupt the reticulospinal tracts for breathing.
   a. A **sagittal** cut, a few millimeters long and a few millimeters deep, through the obex divides the tracts as they decussate.
   b. A **transverse** cut through the ventrolateral quadrant of the spinal cord at C1 or C2 interrupts the reticulospinal tracts as they descend to the LMNs after decussating.
   c. In order to completely abolish RF functions, the transverse cut has to be bilateral because of some nondecussating or double decussating fibers.
   d. Any high cervical cord lesion that interrupts the ventrolateral quadrants of the cord may interrupt the reticulospinal pathways and eliminate automatic breathing (see Ondine's curse, XII H 2).

G. **Afferent pathways to the medullary respiratory centers** arise from the:

1. Remainder of the RF

2. Descending motor pathways
   a. Pyramidal tract collaterals, corticobulbar and corticospinal
   b. Limbic pathways, which are poorly defined, but inferred from functional considerations

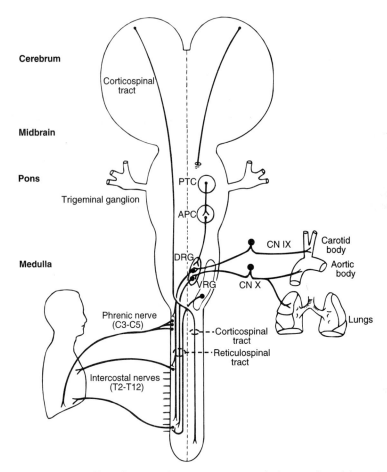

FIGURE 7-40. Neuroanatomy of breathing. By their connections with the spinal cord from C3 to T1, the corticospinal tracts control volitional breathing, and the reticulospinal tracts control automatic breathing. *APC* = apneustic center; *DRG* = dorsal respiratory group of neurons, mainly inspiratory, associated with the nucleus solitarius; *PTC* = pneumotaxic center; *VRG* = ventral respiratory group of mixed inspiratory-expiratory neurons associated with the nucleus ambiguus and retroambigualis.

   3. Ascending sensory pathways to medullary respiratory neurons

      a. Afferent stimulation in general increases RF activity and breathing.

      b. Stimulation of skin afferents increases breathing, while section of thoracic dorsal roots decreases breathing. These two facts suggest an ascending spinal pathway as yet unknown or collaterals from the long ascending tracts.

      c. Pain has a variable effect on breathing. Severe pain may increase or decrease breathing, depending in part on its emotional impact. Pleuritic or chest wall pain always inhibits breathing.

      d. CN IX and CN X afferents from the throat and lungs mediate inhibitory or excitatory respiratory reflexes.

H. **The dichotomy between volitional and automatic breathing**

   1. Pyramidal tract section or sleep abolishes voluntary breathing and the normal drive to breathe that arises in the waking forebrain. The patient survives because the pontomedullary respiratory centers continue to act automatically after the patient goes to sleep. Although the medullary respiratory center acts automatically, the pyramidal system can, for periods, command breathing to produce speech, just as it superimposes control on other autonomic functions (e.g., micturition, defecation).

   2. After destruction of the medullary respiratory centers or section of the reticulospinal pathways, the awake patient maintains breathing through the forebrain and pyramidal tracts, but loses automatic breathing. If the patient sleeps, which removes the forebrain drive to breathe, respiration stops (sleep apnea) and the patient may die. The loss of automatic breathing, called **Ondine's curse**, condemns the patient to remain forever awake in order to breathe.

I. **Sudden infant death syndrome** (SIDS or crib death). Infants with SIDS fail to maintain automatic respiration when they go to sleep. They are found dead the next morning. Even though simply positioning infants on their backs for sleep reduces the incidence of SIDS, postmortem histologic studies indicate that susceptible infants may have predisposing defects in the respiratory centers of the medulla or in their afferent or efferent pathways, which should maintain automatic breathing during sleep.

XIII. CORTICOBULBAR TRACTS

A. **Definition.** Corticobulbar tracts are the efferent fibers that arise in the frontoparietal sensorimotor (paracentral) cortex and provide the upper motor neuron innervation for the RF and cranial nerves. This definition excludes the corticopontine tracts that end on nuclei of the pontine basis. The corticobulbar pathways control voluntary movements and modulate transmission of impulses in sensory nuclei.

B. **Course of corticobulbar tracts**

1. From the paracentral cortex, the corticobulbar fibers descend through the white matter and internal capsule (see Figures 12-6 and 12-7) to enter the midbrain basis. In the midbrain basis, the corticobulbar fibers occupy an intermediate position, between the frontopontine and temporopontine tracts (see Figure 7-21).

2. As they descend caudally through the brain stem basis, groups of corticobulbar fibers veer dorsally into the tegmentum at various levels. Some fibers veer directly into the tegmentum to their synaptic stations, some veer into the tegmentum and travel caudally various distances in the medial lemniscus before ending, and some, after curving dorsally into the tegmentum, recurve rostrally.

3. Only about half of the corticobulbar fibers decussate, in contrast to the corticospinal component of the pyramidal tract, where most decussate.

C. **Termination of corticobulbar tracts**

1. Corticobulbar tracts end in:
   a. RF and satellite nuclei scattered along the brain stem
   b. Cranial nerve motor and sensory nuclei

2. The vast majority of the corticobulbar pathways are routed through RF and satellite nuclei. Only a small minority of corticobulbar axons end directly on the LMNs of the cranial nerve nuclei.

D. **Corticobulbar [upper motoneuron (UMN)] pathways to cranial nerve motor nuclei**

1. **Optomotor nuclei: CN III, CN IV, and CN VI.** Chapter 9 describes the pathways for volitional **horizontal** and **vertical** eye movement.

2. **Motor nuclei: CN V, CN VII, CN IX, CN X, CN XI, and CN XII**
   a. Except for CN VII, the motor nuclei of this group are thought to receive about an equal number of decussated and nondecussated fibers.
   b. Because of bilateral dispersion of the axons from one corticobulbar tract, unilateral corticobulbar tract interruption causes only mild weakness of the bulbar muscles bilaterally. Thus, the patient experiences some difficulty chewing, swallowing, phonating, and articulating (dysphagia, dysphonia, and dysarthria), but usually no significant unilateral paralysis, as occurs after LMN lesions of the brain stem. Mild bilateral weakness of the intercostal muscles and diaphragm occurs, causing a reduction in the maximum inspiratory effort, but not unilateral paralysis.

3. UMN innervation of the nucleus of CN VII

   a. LMNs of CN VII for the facial muscles have a topographic arrangement. The LMNs for the frontalis (forehead) muscles and, to a lesser extent, the orbicularis oculi, receive **bilateral** corticobulbar fibers.

   b. LMNs for the lower facial muscles that retract the angles of the mouth, as in smiling, receive almost exclusively **contralateral** (decussated) corticobulbar fibers.

   c. A UMN lesion of the corticobulbar fibers paralyzes only the lower facial muscles. The patient has a flat nasolabial fold and cannot retract the corner of the mouth but can elevate the forehead and close the eye. The mouth weakness is **contralateral** if the lesion affects the corticobulbar tract prior to its brain stem decussation.

   d. Destruction of the nucleus of CN VII or the trunk of the nerve paralyzes all ipsilateral facial muscles (Bell's palsy), not just the lower part of the face.

E. **Corticobulbar pathways to cranial nerve sensory nuclei**

   1. Corticobulbar fibers end in the sensory nuclei of the brain stem, including the:
   a. Nuclei gracilis and cuneatus
   b. Nucleus of the tractus solitarius
   c. All components of the nucleus of the trigeminal nerve

   2. These corticobulbar fibers are thought to inhibit or enhance sensory transmission through the various sensory relay nuclei, which allows selective attention or selective inattention to various stimuli.

F. **Corticobulbar fibers to the RF** (corticoreticular system)

   1. Corticoreticular fibers depart from the pyramidal tract at various brain stem levels. Most end in the oral pontine RF of the pons or the gigantocellular nucleus of the medulla, and others end in the cerebellar RF nuclei (see Figure 7-38).

   2. From these RF nuclei, pathways ascend and descend to all parts of the nervous system, to the cranial nerve nuclei, and to the cerebellum through the cerebellar nuclei of the RF. The cortico-reticulo-cerebellar projection gives the cerebral motor cortex an alternate route to the cerebellum, in parallel with the cortico-ponto-cerebellar system.

XIV. CLINICAL SYNDROMES OF BRAIN STEM AND INTRA-AXIAL CRANIAL NERVE LESIONS

A. **The symptoms and signs of a brain stem lesion** depend on the **longitudinal site** along the brain stem, in the midbrain, pons, or medulla, and the **cross-sectional site,** in the basis or tegmentum.

B. **Classical brain stem syndromes characteristic of the lesion site**

   1. Alternating right- and left-sided signs of unilateral brain stem lesions
   a. Interruption of a cranial nerve in the brain stem causes ipsilateral LMN paralysis or ipsilateral loss of sensation.
   b. Interruption of the pyramidal tract, which will decussate, or of a long sensory tract, which has decussated, causes contralateral signs.
   c. The term **alternating** refers to the fact that the signs of interruption of the long tract alternate with (i.e., are on the opposite side of) the cranial nerve signs.

   2. Alternating hemiplegia, hemianesthesia, and hemihyperkinesia
   a. Alternating hemiplegia. A frequent syndrome involves a somite cranial nerve palsy such as CN III, CN VI, or CN XII palsy, and contralateral hemiplegia because the somite nerves exit ventrally in the paramedian plane and run near the pyramidal tract (Figure 7-41 A, C).

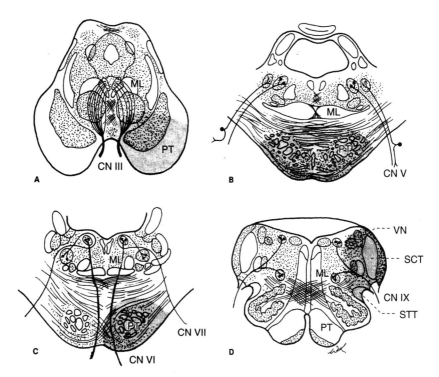

FIGURE 7-41. The shaded areas depict lesions of various brain stem levels. See also Figures 7-10 through 7-21. (*A*) Midbrain, CN III level. (*B*) Rostral pons, CN V level. (*C*) Caudal pons, CN VI and CN VII level. (*D*) Medulla, CN IX level. *ML* = medial lemniscus; *PT* = pyramidal tract; *SCT* = spinocerebellar tract; *STT* = spinothalamic tract; *VN* = vestibular nuclei.

   b. Alternating hemianesthesia. Interruption of the medial lemniscus along with the cranial nerve palsy, with or without pyramidal tract involvement, causes contralateral hemianesthesia.

   c. A midbrain lesion (see Figure 7-41A) may cause a palsy of CN III and contralateral tremor or ataxia (see XIV E 3).

C. **Special medullary syndromes**

  1. Lateral medullary syndrome of Wallenberg

   a. A lesion of the lateral part of the medulla produces a classical syndrome with alternating signs. This region, irrigated by the **posterior inferior cerebellar artery** (see Chapter 15 III), frequently undergoes infarction in patients with cerebrovascular disease (PICA syndrome).

   b. Like the Brown-Séquard syndrome of spinal cord hemisection (see Table 6-4), the lateral medullary syndrome critically tests your knowledge of neuroanatomy (Table 7-5 ; see Figure 7-41D).

  2. Bulbar palsy

   a. The medulla, a bulb-like expansion of the spinal cord, innervates the muscles of the tongue, palate, pharynx, and larynx through CN IX, CN X, and CN XII.

   b. LMN paralysis of these muscles, resulting in dysphagia, dysphonia, and dysarthria, is called "true" bulbar palsy.

  3. Pseudobulbar palsy

   a. Definition. Pseudobulbar palsy is a syndrome of weakness of volitional facial and oropharyngeal movements and consequent dysphagia, dysphonia, dysarthria, and emotional lability, characterized by exaggerated laughing or crying. It is caused by bilateral, partial interruption of the corticobulbar tracts. Bilateral, complete destruction of the corticobulbar and corticospinal tracts results in the **locked-in syndrome** (see XIV D 1).

TABLE 7-5. Lateral Medullary Syndrome of Wallenberg (Compare to Figure 7-41D)

Signs and Symptoms	Structure Involved
Ipsilateral	
Facial pain; dysesthesia or anesthesia; reduced corneal reflex	Descending root of CN V
Dysphagia and dysarthria	CN IX, X, or the nucleus ambiguus
Paralysis of palatal elevation, pharyngeal constrictors, and vocal cord	
Ataxia, dysmetria, and intention tremor	Spinocerebellar tract (SCT) or cerebellar hemisphere
Horner syndrome of miosis, ptosis, and anhidrosis of the face	Descending autonomic tract in the lateral reticular formation
Contralateral	
Loss of pain and temperature in the body and extremities (may be combined with ipsilateral sensory loss in the face)	Spinothalamic tract (STT)
General	
Nausea, vomiting, vertigo, and hiccuping	Reticular formation and vestibular connections [e.g., vestibular nuclei (VN)]

    b. Patients with pseudobulbar palsy laugh or cry involuntarily in response to slight provocation, and they switch rapidly from one to the other if the examiner suggests a humorous or sad situation.

    c. Because the lesion is in the motor cortex or somewhere along the corticobulbar tracts, not in the bulbar nerves, the syndrome is referred to as "pseudobulbar palsy," in contrast to "true" LMN bulbar palsy.

    d. The neurophysiologic mechanism for the exaggerated emotional expression released by the corticobulbar lesion is unclear, but presumably involves limbic or extrapyramidal centers.

D. **Special pontine syndromes** (other than alternating syndromes)

    1. Locked-in syndrome of the pontine basis

        a. Definition. The locked-in syndrome consists of complete quadriplegia and bulbar and facial palsy caused by complete interruption of both pyramidal tracts. The lesion is usually in the basis pontis, consisting of an infarct, neoplasm, trauma, or demyelination (see Figure 7-41B).

        b. The patient is conscious, but can make only vertical eye movements. All other voluntary movements, including horizontal eye movements, are completely paralyzed. The patient retains **vertical** eye movements because the corticobulbar pathway for vertical movements runs directly from the cerebrum into the pretectal region and midbrain. In contrast, the corticobulbar pathway for **horizontal** eye movements loops caudally into the pons, where the lesion interrupts it (see Figure 9-20).

        c. Because the lesion spares the pontine and the midbrain tegmentum, the patient retains consciousness and can see, hear, and communicate by moving the eyes up and down for yes and no. Thus, the patient, although conscious and mentally intact, is "locked-in" to himself by the complete paralysis of all other movements.

    2. Caudal pontine respiratory syndrome. Caudal pontine tegmental lesions may cause apneustic breathing (see Figure 7-39C) along with interruption of CN VI or CN VII.

    3. Extensive pontine tegmental lesions may damage the superior olivary nuclei and trapezoid body, causing impaired hearing.

E. **Special midbrain syndromes** (other than loss of consciousness-alternating syndromes)

1. Decerebrate rigidity
   a. Definition. Decerebrate rigidity is a characteristic driven posture that follows anatomic or physiologic transection of the midbrain. The patient is comatose and assumes a position dictated by the pull of the antigravity muscles (Figure 7-42).
   b. Experimentally, the syndrome is produced by a surgical transection of the midbrain at the midcollicular level. This lesion effectively disconnects the cerebrum or decerebrates the individual.
   c. Any driven posture or release phenomenon requires two conditions:
      (1) A lesion that "releases" a subordinate mechanism to display an action
      (2) Integrity of a subordinate mechanism to produce the drive that is released and causes the posture
   d. Midbrain transection incites or releases decerebrate rigidity.
   e. The vestibular system drives the decerebrate rigidity, which disappears after:
      (1) Destruction of the vestibular nerves, vestibular nuclei, or transection of the vestibulospinal tracts
      (2) Division of the dorsal roots
      (3) Division of the ventral roots (eliminates all neurally driven muscular activity)

2. Parkinson's disease (paralysis agitans)
   a. Definition. Parkinson's disease is a syndrome of tremor at rest and rigidity of the muscles and overall bradykinesia. It is caused by a lesion, usually degeneration, of the substantia nigra, which deprives the striatum of dopaminergic fibers.
   b. If the lesion is unilateral, the patient shows only contralateral parkinsonism.

3. Miscellaneous hyperkinesias. Rostral midbrain lesions, interrupting connections with the diencephalon and basal motor nuclei, result in a variety of contralateral involuntary movements varying from tremor to hemichorea and hemiballismus.

4. Coma plus oculomotor paralysis and pupillodilation
   a. Bilateral lesions of the midbrain tegmentum, which interrupt the ascending reticular activating system, result in coma.

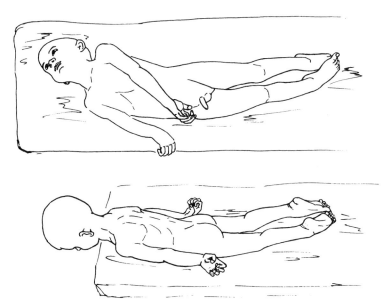

FIGURE 7-42. Posture of a patient with decerebrate rigidity. The patient is arched back (opisthotonos), holds the arms and legs rigidly extended, and shows flexion and pronation of the hands and plantar flexion of the feet. (Redrawn with permission from Penfield W, Jasper H: *Epilepsy and the Functional Anatomy of the Human Brain.* Boston, Little, Brown, 1954, p 380.)

b. The lesion frequently also interrupts the fibers of CN III, causing in addition:
  (1) Paralysis of ocular rotatory muscles
  (2) Pupillodilation from interruption of the parasympathetic fibers to the pupillo-constrictor muscle of the iris
c. The full midbrain syndrome of interruption of the midbrain with quadriparesis; coma; decerebrate rigidity, immobile eyes; and dilated, fixed pupils occurs when lesions that expand in the supratentorial space cause the cerebrum and diencephalon to herniate through the tentorium to compress the midbrain. The patient usually dies.

F. **A localizing diagnosticon for diencephalic and brain stem lesions** (Figure 7-43)

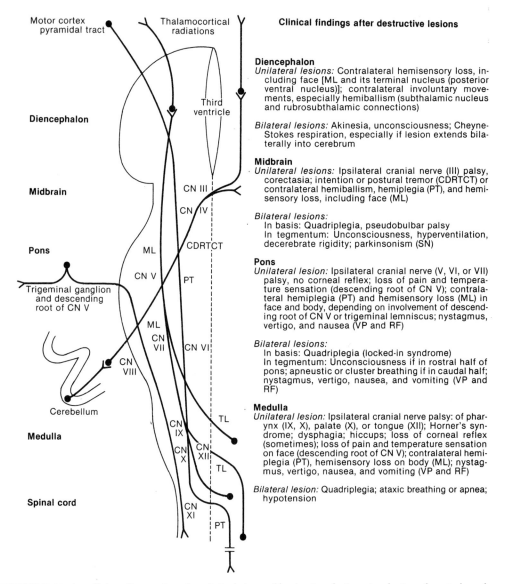

Clinical findings after destructive lesions

Diencephalon
Unilateral lesions: Contralateral hemisensory loss, including face [ML and its terminal nucleus (posterior ventral nucleus)]; contralateral involuntary movements, especially hemiballism (subthalamic nucleus and rubrosubthalamic connections)

Bilateral lesions: Akinesia, unconsciousness; Cheyne-Stokes respiration, especially if lesion extends bilaterally into cerebrum

Midbrain
Unilateral lesions: Ipsilateral cranial nerve (III) palsy, corectasia; intention or postural tremor (CDRTCT) or contralateral hemiballism, hemiplegia (PT), and hemisensory loss, including face (ML)

Bilateral lesions:
  In basis: Quadriplegia, pseudobulbar palsy
  In tegmentum: Unconsciousness, hyperventilation, decerebrate rigidity; parkinsonism (SN)

Pons
Unilateral lesion: Ipsilateral cranial nerve (V, VI, or VII) palsy, no corneal reflex; loss of pain and temperature sensation (descending root of CN V); contralateral hemiplegia (PT) and hemisensory loss (ML) in face and body, depending on involvement of descending root of CN V or trigeminal lemniscus; nystagmus, vertigo, and nausea (VP and RF)

Bilateral lesions:
  In basis: Quadriplegia (locked-in syndrome)
  In tegmentum: Unconsciousness if in rostral half of pons; apneustic or cluster breathing if in caudal half; nystagmus, vertigo, nausea, and vomiting (VP and RF)

Medulla
Unilateral lesion: Ipsilateral cranial nerve palsy: of pharynx (IX, X), palate (X), or tongue (XII); Horner's syndrome; dysphagia; hiccups; loss of corneal reflex (sometimes); loss of pain and temperature sensation on face (descending root of CN V); contralateral hemiplegia (PT), hemisensory loss on body (ML); nystagmus, vertigo, nausea, and vomiting (VP and RF)

Bilateral lesion: Quadriplegia; ataxic breathing or apnea; hypotension

FIGURE 7-43. Localizing diagnosticon for clinical signs of brain stem lesions (exclusive of central ocular pathways). *CDRTCT* = cerebello-dentato-rubro-thalamo-cortical tract; *ML* = medial lemniscus; *PT* = pyramidal tract; *RF* = reticular formation; *Roman numerals* = cranial nerve nuclei; *SN* = substantia nigra; *TL* = trigeminal lemniscus; *VP* = vestibular pathways.

XV. CLINICAL SYNDROMES OF EXTRA-AXIAL CRANIAL NERVE LESIONS

A. **Anatomic proximity of cranial nerves.** Two or more cranial nerves may come into conjunction as they leave the brain stem, cross the subarachnoid space, or converge to exit from the skull through a foramen. Lesions at the conjunction sites cause characteristic, localizing syndromes because they affect more than one nerve.

B. **Characteristic sites of conjunction of cranial nerves include the:**

1. **Parasellar region, cavernous sinus,** and **superior orbital fissure,** where the optic chiasm and CN III, CN IV, CN V, and CN VI come into conjunction (see Figure 7-23 and Figure 9-17)

2. **Cerebellopontine angle,** where CN VI, CN VII, and CN VIII run close together and CN V, CN IX, and CN X are nearby (see Figure 7-1 to Figure 7-3)

3. **Jugular foramen,** where CN IX, CN X, and CN XI exit (see Figure 7-23 and Figure 7-35)

STUDY QUESTIONS

DIRECTIONS: Each of the numbered items or incomplete statements in this section is followed by answers or by completions of the statement. Select the ONE lettered answer or completion that is BEST in each case.

1. Testing the sense of taste would be most important in a patient presenting with

(A) loss of hearing
(B) diplopia
(C) dystaxia
(D) dysphagia
(E) hemifacial paralysis

2. The gag reflex involves which of the following cranial nerve pathways?

(A) CN VII afferent and CN VII efferent
(B) CN VIII afferent and CN IX efferent
(C) CN IX or CN X afferent and CN IX or CN X efferent
(D) CN X afferent and CN XI efferent
(E) CN IX afferent and CN XII efferent

3. Assuming support of breathing and blood pressure, if required by the site of the lesion, which surgical lesion would abolish consciousness?

(A) Transection of the rostral part of the cervical cord
(B) Transection of the pontine basis
(C) Hemispherectomy
(D) Transection of the midbrain tegmentum
(E) Removal of the cerebellum

4. Decerebrate rigidity can be abolished by transection of the

(A) diencephalon
(B) cerebellum
(C) corticospinal tracts
(D) vestibulospinal tracts
(E) spinocerebellar tracts

5. A patient with a skull fracture through the floor of the right middle fossa has no tear secretion on that side. The most likely cause is damage to the

(A) ciliary ganglion
(B) chorda tympani
(C) greater superficial petrosal nerve
(D) pericarotid sympathetic plexus
(E) otic ganglion

6. The posterior plane of cutaneous innervation by the trigeminal nerve is at the

(A) occipitocervical junction
(B) lambdoid suture plane
(C) interaural plane
(D) coronal suture plane
(E) intercanthal line

7. The descending root of CN V ends at the

(A) pontomedullary junction
(B) midmedullary level
(C) obex
(D) upper cervical level
(E) upper thoracic level

8. On the right side, a patient shows paralysis of palatal elevation, the vocal cord, and the trapezius and sternocleidomastoid muscles. The gag reflex is absent on the right, and the patient has moderate difficulty swallowing. A site for a lesion that would explain all of these findings is the

(A) left cerebellopontine angle
(B) right cavernous sinus
(C) left pontine tegmentum
(D) right jugular foramen
(E) right cerebral peduncle and interpeduncular fossa

9. The maxillary division of the trigeminal nerve supplies the

(A) helix of the ear
(B) skin of the upper lip
(C) skin over the angle of the mandible
(D) forehead
(E) none of the above

10. A patient with Bell's palsy complains of excessive loudness of sounds. This finding indicates paralysis of which muscle?

(A) Stapedius muscle
(B) Levator palatini
(C) Omohyoid muscle
(D) Lateral pterygoid muscles
(E) Geniohyoid muscle

11. The site at which the smallest lesion can produce complete loss of consciousness with minimal effects on other functions is the

(A) medullary tegmentum
(B) caudal pontine tegmentum
(C) rostral midbrain tegmentum
(D) dorsolateral diencephalon
(E) medial hemispheric wall in the cingulate gyri

12. In the locked-in syndrome, the lesion usually involves the

(A) midbrain tectum
(B) midbrain tegmentum
(C) midbrain or pontine basis
(D) pontine tegmentum
(E) medullary pyramids

13. If the palate fails to elevate on the right side when a patient says "Ah," one would suspect a lesion of the

(A) right vagus nerve
(B) right glossopharyngeal nerve
(C) right spinal accessory nerve
(D) recurrent branch of the ansa hypoglossi on the left
(E) trigeminal nerve on the right

14. An operation that would abolish automatic breathing is

(A) transection of the basis of the midbrain
(B) transection of the pons at a rostral level
(C) transection of the pyramids
(D) a sagittal cut limited to the dorsal part of the cervicomedullary junction
(E) a sagittal cut limited to the pyramidal decussation at the cervicomedullary junction

15. The decerebrate posture generally indicates a lesion of the

(A) pons
(B) medulla
(C) midbrain
(D) cerebellum
(E) diencephalon

16. The corneal reflex involves an afferent and efferent arc, which is mediated by

(A) CN V only
(B) CN III only
(C) CN III and CN VII
(D) CN III and CN VIII
(E) CN V and CN VII

DIRECTIONS: Each set of matching questions in this section consists of a list of four to twenty-six lettered options (some of which may be in figures) followed by several numbered items. For each numbered item, select the ONE lettered option that is most closely associated with it. To avoid spending too much time on matching sets with large numbers of options, it is generally advisable to begin each set by reading the list of options. Then, for each item in the set, try to generate the correct answer and locate it in the opinion list, rather than evaluating each option individually. Each lettered option may be selected once, more than once, or not at all.

Questions 17–21

Match the anatomic features listed below with the appropriate brain stem level.

(A) Midbrain
(B) Pons, rostral level
(C) Pons, middle level
(D) Pons, caudal level
(E) Medulla, caudal level

17. Largest diameter of the brain stem

18. Smallest diameter of the brain stem

19. Thickest roof plate

20. Narrowest site of communication between the ventricles

21. Largest indentation in the basis, the site of the interpeduncular fossa

Questions 22–26

Match each spinal cord structure listed below with its closest homologous or analogous structure in the brain stem.

(A) Hypoglossal nucleus
(B) Medial longitudinal fasciculus
(C) Edinger-Westphal nucleus
(D) Vestibular nerve
(E) Nucleus ambiguus

22. Nucleus of the spinal accessory nerve

23. Ground bundles

24. Sacral parasympathetic nuclei

25. Ventral somatomotor neurons

26. Dorsal roots

Questions 27–30

Match each ganglion with the cranial nerve to which it contributes sensory axons.

(A) CN I
(B) CN VII
(C) CN V
(D) CN VIII
(E) CN III

27. Gasserian (trigeminal, semilunar) ganglion

28. Olfactory ganglion

29. Geniculate ganglion

30. Vestibular ganglion

DIRECTIONS: Each set of matching questions in this section consists of a list of four to twenty- six lettered options followed by several numbered items. For each numbered item, select the appropriate lettered option(s). Each lettered option may be selected once, more than once, or not at all. EACH ITEM WILL STATE THE NUMBER OF OPTIONS TO SELECT. CHOOSE EXACTLY THIS NUMBER.

Questions 31–34

(A) Reduction in salivary secretion (xero-stomia)
(B) Paralysis and atrophy of one-half of the tongue
(C) Loss of sense of smell (anosmia)
(D) Paralysis of the chewing muscles on one side
(E) Hemifacial paralysis
(F) Difficulty swallowing (dysphagia)
(G) Vocal cord paralysis
(H) Inability to abduct the eye
(I) Hemifacial loss of touch, pain, and tem-perature
(J) Loss of sensation in the skin of the ear, external auditory canal, or ear drum

For each cranial nerve (CN), select the clinical deficit that would occur after a lesion of the trunk or one of the branches of that cranial nerve.

31. CN V (SELECT 3 DEFICITS)

32. CN VII (SELECT 3 DEFICITS)

33. CN IX (SELECT 3 DEFICITS)

34. CN X (SELECT 3 DEFICITS)

ANSWERS AND EXPLANATIONS

1. The answer is E [X C 3]. Testing the sense of taste would be most important in a patient who has hemifacial paralysis, which would indicate a lesion of CN VII. The taste fibers and the motor fibers of the cranial nerve run together through the middle ear. The taste fibers then depart through the chorda tympani nerve, and the motor fibers continue through the facial canal to exit at the stylomastoid foramen. If the lesion is in the facial nerve proximal to the origin of the chorda tympani nerve, loss of taste indicates the location of the lesion. Sparing the sense of taste suggests that the lesion is distal to the takeoff of the taste fibers.

2. The answer is C [X D 5 c (2)]. The gag reflex involves an afferent arc over CN IX or CN X and an efferent arc to the levator palatini muscle, which is supplied by CN X or, in some instances, predominantly by CN IX. Absence of the gag reflex from interruption of the afferent or efferent pathways causes dysphagia and dysarthria.

3. The answer is D [XIV D 1 c; Figure 7-43]. Large parts of the nervous system can be removed or transected without abolishing consciousness. A cerebral hemisphere or the entire cerebellum can be removed. The spinal cord or the brain stem, from the caudal pontine levels on down, can be transected without abolishing consciousness if blood pressure and breathing are supported. A relatively small lesion that damages the midbrain tegmentum permanently abolishes consciousness.

4. The answer is D [XIV E 1 d, e]. Decerebrate rigidity is a postural syndrome that occurs after midbrain transection or compression. It is driven by the vestibulospinal system. Therefore, after the syndrome has been produced, section of the vestibulospinal tracts will abolish it.

5. The answer is C [X C 8 d (1); Table 7-4; Figure 7-31]. The greater superficial petrosal nerve leaves CN VII at the geniculate ganglion and crosses the floor of the middle fossa to reach the sphenopalatine ganglion, where the axons synapse. The ganglionic neurons then innervate the lacrimal glands.

6. The answer is C [X B 1 b (1); Figures 7-29 and 7-30]. The junction between the innerva-

tion of the cranial nerves and the spinal nerves occurs at or near the interaural plane. This is a line roughly connecting the external auditory canals over the vertex of the head. This line does not correspond to any particular underlying bony line marks, such as the coronal or lambdoidal sutures.

7. The answer is D [X B 5 b, c]. The descending root of CN V ends in the upper cervical region, where an expansion of the substantia gelatinosa receives the pain and temperature fibers from the face. The substantia gelatinosa is one continuous nuclear mass representing the entire body from the tip of the coccyx in the caudal region of the cord on up to the lips in the rostral region of the cervical cord.

8. The answer is D [XV B 3; Figure 7-23]. CN IX, CN X, and CN XI exit from the skull through the jugular foramen. A lesion at that foramen would interrupt all three nerves and paralyze the ipsilateral palatal, pharyngeal, sternocleidomastoid, and trapezius muscles. This is one example of several syndromes that occur when a single, often small lesion affects a conjunction of cranial nerves at the base of the skull.

9. The answer is B [VI B 4 C (3); Figure 7-30]. The trigeminal nerve receives its name from its three large sensory divisions. The ophthalmic division innervates the forehead and bridge of the nose; the maxillary innervates the skin over the upper lip, maxilla, and nares; and the mandibular innervates the skin over the mandible, except for the skin over the angle, which is innervated by cervical nerves.

10. The answer is A [X C 7 a; Figure 7-32]. CN VII innervates the stapedius muscle. This muscle dampens the oscillations of the ossicles of the inner ear. This action appears to protect the ear against excessively loud sounds. Stapedius muscle paralysis causes the patient to experience normal sounds as uncomfortably loud (hyperacusis).

11. The answer is C [XI I 2, J 1 a, c]. In general, discrete brain lesions that impair consciousness are found somewhere between the rostral pontine tegmentum and the medial hemispheric wall extending through the midbrain and diencephalon. The lesion site that causes the most severe, enduring loss of consciousness with the least destruction of tissue is in the midbrain tegmentum. The ascending reticular activating system (ARAS) funnels through this region into the diencephalon and the hemispheres. This narrow portion of the brain is appropriately called the cerebral isthmus.

12. The answer is C [XIV D 1]. The locked-in syndrome involves complete paralysis of all voluntary movements except for vertical eye movements, although the patient retains consciousness and normal mental functions. Such a state occurs after bilateral interruption of the pyramidal tracts, usually in the basis pontis, but sometimes in the midbrain. If the lesion were located at the medullary level, the patient would retain some chewing and other facial movements because corticobulbar fibers depart rostral to that level.

13. The answer is A [X E 6; Figure 7-34]. Several cranial nerves innervate the tongue, palate, and pharynx. Of these cranial nerves, the most important one for palatal elevation is generally the vagus nerve (CN X). Interruption of the right vagus nerve would cause paralysis of elevation of the palate on the right side.

14. The answer is D [XII E 2, F 2 a, H 2; Figure 7-40]. To abolish automatic breathing, the experimenter could destroy the caudal medullary tegmentum, which contains the critical respiratory neurons necessary to drive respiration. Section of the reticulospinal tracts that decussate ventral to the obex at the cervicomedullary junction to enter the cord, or of the reticulospinal tracts in the ventrolateral columns of the spinal cord, would accomplish the same end.

15. The answer is C [XIV E 1 a; Figure 7-42]. Lesions at various levels of the brain stem may cause characteristic changes in the patient's breathing or posture. Midbrain transection results in a characteristic driven posture called decerebrate rigidity. The patient has opisthotonos, extension and pronation of the arms, extension of the lower extremities, and plantar flexion of the feet.

16. The answer is E [X B 6 b (2)]. Many of the brain stem reflexes involve an afferent arc over one of the cranial nerves and an efferent arc over another cranial nerve. The corneal reflex with its afferent arc mediated through CN V and its efferent arc through CN VII exemplifies this fact.

17–21. The answers are 17-C, 18-E, 19-A, 20-A, 21-A [II A–C, III A–D; Figures 7-1, 7-2, and 7-3]. The widest part of the brain stem is the midpontine level. The size of the brain stem diminishes, going caudally from the midpontine level into the medulla or rostrally from the midpontine level into the midbrain. The smallest cross-sectional diameter is located at the caudal medullary level. On the dorsal surface of the brain stem, the caudal medullary level has the thinnest roof plate. The roof plate of the caudal medulla consists of the posterior medullary velum, which is a thin membrane consisting of an ependymal lining, a pial covering, and containing a choroid plexus. On the contrary, the tectum, or roof plate, of the midbrain consists of a thick lamina of nerve cells and fibers known as the quadrigeminal plate. Internally, the narrowest site of communication between the ventricles is the aqueduct of the midbrain. In the pons, the aqueduct expands to form the fourth ventricle, which has its widest lateral diameter at the plane of the pontomedullary sulcus. From that point, the fourth ventricle narrows to an apex at the obex, which is at the junction of the medulla and spinal cord. The fourth ventricle then continues into the central canal of the spinal cord.

22–26. The answers are 22-E, 23-B, 24-C, 25-A, 26-D [Table 7-1]. The brain stem as a whole and the medulla in particular can be interpreted as a merely expanded and somewhat elaborated spinal cord. Both the brain stem and spinal cord have a similar embryogenesis, with alar and basal plates, and both have a basically segmental plan, with somites extending from the spinal cord to the midbrain level. Both have a central cavity, the central canal in the spinal cord and the aqueduct and fourth ventricle in the brain stem. The best possible spinal cord homolog for any of the branchial arch nuclei, such as the nucleus ambiguus, is the spinal accessory nucleus in the rostral part of the cervical cord. Several brain stem structures have direct homologs in the spinal cord. The hypoglossal nucleus consists of ventral somatomotor neurons just like the ventral somatomotor neurons of the spinal cord gray matter. The medial longitudinal fasciculus is a brain stem ground bundle, which interconnects the somitic CN III, CN IV, and CN VI in the same way that the ground bundles of the spinal cord convey the short intra- and intersegmental pathways for the cord. The Edinger-Westphal nucleus consists of the preganglionic parasympathetic neurons of CN III in the same way that the sacral parasympathetic nuclei are preganglionic neurons for the pelvic splanchnic nerve. The dorsal roots of the spinal nerves correspond to the ganglia on CN IX and CN X, the gasserian ganglion, and also the special sensory ganglia of CN VIII, with its cochlear and vestibular divisions. The numerous similarities of structure between brain stem and spinal cord stop at the rostral end of the brain stem (the midbrain-diencephalic junction). Rostral to that level, in the diencephalon and cerebrum, the anatomic arrangements differ drastically. The spinal cord has no direct homolog for the cerebral cortex.

27–30. The answers are 27-C, 28-A, 29-B, 30-D [VIII F]. Various cranial nerves have one or more ganglia along their course. CN VIII has two ganglia, the spiral ganglion, which serves the auditory part of the nerve, and the vestibular ganglion, which serves the vestibular component of the nerve. CN V receives its sensory axons from the gasserian ganglion, which is outside the central nervous system (CNS), but it also has a unique ganglion in the CNS called the mesencephalic nucleus of CN V, which also provides sensory axons. No other nerves have a similar arrangement. CN I has the two olfactory ganglia, one on each side of the nasal septum. They produce the shortest cranial nerve of all. Its axons run only from the ganglion beneath the cribriform plate, through the cribriform plate, to synapse on the olfactory bulb. Some cranial nerves that are essentially motor in function lack their own ganglion and probably receive their sensory fibers from the gasserian ganglion. Examples include CN III, CN IV, and CN VI, which innervate the ocular rotatory muscles. The sphenopalatine ganglion of CN VII contributes postganglionic axons that enter a peripheral branch of CN V to reach the lacrimal gland and the nasal mucosa. The geniculate ganglion contributes taste fibers to CN VII, which ultimately run through the lingual branch of CN V.

31. The answers are: D, I, J [X B 1, 2, 7; Figures 7-29 and 7-30]. Cranial nerve (CN) V provides sensation for half of the face and head, back to the interaural line. It also provides sensory afferents to the sinuses, nasal mucosa, and teeth. Its afferents thus conduct some of the most severe pain, such as from toothache, sinusitis, temporal arteritis, and other forms of headache. The motor axons of CN V innervate the chewing muscles. The clinician can directly assay masseter function by asking the patient to clamp the teeth to-

gether and palpating the contraction of the muscle. After prolonged interruption of the motor axons, atrophy of the masseter and temporalis muscle will cause the temple and cheek to appear hollow.

32. The answers are: A, E, J [X C 10; XIII D 3; Figures 7-31 and 7-32]. Interruption of cranial nerve (CN) VII causes hemifacial paralysis affecting all of the muscles that activate one side of the face during volitional movements and emotional expression. An upper motoneuron (UMN) lesion causes paralysis only of the lower half of one side of the face because the lower motoneurons (LMNs) of CN VII of those muscles receive only crossed axons. CN VII innervates the sphincters of the mouth (orbicularis oris) and eye (orbicularis oculi) that control the closing of the oral and ocular apertures. Loss of the parasympathetic innervation of the submandibular and sublingual glands via the intermediate nerve of Wrisburg and the chorda tympani causes dryness of the mouth (xerostomia). The clinician directly observes the action of the facial muscles during the neurologic examination. Like other branchial cranial nerves, CN VII sends a twig to the ear because the first three branchial arches contribute to the ear and retain their original nerve supply.

33. The answers are: A, F, J [X D 2 b, 6; Figure 7-33]. Interruption of the parasympathetic axons of cranial nerve (CN) IX for the parotid gland via the otic ganglion results in xerostomia. Interruption of CN IX causes dysphagia because its motor axons innervate palatal and pharyngeal constrictors that process boluses of food or liquid. If the history suggests dysphagia, the clinician can best assess the dynamics of swallowing by radiographic cinematography. Like CN VII, CN IX sends a twig to the ear.

34. The answers are: F, G, J [X E 6; Figure 7-34]. Interruption of cranial nerve (CN) X causes dysphagia and dysphonia because of paralysis of pharyngeal constrictors and the vocal cords. The clinician can directly visualize the vocal cords by laryngoscopy. Interruption of CN X also results in loss of cardioinhibitory reflexes mediated by the carotid sinus. Carotid sinus hypersensitivity may lead to syncope from cardiac inhibition and hypotension. CN X, like CN VII and CN IX, sends a twig to the ear. Stimulation of the auditory canal, as when the clinician inserts an otoscope to visualize the ear drum, may result in vagal syncope because of cardiac inhibition and hypotension. The afferent arc of this vagal reflex enters the brain stem through these twigs and stimulates the preganglionic parasympathetic axons in the dorsal motor nucleus of CN X to inhibit the heart. Many other connections through the reticular formation (RF), such as from the vestibular system, may also activate a vagal reflex and result in syncope.

Chapter 8

The Vestibulocochlear Systems

I. INTRODUCTION TO CRANIAL NERVE VIII, THE VESTIBULOCOCHLEAR NERVE

A. Definition

1. CN VIII is a special sensory afferent (SSA) nerve that serves two systems of the inner ear, the **vestibular** and **cochlear** systems.

2. Older texts call the **vestibulocochlear** nerve the **auditory** nerve, but only the cochlear component of the nerve mediates hearing.

B. The primary neurons

1. Both components of CN VIII originate in bipolar neurons located in ganglia in the inner ear. These ganglia are homologs of the dorsal root ganglia of the spinal nerves.

2. The **vestibular ganglion** (Scarpa's ganglion), located at the distal end of the internal auditory meatus, contains the primary neurons of the **vestibular** system (Figure 8-1).

3. The **spiral** or **cochlear** ganglion, located in the cochlea of the inner ear, contains the primary neurons for **hearing** (Figure 8-2).

4. Most primary neurons of CN VIII synapse on secondary neurons in the **cochlear** or **vestibular** nuclei, respectively. The vestibular nuclei extend from the pontomedullary junction through the medulla (see Figure 7-22).

C. Phylogenetic relation of the vestibular and cochlear systems

1. Phylogenetically, the vestibular system antedates the cochlear system. All vertebrates have a vestibular system, while the cochlear system begins with the amphibians. In accordance with the law of lamination by phylogenesis, the cochlear nuclei are piled on dorsolateral or peripheral to the vestibular nuclei (see Figure 7-15).

2. The peripheral axons of the two systems, although starting in different ganglia for the vestibular and cochlear end organs, unite to travel in a common nerve to the brain stem, where they separate again to follow different central pathways.

3. The cochlear and vestibular divisions of CN VIII mediate only their own special senses. CN V, CN VII, CN IX, and CN X innervate pain and touch for the ear, auditory canal, and drum.

II. THE VESTIBULAR SYSTEM OF CRANIAL NERVE VIII

A. Introduction. The vestibular system commences with receptors in the labyrinth of the inner ear. Head movements and the pull of gravity stimulate the receptors. In the central nervous system (CNS), the cochlear nuclei disperse pathways to the reticular formation (RF), optomotor nuclei, cerebellum, thalamus, and cortex that aid in balance, equilibrium, posture, and the control of eye movements.

B. Two vestibular receptors

1. **The cristae**
   a. Hair cells that act as transducers extend into the fluid of the ampules of the semicircular canals.
   b. When the head moves, the inertia in the fluid in the semicircular canals deflects the hair cells, thus originating nerve impulses. The cristae of the ampules of the semicircular canals detect rotational or angular acceleration of the head.

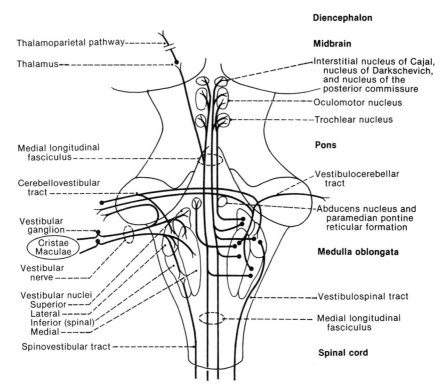

FIGURE 8-1. Dorsal diagram of the brain stem showing the vestibular pathways of the vestibulocochlear nerve. The left side shows the afferents to the vestibular nuclei. The right side shows the efferents from the vestibular nuclei. The diagram omits the profuse to-and-fro connections with the reticular formation.

2. The maculae
   a. The utricle and saccule contain maculae.
   b. In the maculae, small concretions rest against the tip of hair cells. Tilting the head causes these concretions to stimulate the hair cells; thus, they act as tilt receptors. Also, by offering inertia, these concretions detect linear acceleration.

C. **Vestibular ganglion**

   1. The ganglion sits at the distal end of the internal auditory meatus, near the cristae and maculae (see Figure 8-2).

   2. The **distal** processes of the bipolar neurons receive the stimulus from the hair cells.

   3. The **proximal** processes combine into the vestibular nerve (see Figure 8-1).

D. **Extra-axial course of the vestibular nerve**

   1. The vestibular nerve, joined by the cochlear nerve, forms CN VIII. CN VIII travels centrally in the internal auditory canal along with the two components of CN VII, the motor root and the intermediate nerve of Wrisberg (see Figure 7-3).

   2. After crossing the subarachnoid space, CN VIII attaches to the pontomedullary junction near the lateral recess of the fourth ventricle, next to CN VII (see Figure 7-3).

E. **Intra-axial dispersion of primary vestibular afferent fibers**

   1. The vestibular and cochlear fibers split at the caudal cerebellar peduncle (see Figure 7-15).
      a. The **vestibular** fibers split away **ventrally** to reach the vestibular nuclei. Some enter the peduncle.
      b. The **cochlear** fibers split away **dorsally** to enter the cochlear nuclei that drape around the caudal peduncle.

2. **The primary vestibular fibers terminate in:**
   a. **An interstitial nucleus** along the course of the entering vestibular axons and in the **vestibular nuclei**
   b. **Cerebellum** (flocculonodular lobe)
   c. **RF**

3. **No primary vestibular fibers go directly to the spinal cord, other cranial nerve nuclei, diencephalon, or cerebrum.**

F. Connections of the vestibular nuclei

1. **Four vestibular nuclei.** The four nuclei containing the secondary neurons of the vestibular pathway straddle the pontomedullary junction and extend caudally into the medulla (see Figure 8-1).

2. **Afferents to the vestibular nuclei** include the:
   a. Vestibular portion of CN VIII
   b. Spinovestibular tract

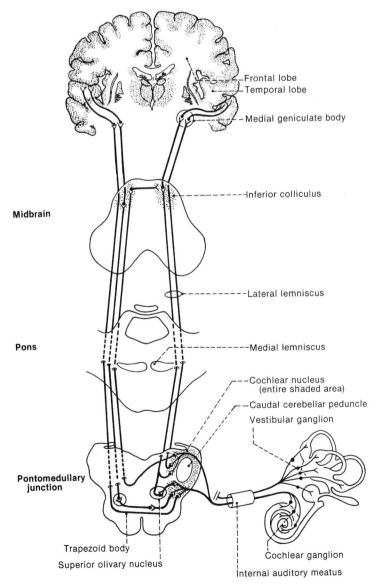

FIGURE 8-2. Diagram of the auditory pathways from periphery to cerebral cortex.

    c. Cerebellovestibular tracts
    d. Reticulovestibular tracts

3. Efferents from the vestibular nuclei
    a. Medial longitudinal fasciculus (MLF)
        (1) The **superior, medial, and spinal** vestibular nuclei send axons into the MLF, which connects the nuclei of CN III, CN IV, and CN VI of the optomotor system. See Chapter 9 VII E 6 for a discussion of the MLF syndrome.
        (2) Axons of the MLF also descend into the cervical spinal cord as the **medial vestibulospinal** tract to coordinate eye movements and head posture.
    b. Vestibulospinal tracts
        (1) Direct tracts descend into the spinal cord from the vestibular nuclei. The main tract, the **lateral vestibulospinal tract**, arises from the **lateral vestibular nucleus**. This nucleus receives the Purkinje axons from the vermian cortex of the cerebellum. These axons bypass the deep cerebellar nuclei.
        (2) These tracts facilitate the contraction of the extensor muscles, which support the body against collapse by the pull of gravity.
    c. Vestibulocerebellar pathways. These afferent and efferent pathways reflect the original derivation of the cerebellum, particularly the flocculonodular lobe, as an integrative center for the vestibular system (see Figure 10-11). These connections coordinate the axial muscles to maintain the upright posture.
    d. Vestibuloreticular pathways. Afferent and efferent connections of the vestibular nuclei with the RF mediate the nausea, vomiting, pallor, and hypotension that accompany vestibular system dysfunctions, such as motion sickness.
    e. Vestibulothalamocortical pathway. The effects of vestibular stimulation reach conscious appreciation in the form of nausea and vertigo and contribute to a sense of balance, verticality or tilt, and spatial orientation.
        (1) Vestibular pathways are thought to ascend through the central tegmental region of the brain stem to the thalamus. A portion of nucleus ventralis posterolateralis of the thalamus receives the vestibular impulses and relays them to the cortex.
        (2) The cortex does not receive vestibular impulses in one discrete, point-to-point specific region as it does for vision, touch, and hearing. Rather, the vestibular impulses reach separate portions of the parietal lobe and subjacent posterior insular and temporal cortex. Positron emission tomography (PET) scans show increased blood flow in these regions during vestibular stimulation.
        (3) Epileptogenic lesions of the parietoinsular vestibular cortex cause vertigo, while destructive lesions disturb the patient's sense of verticality.

G. **Functions of the vestibular system.** The vestibular system serves three major functions: detection of head movement and position, vestibulo-ocular reflexes, and activation of the antigravity muscles.

    1. Detection of head movement and changes in head position. The vestibular hair cells detect linear or angular acceleration or deceleration of the head and the tilt of the head in relation to the pull of gravity (tilt reception). This information aids in:
    a. Coordinating the position of the eyes, head, and neck
    b. Providing a sense of balance (other systems contributing to a sense of balance are the skeletomuscular proprioceptors, visual, and auditory)

    2. Mediation of vestibulo-ocular reflexes
    a. In a word, vestibulo-ocular reflexes **counter-roll** the eyes against the direction of head movement to keep them on their original fixation point. If the head turns to the **right**, vestibulo-ocular reflexes, acting through the MLF, counter-roll the eyes to the **left** to compensate. In effect, the eyes remain on the visual target despite head movement.
    b. Without the vestibulo-ocular reflexes, head movements cause blurred vision and apparent movement of objects viewed.

    3. Control of the tone in the antigravity muscles. The antigravity muscles support the skeleton against collapse by the pull of gravity. Overactivity of the antigravity muscles as a system produces decerebrate rigidity (see Figure 7-42).

H. **Clinical effects of vestibular nerve lesions**

1. An acute lesion of the vestibular nerve causes:
   a. Severe **vertigo** with falling and pastpointing to the side of the lesion, and the inability to maintain a vertical posture (postural instability)
   b. **Nystagmus** (rhythmic to-and-fro eye movements), **oscillopsia** (apparent to-and-fro movements of objects viewed), and **blurred vision**
   c. Autonomic symptoms and signs
      (1) Nausea and vomiting
      (2) Pallor
      (3) Sweating
      (4) Hypotension

2. Lesions of the vestibular system may produce symptoms recurrently, such as in Meniere's disease, which affects both components of CN VIII. In this disease, concomitant involvement of the cochlear component of CN VIII adds tinnitus and deafness.

3. Motion sickness, or "merry-go-round sickness," produces all of the clinical features associated with vestibular nerve lesions.

I. **Clinical testing for vestibular dysfunction by eliciting vestibulo-ocular responses**

1. **Tilt test.** The clinician tilts the patient from the vertical to the horizontal position, looks for positional nystagmus, and asks the patient about vertigo and nausea.

2. **Contraversive head-turning test (counter-rolling test or doll's eye test)**
   a. This test applies to the unconscious patient who has no visual fixation. Fixation reflexes collaborate with the vestibulo-ocular reflexes to keep the eyes on target in the conscious patient (see Chapter 9 VII A 4 b).
   b. The examiner holds the patient's head in a neutral position and then moves it briskly to the right or left and up or down. Normally, the eyes counter-roll to the same degree that the head rotates; hence, the eyes rotate relative to the eye sockets, but remain straight ahead and on the original visual target.

3. **Caloric irrigation**
   a. Syringing the external auditory canal with warm or cold water induces eye deviation and nystagmus because of convection currents set up in the endolymph of the semicircular canals.
   b. The pathway for the vestibulo-ocular reflex leads from the vestibular end organs through the vestibular nuclei and the MLF to activate the motoneurons of CN III, CN IV, and CN VI (see Figure 9-20).
   c. Caloric irrigation tests the integrity of the vestibular receptors and their pathway through CN VIII, the MLF, and the tegmental core of the brain stem to the optomotor nuclei. It is an essential part of the examination of unconscious patients or those suspected of brain death. If the brain stem tegmentum and its contained MLF are dead, vestibular stimulation fails to cause eye movement. Likewise, no other stimuli that act through any cranial nerve receptors will produce any responses.
   d. Caloric irrigation elicits a stronger vestibulo-ocular reflex counter-rolling than the contraversive head-turning test.

4. **Electronystagmography.** An X-Y recorder records the movements or oscillations of the eyes induced by one of the methods of vestibular stimulation, such as rotating the patient on a special chair or caloric irrigation.

III. **THE COCHLEAR COMPONENT OF CRANIAL NERVE VIII**

A. **Cochlear receptor for hearing**

1. The cochlea of the inner ear contains the end organ for hearing, the **organ of Corti**. The cochlea consists of a canal wound into two and one-half turns. Hair-

cell receptors tonotopically organized to detect sound of low to high frequencies line the tectorial membrane in the canal.

2. The **cochlear (spiral) ganglion** in the modiolus, or core of the cochlea, contains the primary bipolar auditory neurons (see Figure 8-2).
   a. The **distal** or **receptor** branches of the bipolar neurons end in contact with the hair cells located along the coiled cochlear duct. The hair cells transduce the various frequencies of sound into nerve impulses.
   b. The tonotopic organization of the hair cells that successively detect sound of low to high frequencies extends through the auditory pathway up to and including the auditory receptive cortex.

B. **Extra-axial course of the cochlear nerve**

1. The **proximal** or **central** processes of the bipolar neurons unite into the cochlear (auditory) nerve in the distal end of the internal auditory canal. The cochlear nerve runs centrally through the internal auditory canal in company with the vestibular nerve and CN VII.

2. After crossing the subarachnoid space, the cochlear nerve enters the brain stem at the lateral recess of the fourth ventricle, in the **cerebellopontine angle** (see Figures 7-2 and 7-3).

C. **Intra-axial course of the cochlear afferent axons** (see Figure 8-2)

1. The nerve divides into two parts that synapse on the **dorsal** and **ventral** cochlear nuclei, respectively.

2. The cochlear nuclei, which contain the secondary neurons of the auditory pathway, drape around the caudal cerebellar peduncle in a manner similar to a saddlebag.

D. **Efferent (secondary) pathways from the cochlear nuclei**

1. Most efferent axons from the cochlear nuclei will synapse in the:
   a. **Nuclei of the auditory pathway**
      (1) Superior olivary complex
      (2) Nuclei of the trapezoid body
      (3) Nuclei of the lateral lemniscus
   b. **Inferior colliculus**
   c. **RF** (Primary and secondary auditory afferents to the RF mediate the auditopalpebral reflex consisting of eyelid closure to sound and the alerting and startle responses to auditory stimuli that activate the ascending reticular activating system.)

2. The secondary cochlear axons and the tertiary and quaternary axons from the auditory nuclei form an interconnecting, trapezoidal configuration in the caudal pontine tegmentum, called the **trapezoid body** (see Figure 8-2).

E. **Efferent tertiary and quaternary pathways from the auditory nuclei**

1. **Lateral lemniscus.** The lateral lemniscus is the main efferent pathway from the superior olivary nuclei and nuclei of the trapezoid body.

2. **Connections with the RF.** These connections mediate the startle response to sound and control the stapedius muscles.

3. **Connections with lower motoneurons (LMNs) of the stapedius and tensor tympani muscles.** These efferent axons from the superior olivary nuclei and RF reflexly control the stapedius muscle via CN VII and the tensor tympani muscle via CN V. These muscles modulate and dampen the vibrations of the ossicles of the middle ear and ear drum, thus protecting the delicate hair cells of the organ of Corti from damage by loud sound.

4. **Efferents back into the organ of Corti.** An olivocochlear efferent tract, crossed and uncrossed, runs from the superior olive via CN VIII to the organ of Corti, where it synapses on the hair cells.
   a. This pathway may influence the reception of sound at the organ of Corti by controlling the receptivity of the hair cells.

b. Because these efferent axons do not end on muscle or gland effectors, they are not generally included in the theory of nerve components.

F. **The lateral lemniscus**

1. The lateral lemniscus forms at the level of the trapezoid body and ascends in the dorsolateral pontine and midbrain tegmentum and conducts auditory impulses rostrally (see Figure 8-2 and Figures 7-16 to 7-19).

2. The lateral lemniscus comes into contact with the medial lemniscus at midbrain levels, making a **lemniscal crescent** in the midbrain tegmentum. The crescent consists of the **medial, lateral, spinal,** and **trigeminal** lemnisci (see Figure 7-18).

3. **Axons of the lateral lemniscus terminate in the:**
   a. Nuclei scattered along its course
   b. Inferior colliculus of the quadrigeminal plate
   c. Medial geniculate body of the thalamus. In common with the thalamic nuclei for the other senses, the medial geniculate body receives no primary afferents from the peripheral nerves, only relayed afferents.

4. Because the lateral lemniscus contains decussated and nondecussated axons, unilateral interruption of one lateral lemniscus or its synaptic stations does not cause unilateral deafness.

G. **Projections of the inferior colliculus of the quadrigeminal plate.** Collicular neurons relay auditory impulses to the medial geniculate body via the brachium of the inferior colliculus (see Figures 7-9A and 7-20).

H. **Projections of the medial geniculate body**

1. The medial geniculate body is the specific thalamic sensory relay nucleus for hearing (see Figure 8-2). It projects axons via a **geniculotemporal tract** through the deep hemispheric white matter to the auditory receptive cortex of the temporal lobe [see Figure 12-6, #7 (auditory radiations)].

2. Two different nuclear groups of the medial geniculate body project axons to the auditory cortex.
   a. Axons that synapse on the primary auditory cortex in a tonotopic order constitute the **core projection** from part of the medial geniculate body.
   b. Axons that synapse on the secondary auditory cortex that surrounds the primary auditory receptive cortex constitute the **belt projection.**

I. **Auditory receptive cortex**

1. The auditory receptive cortex that receives the core and belt projections from the medial geniculate body occupies the **transverse gyri of Heschl** in the temporal lobe.

2. The transverse gyri form part of the floor of the lateral (sylvian) fissure (see Figure 13-7).
   a. The primary tonotopic cortex (see Figure 13-35, area 41 of Brodmann) that receives the **core projection** occupies the middle part of the anterior transverse gyrus and part of the posterior transverse gyrus.
   b. The remainder of the region surrounding the tonotopic cortex receives the **belt projection.** See Chapter 13 VI G 3, 4 for a discussion of the role of the auditory receptive cortex in language.

J. **Clinical effects of lesions of the auditory nerve and central pathways**

1. Damage to the organ of Corti, the hair cells, the spiral ganglion neurons, or the cochlear nerve causes diminished hearing or complete deafness. Irritation may cause tinnitus. Lesions of the auditory association regions of the cortex may cause auditory hallucinations.

2. The bilaterality of representation of auditory axons in the lateral lemnisci means that unilateral lesions of the auditory pathway, from lemniscal origin to and including the receptive cortex, do not cause unilateral deafness. To cause unilateral deafness,

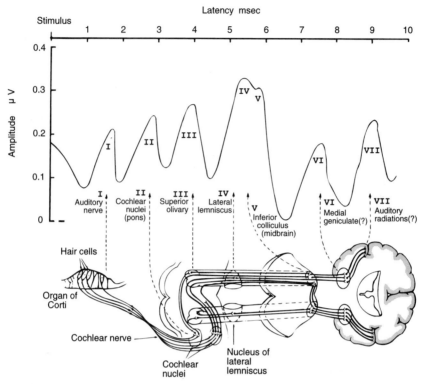

FIGURE 8-3. Diagram relating brain stem auditory evoked potentials as recorded from the surface of the head to the anatomic stations along the auditory pathway. (Adapted with permission from Stockard JJ, Stockard JE, Sharbrough FW. Detection and localization of occult lesions with brainstem auditory responses. *Mayo Clin Proc* 1977;52:761-769. Original drawing by Ellen Grass.)

the lesion has to affect the cochlear nuclei, the cochlear nerve, the organ of Corti, or the middle or inner ear.

3. The site of abnormalities in the conduction of auditory impulses through CN VIII and its brain stem pathways, up to and including the auditory cortex, can be detected by surface electrodes on the head using the brain stem auditory evoked potentials (BAEP) test. The wave forms recorded reflect the electrical activity at specific sites along the auditory pathway (Figure 8-3).

4. Middle ear lesions or stapedius paralysis may cause hyperacusis or diplacusis.

STUDY QUESTIONS

DIRECTIONS: Each of the numbered items or incomplete statements in this section is followed by answers or by completions of the statement. Select the ONE lettered answer or completion that is BEST in each case.

1. On the left side, a patient is found to have diminished hearing, an inactive labyrinth to electronystagmography, hemifacial weakness, loss of taste on the anterior two thirds of the tongue, and absence of tearing. These functions are intact on the right side, and the remainder of the neurologic exam is normal. Select the best interpretation of the clinical findings.

(A) The patient has multiple lesions of the various cranial nerves
(B) The patient has a single lesion in the internal auditory meatus or internal auditory canal
(C) The patient has multiple lesions in the brain stem
(D) A combined lesion of the brain stem and peripheral nerves is necessary to account for all of the findings
(E) None of the above provide an adequate explanation

2. A basic function of the vestibular system is to

(A) counter-roll the eyes against the direction of head movement
(B) detect sounds of low frequency
(C) agitate the eyeballs to prevent visual fatigue of the retinal image
(D) elevate the eyes against the pull of gravity on the eyeballs
(E) none of the above

DIRECTIONS: Each of the numbered items or incomplete statements in this section is negatively phrased, as indicated by a capitalized word such as NOT, LEAST, or EXCEPT. Select the ONE lettered answer or completion that is BEST in each case.

3. All of the generalizations about the primary vestibular afferent fibers are true EXCEPT

(A) primary vestibular afferents may synapse directly in the reticular formation (RF)
(B) primary vestibular fibers split away from the auditory fibers on entering the brain stem
(C) primary vestibular axons reach the cerebellum
(D) primary vestibular axons do not reach the medial geniculate body
(E) primary vestibular afferents all originate in the spiral ganglion

4. Which of the following statements about the lateral lemniscus is NOT true?

(A) It conveys auditory impulses
(B) It ascends in the dorsolateral part of the tegmentum and becomes part of a "lemniscal crescent"
(C) It synapses in the inferior colliculus
(D) It terminates in a specific thalamic relay nucleus
(E) It consists nearly exclusively of crossed axons

5. Select the comparison of the vestibular and cochlear components of CN VIII that is NOT true.

(A) The transducers of both components consist of hair cells

(B) Some primary afferents of both components run into the reticular formation (RF)

(C) Both systems are strongly organized for point-to-point topographic transmission, up to and including the cortex

(D) The primary axons of both components accompany each other in the internal auditory meatus

(E) The primary axons of both components diverge upon entering the brain stem

---

DIRECTIONS: Each set of matching questions in this section consists of a list of four to twenty-six lettered options followed by several numbered items. For each numbered item, select the appropriate lettered option(s). Each lettered option may be selected once, more than once, or not at all. EACH ITEM WILL STATE THE NUMBER OF OPTIONS TO SELECT. CHOOSE EXACTLY THIS NUMBER.

Questions 6-7

(A) Degeneration of the hair cells of the organ of Corti
(B) Degeneration of the hair cells of the cristae of the ampules
(C) Spiral ganglion
(D) Vestibular ganglion
(E) Trigeminal nerve
(F) Vagus nerve
(G) Cochlear division of CN VIII
(H) Vestibular division of CN VIII
(I) Olivocochlear nerve
(J) Cochlear nuclei
(K) Vestibular nuclei
(L) Basis pontis
(M) Transverse temporal gyri bilaterally
(N) Postcentral cortex bilaterally

For each clinical feature, select the anatomic site or sites for the responsible lesion.

6. Pain in the ear (SELECT 2 SITES)

7. Absence of eye deviation or nystagmus to caloric irrigation (SELECT 4 SITES)

ANSWERS AND EXPLANATIONS

1. The answer is B [I B, C 2; III J]. The principle of parsimony requires the clinician to seek a single explanation for neurologic findings. A single lesion in the cerebellopontine angle or obstructing the internal auditory meatus or internal auditory canal can account for all of the findings. The internal auditory canal transmits axons for all of the various components constituting CN VII and CN VIII. Thus, it transmits axons of the facial root proper and the intermediate nerve of Wrisberg with its secretomotor and taste components and the axons of the vestibular and cochlear divisions of CN VIII and the olivocochlear bundle. The common, classical lesion of this region is an acoustic neuroma, which is an overgrowth of Schwann cells that often commences in the internal auditory canal. The clinician would not suspect an intra-axial lesion of the brain stem because the patient showed no evidence of interruption of long tracts (i.e., pyramidal, lemniscal, or cerebellar) and no sixth-nerve palsy. Large tumors of the cerebellopontine angle may also affect CN V and CN IX.

2. The answer is A [II G 2]. A basic function of the vestibular system is to counter-roll the eyes against the direction of head movement. This reflex, in alliance with the fixation reflexes, permits the eyes to remain on target even though the head and body are moving. Otherwise, movement of the head and body might interfere with the continued alignment of the eyes on the visual target and cause blurred vision. Dysfunction of the vestibular system results in oscillation of the eyes, called nystagmus.

3. The answer is D [II E]. In general, primary sensory pathways do not synapse directly on thalamic nuclei, such as the medial geniculate body. After originating in the vestibular ganglion, primary vestibular fibers end in the vestibular nuclei, the reticular formation (RF), the interstitial nucleus of the vestibular nerve, and some pass directly to the flocculonodular lobe of the cerebellum. Among cerebellar afferents, the direct connections of the primary vestibular axons are unique. Other sensory pathways to the cerebellum first synapse at spinal cord or brain stem levels.

4. The answer is E [III F 4]. The lateral lemniscus consists of about an equal number of crossed and uncrossed auditory axons. These are mostly secondary auditory afferent fibers, many of which originate in the superior olivary nucleus. The auditory pathway runs through the lateral lemniscus to the inferior colliculus and to a specific thalamic relay nucleus, the medial geniculate body. Because of the large number of uncrossed axons up and down the whole system to the auditory cortex, unilateral lesions at any level of the lemniscal pathways do not cause contralateral deafness.

5. The answer is C [II F 3 e (2); III A 2 b]. The cochlear and vestibular systems share many features in common, including their hair cell transducers and peripheral course. A major difference is that the cochlear component preserves a strongly tonotopic, point-to-point representation of sound frequencies from periphery to cortex and has a single, topographically-organized receptive cortex, similar to the visual and somatosensory cortices. The vestibular component ends in three areas that do not seem to have the obvious topographic organization of the cochlear component.

6. The answers are: E, F [I C 3]. Several nerves innervate the ear. The cochlear and vestibular divisions of CN VIII mediate the special sensory functions but do not mediate touch and pain. CN V, CN VII, CN IX, and CN X provide touch and pain afferents to the ear drum, auditory canal, or ear itself. The olivocochlear nerve sends axons to the organ of Corti that apparently act to gate or modulate sound reception.

7. The answers are: B, D, H, K [II I 3]. Interruption of the afferent pathway to the lower motoneurons (LMNs) of the ocular muscles will abolish the response to caloric irrigation. This pathway extends from the vestibular end organ through the cochlear nerve, cochlear nuclei, and medial longitudinal fasciculus (MLF) to the nuclei of the ocular muscles. Caloric irrigation tests the entire afferent and efferent arcs of the vestibulo-ocular system. Caloric irrigation is used clinically in conscious and unconscious patients. Irrigation of the external ear with warm or cold water causes slow deviation of the eyes to one side and a reflex kickback to the midline. The clinician can directly observe this action, called nystagmus, or can record the eye movements by electronystagmography for quantitative analysis. Brain-dead patients fail to respond at all to caloric stimulation or the adversive head-turning test. The brain stem auditory evoked potential (BAEP) test also documents the absence of conduction through the cochlear pathways in a brain-dead patient.

Chapter 9

Vision and the Optomotor System

I. MOTOR AND SENSORY COMPONENTS OF THE OPTIC SYSTEM

A. The **sensory**, or **afferent**, component of the optic system produces vision. It acts through CN II, the optic nerve, and its special central pathways to the cerebral cortex.

B. The **motor**, or **efferent**, component selects a target and fixates the eyeballs on it, moves the eyes conjugately to locate or pursue targets, controls the size of the pupil and the focusing of light rays on the retina, and elevates the eyelid. The motor system acts through its own supranuclear central pathways and the lower motoneuron (LMN) nuclei of cranial nerve (CN) III, CN IV, and CN VI, and their peripheral nerves.

C. **Clinical testing of the sensory and motor functions of the optic system.** Only by knowing the neuroanatomy of the optic system can the student understand how the clinician tests it (Table 9-1; see Appendix VI A).

II. ANATOMY OF THE EYEBALL

A. **Frontal aspect of the eye.** Ocular structures seen from the front consist of the **cornea, iris, pupil**, and **conjunctiva**.

  1. The **cornea** is a transparent disc that covers the iris.

  2. The **iris** is an opaque, pigmented diaphragm with a central opening called the **pupil** (Figure 9-1), which varies in size.

  3. The **conjunctiva** is a mucous membrane that covers the exposed surface of the eyeball peripheral to the cornea.

B. **Transverse section of the eyeball** discloses three main layers: the **sclera**, the **choroid**, and the **retina** (see Figure 9-1).

  1. The **sclera** is the outer tunic of the eyeball. It consists of tough, fibrous connective tissue. Seen through the conjunctiva, it is the white of the eye. The sclera continues intracranially through the optic foramen as the **dura mater**.

  2. The **choroid** is a vascular coat that contains capillaries and venules. It extends forward as the **ciliary body** and **iris**.

  3. The **retina** is the neuronal, light-sensitive layer of the eyeball.

C. **Ophthalmoscopic anatomy of the optic fundus**

  1. With an ophthalmoscope, the physician can look through the patient's pupil to examine the living retinal tissue and blood vessels in the back, or **fundus**, of the eye (Figure 9-2).

    a. Notice the **optic disc** (optic papilla) and the **macula lutea** with a **fovea centralis**.

    b. **Arteries** emerge from the optic disc, and **veins** converge on it. The vessels travel across the retinal surface, between it and the entering light rays. The arteries ramify toward, but do not encroach on, the macula, leaving it an avascular area.

    c. The fundus appears reddish because the neuronal layers of the retina are completely transparent and the light reflects off of the pigment cell layer and the rich vascular plexus of the choroid.

  2. **Transverse section of the fundus.** In Figure 9-3, notice the slight elevation of the optic disc margins where the optic axons from the retinal neurons converge on the optic disc. These axons form the **optic nerve** after piercing the **lamina cribrosa** of the **sclera**.

    a. The optic disc and macula each show a depression, the **physiologic cup** and the **fovea centralis**, respectively.

TABLE 9-1. Outline of Clinical Tests for Central Eye Movement Disorders

Type of Eye Movement	Method of Examination
Spontaneous and volitional movements that accompany ordinary behavior and ordinary environmental stimuli	Inspection while taking the history
Volitional fixation and volitional movements	The examiner observes steadiness and range of eye movements after requesting the patient to fixate on a distant, straight-ahead object and then to move the eyes right, left, up, and down; test for impersistence of gaze.
Visual reflex ocular movements	
Smooth pursuit	The patient's eyes pursue the examiner's finger as it moves through the full range of ocular movements
Vergences	The examiner directs the patient to look at near and distant objects and to follow the examiner's moving finger in toward the patient's nose (convergence)
Reflex fixation	The patient fixates straight ahead, and the examiner turns the patient's head to the right, left, up, and down
Alignment lock	As the patient fixates straight ahead, the examiner alternately covers and uncovers first one, then the other eye and looks for deviation in alignment, resulting from monocular occlusion of vision (cover–uncover test)
Optokinetic nystagmus	The examiner rotates a drum or moves a striped strip. The patient's eyes pursue the drum to one side slowly, and then a saccade kicks them back to the primary position
Nonvisual reflex ocular movements	
Caloric nystagmus	Irrigate the ears with hot or cold water
Positional nystagmus	The examiner places the patient's head in various positions
Contraversive eye-turning test (doll's eye test, oculocephalic test)	The examiner grasps the patient's head and rapidly turns it to the right and left and up and down
Associated eye movement (Bell's phenomenon)	The examiner holds the patient's eyelids open and observes the upward movement of the eyes that occurs when the patient attempts to close the lids

FIGURE 9-1. Horizontal section of the right eyeball as seen from above. Note that the optic papilla and optic nerve are medial to the fovea.

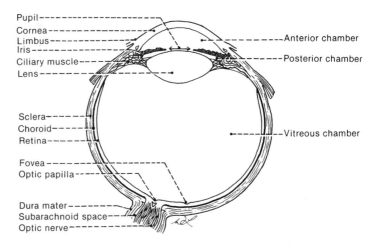

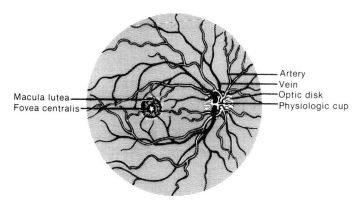

FIGURE 9-2. Anatomy of the optic fundus as seen by ophthalmoscopy. The macula is the visual center of the retina. The area surrounding the macula is called the periphery of the retina.

Artery
Vein
Optic disk
Physiologic cup

Macula lutea
Fovea centralis

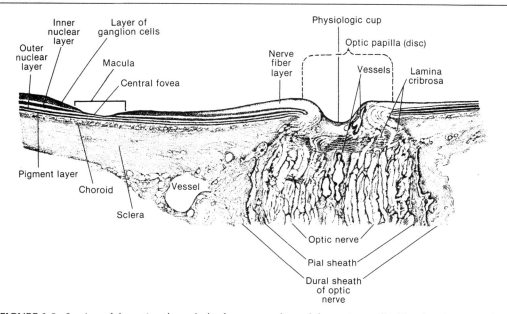

FIGURE 9-3. Section of the retina through the fovea centralis and the optic papilla. The drawing omits the blood vessels on the retinal surface and traversing the physiologic cup. (Reprinted with permission from Bloom W, Fawcett D: *A Textbook of Histology.* Philadelphia, WB Saunders, 1970, p 795.)

   b. Upon ophthalmoscopic examination, the **optic disc** appears pink in the region around the physiologic cup, where the optic nerve axons perforate the outer, peripheral part of the disc. The pinkness comes from the capillaries that accompany the otherwise transparent axons.
   c. Contrarily, the physiologic cup, located in the center of the optic disc, appears white. Large vessels perforate the cup, but no nerve fibers; hence, it lacks a covering of capillaries, allowing the scleral white of the lamina cribrosa to shine through, untinted.
 3. Ophthalmoscopic anatomy of optic atrophy and papilledema
   a. Optic atrophy refers to degeneration of optic nerve fibers.
      (1) The optic nerve fibers may undergo **anterograde degeneration** after lesions that destroy the neurons of origin in the retina.
      (2) The optic nerve fibers may also undergo **retrograde degeneration** back into the retina after lesions interrupt the optic nerve axons distal to the eyeball.
      (3) In either event, if the axons disappear, the capillaries that give the nerve fiber layer of the disc its normal pink color also disappear. The entire optic disc then appears white because the loss of axons and capillaries exposes the white sclera and its lamina cribrosa.

    b. Papilledema refers to swelling of the nerve fiber layer of the optic papilla (disc).
      (1) The subarachnoid space extends out along the optic nerve to the eyeball (see Figures 9-1 and 9-3). The ophthalmic artery and ophthalmic vein run with the optic nerve.
      (2) Increased pressure from a lesion in the cranial cavity will reflect out into the subarachnoid space and collapse the ophthalmic vein. Fluid leaks into the optic papilla and surrounding retina from the dammed-up blood vessels. Ophthalmoscopy shows an elevated, swollen optic papilla with obliteration of the physiologic cup and engorged retinal veins.

D. **The retinal neurons and layers**

    1. The retina contains six types of neurons distributed in three layers (Figure 9-4; Table 9-2).

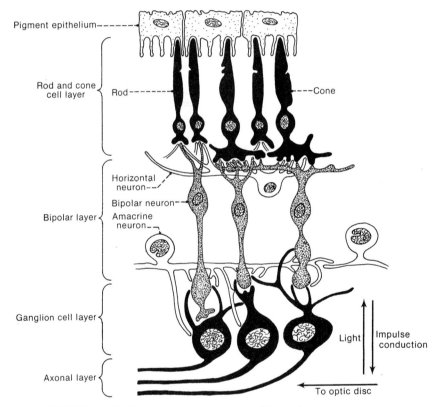

FIGURE 9-4. Retinal neurons as diagrammed from electron microscopy.

TABLE 9-2. Three Layers and Six Neuronal Types of the Retina

Layers and Neurons	Function
Outer layer (scleral side of the retina) Rod neurons Cone neurons	Receptor layer for light rays
Middle layer Bipolar neurons Horizontal neurons Amacrine neurons	Layer of retinal interneurons
Inner layer (corneal side of the retina) Ganglionic neurons	Efferent layer, originating axons of the optic nerve

2. **Rod and cone (receptor) layer of the retina**
   a. The **rods** and **cones** are the receptors for light. They occupy the **scleral** side of the retina; thus, light must penetrate the overlying retinal layers to reach the rods and cones.
      (1) **Cones** concentrate at the macula and fovea centralis, where they are not covered by overlying retinal elements or blood vessels (see Figure 9-3). The eyeballs align so that the cones receive the central ray of light from the object viewed (see Figure 9-6).
      (2) The retinal receptors peripheral to the macula are mainly **rods**.
   b. Rods and cones make the retina a **dual organ**. The retina mediates two types of vision, **central** and **peripheral**, based on the location of the rods and cones.
      (1) **Central vision** is mediated by the **cones**, which concentrate in the maculae. The cones serve two functions: **acuity** and **color vision**.
         (a) **Acuity** refers to the ability to discriminate lines or points at a distance, which is tested by reading letters.
         (b) **Color vision** is tested by color recognition.
         (c) **Mnemonic.** The Cones Cluster in the retinal Center (maCula) and mediate aCuity and Color.
      (2) **Peripheral vision** is mediated by the **rods**, which occupy the peripheral retina around the macula. The peripheral retina has three functions:
         (a) Registration of the periphery of the visual field around the macula
         (b) Night vision
         (c) Motion detection

3. **Bipolar (internuncial) layer of the retina**
   a. The middle retinal layer contains three types of neurons: **bipolar**, **horizontal**, and **amacrine neurons** (see Figure 9-4).
      (1) **Bipolar** neurons predominate in this layer of the retina. They connect the rods and cones with the ganglion cell layer.
      (2) **Horizontal** neurons have their perikarya in the outer part (scleral side) of the bipolar layer.
      (3) **Amacrine** neurons have their perikarya in the inner part (antiscleral side) of the bipolar layer.
   b. Horizontal and amacrine cell processes defy classification as dendrites or axons.
      (1) Horizontal cell processes contact the axodendritic synapses of the rod and cone cells with the bipolar cells (see Figure 9-4).
      (2) Amacrine cell processes contact the synapses of bipolar neurons with the dendrites of the ganglion layer neurons (see Figure 9-4).
      (3) Because the processes of the bipolar, horizontal, and amacrine neurons all remain in the retina, they constitute the **internuncial** layer.

4. **Ganglionic (efferent) layer of the retina**
   a. The efferent layer, which is on the antiscleral surface of the retina, consists of multipolar neurons with standard dendrite to axon polarization.
   b. The neurons of the ganglionic layer originate the optic nerve axons. They travel across the antiscleral surface of the retina to converge on the optic papilla in a specific pattern (Figure 9-5).
   c. **Course of ganglionic axons across the retina**
      (1) The axons from the maculae converge directly on the optic papilla, forming a **maculopapillary** bundle.
      (2) The axons of the ganglion cells surrounding the macula take an increasingly curved course to the optic papilla (see Figure 9-5).
      (3) Macular degeneration results in the loss of the maculopapillary bundle axons and their capillaries, which causes the optic disc to appear pallid or white on its **lateral** side.

5. **Myelination of the optic nerve**
   a. After exiting through the cribriform plate of the sclera, the retinal axons immediately enter the optic nerve and acquire a myelin sheath.
   b. Because the retina and the optic stalk (into which the retinal axons grow) arise by evagination of the diencephalon, the myelin comes from oligodendroglia, not Schwann cells, as in true peripheral nerves.

FIGURE 9-5. Fundus of the right eye. The fibers from the macula (*M*) run straight to the optic papilla (*OP*), forming a straight maculopapillary bundle. The fibers peripheral to the macula take an increasingly curved course.

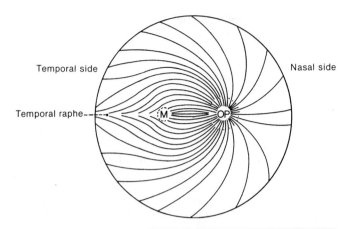

FIGURE 9-6. Retinal image formed by monocular (*A*) and binocular (*B*) fixation.

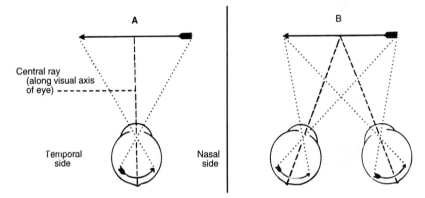

    c. Normally, myelination starts only after the axons have perforated the lamina cribrosa and entered the optic nerve. If the optic axons were myelinated as they crossed the retina, the myelin would cover the retinal light receptors and block vision.

    d. Sometimes oligodendroglia creep for a short distance from the disc into the retina. Ophthalmoscopy then discloses them as a whitish patch on the disc margin. They then create a "blind spot," which the clinician can disclose by mapping out the patient's central visual field.

III. THE VISUAL PATHWAY (RETINO-GENICULO-CALCARINE PATHWAY)

 A. **Physical optics of image formation on the retina**

    1. The physical optics of the eye invert the retinal image (Figure 9-6).

    2. The actual retinal image is a real image based on physical optics. Neural events then translate this physical image into a physiologic event, called a **visual image**. The mind learns to project the visual image back to the original site of the visual stimulus.

        a. If a light ray strikes the **nasal** half of the retina, the mind projects, perceives, or interprets the object correctly as located in the **temporal** half of space (see Figure 9-6).

        b. If a light ray strikes the **superior** half of the retina, the mind projects the visual image to the **inferior** half of space.

3. Figure 9-6 depicts image formation as if it were simply a pinhole camera effect. In reality, the cornea and lens refract the light rays to focus them on the retina. Only the central ray, which strikes the macula, does not undergo refraction, making the macula the site of maximum visual acuity.

B. **Representation of the visual fields**

1. The phylogeny of vision best explains the arrangement of axons in the visual pathways.

   a. The eyes of **lower mammals** and **submammalia** angle to the sides. These animals view an arrow by **panoramic vision**, in which the fields of the two eyes do not overlap. In order to represent the fields from the two eyes as a continuous, panoramic field, the optic nerve fibers undergo a total decussation (Figures 9-7 and 9-8).

   b. In primates, both eyes angle forward. These animals view an arrow by means of **stereoscopic binocular vision**. The axonal arrangement must integrate the **nasal** half of the visual field of one eye with the **temporal** half of the visual field of the

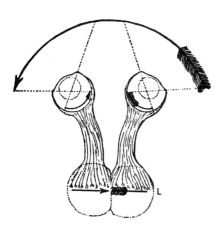

FIGURE 9-7. Discontinuous representation of the visual image if the optic nerve does not decussate. *L* = visual center. (Reprinted with permission from Ramón y Cajal S: *Recollections of My Life, Memoirs of the American Philosophical Society*, vol 8. Cambridge, MA, MIT Press, 1937, p 472.)

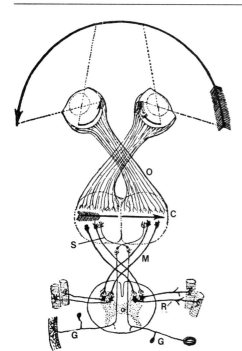

FIGURE 9-8. Continuous representation of the visual image resulting from decussation of the optic nerve in a lower animal with panoramic vision. Compare with Figure 9-9, which represents binocular stereoscopic vision. *C* = visual center; *G* = ganglion; *M* = crossing motor fibers; *O* = decussated optic nerve; *R* = motor root of spinal nerve; *S* = decussated central sensory pathway. (Reprinted with permission from Ramón y Cajal S: *Recollections of My Life, Memoirs of the American Philosophical Society*, vol 8. Cambridge, MA, MIT Press, 1937, p 473.)

other eye. This representation requires a shift from total decussation of the optic-nerve fibers at the optic chiasm (the primitive arrangement) to partial decussation (the advanced arrangement) [Figure 9-9].

2. In **submammalia**, the midbrain tectum, which corresponds to the superior colliculus, receives the retinal fibers; thus, a **retinocollicular** tract mediates vision. Because these animals lack a cerebral cortex as such, they have no primary visual receptive cortex.

3. In **higher animals**, the lateral geniculate body, which is a thalamic nucleus, receives the retinal axons, forming a **retinogeniculate tract**. A **geniculocalcarine tract** then relays visual impulses to the calcarine region of the occipital lobe (see Figures 9-9 and 9-11).

4. To reach the geniculate body, the retinogeniculate axons, which begin in the ganglionic layer of the retina, cross the retina (see Figure 9-5) and traverse the **optic nerve**, **optic chiasm,** and **optic tract**. In Figure 9-9, study the different visual-field defects caused by lesions at these three sites.

C. Course of optic nerve fibers through the chiasm

1. The optic nerve exits from the orbit into the intracranial cavity through the **optic foramen**, in company with the ophthalmic artery and vein. At the optic chiasm, approximately half of the axons of each optic nerve decussate (see Figure 9-9).

2. Figure 9-10 presents the actual course of the axons as they run through the chiasm and illustrates the following facts.
   a. The fibers from the **temporal** half of the macula and peripheral retina do not decussate, but run in the **ipsilateral** optic tract. Recall that the **temporal** half of the retina mediates the visual field in the **nasal** half of space (see Figure 9-6).
   b. Fibers from the **nasal** half of each retina decussate in the chiasm to reach the **contralateral** optic tract.
   c. The decussating axons form two knees (Figure 9-10, K_1 and K_2).
      (1) The knee (K_1) of axons from the **inferior** nasal retinal quadrant serves the **superior** temporal fields.

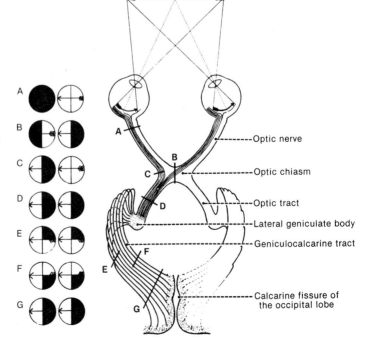

FIGURE 9-9. Visual pathway from the retina to the calcarine cortex, showing the visual-field defects resulting from lesions at sites *A–G*. The optic axons synapse in the lateral geniculate body, a feature not shown because of the scale of the drawing. *A* = complete blindness, left eye; *B* = complete bitemporal hemianopia; *C* = complete left nasal hemianopia; *D* = complete right homonymous hemianopia; *E* = complete right superior homonymous quadrantanopia; *F* = complete right inferior homonymous quadrantanopia; *G* = complete right homonymous hemianopia.

Optic nerve
Optic chiasm
Optic tract
Lateral geniculate body
Geniculocalcarine tract
Calcarine fissure of the occipital lobe

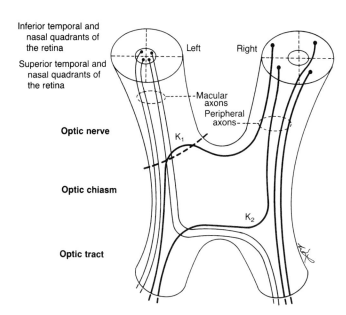

Inferior temporal and nasal quadrants of the retina

Superior temporal and nasal quadrants of the retina

Optic nerve

Optic chiasm

Optic tract

Left   Right

—Macular axons
Peripheral axons—

K_1

K_2

FIGURE 9-10. Actual pattern of decussation of the optic axons in the optic chiasm as viewed from above. Macular projection shown on *left*; peripheral retinal projection on *right*.

    (2) The knee (K_2) of axons from the **superior** nasal retinal quadrant serves the **inferior** temporal fields.

  d. Notice that the macular fibers (maculopapillary bundle) decussate posteriorly in the chiasm, forming a chiasm within a chiasm.

  e. Lesions that encroach on the chiasm may selectively affect these knees or certain groups of fibers, producing different field defects. For example, a lesion could affect the junction of the optic nerve and chiasm (see the dashed line in Figure 9-10). This lesion causes complete blindness of the **ipsilateral** eye (interruption of the optic nerve) and a **contralateral** superior temporal quadrantanopia (interruption of the knee formed by the inferior nasal retinal fibers of the contralateral eye).

D. **Relation of the optic chiasm to the surrounding structures**

  1. The optic chiasm sits just **below** the third ventricle and floor of the diencephalon, to which it attaches. The chiasm is just **above** the pituitary gland (see Figures 12-10 and 12-17).

  2. Obstruction of cerebrospinal fluid (CSF) through the cerebral aqueduct or out of the foramina of Luschka or foramen of Magendie causes the ventricular system to enlarge. In this case, the floor of the diencephalon balloons **downward** onto the chiasm, producing visual impairment and visual-field defects.

  3. Pituitary tumors expand **upward** from the sella turcica and encroach on the bottom of the chiasm. The tumor initially encounters and interrupts the decussating axons of the inferior nasal quadrants, producing a superior bitemporal quadrantanopia that may progress to a complete bitemporal hemianopia (see Figures 9-9 and 9-10).

  4. Aneurysms of the internal carotid artery (ICA) and circle of Willis may also encroach on the chiasm. Study the relationship of the blood vessels to the chiasm in Figure 15-9.

E. **Optic tract**

  1. The optic tract runs from the optic chiasm to the lateral geniculate body by encircling the midbrain-diencephalic junction (see Figures 7-1 and 7-2).

  2. The axons of the optic tract separate into two streams: a **retinogeniculate** tract and a **retinopretectal** tract.

    a. The **retinogeniculate** tract enters the lateral geniculate body. These axons mediate vision.

b. The **retinopretectal** tract continues past the genticulate body to enter the pretectal region, a region of the diencephalon just rostral to the midbrain tectum. These axons mediate the pupillary light reflexes.

The lateral geniculate body and geniculocalcarine tract

1. The lateral geniculate body, a thalamic sensory-relay nucleus, retains the topographic representation of the visual fields by the retinal axons. Its axons form the **geniculocalcarine tract**, which skirts the ventricular wall as the **external sagittal stratum** (Figure 9-11).

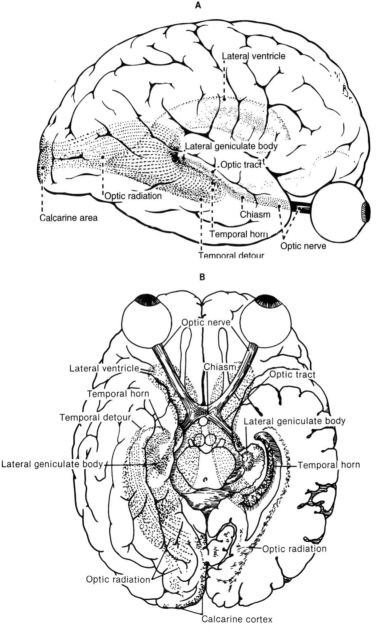

FIGURE 9-11. Phantom view of the cerebrum to show the anatomic relationship of the optic pathways to the cerebral wall. (*A*) Lateral view of the cerebrum. (*B*) Ventral view of the cerebrum. On the left, the temporal lobe is sectioned. (Reprinted with permission from Cushing H: *Trans Am Neurol Assoc* 47:374–423, 1921.)

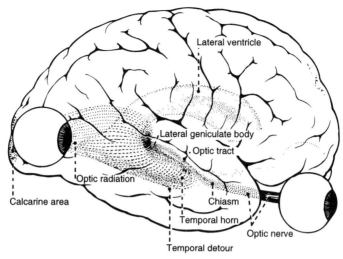

Lateral ventricle

Lateral geniculate body

Optic tract

Optic radiation

Calcarine area

Chiasm

Temporal horn

Optic nerve

Temporal detour

FIGURE 9-12. Superimposition of the eyeball on the occipital lobe provides a mnemonic for remembering the topographic representation of the retina and visual fields. (Reprinted with permission from Cushing H: *Trans Am Neurol Assoc* 47:374–423, 1921.)

2. The geniculocalcarine tract preserves the topographic representation of the visual fields, as does the calcarine cortex.
   a. Interruption of the **superior** fibers of the geniculocalcarine tract or the **superior** bank of the calcarine fissure causes contralateral **inferior** homonymous quadrantanopia (see Figure 9-9).
   b. Interruption of the **inferior** fibers of the tract or inferior bank of the calcarine cortex causes contralateral **superior** homonymous quadrantanopia (see Figure 9-9).
   c. Complete interruption of one geniculocalcarine tract or calcarine cortex causes complete contralateral homonymous hemianopia (see Figure 9-9).
   d. To remember the topography of the retina in the optic tract, geniculocalcarine tract, and calcarine cortex, merely set the eyeball back along the tract (Figure 9-12). Then recall the inversion of the visual field in relation to the retinal image (see Figure 9-6).
   e. With the eyeball superimposed on the occipital pole, the macula is represented posteriorly and the periphery of the retina more **anteriorly** (see Figure 9-12).

IV. THE EXTRAOCULAR MUSCLES AND THEIR ACTIONS

A. Classification of ocular muscles

1. Each eye has eleven muscles, classified as **smooth** or **striated** and **intraocular** or **extraocular** (Figure 9-13).
2. The **orbicularis oculi**, a striated sphincter muscle, closes the eyelids. Similar to the orbicularis oris that closes the mouth, it belongs to the facial, rather than the ocular muscles, because of its branchial origin and innervation by CN VII. The extraocular muscles proper all derive from somites.

B. Extraocular striated muscles

1. One of the seven extraocular muscles, the levator palpebrae, elevates the eyelid. The remaining six rotate the eyeball around one of its three axes (Figure 9-14).
2. **Origin and insertion of the ocular rotator muscles**
   a. Five of the six ocular rotator muscles **originate** from the annulus of Zinn. The inferior oblique muscle originates from the anterior rim of the orbit.

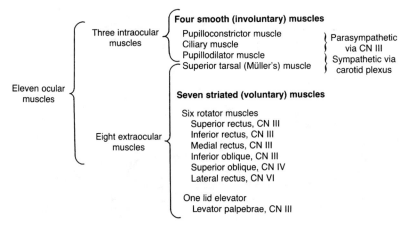

FIGURE 9-13. The eleven ocular muscles and their innervation.

FIGURE 9-14. The three rotational axes of the eye. *A-P* = anteroposterior; *L* = lateral; *V* = vertical.

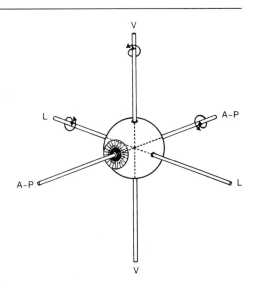

    b. All six rotator muscles **insert** on the sclera (Figure 9-15).

    c. The muscles of each eyeball act in agonist–antagonist pairs, or sets of muscles. The muscle or muscles that rotate the eyeball in one direction oppose the muscle or muscles that rotate it in the opposite direction. Table 9-3 lists the actions of the individual muscles.

C.   **Action of medial and lateral recti**

    1. The lateral rectus muscle **abducts** the eye, rotating the cornea **laterally**. Its paired antagonist, the medial rectus muscle, **adducts** the eye, rotating the cornea **medially**. Both muscles rotate the eye only around its vertical axis (see Figure 9-14).

TABLE 9-3. Movements of Individual Ocular Muscles

Muscle	Primary Action	Secondary Action	Tertiary Action
Medial rectus	Adduction		
Lateral rectus	Abduction		
Superior rectus	Elevation	Adduction	Intorsion
Inferior rectus	Depression	Adduction	Extorsion
Superior oblique	Depression	Abduction	Intorsion
Inferior oblique	Elevation	Abduction	Extorsion

2. A medial or lateral rectus muscle has only a **primary** action because it pulls "on center" and only **adducts** or **abducts** the eye.

3. The remaining ocular muscles, depending on the position of the eye, may pull "off center," which produces additional **secondary** and **tertiary** rotations (see Table 9-3).

D. Action of superior and inferior recti

1. The primary action of the superior and inferior recti is to elevate or depress the eyeball by rotating it around its **lateral** or **transverse** axis.

2. With the eye **abducted**, the superior rectus acts only as an elevator and the inferior rectus acts only as a depressor.

3. With the eye **adducted**, the elevator action converts to **adduction** and **intorsion** for the superior rectus, and **adduction** and **extorsion** for the inferior rectus. Torsions, intorsion or extorsion, rotate the eyeball around its **anterior–posterior** axis.

E. Action of superior and inferior oblique muscles

1. The primary action of the superior and inferior oblique muscles is to **depress** and **elevate** the eye when it is **adducted** by the medial rectus muscle.

2. With the eye **abducted** by the lateral rectus muscle, the depressor action of the superior oblique converts to **intorsion** and **abduction**.

3. With the eye **abducted** by the lateral rectus muscle, the elevation by the inferior oblique converts to **extorsion** and **abduction**.

4. Thus, with adduction, elevation or depression of the eye by the superior or inferior recti **decreases**. To compensate, the power of the obliques to elevate or depress the eye **increases** with the eye adducted.

F. Law of tonic oppositional action of ocular muscles

1. In any still position of the eyes, when looking straight ahead (primary position), or looking in any direction, all of the ocular muscles receive active tonic innervation.

2. With the eyes still, either straight ahead or deviated, the agonist and antagonist sets of muscles receive equal tonic innervation that cancels out their opposing actions and acts to keep the eyeball in place. Thus, positive tonic muscular activity maintains the position of the eyes.
   a. Two lines of evidence demonstrate the tonic innervation: electromyography and deviation of an eye after paralysis of a muscle.
      (1) An electromyographic needle inserted into any ocular rotatory muscle when the eyeball is not moving records a continuous play of muscular contraction (tonic innervation). Other skeletal muscles receive no nerve impulses and are electrically silent when the part they act on is not engaged in a volitional or postural action.
      (2) After paralysis of an ocular muscle, the tonic innervation of the intact antagonistic muscle rotates the eyeball toward its direction of action. For example, after **lateral** rectus palsy, the **medial** rectus muscle pulls the eye into adduction.

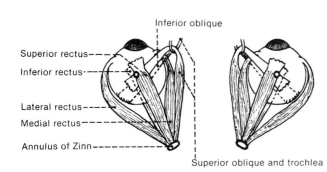

Inferior oblique

Superior rectus

Inferior rectus

Lateral rectus

Medial rectus

Annulus of Zinn

Superior oblique and trochlea

FIGURE 9-15. The eyeballs as seen from above, showing the origin and insertion of the ocular rotator muscles. All ocular rotator muscles originate from the annulus of Zinn, except for the inferior oblique muscle, which originates from the anterior rim of the orbit.

     b. After ocular-muscle paralysis and the resultant ocular malalignment, the retinal image is displaced off of the macula of the affected eye. The unaffected eye remains on target. The mind then sees two visual images, a condition called **double vision** or **diplopia**.

G. **Muscles that elevate the eyelid**

    1. The **levator palpebrae muscle**, a striated muscle innervated by CN III, originates from the optic foramen. It inserts into the tarsal plate of the upper eyelid. It holds up the eyelid tonically and further elevates it by involuntary or reflex actions when the person looks upward.

    2. The **superior tarsal muscle**, a smooth muscle innervated by the carotid sympathetic nerve, originates from connective tissue of the orbit and inserts into the tarsal plate. It acts tonically and involuntarily to set the height of the palpebral fissure; for example, the muscle further elevates the eyelid during fright, giving a wide-eyed appearance. The levator palpebrae muscle elevates the lid during voluntary gaze upward.

V. PERIPHERAL INNERVATION OF THE EYES

A. **Six nerves innervate the eyes** (Table 9-4)

TABLE 9-4. Innervation of the Eye by Its Six Nerves: Cn II, III, IV, V, VI, and Carotid Sympathetic

Number and Name of Nerve	Innervation	Clinical Effects of Interruption of Nerve
Efferent		
CN III (oculomotor nerve)	Striated muscle: superior, medial, and inferior recti; inferior oblique	Diplopia, eye abducted and turned down
	Levator palpebrae	Ptosis (paralysis of volitional lid elevation)
	Smooth muscle: pupilloconstrictor	Pupil dilated and fixed to light
	Ciliary muscle	Loss of lens thickening
CN IV (trochlear nerve)	Striated muscle: superior oblique	Diplopia, most severe on looking down and in; eye extorted; head tilted to side opposite paralyzed eye
CN VI (abducens nerve)	Striated muscle: lateral rectus	Diplopia, most severe on looking to side of paralysis; eye turned in (adducted)
Carotid sympathetic nerve	Smooth muscle: superior tarsal and pupillodilator	Bernard-Horner syndrome (ptosis, cormiosis, hemifacial anhidrosis, vasodilation)
Afferent		
CN II (optic nerve)	From retina	Blindness
CN V (trigeminal nerve)	Proprioceptive afferent	No known clinical effect
	Corneal/conjunctival afferents	Anesthesia of cornea with loss of corneal reflex

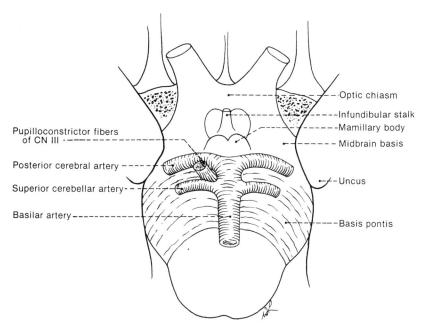

FIGURE 9-16. The parasympathetic pupilloconstrictor axons occupy the dorsomedial sector of CN III as it exits into the interpeduncular fossa and encounters the posterior cerebral artery.

B. **CN III, the oculomotor nerve** (see Figure 7-27)

1. Functional components

    a. The general somatic efferent (GSE) axons for the ocular rotatory muscles and the levator palpebrae originate in the oculomotor nucleus of the rostral midbrain tegmentum, just ventral to the periaqueductal gray matter. Longitudinally, the nucleus coincides with the superior colliculus.

    b. The general visceral efferent (GVE), parasympathetic axons for the pupilloconstrictor and ciliary muscles arise in the Edinger-Westphal nucleus, which forms a rostrodorsal cap over the oculomotor nucleus proper.

2. Course of CN III

    a. Intra-axially, CN III runs ventrally to exit into the subarachnoid space of the interpeduncular fossa (see Figures 7-20 and 12-9).

    b. Extra-axially, as it enters the interpeduncular fossa, CN III encounters the posterior cerebral artery (PCA) in the interpeduncular fossa (see Figures 9-16 and 15-9).

      (1) At the site of exit of CN III into the interpeduncular fossa from the midbrain basis, the parasympathetic axons of CN III cluster in the dorsomedial sector of the nerve (Figure 9-16).

      (2) The PCA may impinge on the pupillodilator fibers first if it is enlarged by an aneurysm, or displaced by herniation of a cerebral hemisphere (see Figure 1-12). In this case, pupillodilation precedes paralysis of the ocular-rotator muscles and warns the clinician of a life-threatening change in the patient.

    c. After passing the PCA, CN III enters the lateral dural leaf of the cavernous sinus (Figure 9-17).

    d. From the cavernous sinus, CN III enters the orbit through the superior orbital fissure (see Figure 7-23).

      (1) The **GSE axons** innervate the four rectus muscles and the inferior oblique muscle (see Figure 7-27).

      (2) The **parasympathetic axons** follow the inferior oblique branch of CN III and reach the ciliary ganglion through its short root (Figure 9-18).

3. The **ciliary ganglion** contains the parasympathetic, postganglionic neurons for the pupilloconstrictor and ciliary muscles. The postganglionic axons from the ciliary ganglion reach the eyeball in the **short ciliary** nerves (see Figure 9-18).

FIGURE 9-17. (*A*) Transverse (coronal) section through the cavernous sinus and sella turcica. CN III, CN IV, and the two sensory branches of CN V run through the lateral wall of the cavernous sinus; CN VI runs through the lumen. (*B*) Interior view of the base of the skull. The rectangle represents the section shown in Figure 9-17A. *ICA* = internal carotid artery; *V1* = ophthalmic division of CN V; *V2* = maxillary division of CN V.

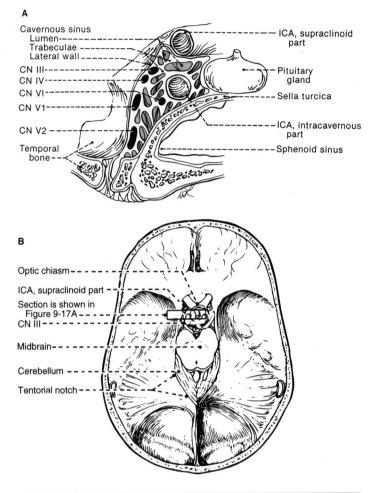

FIGURE 9-18. Lateral aspect of the right eye showing its innervation. Muscular branches of CN III: *IO* = inferior oblique; *IR* = inferior rectus; *LP* = levator palpebrae; *MR* = medial rectus; *SR* = superior rectus.

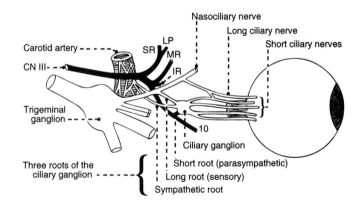

4. **Short ciliary nerves** convey three types of axons, including:
   a. **Postganglionic, parasympathetic axons** for the pupilloconstrictor and ciliary muscles (These are the only axons of the three types that actually synapse in the ciliary ganglion.)
   b. **Postganglionic, sympathetic vasomotor axons** to smooth muscle of the intraocular blood vessels
   c. **Afferent fibers** from the nasociliary branch of CN V for the interior of the eyeball

5. **The long ciliary nerve** (see Figure 9-18) conveys two types of axons, including:
   a. **Afferents**, mainly **pain afferents**, from the cornea and iris through the nasociliary branch of CN V (These axons mediate the corneal reflex.)
   b. **Sympathetic efferents** for the pupillodilator muscle

6. **Signs of CN III interruption** consist of lateral and downward deviation of the eyeball, pupillodilation, ptosis, and absence of lens thickening during accomodation for near vision.
   a. **Lateral and downward rotation of the eye** results from paralysis of the ocular rotatory muscles of CN III and the unopposed tonic innervation of the lateral rectus and superior oblique muscles. The patient experiences diplopia. Paralysis of the medial rectus muscle prevents adduction. If the patient attempts to adduct the eye and look down, the eye intorts because of the action of the superior oblique, but the superior oblique will not cause the eye to rotate down with the eye abducted.
   b. **Pupillodilation and absence of pupilloconstriction** in response to light or in accommodation results from paralysis of the pupilloconstrictor muscle.
   c. **Ptosis.** Paralysis of the levator palpebrae muscle causes severe ptosis that does not correct when the patient looks up. The usually mild ptosis caused by sympathetic paralysis corrects when the patient looks up, if the levator palpebrae muscle is intact.
   d. **Absence of lens thickening** causes blurred vision for near objects and occurs because of ciliary-muscle paralysis.

C. **CN IV, the trochlear nerve**

1. **Functional components.** CN IV contains GSE and general somatic afferent (GSA) axons for proprioception only.

2. **Course**
   a. **Intra-axially**, the axons originate in the trochlear nucleus, which is embedded in the medial longitudinal fasciculus (MLF) ventral to the inferior colliculus and aqueduct. The axons undergo a complete internal decussation and exit **dorsally** into the subarachnoid space, just caudal to the inferior colliculus (see Figure 7-3).
   b. **Extra-axially**, CN IV wraps around the midbrain and continues ventrally between the PCA and superior cerebellar artery (SCA) [see Figure 15-9]. After entering the lateral wall of the cavernous sinus (see Figure 9-17), CN IV runs through the superior orbital fissure to end on the superior oblique muscle, its only muscle.

3. **Unique anatomic features of CN IV**
   a. It undergoes complete internal decussation.
   b. It exits from the dorsal aspect of the brain stem.
   c. It has the smallest diameter of the 12 pairs of cranial nerves, and is the least myelinated.

4. **Signs of CN IV interruption.** The eye is extorted and elevated because of the unopposed action of the intact inferior oblique muscle. The patient has diplopia, which worsens when trying to look down with the eye adducted.

D. **CN VI, the abducens nerve**

1. **Functional components.** CN VI contains GSE and GSA axons for proprioception only.

2. **Course**
   a. **Intra-axially**, CN VI commences in the abducens nucleus beneath the floor of the fourth ventricle near the pontomedullary junction. Coursing ventrally, the axons enter the subarachnoid space at the pontomedullary sulcus. CN VI exits between the internal auditory artery and the anterior inferior cerebellar artery (AICA) [see Figure 15-9].
   b. **Extra-axially**, CN VI takes a long intracranial course. It turns rostrally, running along the length of the belly of the pons to enter the cavernous sinus where it runs in the lumen, in contrast to CN III, CN IV, and CN V, which run in the

lateral, dural wall of the sinus (see Figure 9-17). CN VI enters the orbit through the superior orbital fissure to innervate the lateral rectus muscle, its only muscle.

3. **Signs of CN VI interruption.** The eye remains adducted because of unopposed tonus of the medial rectus muscle. The patient complains of diplopia, which is most severe when the patient trys to abduct the affected eye to look to the side.

VI. ACTION AND INNERVATION OF THE SMOOTH MUSCLES OF THE EYE

A. The four **smooth muscles** of the eye consist of three **intraocular** muscles (the pupilloconstrictor, pupillodilator, and ciliary) and one **extraocular** muscle (the superior tarsal).

1. The pupillary muscles adjust the size of the pupil. The ciliary muscle adjusts the thickness of the lens. The superior tarsal muscle adjusts the height of the palpebral fissure.

2. **Parasympathetic axons** via CN III and the ciliary ganglion innervate the pupilloconstrictor and ciliary muscles.

3. **Sympathetic axons** via the carotid sympathetic nerve innervate the pupillodilator and superior tarsal muscles.

B. **The pupillary muscles**

1. The **iris**, a diaphragm between the cornea and lens, contains a central aperture of variable diameter, the pupil (see Figure 9-1).

2. **Pupillodilator muscle fibers** originate in the outer part of the iris and run radially to insert into the pupillary margin. Their contraction **enlarges** the diameter of the pupil.

3. **Pupilloconstrictor muscle fibers** encircle the pupillary border of the iris, forming a sphincter. Their contraction **reduces** the diameter of the pupil.

4. **Control of pupillary size**
   a. The pupils are almost exactly round, equal in size, and centered in the iris. They continuously change size.
      (1) Light, accommodation for near vision, and drowsiness or sleep **reduce** pupillary size.
      (2) Alertness, fright, pain, and strong emotion **increase** pupillary size. In fact, almost any pathway through the limbic system/hypothalamus or reticular formation (RF) may influence pupillary size.
   b. The pupil may constrict because of **increased** stimulation of the pupilloconstrictor muscles or **decreased** stimulation of the pupillodilator muscle. The reverse holds true for dilation of the pupil.
   c. Both the constrictor and dilator muscles receive tonic innervation. Paralysis of one of the two muscles will allow its antagonist to act unopposed. The pupil assumes the size dictated by the pull of the intact muscle; for example, after interruption of the sympathetic axons, the tonic innervation of the pupilloconstrictor muscle **decreases** the size of the pupil.

5. **Direct and consensual pupillary light reflexes**
   a. Either pupil constricts directly when its eye is illuminated, the **direct** pupillary light reflex. Either pupil also constricts equally when the opposite eye is illuminated, the **consensual** pupillary light reflex.
   b. Normally, both pupils constrict equally during either the direct or consensual reflex. Thus, illumination of one eye causes equal constriction of both pupils.

6. **Arc of the pupillary light reflex**
   a. The **afferent** arc is CN II; the **efferent** arc is CN III (Figure 9-19).

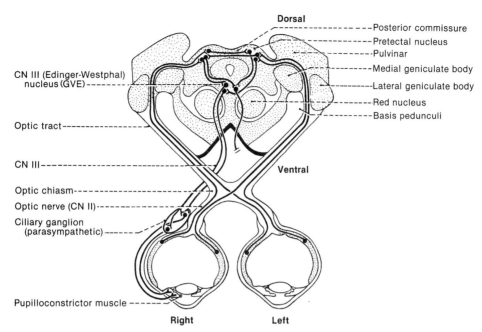

Dorsal
- Posterior commissure
- Pretectal nucleus
- Pulvinar
- Medial geniculate body
- Lateral geniculate body
- Red nucleus
- Basis pedunculi

CN III (Edinger-Westphal) nucleus (GVE)

Optic tract

CN III

Ventral

Optic chiasm

Optic nerve (CN II)

Ciliary ganglion (parasympathetic)

Pupilloconstrictor muscle

Right   **Left**

FIGURE 9-19. Pathway for the pupillary light reflex from the retina to the pretectum and Edinger-Westphal nucleus and back to the pupilloconstrictor muscle. *GVE* = general visceral efferent. (Redrawn with permission from Crosby E, Humphrey T, Lauer E: *Correlative Anatomy of the Nervous System.* New York, Macmillan, 1962, p236.)

b. The afferents for the pupillary light reflex presumably are collaterals of the axons that synapse in the lateral geniculate body. They depart from the optic tract as the **retinopretectal tract**.

c. These fibers or their pretectal connections disperse bilaterally from the pretectal region to the Edinger-Westphal nucleus. The bilateral dispersion of the pathway accounts for the normal equality of the direct and consensual pupillary light reflexes.

7. Effects of optic and CN III nerve lesions on pupillary light reflexes

    a. Consider a patient who is blind in one eye after interruption of one optic nerve.

        (1) Both pupils remain equal and will still constrict equally when the intact eye is illuminated. The consensual pupillary reflex of the affected eye during illumination of the other eye will remain intact.

        (2) Interruption of the afferent arc of the pupillary light reflex will abolish the direct pupillary light reflex of the affected eye **and** the consensual reflex of the opposite eye.

    b. Interruption of CN III (parasympathetic component) abolishes both the direct and consensual pupillary reflex of the affected eye.

        (1) The direct pupillary light reflex of the opposite eye and its consensual reflex to illumination of the affected eye remain intact.

        (2) The pupil of the affected eye is larger than the other because of unopposed action of the pupillodilator muscle.

C. **Brain stem pathways for pupillary control**

    1. Hypothalamic centers and their descending pathways

        a. Stimulation of the hypothalamus demonstrates overlapping areas that cause pupillodilation by sympathetic stimulation or by parasympathetic inhibition.

        b. The **parasympathetic inhibitory pathway** runs directly from the hypothalamus through the periventricular region and periaqueductal gray matter to the Edinger-Westphal nucleus.

    c. The **sympathetic excitatory pathway** takes a lateral course.
        (1) It enters the midbrain by running through the substantia nigra.
        (2) It then shifts to descend through the brain stem in proximity to the lateral spinothalamic tract. Its interruption in the medullary tegmentum accounts for the Horner syndrome component of the lateral medullary wedge syndrome (see Table 7-5).
        (3) In the cervical cord, the descending sympathetic pathway shifts to the lateral white column, near the plane of the denticulate ligaments. The axons end in the ciliospinal center of Budge, which contains the preganglionic neurons for the cervical sympathetic chain (see Figure 5-4).

2. Ascending brain stem pathways for pupillodilation. Two ascending pathways cause pupillodilation by inhibition of the Edinger-Westphal nucleus.
    a. One ascends in the paramedian RF, near the MLF.
    b. The other runs in or is identical with the lateral spinothalamic tract. It is in close proximity to the descending excitatory sympathetic pupillodilator pathway. This pathway, in part at least, mediates the spinociliary pupillodilation reflex to pain.

D. The ciliary muscle and the accommodation reflex for near vision

1. Accommodation for near vision requires the integration of three actions: **convergence** of the eyes, **pupilloconstriction**, and **lens thickening**.
    a. **Convergence** requires contraction of the medial recti, an act that occurs reflexly when the eyes pursue an object moving toward the observer. One can also volitionally look "cross-eyed." Either reflex or volitional convergence automatically triggers reflex pupilloconstriction and lens thickening.
    b. **Pupilloconstriction** blocks off the more peripheral rays that strike the cornea and iris, reducing spherical and chromatic aberration, thus promoting visual acuity during near vision.
    c. **Lens thickening** follows contraction of the ciliary muscle, an intraocular sphincter (see Figure 9-1).
        (1) Reduction of the sphincter diameter **relaxes** the suspensory ligaments of the lens.
        (2) The inherent elasticity of the lens causes it to thicken, increasing its refractive power to accommodate for near vision.

2. Supranuclear pathways for accommodation
    a. Cortical projection systems for accommodation arise in the occipital and frontal regions, pass through the deep white matter of the cerebrum, and synapse in the pretectal area for relay to the Edinger-Westphal nucleus.
    b. In the pretectal region, the fibers for accommodation are thought to run ventral to the retinopretectal pupilloconstrictor tract.
    c. Compression of the pretectal area from above, as from a pineal tumor, may abolish the pupillary light reflex, leaving pupilloconstriction in accommodation intact. Central nervous system (CNS) syphilis may also cause loss of the pupillary light reflex, with preservation of pupilloconstriction during accomodation. This feature, along with small, irregular pupils and iris atrophy, constitute the so-called **Argyll Robertson pupil**.

E. Carotid sympathetic nerve and central pathways (see Figure 5-4)

1. The carotid sympathetic nerve innervates the following:
    a. Superior tarsal muscle
    b. Pupillodilator muscle
    c. Smooth muscles of the carotid arteries and their intracranial and extracranial branches
    d. Sweat glands of the face
    e. Mucosal, salivary, and lacrimal glands of the head

2. Supranuclear pathways for the carotid sympathetic nerve descend from the hypothalamus to the preganglionic neurons (see Figure 5-4).

3. **Preganglionic neurons** are located in the intermediolateral column of the spinal cord gray matter from C8 to T2 or T3 (ciliospinal center of Budge). The axons leave the spinal cord with the T1 to T3 nerve roots, and ascend to the cervical sympathetic ganglia.

4. **Postganglionic neurons** are located in the superior cervical ganglion (see Figure 5-4).
   a. The postganglionic axons ascend at first along the carotid artery.
   b. In the middle ear, some sympathetic axons detour across the eardrum, forming a **corticotympanic plexus** with branches of CN IX. The sympathetic axons then rejoin the carotid artery.
   c. The neurons are adrenergic, except for most axons to sweat glands, which are cholinergic.

5. The sympathetic axons for the orbit leave the carotid artery, enter the orbit through the superior orbital fissure, and reach their terminal smooth muscles in the eye by the following three routes:
   a. Anastomosis with the nasociliary branch of CN V and, thus, via the **long ciliary nerves** to the pupillodilator muscle (see Figure 9-18)
   b. Anastomosis with the **short ciliary nerves** after passing through, but not synapsing in, the ciliary ganglion of the orbit (see Figure 9-18)
   c. Continuation with the ophthalmic artery after it branches from the carotid artery (see Figure 15-13)

6. **Horner's (Bernard-Horner) syndrome of sympathetic paralysis.** Interruption of the sympathetic excitatory pathway in the CNS or peripheral nervous system (PNS) results in characteristic signs **ipsilateral** to the lesion, including:
   a. **Miosis** (pupilloconstriction)
   b. **Ptosis** (mild and corrected when the patient uses the intact levator palpebrae muscle to look up)
   c. **Anhidrosis** of half of the face
   d. **Vasodilation** of half of the face

7. **Spinociliary reflex (often misnamed the ciliospinal reflex).** Pinching the skin of the neck or face results in bilateral pupillodilation. CN V or the dorsal roots of C2 or C3 convey the afferents to the RF and hence to the ciliospinal center of Budge or via inhibitory pathways to the Edinger-Westphal nucleus.

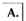

VII. **CENTRAL OR SUPRANUCLEAR PATHWAYS FOR THE CONTROL OF EYE MOVEMENTS**

A. Basic clinical neurophysiology of eye movements

1. **The supranuclear optomotor systems are designed to aim and align the eyes and control refraction.**
   a. **Aiming** enables each eye to find, fixate on, and pursue visual targets.
   b. **Binocular alignment** of the eyes produces stereopsis (binocular stereoscopic vision). It causes each of the eyes to receive the central rays from the visual target on the fovea centralis, and to receive the entire retinal image on corresponding points of each retina, allowing the mind to fuse the two retinal images into one visual image.
   c. **Refraction control** ensures maximum visual acuity in each eye.

2. **Conjugate eye movements and fusion.** Unless the eyes align when they are still and move conjugately during horizontal and vertical movements, the retinal images fall on noncorresponding retinal points. Because the mind cannot fuse the two noncorresponding retinal images into one visual image, the patient experiences diplopia.

3. **Vergences and accommodation.** The two eyes **converge** (cross) to accommodate for viewing near objects and **diverge** to be parallel to view distant objects. When the eyes align and view a distant object straight ahead, they are said to be in the **primary position**.

4. Volitional control and the fixation and visual-pursuit reflexes
   a. The act of finding a visual target is volitional. It depends on the mental set of the person and the attractiveness of the visual target. Volitional movements depend on **frontal** pathways to the brain stem.
   b. After the eyes find a visual target, **fixation reflexes** tend to lock the eyes onto the target. Then volition can override the fixation reflexes to select another target.

5. Volitional versus reflex control of eye movements and eye position
   a. If the visual target moves and the eyes reflexly pursue it from the primary position, **optokinetic** reflexes tend to kick the eyes back to the primary position. Optokinetic reflexes (i.e., pursuit and the kickback therefrom) depend on **occipital** and **occipitofrontal** pathways to the brain stem.
   b. If the head moves, reflexes tend to counter-roll the eyes against the direction of head movement to keep the eyes on the visual target. Thus, if the head moves to the **right**, the eyes counter-roll in equal degree to the **left**, staying aligned where they were. In the conscious person, these **doll's eye reflexes** depend on the vestibular system, abetted by the fixation reflexes (see Chapter 8 II G 2, I 2).
   c. Speed of eye movements
      (1) Eye movements are classified as **fast** or **slow**. All volitional eye movements, except vergences, are fast (saccadic).
      (2) The **deviation phase** of most reflex eye movements, particularly optokinetic and vestibular reflexes, is slow, but the kickback is saccadic. The phenomenon of repeated, rhythmic, slow deviations of the eyes and quick jerks back is called **jerk nystagmus**. It reflects derangement of the brain-stem pathways for optomotor control via vestibular and cerebellar systems.
      (3) Frontal efferent pathways mediate the saccades of volitional movements and are presumed to mediate the kickback saccades of reflexes.

B. **Basic clinical laws of the central and peripheral optomotor systems** (Table 9-5)

1. The law of tonic oppositional innervation of intra- and extraocular muscles. This law explains the positive positioning of the eyes in the normal person, and explains the deviation of the eyeball after paralysis of an extraocular muscle. It also explains why the pupil enlarges or constricts after interruption of its sympathetic or parasympathetic innervation (see IV F).

2. Law of conjugate alignment of the eyes. The eyes remain conjugate at rest and during horizontal and vertical movements, but they angle in or out during vergences.

3. The law of equal innervation (yoking) of corresponding ocular muscles of the two eyes during movement (Hering's law). The eyes move conjugately during reflex or volitional horizontal or vertical movements because of equal activation of the muscles that move the two eyes in the designated direction. When a person looks to the side, the **lateral** rectus muscle of the leading eye and the **medial** rectus muscle of the following eye receive equal innervation. Otherwise, the eyes would not remain aligned and the person would experience diplopia. Similarly, when looking to the right and then down, the medial and lateral recti are yoked to rotate the eyes to the right, and the right inferior rectus muscle and the left superior oblique muscles are yoked to rotate the eyeballs down.

4. The law of automatic return or kickback of the eyes to the primary position. The eyes tend to remain in the primary position or automatically return to it if deviated.
   a. Deviation of the eyes vertically, horizontally, or during convergence triggers a kickback reflex that tends to return them to the primary position (null point).
   b. The return of the eyes to the null point suggests the presence of an eye (and head) centering mechanism based on opposing vectors.
      (1) Although no single eye- and head-centering center exists as such, tonic innervation vectors that originate at various levels of the right half of the brain tend to drive the eyes to the left and are equally opposed by vectors from the left half of the brain.
      (2) Upward vectors counteract **downward** vectors.

TABLE 9-5. Summary of the Laws of Ocular Movements

The eyes align, fixate, and move conjugately, and the yoke muscles involved in conjugate deviation of each eye receive equal innervation (Hering's law). **Corollary:** If the eyes fail to act conjugately in aligning on visual targets, a lesion is present in the optomotor system at the level of the internuclear neurons or lower motoneurons, neuromuscular junction, or muscle.

The extraocular muscles and pupillomotor muscles act in agonist-antagonist pairs. Each muscle of the pair receives tonic innervation (i.e., a continuous flow of nerve impulses) that causes the pairs to balance each other's pull when the eyes are not moving. Thus, the position of the eyes is always positively determined. **Corollary:** Interruption of the nerve to an ocular rotatory or pupillomotor muscle causes the eye to deviate in the direction of pull of the intact muscle that opposes (antagonizes) the paralyzed muscle; or the pupil assumes the size dictated by the pull of the intact pupilloconstrictor or pupillodilator muscle.

The eyes and head tend to return to the primary, neutral position because of an active neurophysiologic centering mechanism. **Corollary:** Persistent (forced) or recurrent conjugate deviation of the eyes or head in any direction from the primary position is abnormal, indicating an imbalance in the drives that tends to keep the head and eyes in a neutral position.

The pathways for horizontal and vertical conjugate eye movements take different courses. **Corollary:** Central nervous system lesions may selectively paralyze conjugate eye movements in only one plane, horizontal or vertical.

Fast and slow eye movements originate in different sites and are mediated by different pathways. Saccadic (quick) movements require an intact frontotegmental pathway. **Corollary:** Central nervous system lesions may affect each form of movement separately.

When a conscious patient turns his or her head, the optic fixation reflexes and vestibular reflexes counter-roll the eyes against the direction of the turn, thus keeping the eyes on target. **Corollary:** When unconsciousness negates fixation, counter-rolling of the eyes depends solely on the vestibular system. The doll's eye test or head-turning test for counter-rolling enables the examiner to test the integrity of the vestibulo-optomotor system from CN VIII to CN III and, hence, the integrity of the MLF and tegmental core of the brain stem in a comatose patient.

Fixation, fusion of two images, pursuit, and vergences operate reflexly but can also be subordinated by volition, as can some forms of nystagmus. **Corollary:** A competition exists between reflex demand and volitional intent. Volitional movements tend to dominate or inhibit reflex ocular movements (e.g., induced nystagmus); or, if volitional pathways for eye movements are interrupted, certain optic reflexes (e.g., fixation) become exaggerated or "released" and the patient cannot voluntarily move the eyes from a point of fixation.

---

(3) The resultant of all of the vectors maintains the tonic oppositional innervation of ocular muscles and the tendency of the eyes to return to and remain in the primary position.

   c. An imbalance or instability in the deviation-kickback forces results in a to-and-fro oscillation of the eyes called **nystagmus.**

C. **Hierarchy of the optomotor system**

   1. The optomotor system has the same hierarchical plan as other motor systems with **supranuclear, internuclear, nuclear,** and **infranuclear** levels. The clinician systematically "thinks through" the levels to analyze abnormal eye movements.

   2. Supranuclear (cortical) pathways originate in nonlimbic and limbic cortex.

      a. Stimulation of almost any cortical or brain-stem area influences the position or movement of the eyes.

      b. Unilateral stimulation usually causes the eyes to move **contralateral** to the side of stimulation.

      c. Bilateral stimulation of mirror-image points of the right and left cerebral hemispheres, brain stem, or vestibular system produces **vertical** eye movements.

      d. Supranuclear pathways typically end on intermediate nuclei, which produce internuclear pathways to the LMNs, rather than directly on LMNs.

3. **Internuclear pathways** that influence the position or movement of the eyes arise in basal ganglia, the diencephalon, the brain stem tegmentum, the cerebellum, and the rostral part of the spinal cord.
    a. The major named internuclear pathway is the MLF (see VII E 5).
    b. In addition to the RF at large and the paramedian pontine RF (PPRF), several satellite or accessory nuclei of the pretectum, rostral brain stem tegmentum, and superior colliculi coordinate eye movements.

4. **The LMN optomotor nuclei** are CN III, CN IV, and CN VI. Their motoneurons provide the only axons to eye muscles and serve as the final common pathway for all reflex and volitional eye movements.

D. **Optomotor control systems and their clinical testing.** Eye movements result from the action of one of five systems (Table 9-6), each of which clinicians routinely test during a neurological examination (see Table 9-1 and Appendix VI A 3).

E. **Frontotegmental pathway for volitional horizontal conjugate eye movements** (Figure 9-20)

1. **Origin and course.** The posterior frontal cortex, or frontal eye field, originates axons for horizontal conjugate deviation of the eyes and head to the opposite side.
    a. The axons descend through the white matter of the hemisphere, through the internal capsule (and perhaps in the zona incerta slightly medial to the capsule), to enter the midbrain tegmentum.
    b. The pathway decussates between the caudal part of the midbrain and the rostral part of the pons (see Figure 9-20).

2. **Termination.** The decussated axons synapse near the abducens nucleus in the **PPRF**, a region sometimes called the **para-abducens nucleus**.

3. **Internuclear pathways for horizontal conjugate gaze**
    a. From the para-abducens region, internuclear pathways run:
        (1) **Ipsilaterally** to the LMNs of the abducens nucleus for the **lateral** rectus muscle
        (2) **Contralaterally** to ascend in the MLF to the LMNs of the **medial** rectus muscle in the nucleus of CN III (see Figure 9-20)
    b. These two pathways fulfill Hering's law of providing equal innervation to yoked muscles (e.g., the medial and lateral recti).

4. **Syndrome of interruption of the frontal horizontal gaze pathways**
    a. After destruction of the one frontal pathway, the eyes and head deviate to the side of the lesion because of the tonic innervation from the contralateral frontal region.
    b. Because of the proximity of the frontal eye field to the motor cortex that originates the pyramidal tract, the lesion usually also involves the motor cortex, causing contralateral hemiplegia. Thus, the hemiplegia is **contralateral** to a cerebral

TABLE 9-6. Five Major Eye Movement Systems

System	Function or Characteristic
Saccadic	Produces all volitional movements and the fast phase of reflex eye movements (frontal lobe)
Fixation (position maintenance)	Fixates eyes on target, maintains them on target, and locks the eyes in unison to fuse the two retinal images into one visual image (occipital lobe)
Smooth pursuit	Keeps eyes on moving target (occipital lobe)
Vergence	Converges or diverges eyes for near or distant targets (occipital lobe)
Counter-rolling	Vestibular and neck proprioceptive system; counter-rolls the eyes to keep them fixed on the visual target to compensate for head movement

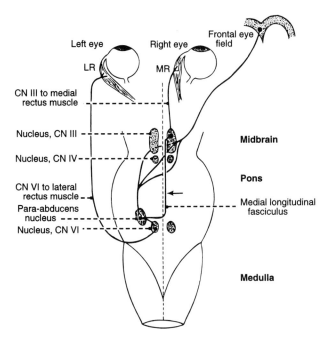

FIGURE 9-20. Frontotegmental pathway for volitional horizontal conjugate eye movements. Start at the frontal eye field of the cerebral cortex and trace the pathway down into the pons and to the medial and lateral rectus muscles. *LR* = lateral rectus; *MR* = medial rectus.

lesion, but the eyes and head deviate **ipsilaterally**. The deviation recovers within hours or days.

c. The frontotegmental horizontal gaze pathway (see Figure 9-20) mediates both the **volitional** and the **reflex** saccades. Reflex saccades kick the eyes back to the straight-ahead position in response to deviation.

  (1) **Unilateral destruction** of this pathway reduces or abolishes the kickback saccades that should occur after the slow phase of vestibular or optokinetic reflexes has deviated the eyes to the side of the relevant frontal eye field (think through Figure 9-20 to understand this statement). If the vestibular system or smooth pursuit system have deviated the eyes to the **right**, the right frontal eye field corrects the deviation by jerking the eyes back to the **left**, the primary position.

  (2) **Bilateral destruction** of the frontal horizontal gaze pathway causes paralysis of volitional movements of the eyes, but the eyes still deviate reflexly in response to vestibular stimulation during the counter-rolling test (doll's eye test) or during smooth pursuit.

5. **Syndrome of the MLF.** A unilateral lesion of the MLF (see Figure 9-20, arrow) causes a definite syndrome when the patient volitionally looks contralaterally.

  a. **Signs on neurologic examination** include:

    (1) Paresis or paralysis of adduction of the eye ipsilateral to the lesion when the patient attempts to look contralaterally, in this case to the left

    (2) Monocular nystagmus of the abducting eye (a feature that cannot be deduced from Figure 9-20)

    (3) Preservation of volitional eye movements in all other directions, including vertical gaze and convergence

  b. **Symptoms** of the MLF syndrome include:

    (1) **Diplopia** on contralateral gaze (from inaction of the medial rectus, which precludes fulfillment of Hering's law)

    (2) **Oscillopia**, an apparent oscillation of objects viewed (caused by nystagmus)

  c. **Neuroanatomic correlation.** Interruption of the frontal pathway through the MLF paralyzes adduction by the medial rectus muscle during volitional horizontal lateral gaze; however, the medial rectus muscles act during convergence because the convergence pathway, like the vertical gaze pathway, enters the midbrain directly, without looping down into the pons and back through the MLF (see VII F 3)

d. The most **common causes** of the MLF syndrome are multiple sclerosis, infarcts, and pontine neoplasms.

F. **Supranuclear pathway for volitional vertical eye movements** (Figure 9-21)

1. Origin. The volitional vertical gaze pathway apparently arises diffusely from the cerebral cortex, but mainly from frontal and occipital lobes.

2. Course and termination of the vertical gaze pathway
   a. From their diverse cortical origin, the axons converge on the pretectal region at the junction of the diencephalon and midbrain. The rostral interstitial nucleus of the MLF is an important way-station in the internuclear pathway for vertical gaze, similar to the PPRF in the horizontal gaze pathway, and also is involved in smooth pursuit and rotatory eye movements.
   b. **For vertical upward movements,** the pathway from the pretectal nuclei runs to the appropriate LMNs of CN III. The convergence pathway is similar.
   c. **For vertical downward movements,** the pathway runs through the RF dorsomedial to the red nucleus and then to the nucleus of CN III, directly or through synapse, in other accessory nuclei of the midbrain tegmentum or periaqueductal gray matter, probably the rostal interstitial nucleus of the MLF. A lesion in the tegmentum dorsomedial to the red nucleus selectively impairs volitional downward gaze.

3. Difference in the vertical and horizontal pathways for conjugate eye movements
   a. **The horizontal gaze pathway** has a recurrent loop down into the pons and back through the MLF to the midbrain (see Figure 9-20).
   b. **The vertical gaze pathway** runs directly to the pretectal-midbrain region without showing a recurrent loop (see Figure 9-21).
   c. Interruption of cortical efferent fibers in the midbrain or pontine basis may cause paralysis of horizontal gaze with complete preservation of vertical gaze (see the **locked-in syndrome** in Chapter 7 XIV D 1).

4. Syndromes of vertical gaze paralysis
   a. Diffuse cortical or white matter disease impairs volitional vertical eye movements before lateral movements.
   b. Downward compression of the pretectal area from above, as by a pineal tumor, initially causes selective paralysis of **upward** gaze, with **downward** gaze spared (Parinaud's syndrome).

FIGURE 9-21. Cortico-pretecto-midbrain pathway for volitional vertical conjugate vertical eye movements. Notice the bilaterality of connections in the pretectal region at the midbrain-diencephalic junction.

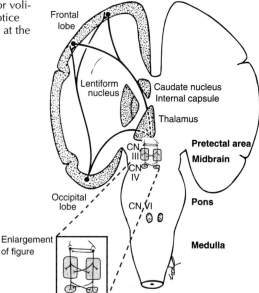

  c. Further compression may also paralyze downward gaze. Lesions confined to the region dorsomedial to the red nucleus may selectively paralyze downward gaze.

G. **Occipital pathways for visually mediated optomotor reflexes**

  1. The visually mediated optomotor reflexes are **fixation, fusion, pursuit, vergences,** and **optokinetic nystagmus.** They require an intact afferent arc through the retino-geniculo-calcarine pathway and an efferent arc from occipitofrontal cortex back to the pretectum and brain stem.

  2. From calcarine cortex, intracortical association pathways connect with the surrounding occipital, parietal, and frontal cortex, which originates the efferent fibers.

  3. The efferents from the cortex descend through the cerebral white matter to the pretectum or tegmentum, where they share the same internuclear pathways for horizontal and vertical movements already depicted (see Figures 9-20 and 9-21).

  4. Many of the pathways for visually mediated optomotor reflexes are poorly understood. For example, the **right** hemisphere is thought to mediate smooth pursuit of a target moving to the patient's **right,** while the right frontotegmental pathway mediates the leftward saccadic kickback toward the midline, as in optokinetic nystagmus. The occipitofrontal connections that would underly this action are not clearly identified.

  5. The superior colliculus coordinates eye and head position through the tectospinal tracts that act on the axial muscles that control the neck.

H. **Comparison of upper motoneuron (UMN) and LMN lesions of the optomotor pathways**

  1. Lesions of the LMNs, the final common pathway for all movements, paralyze the individual muscles and their actions in response to reflex and volitional movements.

  2. UMN (supranuclear) lesions do not paralyze the movements of the individual muscles, but affect **conjugate** movements by the yoked muscles of the two eyes.

  3. Because supranuclear and internuclear pathways arise from several sources, one or more pathways will remain intact after a central lesion. The clinician can use one of these alternative pathways to demonstrate the integrity of the LMNs; thus, if the patient cannot move the eyes to one side volitionally but can do so reflexly, the integrity of the LMNs is established. The lesion must affect the supranuclear or internuclear pathways, not the LMNs.

  4. In analyzing weakness of ocular movements, the clinician has to think through the entire optomotor pathway from the cortex to the brain stem and out through the neuromyal junction and the muscle itself. For example, weakness of lateral rotation of the eye (i.e., the action mediated by CN VI) requires thinking through the LMN system from the nucleus of CN III out along the path of the nerve, the neuromyal junction, and the muscle itself. Various lesions may cause loss of the motoneurons in the nucleus, interruption of the nerve, a chemical defect in cholinergic transmission at the neuromyal junction (myasthenia gravis), or primary muscle diseases (one of the muscular dystrophies). Any such lesion may cause weakness of an ocular rotatory muscle or of the levator palpebrae muscle.

STUDY QUESTIONS

DIRECTIONS: Each of the numbered items or incomplete statements in this section is followed by answers or by completions of the statement. Select the ONE lettered answer or completion that is BEST in each case.

1. Contraction of the lateral rectus muscle causes the eyeball to rotate

(A) laterally
(B) medially
(C) upward
(D) downward
(E) inward (intort)

2. A patient, after a head injury that contused the right orbit, complains of diplopia when looking down and to the left. The diplopia most likely represents weakness of

(A) the right superior rectus or left inferior oblique muscle
(B) the right superior oblique or left inferior rectus muscle
(C) the right lateral rectus or left medial rectus muscle
(D) the right inferior oblique or left superior rectus muscle
(E) none of the above

3. If a patient's left eye fails to adduct when attempting to look to the right, but the eye adducts during convergence, the lesion is in the

(A) left dorsal longitudinal fasciculus
(B) right medial lemniscus
(C) left medial longitudinal fasciculus (MLF)
(D) left side of the nucleus of CN IV
(E) left medial forebrain bundle

4. A patient with unilateral miosis, ptosis, and facial anhidrosis would most likely have a lesion of

(A) CN III
(B) CN VII
(C) the carotid artery
(D) the ciliary ganglion
(E) the greater superficial petrosal nerve

5. If the other cranial nerves remain intact, interruption of CN III results in rotation of the eyeball

(A) medially and upward
(B) medially and downward
(C) laterally and upward
(D) laterally and downward
(E) upward in the midline

6. A light ray striking the nasal side of the retina causes the person to experience a visual image as if coming from the

(A) opposite eye
(B) temporal side of space
(C) midpoint of the horopter
(D) visual axis
(E) none of the above

7. When a patient voluntarily deviates the eyes to the left, the cortical efferent pathway comes from the

(A) right frontal lobe
(B) left frontal lobe
(C) right occipital lobe
(D) left occipital lobe
(E) left temporal lobe

8. Ptosis in Horner's syndrome (Horner-Bernard sympathetic denervation syndrome) is characterized by

(A) disappearing or improving when the patient looks up
(B) being more pronounced when the patient looks up
(C) not changing when the patient looks up
(D) being better after rest
(E) none of the above

9. After CN III enters the subarachnoid space of the interpeduncular fossa, it immediately encounters

(A) CN IV
(B) the infundibular stalk of the pituitary gland
(C) the posterior cerebral artery (PCA)
(D) the dura mater
(E) the posterior clinoid process

10. A lesion that would affect CN III, CN IV, CN VI, and the ophthalmic division of CN V would most likely be in the

(A) pontine tegmentum
(B) cerebellopontine angle
(C) midbrain tegmentum
(D) cavernous sinus
(E) nasopharynx

11. A large acute destructive lesion of the left posterior frontal region would result in

(A) deviation of the eyes to the left
(B) deviation of the eyes to the right
(C) deviation of the eyes upward
(D) deviation of the eyes downward
(E) no deviation of the eyes

12. Which of the following statements about CN IV is true?

(A) It is one of the larger cranial nerves
(B) It innervates the superior and inferior oblique muscles
(C) It courses within the lumen of the cavernous sinus
(D) It wraps around the midbrain
(E) It conveys parasympathetic axons to the ciliary muscle

13. Select the one true statement about the cortical efferent pathway for vertical eye movements.

(A) The vertical pathway loops down into the pons and back up to the nucleus of CN III in the midbrain
(B) Most axons of the vertical pathway end directly on the lower motoneurons (LMNs) of the optomotor nuclei
(C) The vertical pathway acts unilaterally so that the left hemisphere pathway elevates the left eye, and the right the right eye
(D) The vertical pathway runs to all three optomotor nuclei, CN III, CN IV, and CN VI
(E) The vertical pathway for upward movements runs through the pretectum, separate from the pathway for downward movements

14. Select the one true statement about the consequences of optic atrophy.

(A) After optic nerve compression, the optic axons at the optic disc atrophy because of anterograde (Wallerian) degeneration
(B) The optic disc appears whiter than usual
(C) The borders of the disc become elevated
(D) The physiologic cup becomes smaller
(E) The direct pupillary light reflex remains in the affected eye

15. The optic nerve contains fibers from which one of the following sources?

(A) Lateral geniculate body
(B) Amacrine neurons
(C) Rods or cones
(D) Calcarine cortex of the occipital lobe
(E) Ganglion cell layer of the retina

16. A patient with Bell's palsy (acute inflammation of CN VII) would have paralysis of which of these ocular-related muscles?

(A) Pupillodilator
(B) Levator palpebrae
(C) Superior tarsal
(D) Orbicularis oculi
(E) Inferior oblique

17. A patient who complained of night blindness and inability to see objects in the periphery of the visual fields would have a lesion affecting which retinal-cell type?

(A) Cone cells of the macula
(B) Rod cells
(C) Amacrine cells
(D) Bipolar cells
(E) Horizontal cells

DIRECTIONS: Each of the numbered items or incomplete statements in this section is negatively phrased, as indicated by a capitalized word such as NOT, LEAST, or EXCEPT. Select the ONE lettered answer or completion that is BEST in each case.

18. Which of the following ocular actions or reflexes is NOT mediated through the occipital lobe?

(A) Vergences
(B) Smooth pursuit
(C) Binocular fixation
(D) Saccadic kickbacks
(E) Counter-rolling of the eyes with the eyes open and fixating

DIRECTIONS: Each set of matching questions in this section consists of a list of four to twenty-six lettered options (some of which may be in figures) followed by several numbered items. For each numbered item, select the ONE lettered option that is most closely associated with it. To avoid spending too much time on matching sets with large numbers of options, it is generally advisable to begin each set by reading the list of options. Then, for each item in the set, try to generate the correct answer and locate it in the option list, rather than evaluating each option individually. Each lettered option may be selected once, more than once, or not at all.

Questions 19–23

Match each lesion listed below with the resultant visual-field defect.

(A) Contralateral superior homonymous quadrantanopia
(B) Inferior altitudinal hemianopia (blindness in the inferior half of the visual field of both eyes)
(C) Partial contralateral inferior homonymous quadrantanopia
(D) Complete contralateral homonymous hemianopia without macular sparing
(E) Complete blindness

19. Bilateral destruction of the occipital lobes

20. Unilateral destruction of the inferior part of one parietal lobe

21. Destruction of the anterior two-thirds of the temporal lobe

22. Complete destruction of the calcarine cortex of one occipital lobe

23. Bilateral destruction of the superior bank of the calcarine fissure

DIRECTIONS: Each set of matching questions in this section consists of a list of four to twenty-six lettered options followed by several numbered items. For each numbered item, select the appropriate lettered option(s). Each lettered option may be selected once, more than once, or not at all. EACH ITEM WILL STATE THE NUMBER OF OPTIONS TO SELECT. CHOOSE EXACTLY THIS NUMBER.

Questions 24-25

(A) Cranial nerve (CN) II
(B) CN III
(C) CN IV
(D) CN V
(E) CN VI
(F) CN VII
(G) CN VIII
(H) Ciliary ganglion or short ciliary nerves
(I) Long ciliary nerves
(J) Carotid sympathetic nerve
(K) Greater superficial petrosal nerve
(L) Edinger-Westphal nucleus
(M) Caudal pontine basis near the pontomedullary sulcus
(N) Medial longitudinal fasciculus (MLF)

For each clinical deficit, select the nerve or anatomic site that could be responsible for its occurrence.

24. Unilateral pupillodilation (SELECT 3 CAUSES)

25. Double vision (SELECT 5 CAUSES)

ANSWERS AND EXPLANATIONS

1. The answer is A [IV C 1]. The lateral rectus muscle causes the eyeball to abduct or rotate laterally. No matter which position the eyeball is in, the lateral rectus can only abduct the eye when it contracts. Its antagonist, the medial rectus muscle, can only adduct the eye. Thus, these two muscles have only one action each. The other eye muscles have a variable action, depending on the position of the eyeball when the muscle contracts.

2. The answer is B [IV D, E; Figure 9-15]. When a person looks downward and to the left, the right superior oblique muscle is yoked with the left inferior rectus muscle. When the eyes look conjugately in any direction, the muscle that is the prime mover of the leading eye acts in unison with (i.e., is yoked to) a muscle of the following eye, which corresponds. Both muscles receive equal innervation in order to move the eyes equally to maintain the visual axes of both eyes on the target, thus avoiding diplopia. Orbital injuries often impair the action of the superior oblique muscle because of displacement of the trochlea, which attaches to the anterior rim of the orbit and acts as a sling for the recurrent course of the trochlear tendon.

3. The answer is C [VII E 5 a; Figure 9-20]. When an eye fails to adduct on voluntary horizontal gaze, but it does adduct during convergence, the lesion interrupts the medial longitudinal fasciculus (MLF). This internuclear bundle conveys the voluntary pathway from the paramedian pontine reticular formation (PPRF) to the lower motoneurons (LMNs) of the medial rectus muscle. These LMNs reside in the nucleus of CN III. A lesion of the LMNs themselves or of their axons in CN III would paralyze adduction during volitional movements, convergence, and all other optomotor reflexes. The upper motoneuron (UMN) pathway from the cortex that activates the medial rectus during convergence runs directly into the midbrain and nucleus of CN III, rather than looping down into the pons and returning to the midbrain via the MLF. The common causes of the MLF syndrome are brain stem infarcts and multiple sclerosis.

4. The answer is C [VI E 6 a-c]. Unilateral miosis, ptosis, and anhidrosis indicate interruption of the sympathetic innervation of that half of the face. Because the sympathetic axons travel along the carotid artery, lesions of that vessel, such as aneurysms, may interrupt the sympathetic axons.

5. The answer is D [V B 6 a]. After interruption of CN III, the eyeball turns laterally and down. The tonic contraction of the intact lateral rectus muscle will turn the eyeball laterally, and that of the superior oblique muscle will turn the eyeball down and intort it. CN III innervates the muscle that would normally counteract the foregoing two muscles.

6. The answer is B [III A 2 a; Figure 9-6]. The retinal image is inverted in relation to the origin of light rays. Thus, a light ray that comes from the temporal side of the visual field would strike the nasal side of the retina. The person learns to interpret a stimulus on the nasal side of the retina as coming from the temporal half of space.

7. The answer is A [VII E 1; Figure 9-20]. The law of contralateral innervation of movements by the upper motoneuron (UMN) pathways applies to horizontal eye movements. Thus, the motor area of the right frontal lobe sends impulses to the lower motoneurons (LMNs) for voluntary deviation of the eyes to the left. The cortical efferent axons terminate in the paramedian pontine reticular formation (PPRF), also known as the para-abducens center, which relays to the LMNs per se.

8. The answer is A [VI E 6 b]. Sympathetic denervation paralyzes the superior tarsal muscle. This muscle acts tonically and involuntarily to elevate the eyelid and set the height of the palpebral fissure, but it does not further contract during voluntary movements. The levator palpebrae muscle acts to elevate the lid further during voluntary upward gaze. Because the levator palpebrae muscle receives its innervation from CN III, it will still act to elevate the lid, even after paralysis of the superior tarsal muscle.

9. The answer is C [V B 2 b; Figure 9-16]. After CN III enters the subarachnoid space of the interpeduncular fossa, it loops under the posterior cerebral artery (PCA). Downward traction on the PCA by herniation of the adjacent temporal lobe may cause the artery to impinge on CN III. It first compresses the pupilloconstrictor axons in the dorsomedial sector of CN III. As a result of compression of the pupilloconstrictor axons, the tonic action of the pupillodilator muscle enlarges the pupil. As the midbrain compression increases, the extraocular muscles innervated by CN III become paralyzed. Unilateral pupillary dilation in the comatose patient is an important clinical sign of progressive brain herniation, which may kill the patient unless treated.

10. The answer is D [Figure 9-17]. The cavernous sinus syndrome involves varying combinations of paralysis of CN III, CN IV, and CN VI and sensory loss in the ophthalmic division of CN V. These nerves come into conjunction in the lateral wall of the cavernous sinus. Lesions that would commonly cause the syndrome are aneurysmal dilations of the intracavernous portion of the internal carotid artery (ICA), cavernous sinus thrombosis, or neoplasms of the base of the skull. Involvement of the carotid artery might also cause Horner's syndrome, owing to interruption of the postganglionic sympathetic axons that travel along the artery.

11. The answer is A [VII E 4]. An acute, large destructive lesion of the left frontal lobe will result in deviation of the head and eyes to the left. Under normal circumstances, the left side of the brain acts to turn the eyes to the right, and the right side acts to turn the eyes to the left. When a lesion destroys an area of special significance for eye deviation, such as the posterior frontal eye fields, the eyes will deviate to the side of the lesion because the intact, opposite side of the brain acts unopposed, whereas the damaged side cannot generate a saccade or tonic innervation to move the eyes to the opposite side. Unilateral cerebral lesions do not paralyze vertical eye movements.

12. The answer is D [V C 2 b]. CN IV is unique in many ways. It is the smallest of the cranial nerves. It undergoes complete internal decussation in the brain stem and exits dorsally from the midbrain just caudal to the inferior colliculus. It then wraps around the midbrain, crosses the subarachnoid space (in common with all cranial nerves), and enters the lateral wall of the cavernous sinus. Neither CN IV nor CN VI of the optomotor group of nerves convey autonomic axons.

13. The answer is E [VII F 1–4; Figure 9-21]. The vertical eye movement pathways run directly into the pretectum and midbrain without looping down through the pons. The pathway

for vertical downward eye movements run just dorsomedial to the red nucleus. The pathway for vertical upward movements runs more dorsally, through the pretectal region, and thence to the midbrain tegmentum. Thus, lesions may selectively paralyze upward or downward movements of the eyes. Horizontal eye movements, having a separate pathway, may be spared in spite of vertical paralysis. Conversely, lesions may interrupt the horizontal gaze pathway, as in the locked-in syndrome, but vertical eye movements remain intact.

14. The answer is B [II C 3 a]. Optic nerve fibers originate in the retina. After compression of the optic nerve or chiasm, the optic nerve axons undergo retrograde degeneration back into the retina, toward their perikarya of origin. Because the axons degenerate back into the retina, they disappear from the optic disc. The capillaries that had given the disc its pink color also disappear. The entire optic disc appears white because the lamina cribrosa of the sclera has been denuded of capillaries. The physiologic cup disappears because it is only a depression in the middle of the ring of nerve fibers that converge on and penetrate the optic disc from the retina. The consensual pupillary light reflex, initiated by the opposite eye, remains intact, but the direct light reflex disappears.

15. The answer is E [II D 5 b]. The optic nerve contains axons that arise in the ganglion cell layer of the retina. The rods and cones and amacrine neurons of the retina do not send fibers into the optic nerve, nor does the lateral geniculate body in which the optic nerve fibers end, nor does the calcarine cortex. Although the optic nerve may contain a few efferent fibers, their origin and functional significance are unknown.

16. The answer is D [IV A 2]. The muscles in and around the eyes receive their innervation from a variety of different nerves. The facial nerve innervates the orbicularis oculi muscle. Thus, in Bell's palsy, the patient cannot close or blink the eye. All the rest of the intra- and extraocular striated muscles receive their innervation from CN III, CN IV, or CN VI. Autonomic nerves innervate the smooth muscles, the pupilloconstrictor and dilator ciliary muscles, and the superior tarsal muscles.

17. The answer is B [II D 3]. The retina functions as a dual organ. The macula mediates central vision (i.e, visual acuity, color, and the central part of the visual field). The periphery of the retina mediates night vision and motion detection. The rod cells dominate in the periphery, and the cones dominate in the macula. Specific degenerative diseases can affect either the rods or the cones, causing defects specific to their functions. The amacrine, horizontal, and bipolar cells, as well as the ganglion cells, occur throughout the retina.

18. The answer is D [VII G 1–4; Table 9-6]. Several ocular movements or actions require an intact afferent arc from the retina to the occipital lobe. These include vergences, smooth pursuit, and binocular fixation. When the eyes counter-roll in response to head movement in the awake patient, the ocular fixation reflexes act to hold the eyes on target, along with the vestibular system. In the unconscious patient who cannot fixate, the vestibular system can still counter-roll the eyes. On the other hand, saccadic movements (i.e., the normal voluntary movements of the eyes) originate in frontal lobe pathways. The saccades, such as in response to evoked nystagmus, do not require an intact retino-occipital pathway.

19–23. The answers are 19-E, 20-C, 21-A, 22-D, 23-B [III C 2 e, F 2 a–c; Figure 9-9]. The topographic representation of the visual fields is very strict. For this reason, lesions affecting particular sites along the optic path cause very characteristic and reproducible field defects. Lesions of the parts of the geniculocalcarine pathway as it courses through the hemispheric wall cause different field defects, depending on the location. Because the geniculocalcarine fibers course deep in the white matter, in the external sagittal stratum (which is a few millimeters lateral to the ventricular wall), the cerebral lesions that cause field defects may be deep within the white matter rather than limited to the cortex or immediately subjacent white matter. A lesion of the more anterior loops of the geniculocalcarine tract around the temporal horn causes a contralateral superior quadrantanopia, which is more or less complete, depending on the number of fibers affected.

As the geniculocalcarine tract proceeds backward, the fibers that represent the inferior visual fields course through the inferior part of the parietal lobe. Hence, lesions of the inferior parietal region that interrupt these fibers give rise to a contralateral inferior homonymous quadrantanopia.

Unilateral lesions of the calcarine regions of the occipital lobe likewise cause contralat-eral defects, which may vary from partial quadrantanopia to a complete contralateral hemianopia. Bilateral occipital lobe destruction causes double hemianopia or, in essence, complete blindness.

Lesions of the superior or inferior banks of the calcarine fissure, either unilateral or bilateral, cause quadrantanopias or hemianopias, depending on the extent of the tissue destroyed. Destruction of either the superior banks or the inferior banks on both sides causes an altitudinal hemianopia. Destruction of the superior banks causes an inferior altitudinal hemianopia in both eyes; destruction of the inferior banks causes a superior altitudinal hemianopia.

Lesions of the cerebral white matter beyond the actual course of the geniculocalcarine tracts do not cause field defects, nor do lesions of the corpus callosum, the tract of axons that connects the two hemispheres. Interruption of the corpus callosum interferes with transfer of visual information from one hemisphere to the other, but does not cause field defects.

24. The answers are: B, H, L [VI B 6, 7; Figures 9-18 and 9-19]. Unilateral pupillodilation may result from lesions of the preganglionic parasympathetic neurons of the Edinger-Westphal nucleus, in the intra- or extra-axial course of cranial nerve (CN) III to the ciliary ganglion, and from the ganglion through the short ciliary nerves to the pupilloconstrictor muscle of the iris. After paralysis of the pupilloconstrictor muscle, the pupil dilates because of the tonic innervation of the pupillodilator muscle, conveyed by the carotid sympathetic nerve. Both the intra- and extraocular muscles receive constant, tonic innervation. Thus, after interruption of the nerve to one muscle, the other muscle (i.e., its antagonist) continues to operate unopposed. Interruption of one optic nerve does not change pupil size. The size remains the same because the afferent optic axons from each eye disperse equally in the pretectal region and Edinger-Westphal nucleus.

25. The answers are: B, C, E, M, N [VII B 3, E 3 a, b; Figure 9-20]. The normal conjugate alignment of the eyes causes the central rays from the visual target to fall on corresponding retinal regions. The mind then fuses the two separate retinal images into one visual image. Interruption of cranial nerve (CN) III, CN IV, and CN VI, which activate the extraocular muscles, will result in disconjugate alignment. A lesion may affect the intra-axial course of CN III, CN IV, or CN VI, such as in the caudal pontine basis traversed by CN VI, or the lesion may occur in the extra-axial course.

Anatomical connections in the brain ensure that each ocular muscle that participates in a given conjugate movement receives equal innervation, guaranteeing correct alignment. Thus, when the patient looks to one side, the lateral rectus muscle of one eye and the medial rectus muscle of the opposite eye receive equal innervation (Hering's law) and rotate each eye the same degree (i.e., conjugately). The medial longitudinal fasciculus (MLF) conveys the impulses from the parabducens eye region that fulfills Hering's law during conjugate horizontal eye movements. The parabducens center sends equal impulses ipsilaterally to the lower motoneurons (LMNs) of the lateral rectus muscle in CN VI and contralaterally through the MLF to the LMNs of the medial rectus muscle in CN III. After interruption of the MLF, the medial rectus does not receive the same innervation as the lateral rectus. The patient will experience diplopia, particularly when looking to the side opposite of the weak muscle, because the medial rectus does not rotate the eye to preserve conjugate alignment.

Chapter 10

Cerebellar System

I. GROSS ANATOMY OF THE CEREBELLUM

A. **Definition.** The cerebellum is a fist-sized, transversely fissured mass of central nervous system (CNS) tissue attached to the dorsum of the pons by peduncles (Figure 10-1; see Figure 1-3).

B. **Composition.** The cerebellum basically consists of the following:

1. Cortex sulcated into numerous parallel transverse **folia** (see Figures 1-8B and 10-1)

2. Deep white matter

3. Paired deep nuclei

4. Paired peduncles that convey afferent and efferent nerve fibers (see Figure 10-10)

C. **Location and anatomical relationships of the cerebellum**

1. The cerebellum occupies the posterior fossa, along with the medulla, the pons, and most of the midbrain.

2. The **cerebellar tentorium**, a dural partition, roofs the posterior fossa, separating the cerebellum from the overlying temporo-occipital lobes of the cerebrum (see Figures 1-12 and 1-13).

3. Supported by its peduncles, the cerebellum overhangs the anterior and posterior medullary vela (the tectal roof of the fourth ventricle) [see Figure 10-3].

4. By slicing the peduncles transversely, the cerebellum falls free from the pons and thus from the neuraxis (see Figure 10-10).

5. Removing the cerebellum fully exposes the rhomboid fossa, the floor of the fourth ventricle.

D. **Transverse subdivision of the cerebellum into three lobes**

1. Transverse clefts or fissures, which are much deeper than the folia, separate the groups of folia into **lobes** and **lobules**. The three cerebellar lobes are (Figures 10-2 and 10-3; see Figure 10-1):
   a. **Anterior lobe**
   b. **Posterior lobe**
   c. **Flocculonodular lobe**

2. Figure 10-2 depicts the cerebellar lobes as if they were flattened out. In reality, the flocculonodular lobe is rolled underneath (compare Figures 10-1, 10-2, and 10-3.)

E. **Three sagittal subdivisions of the cerebellum**

1. Two parasagittal cuts isolate a midline **vermis** from the two **cerebellar hemispheres** (see Figure 10-2).

2. Any sagittal or parasagittal cut reveals the characteristic foliar pattern of the cerebellum and the deeper fissures, which demarcate the three major lobes and minor lobules (see Figure 10-3).

F. **Cerebellar tonsils**

1. A cerebellar tonsil forms the medioventral border of the posterior lobe of each cerebellar hemisphere (see Figure 10-1B).

2. Between the two tonsils is a large subarachnoid space, the **cerebellar vallecula** (cisterna magna cerebelli). In the depths of the vallecula, the following structures can be seen:
   a. The posterior medullary velum, which forms the roof of the fourth ventricle (see Figure 10-3)

   b. The **foramen of Magendie**, a median perforation in the posterior medullary
   velum that allows cerebrospinal fluid (CSF) to exit from the fourth ventricle into
   the subarachnoid space of the vallecula (cisterna magna cerebelli)

3. Dissecting the tonsils off discloses the entire posterior medullary velum.

4. Whenever the intracranial pressure increases, the tonsils tend to herniate downward, out of the posterior fossa and through the foramen magnum (see Figure 1-12).

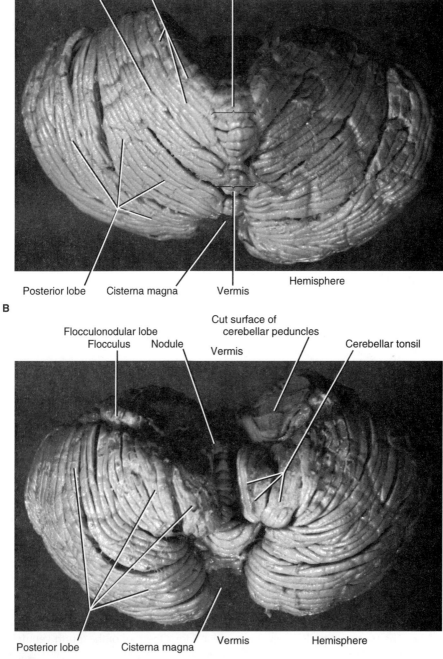

FIGURE 10-1. Gross photographs of the cerebellum. (*A*) Superior surface. (*B*) Inferior surface.

C

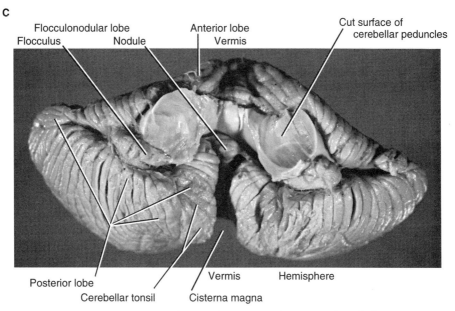

Flocculonodular lobe   Anterior lobe   Cut surface of
Flocculus   Nodule   Vermis   cerebellar peduncles

Posterior lobe   Vermis   Hemisphere
Cerebellar tonsil   Cisterna magna

FIGURE 10-1. (*C*) Anterior view, showing the transversely sectioned cerebellar peduncles.

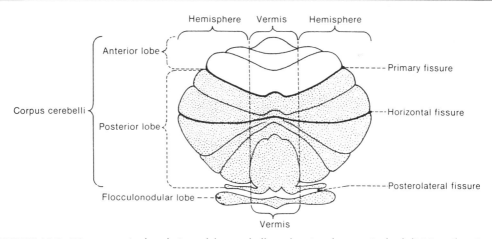

FIGURE 10-2. Diagrammatic dorsal view of the cerebellum showing three sagittal subdivisions (hemisphere, vermis, and hemisphere) and three transverse subdivisions (anterior lobe, posterior lobe, and flocculonodular lobe) [Larsell's nomenclature].

By compressing the medullocervical junction, tonsillar herniation causes quadriplegia and respiratory arrest.

G. **Three deep nuclei of the cerebellum**

1. Three paired nuclear masses, buried in the cerebellar white matter, overlay the fourth ventricle (Figure 10-4).

2. In medial-to-lateral order, the three nuclei are:
   a. **Fastigial nucleus** (nucleus fastigii), whose name comes from its location near the fastigium of the fourth ventricle
   b. **Interpositus nucleus**
      (1) The interpositus nucleus consists of two nuclei: nucleus emboliformis and nucleus globosus.
      (2) It is called the **interpositus** nucleus because of its interposition between the dentate and fastigial nuclei.

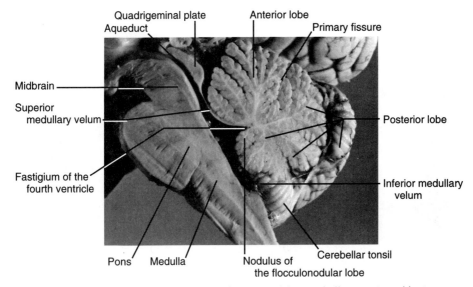

Quadrigeminal plate
Aqueduct
Anterior lobe
Primary fissure
Midbrain
Superior
medullary velum
Posterior lobe
Fastigium of the
fourth ventricle
Inferior medullary
velum
Pons   Medulla
Nodulus of
the flocculonodular lobe
Cerebellar tonsil

FIGURE 10-3. Gross photograph of a sagittal section of the cerebellar vermis and brain stem.

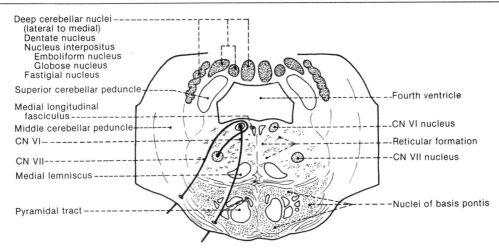

Deep cerebellar nuclei
(lateral to medial)
Dentate nucleus
Nucleus interpositus
Emboliform nucleus
Globose nucleus
Fastigial nucleus
Superior cerebellar peduncle
Medial longitudinal
fasciculus
Middle cerebellar peduncle
CN VI
CN VII
Medial lemniscus
Pyramidal tract
Fourth ventricle
CN VI nucleus
Reticular formation
CN VII nucleus
Nuclei of basis pontis

FIGURE 10-4. Transverse section of the pons, middle cerebellar peduncle, fourth ventricle, and overlying deep cerebellar nuclei in the roof of the fourth ventricle.

    c. Dentate nucleus (nucleus dentatus), which is the largest and most lateral of the cerebellar nuclei (It receives the name **dentate** from its corrugated or tooth-like outline, which closely resembles the inferior olivary nucleus.)

II. ONTOGENY, PHYLOGENY, AND FUNCTION OF THE CEREBELLUM

A. Ontogeny

    1. The cerebellum develops as two hillocks, one in each of the paired rhombic lips of the pons (Figure 10-5).

    2. The hillocks unite in the midline at the roof plate to form the solid cerebellar mass.

    3. Because the cerebellum develops as a thickening in the dorsal wall of the neural tube, not an evagination, it has no ventricular cavity, even though it bulges over the fourth ventricle.

B. **Phylogeny and function**

1. In vertebrates, the flocculonodular lobe appears first.

2. Originally, the flocculonodular lobe developed out of the vestibular nuclei. It retains, even in primates, direct afferent and efferent vestibular connections, reflecting its phylogenetic origin.

3. The flocculonodular-vestibular system coordinated automatic or reflex contractions of the axial muscles to relate the position and movements of the head, eyes, and trunk to each other, to the planes of space, and to the pull of gravity.

4. As the cerebrum came to produce willed movements of the trunk and as the limbs evolved, the cerebellum was adopted to activate the contractions of both the **axial** and **appendicular** muscles during willed postures and willed movements. The cerebropontocerebellar pathway enlarged in parallel with the enlargement of the:
   a. Cerebral motor cortex and pyramidal tracts
   b. Basis pontis
   c. Inferior olivary complex
   d. Cerebellar hemispheres and dentate nucleus

5. The essential clinical sign of cerebellar lesions is **dystaxia**; that is, incoordination of muscular contractions during willed movement or willfully sustained postures.

C. **Phylogenetic/functional nomenclature of the cerebellar lobes**

1. The cerebellum consists of three units of different phylogenetic ages, connections, and function: the **archicerebellum**, the **paleocerebellum**, and the **neocerebellum**. These units correspond to Larsell's lobar subdivisions of the cerebellum (Table 10-1).
   a. The **archicerebellum** (the flocculonodular lobe, or vestibulocerebellum) is the original part of the cerebellum, elaborated in relation to the vestibular nuclei.
   b. The **paleocerebellum** (the anterior lobe, or spinocerebellum) receives the proprioceptive trunk and limb afferents from the spinal cord.
   c. The **neocerebellum** (the posterior lobe, or cerebrocerebellum) receives the corticopontocerebellar pathway and the projection from the inferior olivary nucleus.

2. In turn, each of these three phylogenetic/anatomical/functional subdivisions projects to its own midline nucleus (see Table 10-1).

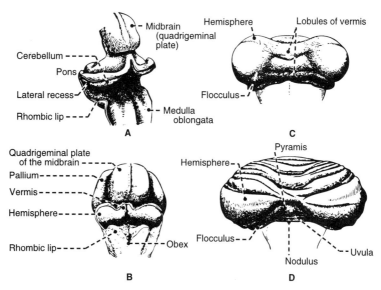

FIGURE 10-5. Dorsal view of the developing cerebellum. (*A*) Six weeks (6 ×). (*B*) Two months (4 ×). (*C*) Four months (3 ×). (*D*) Five months (2.8 ×). (Reprinted with permission from Arey LB: *Developmental Anatomy*. Philadelphia, WB Saunders, 1946, p 441.)

TABLE 10-1. Organization of the Cerebellum into Triads

Larsell's Lobar Subdivisions	Phylogenetic/ Functional Subdivisions	Afferent Peduncle	Efferent Peduncle	Deep (Midline) Nucleus	Olivary Nucleus (Medulla)
Flocculonodular lobe	Archicerebellum (vestibulocerebellum)	Caudal	Caudal	Fastigial	Medial accessory
Corpus cerebelli Anterior lobe	Paleocerebellum (spinocerebellum)	Rostral and caudal	Rostral	Interpositus (emboliform and globose)	Dorsal accessory
Posterior lobe	Neocerebellum (cerebrocerebellum)	Middle	Rostral	Dentate	Inferior

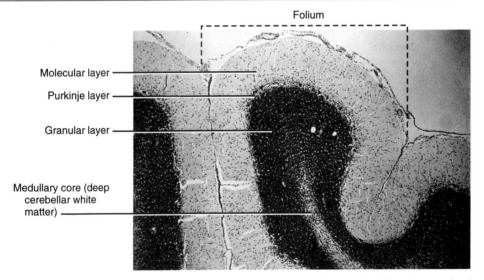

FIGURE 10-6. Photomicrograph of a Nissl-stained transverse section of cerebellar folia, showing the three layers of the cerebellar cortex (40 ×).

III. CEREBELLAR CORTEX

A. Neuronal layers and neuronal types

1. The cerebellar cortex appears the same over the entire surface of the cerebellum and exhibits the same three layers of neuronal perikarya: **molecular, Purkinje cell,** and **granular** (Figure 10-6).

2. The three cortical layers contain five types of neurons (Figure 10-7 and Table 10-2).

3. Although the perikaryon of each neuron occupies only one of the cortical layers, either the dendrites or axons or both extend into or through the other layers.

B. Orientation of cerebellar neurons

1. Many cortical neurons and their processes have a definite spatial orientation to the plane of the folia. Figure 10-7 shows a folium cut across at right angles to its long axis, like slicing a loaf of bread.

2. **Orientation of Purkinje dendrites**
   a. Figure 10-7 shows that the dendrites of the Purkinje neurons and Golgi type II neurons poke up into the molecular layer.

    b. The Purkinje neuron dendrites are flattened to occupy only one plane, a plane **transverse** to the long axis of the folium.

    c. To remember the orientation of the Purkinje cell dendrites, place your hands flat on the sides of your head with your palms on your ears. The plane of your fingers is now across (transverse to) the long axis of the folia and, therefore, represents the actual flat plane of the dendrites of your own Purkinje neurons (and the Golgi type II neurons and stellate neurons).

3. Orientation of granule neuron axons (see Figure 10-7)

    a. The axons of the granule neurons ascend into the molecular layer where they bifurcate.

    b. After they bifurcate, these axons run **parallel** to the long axis of the folia and **parallel** to each other, hence the name **parallel** fibers.

    c. Visualize the parallel axons as electrical wires running across the dendritic trees of several Purkinje, Golgi type II, and stellate neurons, upon which they synapse.

4. Orientation of stellate neuron dendrites and axons (see Figure 10-7)

    a. The dendrites of the inner stellate neurons of the molecular layer occupy the **transverse** plane of the folia, like the dendrites of the Purkinje and Golgi type II neurons.

    b. Their axons also run in the **transverse** plane; thus, they run at right angles to the parallel fibers or tangential to the contour of the folia. Hence, they are called **tangential** fibers. Their terminal axons form **basket** fibers around the perikarya of Purkinje neurons; hence the name basket cells (see Figure 10-7).

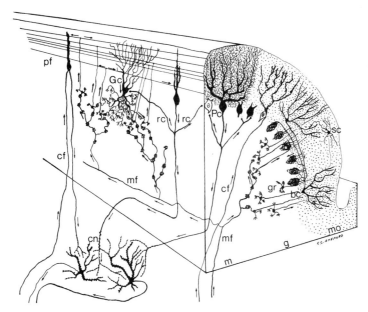

FIGURE 10-7. Stereogram of a transversely cut cerebellar folium, as the neurons and interneuronal connections would appear in Golgi silver impregnations. *bc* = basket cells; *cf* = climbing fiber; *cn* = deep cerebellar nuclei; *g* = granular layer; *Gc* = Golgi cell; *gr* = granule cell; *m* = medullary layer; *mf* = mossy fiber; *mo* = molecular layer; *Pc* = Purkinje cell; *pf* = parallel fiber; *rc* = recurrent collateral; *sc* = stellate cell. (Reprinted with permission from Crosby EC, Humphrey T, Lauer EW: *Correlative Anatomy of the Nervous System.* New York, Macmillan, 1962, p 196.)

TABLE 10-2. Five Types of Neurons in the Cerebellar Cortex and the Layers That Contain Their Perikarya

Neuron	Layer
Outer stellate Inner stellate (basket)	Molecular
Purkinje	Purkinje
Golgi type II (Golgi stellate) Granule	Granular

5. Intrafolial and interfolial connections
   a. The parallel fibers that arise from granule cells run laterally in the molecular layer of the folia. They synapse on the dendrites of the Purkinje, inner stellate, and Golgi type II neurons that extend into the molecular layer, thus forming extended **intrafolial** connections (see Figure 10-7).
   b. The tangential fibers connect the Purkinje neurons in the anterior-posterior plane forming **intrafolial** and **transfolial** or **interfolial** connections.

C. **Mode of termination of the afferent fibers in cerebellar cortex.** The afferents to the cerebellar cortex end as **mossy** or **climbing** fibers.

1. Mossy fibers originate in the spinocerebellar, cuneatocerebellar, vestibulocerebellar, and pontocerebellar systems. The majority of afferents to the cerebellar cortex end as mossy fibers.
   a. After collateralizing to the deep cerebellar nuclei, each axon further produces numerous collaterals that end as tight coils that give the mossy fibers their name.
   b. Each mossy ending forms the core of a glomerulus of the granular layer of the cerebellar cortex. Thus, each axon may affect thousands of granular neurons.

2. Climbing fibers originate from the inferior olivary nucleus.
   a. After collateralizing to the deep cerebellar nuclei, they ascend to the cortex and climb directly up onto the Purkinje neuron dendrites, hence their name.
   b. The relationship of the climbing fibers to the Purkinje cells is nearly one to one.

D. **Cerebellar glomeruli**

1. The mossy fibers end in coiled, rosette-like terminals. Each rosette forms the core of a structure called a **glomerulus**.

2. Each glomerulus consists of a continuous glial capsule that encloses the incoming mossy fiber rosette and its complicated functional contacts with Golgi type II neurons and granule neurons (Figure 10-8). The rosette provides one input to the glomerulus, the Golgi type II neuron provides the other. The **output** is via the axons of granular neurons.
   a. The claw-like dendrites of many granule neurons and the proximal parts of the dendrites of Golgi type II neurons enter the glomerulus to receive the input from the rosette (see Figure 10-8).

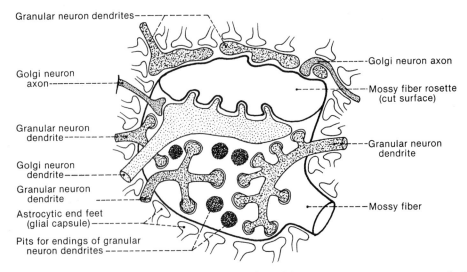

FIGURE 10-8. Reconstruction of electron microscope studies of the synaptic connections in a cerebellar glomerulus.

TABLE 10-3. Five Neuron Types of the Cerebullar Cortex* and Their Synaptic Connections

Neuron Type	Afferent Connections	Axonal Distribution
Outer stellate	Receive parallel fibers from granule neurons	Axons synapse on outer part of Purkinje neuron dendrites
Inner stellate	Receive parallel fibers from granule neurons	Axons form tangential fibers that synapse on Purkinje perikarya via basket collaterals
Purkinje	• Climbing fibers from extracerebellar sources • Parallel fibers from axons of the granule neurons of the cerebellar cortex • Basket fibers from the inner stellate neurons • Axons from the outer stellate neurons • Noradrenergic afferents from nucleus locus coeruleus	Most Purkinje axons run to deep nuclei. A few Purkinje axons, originating in the flocculonodular lobe, bypass the deep nuclei to reach the vestibular nuclei. Purkinje axons also send recurrent collaterals back to themselves and to Golgi type II neurons
Golgi type II	Receive mossy fiber and climbing fiber synapses on dendrites in granular layer and receive parallel axons on dendrites that extend into the molecular layer	Send axons to cerebellar glomeruli to synapse on mossy fiber rosettes
Granule	Receive rosette endings from mossy fibers in cerebellar glomeruli	Send parallel fibers to the Purkinje neuron dendrites and inner and outer stellate neurons of the molecular layer and those parts of Golgi type II neuron dendrites that penetrate the molecular layer

*The neurons are listed in order from superficial to deep as they appear in the cerebellar cortex (see Figure 10-7).

    b. The axons of the Golgi type II neurons also enter the glomerulus.
        (1) They contact the incoming mossy fiber endings, constituting **axo-axonic** synapses.
        (2) The Golgi neuron axons also contact the dendrites of the granular neurons, constituting **axo-dendritic** synapses. Thus, both the axons and dendrites of Golgi type II neurons make contacts with the mossy fibers.

  3. The axons of the granular cells then enter the molecular layer of the cerebellar cortex. The axons bifurcate into parallel fibers that end on the dendrites of Purkinje, Golgi, and stellate neurons (see Figure 10-7 and III B 3).

E. **Synaptic connections of the Purkinje neurons of the cerebellar cortex.** The Purkinje cell is the focal neuron of the cerebellar cortex because of the following.

  1. All afferent pathways ultimately converge on the Purkinje cell.

  2. Purkinje axons are the only way out of the cerebellar cortex, its "final common pathway."
    a. A small minority of Purkinje axons leave the cerebellum. They synapse directly on vestibular nuclei.
    b. The vast majority of Purkinje axons remain in the cerebellum, where they synapse on the deep cerebellar nuclei. The deep nuclei originate most of the efferent fibers that leave the cerebellum.

  3. Purkinje axons, in a curious arrangement, send a recurrent collateral back to adjacent Purkinje cells and to Golgi type II neurons (see Figure 10-7).

F. **Summary of synaptic connections of the cerebellar cortex** (study Table 10-3)

TABLE 10-4. Inhibitory and Excitatory Connections of the Cerebellar Cortex and Deep Nuclei

Inhibitory intrinsic neurons of the cerebellar cortex
    Golgi type II neurons of the granular layer
    Purkinje neurons
    Inner and outer stellate neurons
Excitatory intrinsic neurons of the cerebellar cortex
    Granule neurons
Excitatory extrinsic and intrinsic fibers
    Climbing fibers and mossy fibers, both the direct fibers to the cerebellar cortex and their collaterals to the midline nuclei
    Parallel fibers from granule neurons
Inhibitory intrinsic fibers*
    Basket fibers
    Purkinje fibers
Cerebellar nuclei
    Inhibited by Purkinje fibers
    Excited by collaterals from climbing and mossy fibers and may have their own intrinsic excitatory pacemaker

*There are no inhibitory extrinsic fibers, at least from somatic afferent systems.

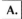

Summary of excitatory and inhibitory synapses of the cerebellar cortex

1. All incoming climbing and mossy fibers produce **excitatory** synapses.

2. Of the intrinsic cerebellar cortical neurons, only the granule neuron axons (parallel fibers), which act by glutamate transmission, produce excitation.

3. Four of the five types of intrinsic neurons of the cerebellar cortex produce **inhibitory** synapses (Table 10-4).

IV. THE CEREBELLAR CIRCUITS

A. **General plan**

1. The cerebellum receives and sends well-defined afferent and efferent pathways.
   a. Its **afferent pathways** arise in sensory systems, motor cortex, and reticular formation (RF).
   b. Its **internal circuitry** converges on the Purkinje cells, most of which relay through the cerebellar nuclei.
   c. Its **efferent pathways** arise from the cerebellar nuclei, which influence parts of the brain stem and thalamus that ultimately act on the lower motoneurons (LMNs).

2. All afferents enter the cerebellum through one of the three cerebellar peduncles, and all efferents leave through either the superior (rostral) or inferior (caudal) cerebellar peduncle.

3. Because the peduncles attach the cerebellum to the pons and only the pons, all afferent and efferent pathways of the cerebellum run through the pons during at least part of their course.

4. The motor and sensory afferent axons turn dorsally in one of the peduncles, send a collateral to a deep cerebellar nucleus, and proceed through the medullary cores of the folia to reach the cerebellar cortex.

B. **Afferent systems to the cerebellum**

1. Sensory system afferents to the cerebellum

a. Proprioceptors provide a major source of cerebellar afferents. Proprioceptive pathways arise in:
(1) Muscle spindles
(2) Joint receptors and Golgi tendon organs
(3) Vestibular end organs

b. The other somatic sensory systems (i.e., special and general) from the spinal cord and brain stem project to the vermis, but the function and clinical significance are unknown.

c. The respective sensory receptive cortices (i.e., somatosensory, auditory, and visual) send cortical efferents to the cerebellar regions that receive impulses from the afferent pathway for that sensory modality. These fibers travel in the corticopontocerebellar pathway that synapses in the basis pontis.

2. Cortical and RF relay systems to the cerebellum

a. In addition to the corticopontocerebellar pathway through the basis pontis, corticobulbar fibers project to the inferior olivary nuclei, cerebellar nuclei of the RF, and vestibular nuclei. These nuclei then project to the cerebellum.

b. The cerebral cortex projects to some RF nuclei classed as "cerebellar nuclei" (see Figure 7-38) because of strong projections to the cerebellum.

c. The nucleus locus coeruleus projects noradrenergic axons to the cerebellum, as it does to all other subdivisions of the CNS (see Chapter 14 II D 1, 2).

3. Topographical distribution of afferents in the cerebellar cortex

a. Vestibular afferents end mainly in the flocculonodular lobe, caudal vermis, and lingula.

b. Spinocerebellar and **trigeminocerebellar afferents** end in the cortex of the vermis, predominantly of the anterior lobe. These cerebellar afferents end somatotopically, with the lower extremity represented most rostrally (Figure 10-9).

c. Basis pontine afferents of the corticopontocerebellar relay system decussate in the basis and end mainly in the cortex of the contralateral cerebellar hemisphere with no overlap in the vermis.

d. Olivary afferents end in a topographical medial-to-lateral manner.
(1) The smaller nuclei of the inferior olivary complex project to the vermian cortex.
(2) The main inferior olivary nucleus projects to the cortex of the contralateral cerebellar hemisphere.

e. Nucleus locus coeruleus afferents project to the cerebellar cortex diffusely.

C. **The pathways through the cerebellar peduncles**

1. On each side of the pons, three peduncles—the **rostral** (superior), **middle**, and **caudal** (inferior)—unite into one stalk of fibers that attach the cerebellum to the pons (Figure 10-10).

2. The caudal and rostral peduncles contain afferent and efferent tracts; the middle peduncle is afferent (Table 10-5).

3. The **caudal** peduncle is largely afferent but conveys some cerebellovestibular connections.

a. The caudal peduncle conveys two components: the **restiform** body and the **juxtarestiform** body (see Table 10-5).

b. The **juxtarestiform** body runs in the medial part of the peduncle, next to the fourth ventricle, and conveys the vestibulocerebellar and cerebellovestibular pathways (Figure 10-11).

c. In Figure 10-11, the uncinate fasciculus (hook bundle of Russell) is so named because it loops or hooks over the rostral cerebellar peduncle as it emerges from

FIGURE 10-9. Sagittal sections through the cerebellar vermis. (*A*) Normal control. (*B*) Cerebellum of alcoholic patient who had dystaxia of the legs and trunk (rostral vermis syndrome). The cerebellar vermis receives the spinocerebellar and trigeminocerebellar tracts in inverted topographic order. The cerebellum in *B* shows atrophy of the culmen, which receives the leg and trunk fibers. *A* = arm; *F* = face; *L* = leg area; *T* = trunk. (Courtesy of Dr. Jans Muller, Indiana University School of Medicine, Indianapolis, IN.)

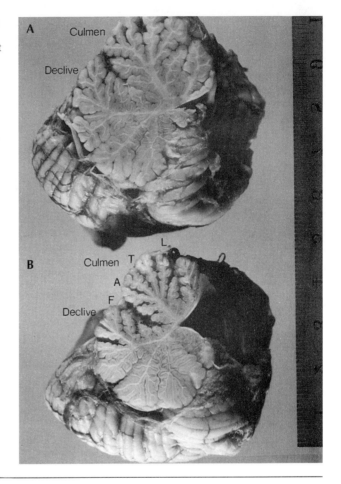

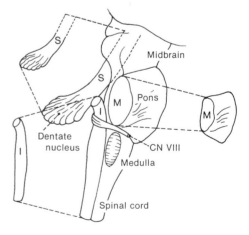

FIGURE 10-10. Exploded lateral view of the cerebellar peduncles. *I* = inferior or caudal cerebellar peduncle; *M* = middle cerebellar peduncle; *S* = superior or rostral cerebellar peduncle.

the dentate nucleus and deep cerebellar white matter. The hook bundle then synapses in the vestibular nuclei and RF.

    d. The **dorsal** spinocerebellar tract enters the cerebellum via the restiform body.

  4. The **middle** peduncle is afferent. It conveys the pontocerebellar pathway.

    a. It is the largest and most lateral of the cerebellar peduncles.

    b. It mainly consists of decussated fibers from the nuclei of the contralateral half of the basis pontis.

5. Rostral peduncle
   a. The rostral peduncle conveys two major efferent pathways from the dentate nucleus: the **dentatothalamic** and the **dentatorubral** tracts.
   b. The ventral spinocerebellar tract, an afferent pathway, curves dorsally to enter through the rostral peduncle.

D. | **Summary of the connections of the deep cerebellar nuclei**
   1. The Purkinje cells provide the largest input to the cerebellar nuclei.
      a. The Purkinje cells of the **median** or **vermian** cortex project to the fastigial nuclei. These nuclei connect with the vestibular nuclei, which produce a vestibulospinal tract. Stimulation of the fastigiovestibular pathway inhibits the vestibular nuclei, which in turn reduces extensor muscle tone.
      b. The **paramedian** or **paravermian** zone projects to the interposed nuclei (globose and emboliform). The emboliform nucleus projects to the red nucleus, which sends axons back to the emboliform nucleus and the decussated **rubrospinal** tracts to the spinal cord. Stimulation of this pathway facilitates flexor muscle tonus.

TABLE 10-5. Major Tracts in the Cerebellar Peduncles

Peduncle	Tracts	Afferent/Efferent
Caudal (inferior)	Restiform body	
	Dorsal spinocerebellar tract	A
	Olivocerebellar tract	A
	Arcuatocerebellar tract	A
	Reticulocerebellar tract	A
	Cuneocerebellar tract	A
	Juxtarestiform body	
	Direct and secondary vestibulocerebellar tracts	A
	Cerebellovestibular tracts	E
Middle	Pontocerebellar tracts	A
Rostral (superior)	Ventral spinocerebellar tract	A
	Trigeminocerebellar tract	A
	Tectocerebellar tract	A
	Brachium conjunctivum (dentatorubrothalamic tract)	E

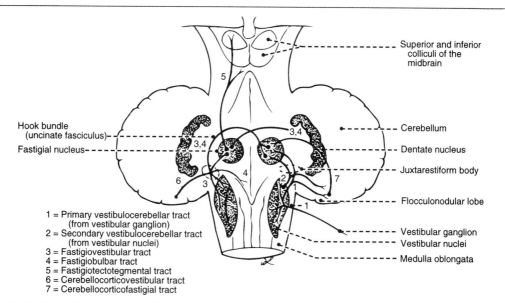

1 = Primary vestibulocerebellar tract (from vestibular ganglion)
2 = Secondary vestibulocerebellar tract (from vestibular nuclei)
3 = Fastigiovestibular tract
4 = Fastigiobulbar tract
5 = Fastigiotectotegmental tract
6 = Cerebellocorticovestibular tract
7 = Cerebellocorticofastigial tract

Hook bundle (uncinate fasciculus)
Fastigial nucleus

Superior and inferior colliculi of the midbrain
Cerebellum
Dentate nucleus
Juxtarestiform body
Flocculonodular lobe
Vestibular ganglion
Vestibular nuclei
Medulla oblongata

FIGURE 10-11. Dorsal diagram of the cerebellum and brain stem showing the vestibulocerebellar connections.

c. The **lateral** or **hemispheric** cerebellar cortex projects to the dentate nuclei. These nuclei project to the red nucleus, the thalamus (nuclei ventralis lateralis, ventralis posterolateralis, and rostral intralaminar), and the inferior olivary nuclei. This pathway assists in the coordination of willed movements.

2. In addition to Purkinje axons, other afferents to the deep nuclei arise from:
   a. Collaterals of pontocerebellar fibers
   b. Collaterals from climbing fibers of the olivary complex and the mossy fibers
   c. Collaterals from the trigeminal nuclei
   d. Direct or collaterals from RF nuclei, nucleus locus coeruleus, and raphe of the brain stem

3. The output from the deep cerebellar nuclei is mainly excitatory.

V. THE CEREBRO-CEREBELLO-PYRAMIDAL PATHWAY

A. Clinical importance

1. The single most important cerebellar circuit connects the cerebellum with the cerebral motor cortex and, through the pyramidal tract of the latter, to the LMNs. In its entirety, it consists of a cerebrocortico-ponto-cerebellocortico-dentato-thalamo-cortico-pyramido-LMN circuit (Figure 10-12).

2. Interruption of the coordinating influence of the cerebellum on the motor cortex causes the outstanding clinical sign of cerebellar dysfunction, the incoordination of willed movements and willed postures (**ataxia**).

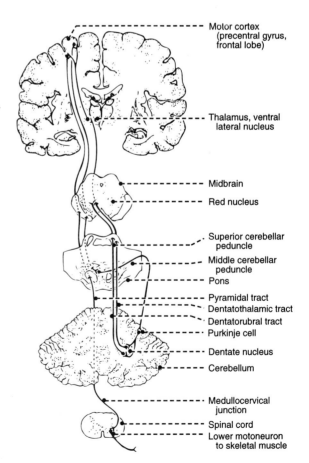

FIGURE 10-12. Diagram of the cerebrocerebellocerebral circuit. Commence at the cerebral motor cortex and trace through the circuit, noting the sites of the decussations. Decussation 1 is in the pons; decussation 2 is in the midbrain; and decussation 3 is the pyramidal tract at the medullocervical junction.

Motor cortex (precentral gyrus, frontal lobe)

Thalamus, ventral lateral nucleus

Midbrain

Red nucleus

Superior cerebellar peduncle

Middle cerebellar peduncle

Pons

Pyramidal tract

Dentatothalamic tract

Dentatorubral tract

Purkinje cell

Dentate nucleus

Cerebellum

Medullocervical junction

Spinal cord

Lower motoneuron to skeletal muscle

B. **Decussations and laterality of cerebellar signs**

1. Notice in Figure 10-12 the two decussations of the cerebrocerebellar circuit.
   a. One decussation is in the pontocerebellar pathway through the basis pontis and the middle cerebellar peduncle.
   b. The other decussation is in the pathway through the rostral cerebellar peduncle as it passes through the caudal midbrain tegmentum on its way to the thalamus.

2. Notice that the circuit brings the coordinating influence of one cerebellar cortex to bear upon the **contralateral** motor cortex. The pyramidal tract from that motor cortex will then decussate before reaching the LMNs. Thus, the entire circuit has three significant decussations, which you should know.

3. Because of the three decussations, a lesion in one cerebellar hemisphere will impair coordination in the **ipsilateral** extremities.

4. Thus, the clinical aphorism is that cerebral hemisphere lesions cause **contralateral** motor signs [the pyramidal syndrome (see Table 6-3)] and cerebellar hemisphere lesions cause **ipsilateral** motor signs.

5. Interruption of the dentatothalamic pathway **before** it decussates causes ipsilateral signs; interruption **after** it decussates causes contralateral signs. Think through the circuit in Figure 10-12 to understand the laterality of cerebellar signs.

VI. CLINICAL EFFECTS OF CEREBELLAR LESIONS

A. **Conditions under which cerebellar signs occur**

1. The cerebellum functions to coordinate the sequence, strength, and velocity of muscular contractions during:
   a. Willed movements of trunk, limbs, and bulbar muscles
   b. Willed postures, such as the vertical posture or holding the hands out

2. Unless the patient can make a voluntary muscular contraction (i.e., mediated through the pyramidal pathways), the cerebellum and its pathways cannot be tested clinically. Therefore, the clinician cannot test the patient's cerebellar pathways during:
   a. Sleep
   b. Coma
   c. Paralysis caused by an interrupted pyramidal tract or neuromuscular system

3. Cerebellar lesions have no clinically explicit effect on mentation, consciousness, memory, sensory perception, or autonomic functions.

B. **Signs and syndromes of cerebellar lesions**

1. Major clinical signs of a cerebellar lesion consist of:
   a. **Dystaxia** and **dysmetria** [Due to incoordinated volitional contractions of axial and appendicular muscles. Dystaxia of axial (truncal) and leg muscles leads to a broad-based, unsteady or staggering gait.]
   b. **Dysarthria** (due to incoordination of speech muscles)
   c. **Nystagmus** (due to incoordination of eye muscles)
   d. **Hypotonia** (the physiologic basis of hypotonia after cerebellar lesions is unclear)

2. Clinicians recognize four cerebellar syndromes, based on the location of the lesion in the cerebellum (Figure 10-13).
   a. The **cerebellar hemisphere syndrome** consists of dystaxia and hypotonia of the ipsilateral extremities. The most common causes are neoplasms and infarcts of a cerebellar hemisphere.
   b. The **rostral vermis syndrome** consists of dystaxia of the legs and trunk during walking, but little or no involvement of upper extremities or of the speech or eye muscles. This syndrome occurs most frequently in chronic alcoholic patients. Alcoholism causes selective degeneration of the "leg region" of the anterior vermis (see Figure 10-9).

Distribution of deficits	Dysarthria	Arm overshoot	Hypotonia	Dystaxia of			Nystagmus	Clinical syndrome	Lobe or lobes affected
				Arms	Gait and trunk	Legs			
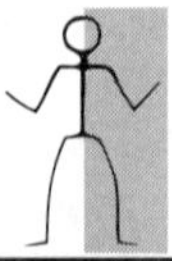	+	+	+	+	+	+	Bidirectional, coarser to side of lesion Fast component to sides of gaze	Cerebellar hemisphere syndrome	Unilateral lesion of the posterior lobe
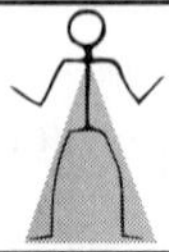	0	±	+	±	+	+	0	Rostral vermis syndrome	Anterior lobe
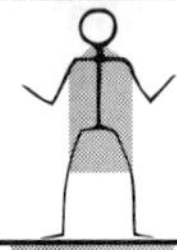	0	0	±	0	+	±	Variable	Caudal vermis syndrome	Flocculonodular and posterior lobes
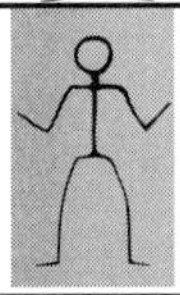	+	+	+	+	+	+	Variable	Pancerebellar syndrome	All lobes bilaterally

FIGURE 10-13. Summary of the four cerebellar syndromes. (Adapted with permission from DeMyer W: *Technique of the Neurologic Examination*, 4th ed. McGraw-Hill Inc., 1994, p 299.)

c. The **caudal vermis syndrome** (flocculonodular lobe syndrome) consists of the inability to maintain the upright posture due to truncal dystaxia. Nystagmus may also be present. This syndrome occurs most commonly with tumors of the vermis (e.g., ependymoma of the fourth ventricle, astrocytoma, or medulloblastoma).

d. The **pancerebellar syndrome**, in which the lesion affects the entire cerebellum, consists of the full picture of bilateral dystaxia, dysarthria, nystagmus, and hypotonia of all voluntary muscles. The most common causes are degenerative diseases, multiple sclerosis, and intoxications. Acute alcoholic intoxication, for example, causes the complete pancerebellar syndrome.

3. Since the causes of the various syndromes differ, identifying the syndrome is nearly tantamount to recognizing the cause.

4. **Signs of interruption of cerebellar pathways**
   a. Interruption of dentatothalamic and dentatorubral pathways may cause a **terminal tremor** (i.e., a tremor of an extremity, which increases as the part nears its endpoint). For example, such a tremor may occur when the fingertip is brought in to touch the nose (see Appendix VI H).
   b. Interruption, even surgical transection, of either spinocerebellar or cerebropontocerebellar pathways causes little or only transient cerebellar dysfunction.

VII. **SUMMARY OF THE CEREBELLAR TRIADS.** As a mnemonic, review the cerebellar triads listed here and in Table 10-1.

A. **Three sagittal divisions:** vermis and two hemispheres

B. **Three transverse divisions** into lobes: anterior, posterior, and flocculonodular

C. **Three phylogenetic/functional subdivisions**, which correspond to the lobes: archicerebellum (vestibulocerebellum, the flocculonodular lobe), paleocerebellum (spinocerebellum, the anterior lobe), neocerebellum (cerebrocerebellum, the posterior lobe)

D. **Three layers of cortex:** molecular, Purkinje cell, and granular, from superficial to deep

E. **Three pairs of midline nuclei:** fastigial nucleus, nucleus interpositus (composed of the emboliform and globose nuclei), and dentate nucleus, in medial-to-lateral order, and the corresponding vermian, paravermian, and hemispheric projections of Purkinje axons from the cerebellar cortex

F. **Three endings of the Purkinje axons:** to a midline nucleus, to a vestibular nucleus, or by means of a recurrent collateral to itself

G. **Three neuronal sources of connections in the cerebellar glomeruli:** mossy fiber endings, dendrites of granule cells, and dendrites and axons of Golgi type II neurons

H. **Three peduncles on each side:** caudal (inferior), middle, and rostral (superior)

I. **Three olivary nuclei:** medial accessory, dorsal accessory, and inferior olivary nuclei

J. **Three major decussations**, which bring the cerebellar influence back to the ipsilateral LMNs (see Figure 10-12).

STUDY QUESTIONS

DIRECTIONS: Each of the numbered items or incomplete statements in this section is followed by answers or by completions of the statement. Select the ONE lettered answer or completion that is BEST in each case.

1. Most efferent axons in the superior cerebellar peduncles arise in

(A) deep nuclei of the cerebellum
(B) stellate neurons of the cerebellar cortex
(C) Purkinje cells
(D) Golgi type II neurons of the cerebellar cortex
(E) none of the above

2. A middle-aged patient of questionable sobriety shows dystaxia of the lower extremities; he has little or no arm dystaxia, dysarthria, or nystagmus. He most likely has a lesion of

(A) the spinocerebellar tracts in the cord
(B) the vermis of the anterior lobe of the cerebellum
(C) the central tegmental tract
(D) the tuber and pyramis
(E) the dentatorubrothalamic tract at the midbrain level

3. Dystaxia resulting from lesions of the cerebellar hemisphere reflects dysmodulation of impulses relayed through which pathway?

(A) Dentatovestibulospinal
(B) Olivocerebellar
(C) Dentatorubral
(D) Dentato-thalamo-cerebrocortical
(E) Spinocerebellar

4. The part of the cerebellum that may undergo transforaminal herniation and strangle the medullocervical junction is the

(A) rostral vermis
(B) flocculonodular lobe
(C) caudal (inferior) peduncle
(D) tonsil
(E) anterior medullary velum

5. Select the one type of cerebellar cortical neuron that is excitatory.

(A) Purkinje neurons
(B) Inner stellate (basket) neurons
(C) Golgi type II neurons
(D) Granule neurons
(E) Outer stellate neurons

6. An ependymoma expanding in the lumen of the fourth ventricle would most likely cause symptoms by encroaching on which one of the following structures?

(A) Cerebellar hemispheres
(B) Vermis and nodule
(C) Pyramidal tracts
(D) Middle cerebellar peduncle
(E) Cochlear nuclei

7. The examiner cannot detect cerebellar dysfunction of the arms and legs unless the patient

(A) is asleep
(B) is quadriplegic
(C) is comatose
(D) has a locked-in syndrome
(E) is awake and not paralyzed

DIRECTIONS: Each of the numbered items or incomplete statements in this section is negatively phrased, as indicated by a capitalized word such as NOT, LEAST, or EXCEPT. Select the ONE lettered answer or completion that is BEST in each case.

8. Which of the following lesions would NOT reduce the afferent fibers to the deep cerebellar nuclei?

(A) Transection of the inferior cerebellar peduncle
(B) Section of the auditory nerve
(C) Destruction of Purkinje neurons
(D) Section of the superior cerebellar peduncle
(E) Destruction of the inferior olivary nuclei

9. A cerebellar glomerulus consists of all of the following EXCEPT

(A) mossy fiber rosettes
(B) axons and dendrites of Golgi type II neurons of the cerebellum
(C) dendrites of granule neurons
(D) a glial capsule
(E) climbing fibers

10. Which of the following statements about the cerebellar peduncles is NOT true?

(A) The middle peduncle conveys mostly crossed pontocerebellar axons
(B) All cerebellar peduncles attach the cerebellum to the pons
(C) The middle peduncle is considerably larger than the others
(D) The inferior peduncle conveys mostly efferent fibers
(E) The superior peduncle conveys the cerebellar outflow to the thalamus

11. Select the one neuronal element that is NOT found in the molecular layer of the cerebellar cortex.

(A) Dendrites of Purkinje neurons
(B) Dendrites of Golgi type II neurons
(C) Cerebellar glomeruli
(D) Parallel and climbing fibers
(E) Stellate neurons

12. Which of the followings statements about parallel fibers is NOT true?

(A) They make a T-like bifurcation, with the axons running transverse to the axis of the folia
(B) They arise in the neurons of the granular layer
(C) They synapse in the molecular layer
(D) They do not synapse on the deep cerebellar nuclei
(E) They are excitatory

13. Which of the following statements about Purkinje neurons is NOT true?

(A) They are located in the second layer of the cerebellar cortex
(B) They are tiny neurons with inconspicuous perikarya
(C) They have dendritic trees that run at right angles to the long axis of the folia
(D) They act as the final common pathway out of the cerebellar cortex
(E) They extend their dendrites into the molecular layer and their axons through the granular layer

DIRECTIONS: Each set of matching questions in this section consists of a list of four to twenty-six lettered options (some of which may be in figures) followed by several numbered items. For each numbered item, select the ONE lettered option that is most closely associated with it. To avoid spending too much time on matching sets with large numbers of options, it is generally advisable to begin each set by reading the list of options. Then, for each item in the set, try to generate the correct answer and locate it in the option list, rather than evaluating each option individually. Each lettered option may be selected once, more than once, or not at all.

Questions 14–18

Match the source of the afferent fibers listed below with their characteristic projection sites in the cerebellum.

(A) Cerebellar hemisphere
(B) Anterior lobe of the vermis
(C) Tonsil
(D) Flocculonodular lobe
(E) All parts of the cerebellum more or less equally

14. Spinocerebellar tracts

15. Trigeminocerebellar tract

16. Principal inferior olivary nuclei

17. Vestibular nerve and nuclei

18. Reticular formation (RF) nuclei such as the nucleus locus coeruleus

ANSWERS AND EXPLANATIONS

1. The answer is A [IV A 1 c]. The superior cerebellar peduncle conveys afferent and efferent cerebellar fibers. The majority of efferent fibers that leave the cerebellum arise in the deep nuclei, mainly the dentate nuclei, and exit through the superior peduncle. The largest group of afferents in the superior peduncle consists of the ventral spinocerebellar tract.

2. The answer is B [VI B 2 b; Figure 10-9]. The vermis of the anterior lobe of the cerebellum represents the body parts in an inverted manner, with the feet and legs being most rostral and superior and the upper parts of the body being more caudal and inferior. The rostral vermis region, the leg region, undergoes degeneration in alcoholic patients. Dystaxia predominantly affects the lower extremities and gait; there is relatively little dystaxia of the arms and little or no dysarthria.

3. The answer is D [V A 1; Figure 10-12]. The dentato-thalamo-cerebrocortical pathway brings the coordinating and modulating influence of the cerebellum to the thalamus, which then projects to the motor cortex. Without this modulating influence, the motor cortex fails to contract the muscles in a smooth, coordinated manner when producing voluntary movements.

4. The answer is D [I F 4; Figure 1-12]. In response to increased intracranial pressure, as may result from edema or various space-occupying lesions, the cerebellar tonsils, which are dorsolateral to the fourth ventricle, herniate through the foramen magnum and compress (or strangle) the medullocervical junction. The patient suffers quadriplegia because of compression of the pyramidal tracts and arrest of breathing (apnea) from compression of the reticulospinal tracts.

5. The answer is D [III G 2; Table 10-4]. All of the neurons of the cerebellar cortex apparently are inhibitory, except for the granule neurons. These, however, are the most numerous neuron type in the cerebellar cortex. The neurons of the deep cerebellar nuclei are excitatory.

6. The answer is B [Figures 10-1C and 10-3]. A tumor of the fourth ventricle will encroach on the nodule of the flocculonodular lobe and the overlying vermis. These parts of the cerebellum control the axial muscles during voli-

tional actions such as standing and walking. The patient is most likely to have an ataxic gait as a reflection of the vermian involvement. Early in its course, an intraventricular tumor usually would not cause pyramidal tract signs because the pyramidal tracts run on the ventral surface of the medulla, which is a considerable distance from the neoplasm. An intraventricular tumor would not affect the cochlear nuclei, which drape laterally around the caudal peduncle and are thus removed from immediate compression. Intraventricular tumors may obstruct cerebrospinal flow and result in increased intracranial pressure with headaches, nausea, and vomiting.

7. The answer is E [VI A 2]. Lesions of the cerebellum cause dystaxia (incoordination) of muscular contractions when the patient voluntarily uses the muscles, either to sustain a posture (e.g., the vertical posture) or to move a part of the body. Such actions are only possible in responsive patients with intact pyramidal and peripheral pathways. For example, a patient with severe acute polyneuropathy, as in Guillain-Barré syndrome, may be completely paralyzed and maintained on a respirator but conscious. The paralysis precludes testing for cerebellar dysfunction. A comatose or sleeping patient or one with interrupted pyramidal tracts, as in the locked-in syndrome or quadriplegia, cannot make willful muscular contractions of the arms, legs, or trunk and would not show cerebellar signs.

8. The answer is B [IV B]. Some direct primary vestibular afferent fibers reach the deep cerebellar nuclei, but no other direct primary afferents come from the auditory nerve or other nerve roots. The deep cerebellar nuclei receive collaterals from the afferent fibers that run through the deep cerebellar white matter to the cortex. These include the afferents from inferior olivary nuclei and the proprioceptive sensory systems via spinocerebellar and trigeminocerebellar pathways. The Purkinje neurons, the only efferent neurons of the cerebellar cortex, mostly synapse on the deep nuclei.

9. The answer is E [III D 2 b; Figure 10-8]. Climbing fibers bypass the glomeruli to climb onto the Purkinje cells. The cerebellar glomeruli are peculiar synaptic arrangements consisting of mossy fiber rosettes, axons and dendrites from Golgi type II neurons of the granular layer, and the dendrites of granule neurons themselves. A glial capsule surrounds the whole conglomeration. The axons of the granule neurons, which enter the molecular layer, provide the output from the glomerulus.

10. The answer is D [IV C; Table 10-5]. The various peduncles have different fiber components. The simplest is the middle peduncle, which conveys mostly crossed pontocerebellar axons. The superior peduncle contains both efferents and afferents. The inferior, or caudal, peduncle is mainly afferent like the middle peduncle; the majority of its fibers are olivocerebellar.

11. The answer is C [III B 2 a, 3 c, C 2 a; Table 10-2]. The cerebellar glomeruli occupy only the granular layer. The neuronal elements in the molecular layer of the cerebellar cortex consist of the inner and outer stellate neurons, the dendrites of Purkinje and Golgi type II neurons, the climbing fibers that accompany the Purkinje dendrites, and the parallel fibers from the granular layer.

12. The answer is A [III B 3]. The parallel fibers are axons that arise by T-like bifurcations of axons of the granular layer of the cerebellar cortex. These axons enter the molecular layer and run parallel to the axis of the folia. They synapse on neurons that extend their dendrites into the molecular layer, namely the Purkinje neurons, inner and outer stellate neurons, and Golgi type II neurons of the granular layer. Parallel fibers do not leave the cerebellar cortex.

13. The answer is B [III A 1, B 2 a, c, E 2; Figures 10-6 and 10-7]. The Purkinje neurons are the only type of neuron in the second layer of the cerebellar cortex. They have huge perikarya and extend huge dendrites into the molecular layer that are flattened at right angles to the long axis of the folia. Purkinje axons run through the molecular layer and medullary cores of the folia to the deep nuclei of the cerebellum. Some Purkinje axons bypass the deep nuclei to end in the vestibular nuclei. The proximal portion of the Purkinje axon sends collaterals back to their own perikarya or to neighboring Purkinje

perikarya. The afferent pathways to the cerebellar cortex all ultimately converge on the Purkinje neurons. Its axons are the only ones to leave the cerebellar cortex. Hence, it constitutes the "final common pathway" out to the rest of the brain from the cerebellar cortex.

14–18. The answers are 14-B, 15-B, 16-A, 17-D, 18-E [IV B 3 a, b, d (2), e]. The afferent tracts to the cerebellum generally terminate in specific regions. The anterior vermis receives the bulk of the spinocerebellar tracts and the trigeminocerebellar tract. The hemispheres receive their strongest projections from the principal olivary nuclei and from the basis pontis.

The flocculonodular lobe is the oldest part of the cerebellum phylogenetically and the part from which the whole cerebellum takes its origin. It originally received the vestibular connections through direct connections to the vestibular nerve and through the vestibular nuclei, and it retains these connections even though the phylogenetically newer parts of the cerebellum are much larger in higher animals. From its original role as an integrating center for the vestibular system in controlling the axial muscles, the cerebellum has now accepted the role of coordinating the appendicular, limb, and speech muscles. The parts of the cerebellum that perform this function have increased in size in accordance with the size of the cerebral motor cortex and the cortical efferent system through the pyramidal and corticopontocerebellar tracts. The corticopontocerebellar system has assumed such importance as an afferent source to the cerebellum that the destruction of the system in early life may result in transsynaptic atrophy of the cerebellar hemisphere.

The vermis also receives projections from the visual and auditory systems, although the functional role of these projections is not well understood. Many of the afferent pathways to the cerebellum also send collaterals to the deep cerebellar nuclei as they pass through the deep cerebellar white matter on their way to the cerebellar cortex. The reticular formation (RF), particularly the nucleus locus coeruleus, projects diffusely to the cerebellum just as it projects diffusely to most other parts of the central nervous system (CNS).

Chapter 11

THE BASAL MOTOR SYSTEM AND ITS RELATION TO THE PYRAMIDAL SYSTEM

I. GROSS ANATOMY OF THE BASAL MOTOR NUCLEI

A. Location

1. Sections through the base of a cerebral hemisphere disclose large, paired nuclear masses. These nuclei are the **thalamus, caudate nucleus, putamen, globus pallidus, claustrum,** and **amygdala** (Figures 11-1 and 11-2).

2. Sections that include the junction of the diencephalon with the midbrain show a number of additional grossly visible but smaller nuclei, the **subthalamic nuclei, red nuclei, substantia nigra,** and the midbrain **reticular formation** (RF) [see Figure 11-7].

B. Relation of the large basal nuclei to the internal capsule

1. The large basal nuclei occupy one side or the other of V-shaped zones of white matter called the **internal capsule**. A horizontal section discloses the **three** parts of the internal capsule (see Figure 11-2):
   a. Anterior limb
   b. Genu (knee)
   c. Posterior limb

2. **Medial** to the **anterior limb** is the **caudate** nucleus of the basal motor nuclei.

3. **Medial** to the **posterior limb** is the **thalamus**. The third ventricle separates the thalami of the two sides.

4. **Lateral** to the **anterior** and **posterior limbs** are the **globus pallidus** and **putamen** of the basal motor nuclei. The apex of the globus pallidus points to the genu (see Figures 11-1 and 11-2).

5. In Figure 11-2, notice the reciprocity between the V-shape of the capsule and the diameter of the adjacent nuclei.
   a. Going **forward** from the genu, the head of the caudate nucleus increases in size.
   b. Going **backward** from the genu, the thalamus increases in size.
   c. Going **forward** or **backward** from the genu, the globus pallidus **decreases** in size. At the apex of the globus pallidus, its maximum transverse diameter corresponds to the genu.
   d. The transverse plane through the apices of the globus pallidus and the genu falls just behind the interventricular foramen (of Monro). This foramen connects the lateral ventricles with the third ventricles (see Figure 1-7).

C. Gross anatomy of the caudate-putamen

1. The head of the **caudate** nucleus sits across the anterior limb of the internal capsule from the **putamen** and **globus pallidus**.

2. The anterior limb of the capsule indents the caudate and putamen, but does not sever them. They retain their connection underneath the crevice for the anterior limb in a zone of continuity called the **nucleus accumbens septi** (Figure 11-3).

3. The **head** and the **body** of the caudate nucleus form the **ventrolateral wall** of the anterior horn of the lateral ventricle (see Figure 11-1)

4. The **tail** of the caudate nucleus circles around the body of the lateral ventricle to proceed forward in the **roof** of the temporal horn. The tail terminates in the **amygdala** (see Figure 11-3).

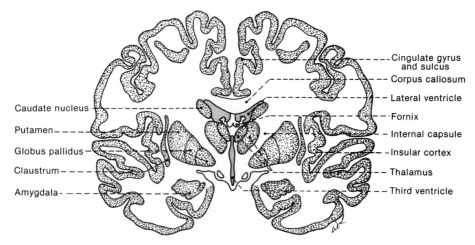

FIGURE 11-1. Coronal section of the cerebral hemispheres through the level of the basal ganglia.

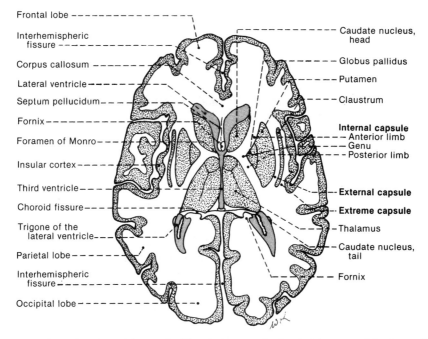

FIGURE 11-2. Horizontal section of the cerebral hemispheres at the level of the genu of the internal capsule.

D. **Naming and defining the basal motor nuclei**

1. Neuroanatomists originally grouped three masses of deep nuclei—the **corpus striatum**, **claustrum**, and **amygdala**—as the **basal ganglia**, before knowing their ontogeny, connections, and functions (Figure 11-4).

2. Now neuroanatomists assign the amygdala of the original basal ganglia to the limbic system, but the function of the claustrum remains unknown. The caudate-putamen and the globus pallidus connect with each other and the other nearby basal nuclei. All of these nuclei mediate motor functions. The basal motor nuclei include cerebral, diencephalic, and midbrain components (Figure 11-5).

3. The names of the basal motor nuclei cause some confusion because the term **corpus striatum** means the combined caudate-putamen-pallidum, whereas the term

striatum means only the caudate-putamen. However, the names can also help to identify structures. For example, the putamen-pallidum has a lens shape, hence the descriptive term, **lentiform nucleus** (see Figures 11-1 and 11-2).

4. The striatum consists of a **dorsal** part, the **caudate-putamen**, and a **ventral** part, the **nucleus accumbens septi** and the **olfactory tubercle** (anterior perforated substance).

   a. The **nucleus accumbens septi** connects the caudate and putamen around the inferior aspect of the anterior limb of the internal capsule (see Figure 11-3).

   b. The **olfactory tubercle** occupies the region just ventral to the nucleus accumbens. It is visible on the inferior aspect of the cerebrum (see Figures 12-9, 13-9, and 13-13).

   c. Some authors call the nucleus accumbens septi and the anterior perforated substance the "limbic striatum" because of their limbic connections (see Chapter 13 II D).

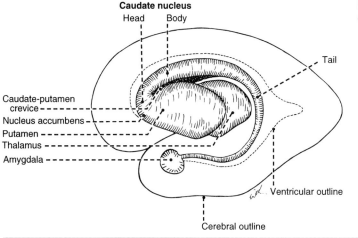

FIGURE 11-3. Phantom drawing of the caudate nucleus in situ.

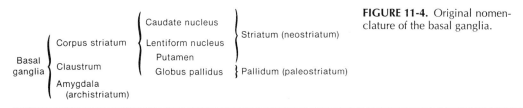

FIGURE 11-4. Original nomenclature of the basal ganglia.

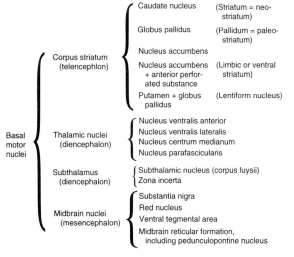

FIGURE 11-5. Current nomenclature of the basal motor nuclei.

TABLE 11-1. Clinicopathologic Correlations between Movement Disorders and Lesions of the Basal Motor Nuclei

Movement Disorder	Lesion
Chorea: multiple quick, randon movements (the "fidgets"), usually most prominent in the appendicular muscles	Atrophy of the striatum, as in Huntington's chorea; may also occur after lesions of the subthalamic-red nucleus region
Athetosis: slow writing movements, usually more severe in the distal appendicular muscles	Diffuse hypermyelinization (status marmoratus) of the corpus striatum and thalamus, as in cerebral palsy
Dystonia: long sustained twisting movements, predominantly of axial muscles	Various genetic, acquired, or pharmacologic lesions of the basal motor nuclei; however, in classic hereditary dystonia, the lesion site is unclear
Hemiballismus: wild flinging movements of half of the body	Hemorrhagic destruction of the contralateral subthalamic nucleus, most commonly seen in hypertensive patients
Parkinsonism (paralysis agitans): pill-rolling tremor (5-6 cycles per second) of the fingers at rest, lead-pipe rigidity, and akinesia	Degeneration of the substantia nigra
Terminal, postural, or **rubral tremor**	Interruption of the dentatothalamic pathway, as in multiple sclerosis

5. **Rationale for the concept of basal motor nuclei**
   a. A series of interconnected nuclei extend contiguously from the base of the cerebrum through the diencephalon to the midbrain.
   b. They all regulate somatomotor activity by means of numerous feedback circuits with each other, and ultimately with the cerebral motor cortex.
   c. Lesions in these nuclei or their pathways result in predictable motor signs, consisting of:
      (1) **Akinesia** and **bradykinesia**, which describe slowness in initiating and executing voluntary movements. Lesions at various sites in the basal motor region, including the striatum, pallidum, and substantia nigra, may result in akinesia-bradykinesia.
      (2) **Rigidity** of the muscles that further impoverishes movement
      (3) **Involuntary movements** (hyperkinesias) that include tremors, tics (Tourette's syndrome), ballismus, chorea, athetosis, and dystonia (Table 11-1)
         (a) Paradoxically, mixtures of hypo- and hyperkinesias occur. In parkinsonism, the patient displays akinesia and bradykinesia, rigidity, and a characteristic hyperkinesia consisting of a five to six cycle per second tremor at rest that disappears when the patient makes a voluntary movement.
         (b) Clinicians classify these distinctive hypo- and hyperkinesias as **extrapyramidal movement syndromes**, in contrast to the pyramidal syndrome.
   d. Lesions of various basal motor nuclei also impair cognitive and affective functions, but not as specifically or predictably as the impairment of motor functions.

II. CONNECTIONS OF THE BASAL MOTOR NUCLEI

A. Overview of connections of the basal motor nuclei

1. The motor and other functions of the basal motor nuclei depend on endless positive and negative feedback circuits among themselves, the cortex, and the motor nuclei of the thalamus. Figure 11-6, a **progressogram**, starts arbitrarily with one link in one

of the most important circuits, the projection of the striatum (caudate-putamen) to the pallidum (globus pallidus).

2. Figure 11-6 depicts only a few of the possible combinations and permutations of connections among the various basal motor nuclei themselves and the cortex. In general, the basal motor nuclei connect with the cortex through thalamic nuclei, not by direct projection.

B. **Myelinated pathways among the basal motor nuclei**

1. Various **capsules, laminae, bundles,** or **fields** of myelinated axons surround, separate, and interconnect the basal motor nuclei (Figure 11-7).

2. **Striatopallidal bundles** run from the striatum, mainly the putamen, to the pallidum (Figure 11-8).

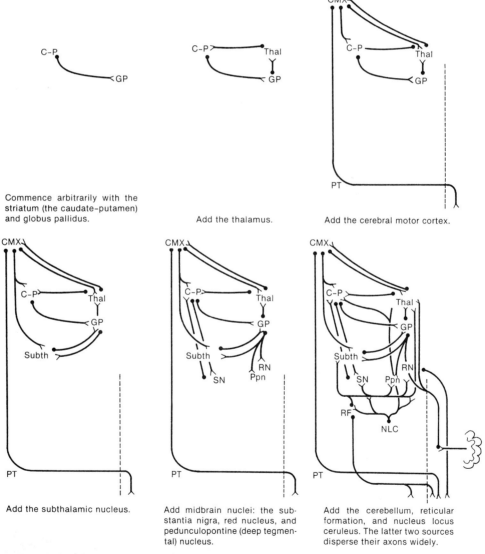

FIGURE 11-6. Progressogram for the conceptual understanding of basal motor circuitry. *CB* = cerebellum; *CMX* = cerebral motor cortex; *C-P* = caudate putamen; *GP* = globus pallidus; *NLC* = nucleus locus coeruleus; *Ppn* = pedunculopontine nuclei of the reticular formation; *PT* = pyramidal tract; *RN* = red nucleus; *SN* = substantia nigra; *Subth* = subthalamic nucleus; *Thal* = thalamus.

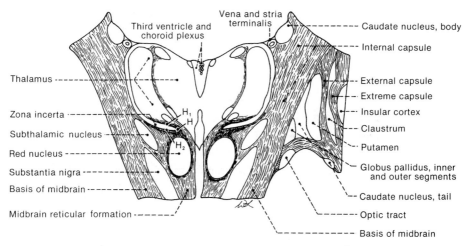

FIGURE 11-7. Drawing of a myelin stained coronal section through the basal motor nuclei, at the level of the red nuclei. *H* = field H of Forel.

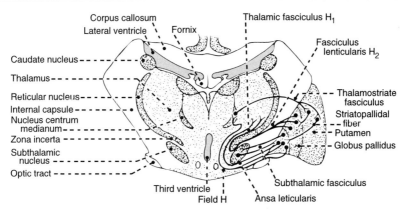

FIGURE 11-8. Diagram of connections of the globus pallidus.

3. **H fields of Forel and the ansa and fasciculus lenticularis**
   a. **Field H.** From the capsule of myelinated fibers that surround the red nucleus, many of which come from the dentatorubral tract, the dentatothalamic tract extends rostrally through field H of Forel.
   b. **Fields H$_1$ and H$_2$.** Field H splits into two laminae: a **dorsal** lamina of fibers, called **field H$_1$**, and a **ventral** lamina of fibers, called **field H$_2$** (see Figure 11-8). A nuclear plate called the **zona incerta** is inserted between these two fields.
      (1) **Field H$_1$** is also called the **thalamic fasciculus**. It conveys three major myelinated pathways to the thalamus:
         (a) Pallidothalamic tract
         (b) Dentatothalamic tract
         (c) Medial lemniscus
      (2) **Field H$_2$** is also called the **fasciculus lenticularis**. It cuts across the internal capsule to convey pallidothalamic axons from the globus pallidus of the lentiform nucleus.
   c. **The ansa lenticularis** (ansa means loop) is a stream of pallidal efferents, mainly pallidothalamic. It loops under the internal capsule, rather than penetrating it like the fasciculus lenticularis, joins field H, and proceeds to the thalamus via H$_1$ (see Figure 11-8).

4. In addition to showing various bundles of fibers, Figures 11-6, 11-7, 11-8, and 12-2 demonstrate the contiguity of the basal motor nuclei at the midbrain-diencephalic junction.

    a. To become oriented to this region, identify the red nucleus in Figure 11-7. This large nucleus is always conspicuous and easy to recognize on magnetic resonance imaging (MRI) scans. Notice the relation of the red nucleus to surrounding structures.

        (1) The substantia nigra is **ventrolateral**.

        (2) The subthalamic nucleus is **dorsolateral**.

        (3) The zona incerta is **dorsal**.

    b. In Figure 11-7, identify the parts of the corpus striatum present at this level:

        (1) Tail of the caudate nucleus (the head of the caudate is on a more anterior coronal plane)

        (2) Putamen

        (3) Pallidum [a lamina of myelinated fibers divides the pallidum into internal and external segments (see Figures 11-1 and 11-7)]

    c. Finally, notice the continuity between the internal capsule and the basis of the midbrain, as well illustrated in Figure 12-5.

C. **Unmyelinated axons**. Numerous unmyelinated catecholaminergic axons, which cannot be demonstrated by standard silver impregnations or myelin stains, course through the basal motor pathways. Chapter 14 II describes these axons, many of which originate in the substantia nigra.

D. **Connections of the caudate-putamen (the striatum)**

    1. Intrinsic neurons of the striatum. The striatum contains neurons ranging in size from small to large.

    a. Most striatal neurons are medium in size and possess spiny dendrites and long axons (Golgi type I). These medium-sized **spiny neurons** provide all axons that extend beyond the striatum to the pallidum and substantia nigra, but they also collateralize in the striatum.

    b. The large neurons have short axons (Golgi type II) and fewer spines. Because their axons synapse in the striatum, they constitute striatal interneurons.

    c. Histochemically, the striatum appears as a mosaic composed of alternating patches of **striosomes** embedded in a **matrix**. The striosomes are acetylcholinesterase poor while the matrix is rich in this enzyme.

    2. Afferents to the caudate-putamen. Afferents arise from the cerebral cortex, thalamus, substantia nigra, and brain stem tegmentum.

    a. Cortical afferents to the striatum

        (1) Most of the cerebral cortex, including limbic cortex, projects to the striatum. The densest projection comes from the sensorimotor cortex of the paracentral region. The sensorimotor areas project to the putamen, while cortical association areas project to the caudate.

        (2) The projection from the general cortex remains mainly ipsilateral, but the sensorimotor cortex and limbic cortex project bilaterally. The axons cross in the corpus callosum (see Figure 13-29).

        (3) The cortex projects directly to the striatum **and** by way of collaterals from the corticothalamic, cortico-olivary, and corticopontine systems.

        (4) Currently, five cortico-striato-thalamo-cortical loops are recognized that connect specific cortical areas with specific striatal areas. These cortical pathways run parallel to each other and loop back to the cortex through the thalamus (see Figure 11-7).

            (a) The **motor loop** connects the putamen and somatosensory areas of the paracentral cortex.

                (i) The striatum receives discrete, topographically organized parallel projections from the face, arm, and leg areas of the cortex. Each cortical area has a "private line."

                (ii) The basal motor nuclei retain this body topography in their afferent and efferent connections.

            (b) The **oculomotor loop** connects the caudate nucleus and cortical eye fields. The caudate then also projects to the superior colliculus.

            (c) The **dorsolateral prefrontal loop** connects the caudate nucleus and the prefrontal cortex (see Figure 13-35, areas 9 and 10 of the frontal pole).

(d) The **lateral orbitofrontal-prefrontal loop** connects the caudate nucleus and the orbitofrontal cortex.

(e) The **limbic loop** connects the ventral striatum and the anterior cingulate cortex (see Figure 13-35, area 24), the medial orbitofrontal cortex, and the temporal lobe.

b. Thalamostriatal afferents. Intralaminar nuclei of the thalamus, including the centrum medianum, send striatal afferents across the internal capsule to the putamen and from the parafascicular nucleus to the caudate nucleus. Probably the ventrolateral and ventral anterior parts of the thalamus also project to the striatum.

c. Nigrostriatal afferents

(1) Unmyelinated dopaminergic axons from the pars compacta of the substantia nigra travel to the striatum via the internal capsule and field H, and as fibers of passage through the medial part of the globus pallidus.

(2) Gamma-aminobutyric acid (GABA) axons travel to the striatum from the pars reticulata of the substantia nigra.

d. Raphe-striatal afferents. The raphe nuclei of the RF send serotonergic axons to the striatum (see Chapter 14 III).

3. Striatal efferents

a. Striatopallidal axons from the spiny, striatal neurons synapse on neurons of the globus pallidus.

b. Striatonigral axons run through the internal capsule to the substantia nigra (pars reticulata).

c. The dorsal striatum (neostriatum) projects to the ventral striatum.

E. **Connections of the globus pallidus (the pallidum)**

1. The globus pallidus contains large, typical multipolar motoneurons. Its "pale globe" appearance results from the large number of myelinated axons that enter and leave it.

2. Pallidal afferents

a. Major afferent sources are the:

(1) Striatum, via the striatopallidal fibers

(2) Subthalamic nucleus, via the subthalamic fasciculus

(3) Cerebral cortex

b. Other afferent sources include:

(1) Substantia nigra

(2) Raphe nuclei and pedunculopontine nuclei of the RF

3. Pallidal efferents

a. The pallidum issues four major bundles of fibers. They depart from its apex and from its dorsomedial and ventral aspects. Figure 11-8 shows three of the bundles: the **ansa lenticularis, fasciculus lenticularis,** and **subthalamic fasciculus.** Figure 11-8 does not include the **pallidotegmental bundle** to the pedunculopontine nucleus nor a projection to the habenular nuclei (Table 11-2).

b. The pallidum acts as a "final common pathway" from the basal motor nuclei to the thalamus (i.e., nuclei ventralis lateralis, ventralis anterior, reticularis, medialis dorsalis, and centrum medianum). The thalamus in turn relays these influences to the motor cortex (i.e., premotor and motor cortex and supplementary motor cortex); thus, it modulates the output of the pyramidal tract to the lower motoneurons (LMNs). Clinically, this is the most important circuit for the motor system.

F. **Connections of the subthalamic nucleus (corpus Luysii)**

1. Afferents come from the pallidum, substantia nigra, pedunculopontine nucleus, and a somatotopic projection from the motor cortex.

2. Efferents of the subthalamic nucleus run across the internal capsule to the ipsilateral pallidum via the subthalamic fasciculus (see Figure 11-8). Some cross to the contralateral pallidum in the dorsal supraoptic commissure of the hypothalamus. Efferents also run to the substantia nigra.

a. Lesions of the subthalamic nucleus result in wild, flinging contralateral movements called **hemiballismus** (see Table 11-1).

TABLE 11-2. Pallidal Efferent Pathways*

Pathway	Course	Destination
Ansa lenticularis	Loops ventromedially under the internal capsule to enter fields H and H_1	Thalamus, nuclei ventralis lateralis and ventralis anterior
Fasciculus lenticularis	Cuts directly through the internal capsule to join field H_2 before recurving dorsally into field H_1	Thalamus, as above
Pallidosubthalamic fasciculus	Cuts directly through the internal capsule	Subthalamic nucleus of Luysii; this pathway also conveys subthalamopallidal fibers
Pallidotegmental tract (not shown in Figure 11-8)	Runs dorsomedially past the subthalamic nucleus and descends into the midbrain tegmentum near the ventrolateral border of the red nucleus	Pedunculopontine nucleus of reticular formation of midbrain tegmentum and substantia nigra

*See Figure 11-8.

      b. Ballistic movements may also result from lesions in the region of the subthalamic nucleus as well as the nucleus itself. Likewise, chorea, while one of the characteristic hyperkinesias resulting from lesions of the striatum, may also occur after lesions of the subthalamic-red nucleus region.

G. **Connections of the red nucleus**

    1. Neuronal types
      a. Small neurons comprise the bulk of the red nucleus (**parvocellular part**).
      b. Large neurons comprise only a small part of the nucleus (**magnocellular part**) and are less prominent in humans than in lower animals.

    2. Afferents come from two main sources: the **cerebral cortex** and **cerebellum**.
      a. Corticorubral fibers come from the ipsilateral precentral gyrus via the **internal capsule**.
      b. Dentatorubral fibers come via the contralateral superior cerebellar peduncle. The tract decussates in the midbrain tegmentum just caudal to the red nucleus (see Figure 7-19).

    3. Efferents from the red nucleus consist of two large pathways and several smaller pathways.
      a. The two major pathways are the **rubro-olivary** and **rubrospinal** tracts.
        (1) The rubro-olivary tract descends ipsilaterally in the central tegmental tract.
        (2) The rubrospinal tract decussates in the ventral tegmental decussation, descends through the brain stem tegmentum, and enters the spinal cord on the ventral border of the crossed lateral corticospinal tract.
      b. Smaller rubral efferent pathways run to the lateral reticular nucleus of the medulla, which, like the inferior olivary nucleus, relays to the cerebellum.
      c. Recent work does not acknowledge the existence of a rubrothalamic tract, as suggested by older studies.
      d. Lesions of the red nucleus or environs result in tremor, ataxia, or sometimes choreiform or ballistic movements. Other midbrain signs, such as a CN III palsy (see Figure 7-20), often accompany the movement disorder.

H. **Connections of the substantia nigra**

    1. The substantia nigra contains large multipolar neurons, which accumulate large amounts of melanin pigment as the brain matures and ages. The neurons form two groups.
      a. The **pars compacta** is located **dorsally**, with its perikarya relatively closely packed. This zone originates most of the efferents.
      b. The **pars reticulata** is located **ventrally**, between the pars compacta and the cortical efferent fibers of the midbrain basis. This zone receives most of the afferents.

2. **Afferents** to the substantia nigra come from the striatum, subthalamic nucleus, pallidum, and, to a lesser extent, the thalamus. The RF of the midbrain tegmentum, particularly the pedunculopontine and raphe nuclei, project to the substantia nigra. No known projections come from the cerebral cortex, cerebellum, or spinal cord.

3. **Efferents** from the substantia nigra that arise mainly in the pars compacta are dopaminergic. The axons from pars reticulata are GABAergic (see Chapter 14 II B). Nigral efferents may follow several different pathways.
   a. Some pass dorsally over the subthalamic nucleus and traverse the globus pallidus to end in the striatum and, to a lesser extent, in the nucleus ventralis lateralis and nucleus ventralis anterior of the thalamus. Some may reach basal forebrain structures and the frontal cortex.
   b. Others synapse in the RF of the midbrain tegmentum and in the superior colliculus of the tectum. Nigral efferents do not run further caudally into the brain stem, spinal cord, or cerebellum.

III. PATHOGENESIS OF MOTOR DEFICITS AFTER LESIONS OF THE BASAL MOTOR NUCLEI

A. The **neurons** of the individual basal motor nuclei vary greatly in biochemistry, structure, and blood supply. Thus, various toxins, medications, viruses, heredofamilial diseases, and anoxia may selectively damage only one population of neurons. The ensuing syndromes of rigidity and involuntary movements differ, depending on the particular nucleus affected (see Table 11-1).

B. Most pathogens act bilaterally, causing **bilateral** signs. Unilateral lesions, such as hemorrhages or infarcts, cause **contralateral** signs. After a unilateral lesion of the basal motor nuclei, the dysmodulation of the ipsilateral thalamus and, in turn, of the ipsilateral motor cortex, results in contralateral involuntary movements because the pyramidal tract, which crosses, conveys abnormal motor impulses to the motoneurons (Figure 11-9).

FIGURE 11-9. Depiction of the pyramidal tract as a funnel or conduit to the lower motoneurons, after the motor and sensory systems have modulated the activity of the motor cortex.

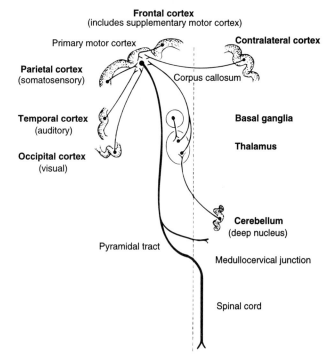

TABLE 11-3. Clinical Syndromes Caused by Lesions at Various Levels of the Motor System

	Type of Lesion				
Syndrome	Pyramidal	Extrapyramidal	Cerebellar	LMN	Muscle
Weakness/paralysis	+		±	+	+
Spasticity	+				
Hypotonia	+*	+†	+	+	+
Extensor toe sign	+				
Increased MSRs	+				
Decreased MSRs	+*			+	+
Severe muscle atrophy				+	+
Dystaxia			+		
Tremor		+	+		
Rigidity		+			
Involuntary movements (patterned)		+			

LMN = lower motoneuron; MSR = muscle stretch reflex.
*Hypotonia and areflexia (neural shock) occur in the acute stage after abrupt pyramidal tract interruption, with spasticity and increased MSRs in the later stages, or if the lesion evolves gradually.
†Hypotonia accompanies chorea, but not the other extrapyramidal movement disorders, which are listed in Table 11-1.

  Role of the corpus striatum in mentation. Although the motor signs of basal ganglia lesions are well known, recent evidence suggests a much broader role of these structures in brain function.

    1. Lesions of the caudate nucleus impair cognitive functions more than lesions of the putamen, which impair motor functions.

    2. Lesions of the nucleus accumbens (ventral striatum) impair the affective and vegetative functions of the limbic system.

    3. Striatal infarcts tend to cause depression or apathy. Patients may also show disinhibited behavior, reduced planning and sequencing skills, and other cognitive and affective disturbances. Lesions of the pallidum may also impair these three functions—cognitive, motor, and limbic or affective.

D. **Summary of the syndromes caused by lesions of the motor system.** Clinically, lesions of the various levels of the motor system—the pyramidal (cortical), extrapyramidal (basal motor), cerebellum, LMN, and muscles—cause distinctive syndromes (Table 11-3).

IV. THE PYRAMIDAL/EXTRAPYRAMIDAL DICHOTOMY AND CONTROVERSY

A. **Definition of the pyramidal system.** Simplistically defined, the pyramidal system consists of those corticobulbar and corticospinal axons that arise in the paracentral cerebral cortex and run directly to interneurons or LMNs in the brain stem tegmentum and spinal cord gray matter to activate LMNs to skeletal muscles.

B. **Definition of the supplementary motor system**

    1. The supplementary motor cortex occupies the medial aspect of the cerebral hemisphere, which is contiguous with the paracentral motor cortex (see Figure 13-36).

    2. The supplementary cortex connects reciprocally with the **ipsilateral** paracentral motor cortex (see Figure 13-36, areas 4 and 6 of the frontal lobe and areas 5 and 7 of the parietal lobe) and with the **contralateral** supplementary cortex.

3. Subcortical projections go to the striatum and to the nuclei ventralis anterior, lateralis, and dorsomedialis of the thalamus. Small numbers of axons project to the spinal cord bilaterally.

4. Functionally, the supplementary motor area may initiate movements, possibly by modulating the paracentral motor cortex. Lesions result in poverty of movement and speech.

5. The supplementary motor cortex does not neatly fit into a pyramidal-extrapyramidal dichotomy. Some authors regard it as a "higher" system, concerned with the planning and initiation of movements.

C. **Definition of the extrapyramidal system**

1. The extrapyramidal system consists of all motor pathways of the brain that ultimately influence LMNs but do not send their axons directly into the pyramidal tract—namely, the circuitry of the basal motor nuclei and the reticulospinal, rubrospinal, olivospinal, vestibulospinal, and tectospinal tracts.

2. Some authors include the cerebellum in the extrapyramidal system and some authors add a cortical extrapyramidal component, that is, those pathways that activate automatic movements after pyramidal tract interruption, such as automatic smiling or crying.

3. Because of the diversity of the extrapyramidal components and the difficulty in extrapolating the results of animal experiments on the two systems to humans, many authors have argued in favor of abolishing the pyramidal/extrapyramidal dichotomy altogether. Yet, clinicians retain it out of necessity because the group of diseases that cause extrapyramidal signs differs from the group that causes pyramidal signs. The crux of the argument is how much of volitional movement is mediated by the pyramidal system and how much is mediated by the extrapyramidal system.

D. **Resolution of the pyramidal/extrapyramidal controversy by phylogeny and clinicopathologic correlation**

1. In **submammalia**, all movements are extrapyramidal because these animals have no cerebral cortex as such and no pyramidal tract.

2. In **lower mammals**, such as marsupials and rodents, the cortex appears but the pyramidal tract remains short and relatively expendable. In fact, the pyramidal tract runs in the dorsal rather than the lateral column of the spinal cord. In lower mammals, pyramidal tract interruption causes less of a deficit than in humans. The animals recover what experimenters interpret as volitional movements better than humans, which indicates that both the pyramidal and extrapyramidal tracts can execute volitional movements in these animals.

3. In **lower primates**, the cortex and pyramidal tract increase in importance, but extrapyramidal pathways can compensate considerably after total pyramidal tract interruption.

4. In **humans**, complete unilateral interruption of the pyramidal tract paralyzes most contralateral volitional movements, particularly of the hand. Recovery usually is minimal. The higher in the phylogenetic series, the more dependent the animal is on the pyramidal tract. Complete bilateral interruption of the pyramidal system, as in the basis pontis in the locked-in syndrome, causes total paralysis of all volitional movements caudal to the level of the lesion (see Chapter 7 XIV D 1). The extrapyramidal pathways cannot substitute. Clinicopathological correlation at autopsy or by computed tomography (CT) or MRI establishes this fact irrefutably.

5. Thus, the phylogenetic series illustrates a gradual increase in the dependence of volitional movement on the pyramidal tract. Volitional somatomotor activity is extrapyramidal in submammalia, mixed pyramidal/extrapyramidal in subhuman mammalia, and essentially pyramidal in humans.

6. **Concept of the pyramidal pathway as an internuncial funnel** (see Figure 11-9)
   a. Clinicopathologic and radiographic correlation of lesions with clinical syndromes discloses the paradoxical fact that in humans pyramidal tract interruption

paralyzes not only voluntary movements but also most involuntary movements that result from lesions of the basal motor nuclei.

b. This observation supports the concept that in humans, movement has become corticalized and pyramidalized, as it were.

c. Various afferent pathways, originating in the RF, cerebellum, basal motor nuclei, and sensory systems, feed through the thalamus and to the paracentral motor cortex to modulate its activity. The motor cortex in turn feeds back to many of these sources.

d. Lesions of the various afferent sensory and motor pathways result in dysmodulation of the motor cortex, which is expressed through an intact pyramidal tract by predictable clinical signs (e.g., chorea, ataxia). These signs have a predictable lesion site and a predictable laterality in relation to that lesion site, based on knowledge of the course of the pathways.

e. Thus, we can view the motor cortex as an internuncial neuronal pool that serves as a funnel, as the final common motor pathway to the LMNs from the diverse sources that modulate motor activity (see Figure 11-9).

7. Clinicians retain the concept of pyramidal and extrapyramidal motor systems for cogent reasons.

a. Interruption of the pyramidal tract causes a distinctive set of clinical features. Interruption of extrapyramidal pathways also causes very distinctive, but different, syndromes (compare Tables 6-3, 11-1, and 11-3).

b. The classic diseases that selectively affect the pyramidal and extrapyramidal systems represent pathogenetically separate disease entities; for example, familial spastic paraplegia in which the pyramidal tract degenerates versus Parkinson's disease in which the substantia nigra degenerates. The treatment, genetics, and management of the disease depend on the correct clinical categorization of the movement disorder.

8. **Caveats about the pyramidal/extrapyramidal dichotomy**

a. The previous statements apply to patients who have an acquired lesion in a relatively mature, previously normal nervous system.

b. Some infants born with congenital malformations or prenatal lesions have no pyramidal tract at all, such as in hydranencephaly, anencephaly, or holoprosencephaly. Although these infants may move their extremities through extrapyramidal pathways, the movements appear to be reflexive, automatic, and nonadaptive rather than volitional in origin. The previously stated rules apply to destruction of the pyramidal tracts in a previously normal, postnatal individual.

c. A few patients recover some degree of volitional movements following severe, unilateral lesions of the pyramidal tract. Such patients might recover because the pyramidal system can function with relatively few remaining crossed axons, or volitional control might develop because of uncrossed fibers of the ipsilateral pyramidal tract or from connections of the supplementary motor cortex.

V. TREATMENT OF INVOLUNTARY MOVEMENTS BASED ON KNOWLEDGE OF PATHWAYS AND NEUROTRANSMITTERS

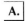

A. Medical treatment

1. Various medications can substitute for neurotransmitters that are lacking after their neurons are destroyed and can block neurotransmission by the neurons in the overactive circuits that drive the abnormal movements.

2. Levodopa (L-dopa), a dopamine precursor, effectively counteracts the loss of the dopaminergic nigrostriatal tract after degeneration of the substantia nigra in parkinsonism.

B. **Stereotaxic surgery and the theory of the countervailing lesion of the basal motor pathways**

1. If a lesion interrupts one part of the maze of inhibitory and excitatory basal motor circuits, another part may become overactive, resulting in tremor, rigidity, involuntary movements, or slowness in initiating movements. In such cases, a countervailing lesion of the overactive circuit may reduce or eliminate the overactivity. Thus, a second lesion counteracts the effects of the original lesion.

2. Neurosurgeons, using anatomical landmarks on x-ray films and stereotaxic coordinates, can selectively direct a needle into a specific basal motor nucleus or tract designated for destruction because the positions of these structures are well-known. Dystonia responds best, athetosis least, to stereotaxic surgery.

C. **Destruction of the pyramidal tract as treatment for involuntary movements**

1. Severe disabling involuntary movements, particularly hemiballismus or severe chorea, may exhaust the patient and threaten life. In the past, neurosurgeons have treated such patients by partial section of the pyramidal tract, either in the motor cortex or by pedunculotomy (i.e., sectioning of the cerebral peduncles).

2. Although interruption of the pyramidal tracts reduces involuntary movements, the concomitant loss of voluntary movements limits the value of the operations to a trade-off between paralysis of voluntary and involuntary movements.

STUDY QUESTIONS

DIRECTIONS: Each of the numbered items or incomplete statements in this section is followed by answers or by completions of the statement. Select the ONE lettered answer or completion that is BEST in each case.

1. An elderly hypertensive patient experiences a sudden onset of violent, flinging, involuntary movements of the left extremities. The lesion most likely involves the

(A) left pontine tegmentum
(B) left caudate nucleus
(C) right subthalamic nucleus
(D) left claustrum
(E) right inferior olivary nucleus

2. A coronal section through the plane of the genu of the internal capsule would almost exactly bisect which structure?

(A) Caudate nucleus
(B) Putamen
(C) Subthalamic nucleus
(D) Thalamus
(E) Globus pallidus

3. The anatomic explanation as to why lesions of the basal motor nuclei on one side cause involuntary movements on the opposite side of the body is that

(A) the basal motor nuclei project to the red nucleus, which sends a crossed rubrospinal pathway to the lower motoneurons (LMNs)
(B) the pallidum sends crossed fibers to the LMNs
(C) the thalamus sends crossed fibers to the LMNs
(D) the motor cortex sends crossed fibers to the LMNs
(E) double-crossed fibers connect the cerebellum with the LMNs via a cerebellospinal tract

4. A structure now excluded from the original definition of "basal ganglia" and from the basal motor nuclei is the

(A) caudate nucleus
(B) subthalamic nucleus
(C) putamen
(D) globus pallidus
(E) amygdala

5. Select the one correct statement about the location of the basal motor nuclei in respect to the internal capsule.

(A) The caudate nucleus is lateral to the anterior limb
(B) The globus pallidus is lateral to the anterior and posterior limbs and genu
(C) The subthalamic nucleus is medial to the anterior limb
(D) The putamen is medial to the anterior and posterior limbs
(E) The substantia nigra abuts on the anterior limb

---

6. All of the following pathways contribute to the H, H₁, or H₂ fields of Forel EXCEPT the

(A) fasciculus lenticularis
(B) ansa lenticularis
(C) lateral lemniscus
(D) dentatothalamic tract
(E) medial lemniscus

7. Fibers enter the thalamic fasciculus (field H₁ of Forel) from all of the following EXCEPT the

(A) medial lemniscus
(B) dentatothalamic tract
(C) fasciculus lenticularis
(D) ansa lenticularis
(E) caudate efferents to the pallidum

8. Which of the following sources does NOT send fibers to the striatum?

(A) Cerebral cortex
(B) Substantia nigra
(C) Nucleus centromedianum of the thalamus
(D) Subthalamic nucleus
(E) Raphe nuclei of the reticular formation (RF)

9. Major numbers of efferent fibers from the pallidum travel in each of the following EXCEPT for the

(A) ansa lenticularis
(B) subthalamic fasciculus
(C) fasciculus lenticularis
(D) tegmental bundle to midbrain reticular formation (RF)
(E) posterior commissure

10. A coronal section through the midbrain-diencephalic junction would show all of the following members of the basal motor nuclei EXCEPT for the

(A) red nucleus
(B) subthalamic nucleus
(C) head of the caudate nucleus
(D) globus pallidus
(E) putamen

Questions 11-15

(A) Amygdala
(B) Supplementary motor cortex
(C) Subthalamic nucleus
(D) Globus pallidus
(E) Vicinity of the red nucleus
(F) Motor cortex
(G) Zona incerta
(H) Substantia nigra
(I) Claustrum
(J) Striatum
(K) Status marmoratus of the corpus striatum and thalamus

For each clinical feature, select the correct site of the lesion.

11. Rigidity and a type of resting tremor that disappears on volitional movement (SELECT 1 SITE)

12. Slowness in the initiation and execution of movements without actual paralysis (SELECT 4 SITES)

13. Ataxia or terminal tremor and CN III palsy (SELECT 1 SITE)

14. Choreiform movements (SELECT 3 SITES)

15. Athetosis (SELECT 1 SITE)

ANSWERS AND EXPLANATIONS

1. The answer is C [II F 2; Table 11-1]. Lesions of the various basal motor pathways tend to cause characteristic syndromes. One such characteristic syndrome, hemiballismus (wild, flinging movements of the extremities on one side), results from a lesion of the contralateral subthalamic nucleus. Because the lesion is usually a hemorrhage in a hypertensive patient, the hemiballismus will have an abrupt onset. If the patient later becomes hemiplegic, the movements disappear.

2. The answer is E [I B 4, 5 c; Figure 11-1]. A coronal section through the plane of the genu will almost exactly bisect the globus pallidus. The globus pallidus has a triangular shape, with the apex fitting into the genu of the internal capsule. As seen in horizontal section, the pallidum diminishes in size as it extends forward or backward from the level of the genu.

3. The answer is D [III B; Figure 11-9]. The thalamus ultimately projects the influence of the basal motor nuclei on one side to the ipsilateral motor cortex. These influences modulate the activity of the pyramidal system. When lesions interrupt basal motor circuitry, the dysmodulation causes the motor cortex to send unwanted (i.e., unwilled) impulses to the lower motoneurons (LMNs) that drive them to produce the involuntary actions. Because the pyramidal tract crosses, the abnormal movements appear on the opposite side of the body. The clinicopathologic support for this theory is that given a patient with chorea, hemiballismus, or tremor arising in the basal motor nuclei, subsequent destruction of the pyramidal tract abolishes or greatly reduces involuntary movement and also causes paralysis of voluntary movements.

4. The answer is E [I D 1, 2; Figure 11-4]. Unfortunately, the definitions of the basal ganglia and extrapyramidal system have changed over the years. The nuclei originally included in the definition were the caudate nucleus, putamen, globus pallidus, and amygdala. The amygdala is currently regarded as part of the limbic system. Various later authors included the subthalamic and other basal motor nuclei with the basal ganglia because they considered all such nuclei as part of an extrapyramidal motor system.

5. The answer is B [I B]. The internal capsule, which has a V-shape on coronal sections, sharply demarcates some of the basal motor nuclei. The globus pallidus is lateral to the genu and the anterior and posterior limbs. The caudate nucleus and thalamus are medial to the anterior and posterior limbs, respectively. The putamen is lateral to the pallidum and, hence, to both the anterior and posterior limbs. The subthalamic nucleus abuts the posterior limb of the capsule at its transition to the midbrain basis.

6. The answer is C [II B 3]. The lateral lemniscus conveys auditory impulses to the inferior colliculus and medial geniculate body, thus bypassing the fields of Forel to reach its relay nucleus to the cerebral cortex. Numerous other pathways run through the laminae of myelinated fibers designated as H fields of Forel. These include afferents to the thalamus from the pallidum, cerebellum, and somatosensory systems via the medial lemniscus.

7. The answer is E [II B 3 c; Figure 11-8]. Field H_1 of Forel, also known as the thalamic fasciculus, consists mainly of fibers from the medial lemniscus, the dentatothalamic tract, and the pallidothalamic tracts of the ansa and fasciculus lenticularis. The ansa lenticularis from the pallidum loops under the internal capsule to enter fields H and H_1, and the fasciculus lenticularis cuts through the capsule to enter field H_2. It then curves dorsally through field H and then laterally through field H_1 to disperse to the ventral-anterior region of the thalamus. The pallidum, not the thalamus, is the major target of striatal efferents.

8. The answer is D [II D 2]. The striatum, which is a huge nuclear mass, receives significant numbers of afferents from the cerebral cortex and from the nucleus centrum medianum of the thalamus. Its best known afferent pathway comes from the substantia nigra. The subthalamic nucleus connects by strong to-and-fro connections with the globus pallidus, but has few, if any, connections with the striatum. The raphe nuclei of the reticular formation (RF) send a strong serotonergic projection to the striatum.

9. The answer is E [II E 3 a; Table 11-2; Figure 11-8]. Two of the four major efferent pathways from the pallidum—the ansa and fasciculus lenticularis—terminate in the nucleus ventralis lateralis and ventralis anterior of the thalamus. These nuclei relay to the cerebral motor cortex, which in turn sends efferents to the striatum. These connections link the cortex and basal ganglia into feedback circuits. The third pathway, the subthalamic fasciculus, conveys reciprocal pallido-subthalamic and subthalamic-pallidal connections. The fourth pathway, the pallidotegmental tract, connects the pallidum with the midbrain reticular formation (RF), especially the pedunculopontine nucleus, which causes walking movements when stimulated (locomotor center) and regulates the onset of rapid eye movement (REM) sleep.

10. The answer is C [II B 4 a, b; Figure 11-7]. A coronal section at the level of the red nucleus illustrates most of the basal motor nuclei of the so-called extrapyramidal system. The tail of the caudate nucleus is present, but not the head. The importance of understanding the propinquity of the basal motor nuclei at the midbrain-diencephalic junction arises from the fact that lesions in this region (i.e., small infarcts, hemorrhages, tumors, or degenerative diseases) cause a variety of movement disorders such as tremors, hemiballismus, and parkinsonism with bradykinesia, tremor, and rigidity. Thus, the clinician should examine this region very carefully in the magnetic resonance imaging (MRI) scan of a patient who has "extrapyramidal" signs.

11. The answer is H [I D 5 c; Table 11-1]. Lesions of the substantia nigra cause parkinsonism, characterized by rigidity and a particular type of resting tremor that suppresses during volitional movements. The rigidity and tremor both result from overactivity of some circuits that an intact substantia nigra suppresses or counterbalances. Parkinsonism usually results from degeneration or viral damage of the substantia nigra neurons. Such lesions generally affect both sides of the midbrain equally. Sometimes isolated, unilateral lesions of the substantia nigra, such as from infarction, neoplasm, or trauma, may cause hemiparkinsonism. The crossing of the pyramidal tract projects the abnormal neural activity to the lower motoneurons (LMNs) of the opposite side of the body.

12. The answers are: B, D, H, J [I D 5 c (1); Table 11-1]. Lesions at several sites in the circuits of the basal motor nuclei result in poverty of movement in the form of akinesia and bradykinesia. The patient initiates movements slowly and executes them slowly, but is not paralyzed or significantly weak. Lesion sites include the supplementary motor cortex, striatum, pallidum, and substantia nigra.

13. The answer is E [II G 3 d]. Lesions of the dentatothalamic tract, which decussates in the caudal midbrain, may cause ataxia (intention tremor) or some other forms of tremor. If one of these features occurs with a CN III palsy, the clinician knows that the lesion must occupy the junction zone between the dentatothalamic tract and CN III; thus, it is in the vicinity of the red nucleus (see Figure 7-20).

14. The answers are: C, E, J [II F 2 b; Table 11-1]. Choreiform hyperkinesia may follow lesions of the striatum as in Huntington's or Sydenham's chorea, the subthalamic-red nucleus region, or rarely even the thalamus. Lesions of the subthalamic-red nucleus region characteristically cause more severe, flinging or ballistic movements of the contralateral extremities. Choreiform movements are random, less severe fragments of movements that resemble the choreographed limb actions of dancers.

15. The answer is K [Table 11-1]. Athetoid movements are slow, writhing movements predominantly of the hand and wrist, but can also involve axial muscles. Contrarily, dystonia characteristically affects axial muscles. These two clinical types of movement disorder overlap in the same way that chorea and hemiballismus represent more or less of a continuum rather than discrete entities. The lesion, status marmoratus, characterizes one form of cerebral palsy. It consists of a marbled appearance (marmor means marble) of the corpus striatum and thalamus, caused by perinatal hypoxia. Hypoxic damage to these regions causes overgrowth of astrocytic processes as part of the healing process. Oligodendrocytes then mistakenly myelinate the astrocytic processes and cause patches of apparent white matter to appear in the nuclei, giving the regions a marbled appearance. Damage to the region from other causes, such as infarcts, may also result in athetosis.

Chapter 12

THE DIENCEPHALON

I. EMBRYOLOGY OF THE DIENCEPHALON AND BASAL MOTOR NUCLEI

A. **Diencephalic development** is characterized by several events (Figure 12-1).

1. Four longitudinal nuclear zones differentiate in the diencephalic wall on each side.

2. The pineal body, neurohypophysis, and optic bulbs arise as separate evaginations from the diencephalon (see Figure 3-5).

3. The diencephalon retains the original lumen of the neural tube as the third ventricle, which has a membranous roof.

B. **Nuclear derivatives of the diencephalon**

1. Masses of neuroblasts proliferate in the periventricular matrix zone and condense into four longitudinal zones of nuclei [Table 12-1 (compare with Figure 12-1)].

2. The subthalamic nucleus and globus pallidus both arise from the hypothalamus (see Table 12-1). Their common origin may explain their similar fiber connections and similar susceptibilities to pathogens. For example, in kernicterus, bilirubin leaks through the blood-brain barrier and stains these nuclei yellow. The neuronal damage results in ballistic or choreiform hyperkinesias.

3. In contrast, the caudate nucleus and putamen arise from the ganglionic hillock of the telencephalon (see Figure 3-10). The amygdala and the claustrum of the four original basal ganglia also arise from the telencephalon.

II. THE THALAMUS DORSALIS

A. **Gross anatomy**

1. **Definition.** The thalamus is an egg-shaped, small egg-sized mass of diencephalic neurons arranged into nuclei. A thalamus develops on each side as the second and by far the largest of the four longitudinal nuclear zones of the diencephalic walls (see Figure 12-1, #2).

2. **Location**
   a. Each thalamus is **medial** to the posterior limb of the internal capsule. Observe this fact in the **horizontal** section in Figure 11-2 and in the **coronal** section in Figure 12-2.
   b. The two thalami form the lateral walls of the third ventricle, superior to the hypothalamic sulcus (see Figure 12-2). The hypothalamus forms the inferior walls of the third ventricle and its floor.

B. **Boundaries of the thalamus.** Each thalamus has **rostral** and **caudal** poles and **dorsal**, **medial**, **ventral**, and **lateral** surfaces.

1. **Rostral and caudal thalamic poles**
   a. The **rostral** pole commences just behind the plane of the foramen of Monro at the genu of the internal capsule (see Figure 11-2).
   b. The **caudal** pole, the pulvinar ("cushioned seat"), overhangs the geniculate bodies and superior colliculi (Figure 12-3).

2. **Dorsal boundary of the thalamus**
   a. **Dorsolaterally**, the thalamus borders on the body and tail of the caudate nucleus and the vena and stria terminalis (see Figure 12-2).

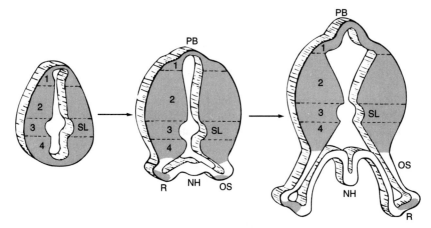

FIGURE 12-1. Cross sections of the diencephalic part of the neural tube. *1* = epithalamus; *2* = thalamus dorsalis; *3* = thalamus ventralis; *4* = hypothalamus; *NH* = neurohypophysis; *OS* = optic stalk; *PB* = pineal body; *R* = retina; *SL* = sulcus limitans (hypothalamic sulcus), in the wall of the third ventricle.

TABLE 12-1. Embryonic and Adult Derivatives of the Diencephalon

Embryonic Subdivision (Dorsal-to-Ventral Order)	Adult Derivative
Epithalamus	Habenular nuclei and commissure and the stria medullaris and taenia tectae, which suspend the membranous roof of the third ventricle, and an evagination, which forms the pineal body
Thalamus dorsalis	Large nuclear masses consisting of the "thalamus" and the metathalamus (the medial and lateral geniculate bodies)
Thalamus ventralis	Zona incerta and nucleus reticularis thalami
Hypothalamus	Evaginations: neurohypophysis and optic bulbs, nerves, and chiasm
	Dorsal nuclear group: globus pallidus, subthalamic nucleus, interstitial nuclei of the inferior thalamic peduncle, and entopeduncular nucleus
	Ventral nuclear group: nuclei of the hypothalamus proper

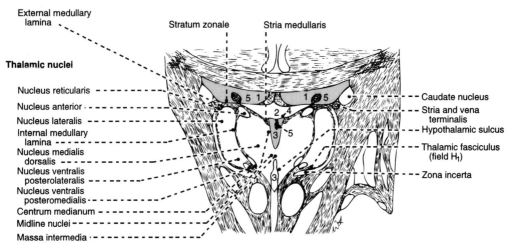

FIGURE 12-2. Myelin-stained coronal section through the thalamus. *1* = lateral ventricle; *2* = cavum veli interpositi; *3* = third ventricle; *4* = tela choroidea; *5* = choroid plexus.

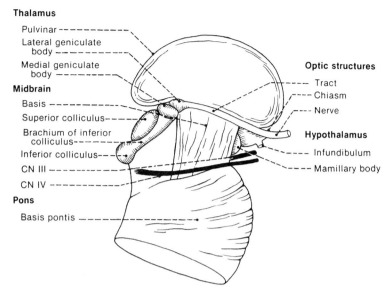

Thalamus
- Pulvinar
- Lateral geniculate body
- Medial geniculate body

Midbrain
- Basis
- Superior colliculus
- Brachium of inferior colliculus
- Inferior colliculus
- CN III
- CN IV

Pons
- Basis pontis

Optic structures
- Tract
- Chiasm
- Nerve

Hypothalamus
- Infundibulum
- Mamillary body

FIGURE 12-3. Lateral view of the brain stem and thalamus, dissected free from the cerebrum and cerebellum.

    b. Dorsomedially, the thalamus forms the floor of the body of the anterior horn of the lateral ventricle.

        (1) The **tela choroidea** covers the dorsomedial aspect of the thalamus and bridges across the lumen of the third ventricle as its roof (see Figure 12-2).

        (2) The tela choroidea consists of an **inner** lining of ependyma and an **outer** layer of pia. The blood vessels that constitute the **choroid plexus** ramify between these two layers.

  3. Medial boundary of the thalamus

    a. The **medial** edge of the thalamus forms the **lateral** boundary of the third ventricle, superior to the hypothalamic sulcus (see Figure 12-2).

    b. A nuclear mass, the **massa intermedia**, may connect the two thalami across the lumen of the third ventricle (see Figure 12-2). Inconstant in size, it is sometimes missing.

  4. Ventral boundary of the thalamus. Ventrally, the thalamic fasciculus (field H_1) separates the thalamus from the zona incerta of the subthalamus (see Figure 12-2).

  5. Lateral boundary of the thalamus. Laterally, a wafer-thin extension of the zona incerta, called the **nucleus reticularis thalami**, separates the thalamus proper from the posterior limb of the internal capsule (see Figure 12-2).

C. Capsules and laminae of myelinated axons that delineate the thalamus and some of its nuclei

  1. The medial thalamic wall that borders the third ventricle consists of a myelin-free zone of so-called midline thalamic nuclei, which are actually **paramedian,** not midline.

  2. On the **dorsal** border of the myelin-free zone, a continuous myelinated capsule commences with the **stria medullaris** (see Figure 12-2). The myelinated capsule extends laterally, ventrally, and medially, surrounding the thalamus in the shape of a C. In sequence, it consists of the following regions (see Figure 12-2).

    a. The **stria medullaris** is a tiny bundle of axons that extends longitudinally along the dorsomedial margin of the thalamus. It suspends the tela choroidea, which bridges the third ventricle.

    b. The **stratum zonale**, a thin myelinated sheet, extends laterally over the dorsum of the thalamus as far as the caudate nucleus.

    c. The **stria** and **vena terminalis** overlie the lateral extent of the stratum zonale.

d. The **external medullary lamina**, a thin, myelin-rich layer, extends in a curve **lateroventrally** from the stratum zonale to become continuous ventrally with the thalamic fasciculus. Nucleus reticulosis separates it from the internal capsule.

e. The **thalamic fasciculus** extends **ventromedially** from the external medullary lamina. It ends at the midline thalamic nuclei in the plane of the hypothalamic sulcus.

f. The posterior limb of the **internal capsule** is the largest myelinated capsule.

3. Internal medullary lamina. An internal medullary lamina cleaves the thalamus into two roughly equal **medial** and **lateral** nuclear groups. It splits dorsally to form a capsule around the anterior nucleus of the thalamus (see Figure 12-2).

D. **Anatomic classification of thalamic nuclei**

1. The **internal** medullary lamina separates the thalamic nuclei into obvious **medial** and **lateral** nuclear groups.

2. Anterior and **posterior** nuclear groups occupy the anterior and posterior poles of the thalamus, respectively. (Study Table 12-2 in relation to Figures 12-2 and 12-4 C and D.)

E. **Functional classification of the thalamic nuclei**

1. Each thalamic nucleus, after receiving impulses from designated subcortical pathways, relays the impulses to designated areas of the cerebral cortex. Each cortical area, in turn, projects back to the nucleus that projects to it. These to-and-fro thalamocortical and corticothalamic circuits allow the thalamus to censor or modulate the motor, sensory, and mental functions of the nervous system.

2. The pathways received by the thalamic nuclei for relay to the cerebral cortex include:

a. The great afferent pathways (lemnisci and optic tract) from the sensory receptors (olfaction excepted)

TABLE 12-2. Topographic Grouping of Thalamic Nuclei*

Anterior group
N. anterior dorsalis
N. anterior ventralis (largest component)
N. anterior medialis
Posterior group
N. pulvinaris
N. corpus geniculatum laterale
N. corpus geniculatum mediale
Medial group
N. medialis (n. medialis dorsalis, n. dorsomedialis)
N. parafascicularis
Ventrolateral group
N. ventralis anterior
N. ventralis lateralis
N. ventralis posterolateralis
N. ventralis posteromedialis (arcuate, or semilunar n.)
Dorsolateral group
N. lateralis dorsalis
N. lateralis posterior
Intralaminar and midline group
N. centrum medianum of Luysii and n. parafascicularis may be included here
Pretectal group

N. and n. = nucleus.
*Partial listing.

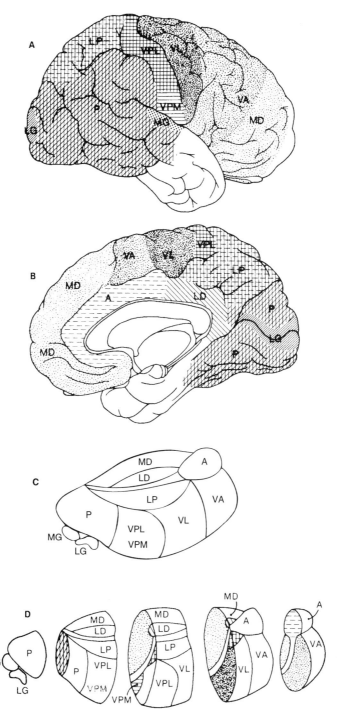

FIGURE 12-4. Pattern of projection of the thalamic nuclei to the cerebral cortex. (*A*) Lateral view of the right cerebral hemisphere showing the cortical areas to which the thalamic nuclei project. (*B*) Medial view of the right cerebral hemisphere showing the cortical areas to which the thalamic nuclei project. (*C*) Lateral view of the right thalamus. Reverse illustrations *C* and *D* to match *B*. (*D*) Exploded lateral view of the right thalamus. *A* = nucleus anterior; *LD* = nucleus lateralis dorsalis; *LG* = lateral geniculate body; *LP* = nucleus lateralis posterior; *MD* = nucleus medialis dorsalis; *MG* = medial geniculate body; *P* = nucleus pulvinaris; *VA* = nucleus ventralis anterior; *VL* = nucleus ventralis lateralis; *VPL* = nucleus ventralis posterolateralis; *VPM* = nucleus ventralis posteromedialis.

    b. Somatomotor pathways of the basal motor nuclei and cerebellum
    c. Reticular formation (RF) pathways
    d. Rhinencephalic and limbic system pathways

3. **Five functional nuclear groups.** Although a nucleus may mediate more than one function, the main groups are:
    a. Sensory relay nuclei (nucleus ventralis posterior, medial geniculate body, and lateral geniculate body)
    b. Motor relay nuclei (nucleus ventralis anterior and nucleus ventralis lateralis)
    c. Ascending reticular activating system (ARAS) relay nuclei (midline and intralaminar) and nucleus ventralis anterior
    d. Limbic system relay nuclei (nucleus anterior, nucleus lateralis dorsalis, and part of nucleus medialis dorsalis)
    e. Association (ectocortical) relay nuclei (part of nucleus medialis dorsalis, nucleus lateralis posterior, and nucleus pulvinaris)

F. **Overview of thalamic connections** (see Figure 12-4). The projection targets of the thalamic nuclei virtually all lie in the forebrain, mostly in the cerebral cortex. The olfactory tubercle, amygdala, and striatum are the only subcortical structures known to receive thalamic projections. Few if any thalamic efferents run to the hypothalamus or caudally to the brain stem, cerebellum, or spinal cord.

1. **Ventral (ventrolateral) tier of thalamic nuclei.** Nuclei of the ventrolateral underbelly of the thalamus relay **somatomotor**, **general somatosensory**, and **special somatosensory** pathways in an orderly anterior-to-posterior sequence.
    a. **Nucleus ventralis anterior** and **nucleus ventralis lateralis** receive somatomotor pathways from the basal motor nuclei and cerebellum.
      (1) **Nucleus ventralis anterior** receives afferents from the substantia nigra, pallidum, intralaminar nuclei (particularly centrum medianum), and frontal cortex. It projects to the intralaminar nuclei and frontal cortex, including the medial orbitofrontal, but excluding area 4 (see Figure 12-2, #4; see Figure 13-35 for cortical areas identified by number). Some doubt exists as to the connections and functions of nucleus ventralis anterior in humans. Although once regarded as a motor relay nucleus, recent evidence suggests that it functions as part of the ARAS.
      (2) **Nucleus ventralis lateralis** receives afferents from the cerebellum, pallidum, and motor cortex. It projects to the motor cortex, essentially area 4 (see Figure 12-2, #4).
    b. **Nucleus ventralis posterior** receives the general somatic afferent (GSA) and taste pathways via medial and trigeminal lemnisci and forms reciprocal connections with the somatosensory cortex of the postcentral gyrus. Nucleus ventralis posterior consists of two parts: nucleus ventralis posterolateralis and nucleus ventralis posteromedialis. These two nuclei maintain the topographic order of the lemnisci.
      (1) Nucleus ventralis posterolateralis receives the medial lemniscus and represents the feet up through the legs, body, and arms, in inverted sequence. It projects the inverted sequence to the postcentral cortex (see Figure 13-37A).
      (2) Nucleus ventralis posteromedialis receives the trigeminal lemniscus (see Figure 7-30) and the taste pathway from nucleus solitarius. The taste pathway projects to the parietal operculum.
    c. The **medial geniculate bodies** receive the auditory pathway and relay to the transverse temporal gyri (see Figure 13-7).
    d. The **lateral geniculate bodies** receive the visual pathway and relay to the calcarine cortex of the occipital lobe. The auditory and visual receptive cortices return fibers to their respective geniculate bodies.

2. **Dorsal tier of thalamic nuclei**
    a. Anteriorly, **nucleus anterior** caps **nucleus anterior ventralis**. It receives afferents via the mammillothalamic tract from the mammillary body of the hypothalamus, which in turn receives the fornix from the hippocampus (see Figures 12-13 and 12-14). Nucleus anterior reciprocally connects with the overlying cingulate gyrus. Nucleus anterior is a way station of the Papez circuit (see Figure 13-16).

   b. Nucleus lateralis dorsalis, just behind nucleus anterior, receives connections from the amygdala and fornix. It reciprocally connects with the overlying cingulate gyrus.

   c. Nucleus lateralis posterior and **nucleus pulvinaris** cover the ventral tier of thalamic nuclei, including the geniculate bodies posteriorly (see Figure 12-3). They belong to the nuclei that reciprocally connect with association cortex. Afferents to these nuclei from infracortical pathways are not as well understood as are those to the ventral tier. Some afferents to these nuclei arise in the thalamus itself.

   (1) Nucleus lateralis posterior reciprocally connects with the parietal lobe behind the somatosensory receptive cortex.

   (2) Nucleus pulvinaris reciprocally connects with the remaining cortex of the parietal lobe and the adjacent cortex of the occipital and temporal lobes (see Figure 12-4).

3. Medial group of thalamic nuclei

   a. Nucleus medialis (nucleus medialis dorsalis) occupies most of the thalamus medial to the internal medullary lamina. It receives afferents from subcortical and cortical regions.

   b. Subcortical afferents come from the basal olfactory structures, amygdala, periventricular fiber systems, striatum, pars reticulata of the substantia nigra, and cerebellum.

   c. Cortical afferents to the nucleus medialis arise in the cortex of the frontal lobe anterior to the motor region, the "prefrontal cortex," and the orbitoinsular limbic cortex and the temporal lobe neocortex.

4. Midline and intralaminar nuclei and nucleus reticularis thalami

   a. The **midline nuclei** are diffuse groups in the periventricular region that connect with the RF, hypothalamus, and basal rhinencephalic structures.

   b. The brain stem RF projects to the midline and intralaminar nuclei, nucleus ventralis anterior, and nucleus reticularis via the central tegmental tract, the internal capsule, and the medial forebrain bundle.

   c. The **intralaminar nuclei** occupy a split in the internal medullary lamina. The largest of these nuclei, **centrum medianum**, projects strongly to the striatum and receives pallidal efferents. Centrum medianum and the other intralaminar nuclei receive strong projections from the cerebral motor cortex.

   d. Physiologic evidence indicates that the ARAS projects diffusely to the entire cerebral cortex through the midline and intralaminar nuclei and perhaps other thalamic nuclei. The exact synaptic connections have been notably difficult to define. Fibers may bypass the thalamus to form direct, monosynaptic connections with the cortex (see Chapter 14 VI) as well as act through the thalamic nuclei. Stimulation of ventralis anterior produces a stronger recruiting response in the cortex than any other thalamic site. Neuroanatomists have disagreed as to whether the intralaminar and midline nuclei receive reciprocal projections from the cortex; recent evidence strongly supports reciprocal connections.

   (1) The ARAS mediates the sleep-wake cycle, the alerting responses, and consciousness in general.

   (2) This diffusely acting system is called **nonspecific** to contrast it with the very discrete, highly organized, and specific connections mediated through the lemniscal and optic systems.

   e. Nucleus reticularis thalami is a wafer of neurons continuing upward between the external medullary lamina and the internal capsule from the zona incerta of the subthalamus (see Figure 12-2). It receives collaterals from the thalamocortical axons. Its own axons point toward the thalamus and synapse on most of the thalamic nuclei, but its function is unknown.

G. **Mnemonic exercise for the cortical projection zones of the thalamic nuclei**

   1. In general, the thalamic nuclei connect with the cortex that is most convenient to them and that mirrors the location of the nucleus in the thalamus.

   2. Start with **nucleus medialis dorsalis** as the cornerstone of the mnemonic exercise. Nucleus medialis dorsalis projects to the frontal lobe anterior to the motor strip of the precentral gyrus (see Figure 12-4). Its zone extends around to the orbital and medial surfaces of the frontal lobe (see Figure 12-4).

3. Next, consider the **ventral** tier of the lateral nuclear group.
   a. **Nucleus ventralis anterior** and **nucleus ventralis lateralis** project to the overlying motor area of the precentral gyrus.
   b. **Nucleus ventralis posterior** projects to the sensory receptive cortex of the postcentral gyrus.

4. Next, consider the **dorsal** tier of thalamic nuclei.
   a. **Nucleus anterior** projects conveniently to the part of the cingulate gyrus just above and medial to it.
   b. **Nucleus lateralis dorsalis**, which is just posterior to nucleus anterior, projects to the cingulate gyrus just posterior to the zone of nucleus anterior.
   c. **Nucleus lateralis posterior** projects to the parietal lobe immediately overlying it, posterior to the postcentral gyrus.
   d. **Nucleus pulvinaris** projects to the shell of parietal, occipital, and temporal cortex that surrounds or mirrors it.

5. Finally, recall the projection of the **medial geniculate bodies** and **lateral geniculate bodies** to their respective temporal and occipital cortices.

6. Whether the frontal and temporal poles receive thalamic connections is still debated.

H. **Anatomical types of pathways to and from the thalamus**

1. Thalamic pathways form **bundles, laminae** or **capsules,** and **thalamic peduncles** or **thalamic radiations** (Table 12-3).

2. The bundles consist of **lemnisci, fasciculi, tracts, striae,** and the **fornix.** These bundles mostly connect the thalamus with subcortical structures.

3. The **laminae** or **capsules** convey fibers that surround thalamic nuclei as the fibers enter or exit from them.

4. The **thalamic peduncles** or **radiations** mostly convey axons that fan out from the internal capsule or converge down into the capsule from various parts of the cerebral cortex. The peduncles constitute a large part of the corona radiata (Figure 12-5).

TABLE 12-3. Named Pathways to and from the Thalamus

Bundles	**Laminae or capsules**
Lemnisci	Internal medullary lamina
Spinal	External medullary lamina
Medial	Stratum zonale
Lateral	Internal capsule
Trigeminal	**Peduncles or radiations**
Fasciculi and ansae	Anterior (frontal)
Lenticular fasciculus	Superior (centroparietal)
Thalamic fasciculus	Posterior (occipital and optic)
Ansa peduncularis	Inferior (temporal) [includes the ansa peduncularis]
Temporothalamic fascicle of Arnold	
Tracts	
Dentatothalamic tract	
Mamillothalamic tract	
Optic tract	
Geniculocalcarine tract	
Striae	
Stria medullaris	
Stria terminalis	
Fornix	

Internal capsule   Corona radiata

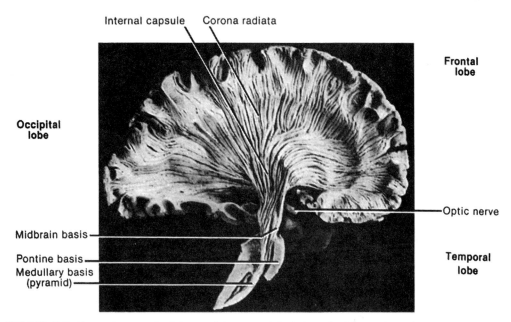

Frontal
lobe

Occipital
lobe

Optic nerve

Midbrain basis

Temporal
lobe

Pontine basis
Medullary basis
(pyramid)

FIGURE 12-5. Gross photograph of the medial aspect of the left cerebral hemisphere dissected to show the fiber bundles of the thalamic peduncles, corona radiata, internal capsule, and basis of the brain stem. (Reprinted with permission from Gluhbegovic N, Williams TH: *The Human Brain: A Photographic Guide.* Philadelphia, Harper and Row, 1980, p 123.)

I. **Sensory pathways to the thalamus**

1. The thalamus receives all lemnisci: **spinal, trigeminal, medial,** and **lateral.** It also receives the **optic lemniscus,** if we choose to call the optic tract a lemniscus (see Table 12-3).

2. Each lemniscus ends in a specific thalamic sensory relay nucleus. Each thalamic sensory nucleus preserves the topographic order of its afferent lemniscus. Then the thalamic projection preserves that topography through to the cortex.

3. A thalamocortical relay apparently is necessary for full conscious appreciation of sensation.

4. Of the senses, only the olfactory has no named lemniscus, but the olfactory bulb is reported to send axons directly to nucleus medialis dorsalis.

5. The vestibular system *a priori* ought to have a lemniscus, but its brain stem route is unclear. A portion of nucleus posterolateralis receives vestibular impulses and relays them to areas of the parietal cortex and the posterior insular region [see Chapter 8 II F 3 e (1)].

J. **Motor pathways to the thalamus**

1. The thalamic somatomotor nuclei are the **nucleus ventralis anterior, nucleus ventralis lateralis,** and **centrum medianum.**

2. Major somatomotor afferent pathways arrive from the cerebral motor cortex, RF, dentatothalamic tract, and globus pallidus via the ansa and fasciculus lenticularis.

K. **Limbic pathways** to the thalamus come from the limbic cortex, periventricular system, hypothalamus (especially the mammillothalamic tract), fornix, striae, and amygdala via the ansa peduncularis.

L. **The internal capsule and thalamic peduncles**

1. The internal capsule requires visualization in **vertical** and **horizontal** sections. (Compare Figures 12-5 and 11-2.)

Anterior limb

1. Anterior thalamic peduncle
2. Frontopontine tract

Genu

Posterior limb

Lenticulothalamic part

3. Superior thalamic peduncle
4. Pyramidal tract

Sublenticular part

5. Ansa peduncularis
6. Thalamotemporal radiations
7. Auditory radiations
8. Optic radiations (geniculocalcarine tract)

Retrolenticular part

9. Posterior thalamic peduncle
10. Temporoparietopontine tract
11. Corticotectotegmental tract

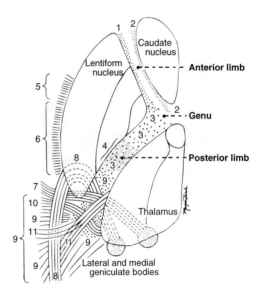

FIGURE 12-6. Horizontal section of the left internal capsule, as seen from above (see Figure 11-2). Dots represent pathways that run in the vertical axis of the capsule or that run radially (see Figures 12-5 and 12-8). Lines, solid or interrupted, represent pathways that run transversely across the vertical axis of the capsule. (Adapted with permission from Crosby E, Humphrey T, Lauer E: *Correlative Anatomy of the Nervous System.* New York, Macmillan, 1962.)

2. The bulk of the fibers in the internal capsule belong to two systems.
   a. Cortical efferent fibers, mostly motor, go to the brain stem and spinal cord.
   b. Thalamic peduncles convey the fibers of the thalamocortical/corticothalamic circuits.
3. The fiber systems of the internal capsule tend to converge into its longitudinal (superior-inferior) axis (see Figure 12-5) or to cut across it transversely (Figure 12-6).
   a. The mainly longitudinal fibers, that is, those radiating to or from the cerebral cortex, consist of:
      (1) Corticobulbar and corticospinal fibers
      (2) Corticopontine fibers
      (3) Majority of corticothalamic/thalamocortical fibers
   b. The bundles that mainly run transversely across the internal capsule consist of:
      (1) A minority of the corticothalamic/thalamocortical connections, including the auditory and optic radiations
      (2) Fasciculus lenticularis
      (3) Subthalamic fasciculus
      (4) Connections with the claustrum and insular cortex
   c. Table 12-4 summarizes specific pathways through the internal capsule (relate it to Figures 12-6 and 12-8).
4. **Location of corticobulbar and corticospinal fibers (pyramidal tract) within the internal capsule**
   a. As the pyramidal tract descends through the internal capsule, the fibers migrate toward the posterior part of the posterior limb before entering the midbrain basis (Figure 12-7).

b. Older texts erroneously depict the fibers more anteriorly in the posterior limb, near the genu. This anterior position holds only for the superior part of the capsule.
c. Because of the restricted location of the pyramidal tract in the internal capsule, a small infarct can cause a pure contralateral hemiplegia, sparing the sensory radiations from the thalamus. Typically, the lesion impairs sensory and motor functions.

 Thalamic peduncles (thalamic radiations). The fibers connecting the thalamus and the cerebral cortex present a continuous, fan-like arrangement as they radiate out from or return to the thalamus (Figure 12-8 and Table 12-5; see Figure 12-5).

 External and extreme capsules

1. These two thin laminae of white matter form a sandwich, with the external capsule medial, the claustrum (a laminae of neurons) in the middle, and the extreme capsule lateral. The insula is lateral to the extreme capsule (see Figure 11-2).

TABLE 12-4. Specific Pathways through Various Parts of the Internal Capsule

Subdivision of the Internal Capsule	Pathway
Anterior limb Lenticulocaudate part of the internal capsule	Anterior thalamic peduncle Frontopontine tract Corticostriatal projections
Genu	Anterior part of superior (centroparietal thalamic) peduncle Corticobulbar tract and frontal eye field projections, according to previous opinions
Posterior limb Lenticulothalamic part of the internal capsule (posterior limb per se)	Posterior part of superior thalamic peduncle Corticospinal tract Corticostriatal, corticorubral, and corticoreticular projections Parietopontine tract
Sublenticular part	Inferior thalamic peduncle Temporothalamic radiations Auditory radiations Origin of optic radiations (geniculocalcarine tract) Ansa peduncularis
Retrolenticular part	Posterior thalamic peduncle Occipitopretectal and occipitotegmental tracts Temporopontine tract

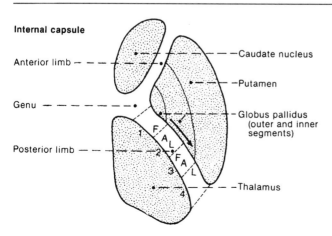

FIGURE 12-7. Horizontal section of the right internal capsule, as viewed from above (see Figure 11-2). At superior levels, the face (*F*), arm (*A*), and leg (*L*) fibers of the pyramidal tract are located anteriorly (*numbers 1 and 2*), while at inferior levels, before the fibers enter the midbrain, they have migrated posteriorly (*numbers 3 and 4*).

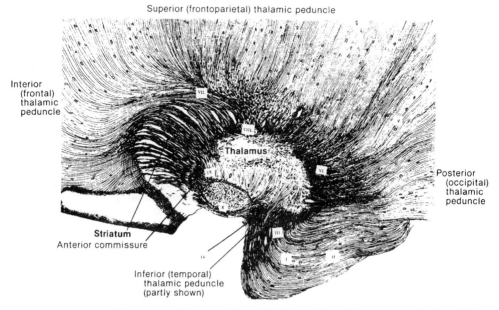

Superior (frontoparietal) thalamic peduncle

Interior (frontal) thalamic peduncle

Thalamus

Posterior (occipital) thalamic peduncle

Striatum
Anterior commissure

Inferior (temporal) thalamic peduncle (partly shown)

FIGURE 12-8. Drawing of a parasagittal section of a cerebral hemisphere demonstrating the fan of fibers that radiate to and from the thalamus. A continuous arc of 300 degrees, the fan is more or less arbitrarily divided into peduncles. *I, II,* and *III* = geniculocalcarine tract of the occipital peduncle (see Figure 10-11); *IV* = transversely cut auditory radiation of the inferior peduncle; *V* and *VI* = superior part of the occipital peduncle; *VII* = subcallosal fasciculus of the frontal peduncle; *VIII* = fibers of the stria terminalis; *IX* and *X* = fibers approaching and surrounding the subthalamic nucleus. (Reprinted with permission from Rosett J: A study of the cerebral fibre systems by means of a new modification of anatomical methods. The lateral wall of the thalamus and the sagittal portion of its cerebral fibre system. *Brain* 45:357–384, 1922. Labels have been added; Roman numerals are original author's.)

2. They convey axons from the longitudinal fasciculi of the cerebrum and the cingulum, connecting the insular cortex and the rest of the cerebrum (see Figures 13-25 and 13-26).

3. Transversely crossing axons interconnect the thalamus and basal ganglia with the claustrum and insula.

4. No known clinical syndrome results from lesions of the external and extreme capsules and the claustrum.

O. **Clinical syndromes resulting from lesions of the thalamus dorsalis.** Because the functions of the thalamus reflect the functions of the whole of the cerebrum, thalamic lesions may impair any of the three great categories of cerebral function: **mental, motor,** and **sensory**.

1. **Unilateral thalamic lesions**
   a. The functions of the left thalamus reflect the functions of the left cerebral hemisphere. Lesions of the left thalamus tend to cause deficits in language production, syntax, word production, prosody, voice volume, and interpretation and expression of words as symbols for communication (thalamic aphasia).
   b. The functions of the right thalamus reflect the functions of the right cerebral hemisphere. Lesions of the right thalamus cause difficulties with spatial relations. The patient neglects tactile, visual, and auditory stimuli from the left half of space and gets lost when going from one place to another. Language functions and mentation are preserved. Right hemisphere lesions tend to cause a defect in the recognition of emotions expressed by others and in the patient's own behavioral expression of affect.
   c. A unilateral lesion of nucleus ventralis posterior, or its projection through the internal capsule, causes contralateral loss of sensation. Because the lesion is usually an infarct, the condition is called "pure thalamic sensory stroke."

(1) Sometimes, along with the loss of sensation, the patient also experiences extreme pain in the affected extremities. This classic thalamic syndrome is called the Dejerine-Roussy syndrome of "painful anesthesia" (anesthesia dolorosa).

(2) Because the lateroventral region of the thalamus shares its blood supply with the internal capsule, the patient with thalamic sensory stroke may also exhibit some degree of hemiparesis.

2. **Bilateral thalamic lesions** impair consciousness and higher mental functions.
   a. The patient becomes demented, amnestic, emotionally labile, and loses orientation to person, time, and place.
   b. The patient may display various degrees of hypokinesia, mutism, or permanent loss of consciousness.

3. **Bilateral lesions of nucleus medialis dorsalis and its frontal connections**
   a. Destruction of nucleus medialis dorsalis, its frontal connections through the anterior thalamic peduncle, or the frontal cortex anterior to the motor region results in loss of drive and initiative, placidity, and a general indifference to stimuli, including pain.
   b. For this reason, neurosurgeons may transect the anterior thalamic peduncle (prefrontal leukotomy or lobotomy) in moribund cancer patients to reduce their reaction to pain. Although lobotomy also has helped some psychotic and severe obsessive-compulsive patients, medications have nearly obviated the operation.

TABLE 12-5. Thalamic Peduncles (Radiations), Their Components, and Their Course Through the Internal Capsule*

Thalamic Peduncle and Course	Thalamic Nucleus	Destination
Anterior thalamic peduncle (through anterior limb of the internal capsule)	N. medialis dorsalis	Frontal granular cortex (prefrontal cortex rostral to motor area)
	N. anterior	Cingulate gyrus
	N. ventralis anterior and lateralis	Areas 4 and 6 (all fibers from n. ventralis are sometimes grouped with superior peduncle)
Superior (centroparietal) thalamic peduncle (through genu and posterior limb per se of the internal capsule)	N. ventralis posterolateralis	Body and extremity area of postcentral gyrus
	N. ventralis posteromedialis	Face area of postcentral gyrus
	N. pulvinaris	Parietal, occipital, and temporal cortex, exclusive of areas served by the thalamic sensory relay nuclei
Posterior thalamic peduncle (through retrolenticular part of the internal capsule)	N. pulvinaris	Occipital cortex, exclusive of calcarine cortex
Inferior thalamic peduncle (through sublenticular part of the internal capsule)		
Anterior component (ansa peduncularis)	Rostromedial thalamic nuclei (exact origin unsettled)	Medial-basal part of temporal lobe: amygdala, piriform lobe, and orbital surface of frontal lobe
Posterior component	Medial geniculate body	Transverse temporal gyri (auditory receptive area)
	Lateral geniculate body (geniculocalcarine tract)	Calcarine cortex of occipital lobe (Area 17, visual receptive area)

N. and n. = nucleus.
*Most of the connections are thalamocortical/corticothalamic circuits.

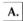 **c.** The neurons of nucleus medialis degenerate in retrograde fashion after prefrontal leukotomy.

III. HYPOTHALAMUS AND PITUITARY BODY

A. **Gross anatomy of the hypothalamus**

1. **Definition.** The hypothalamus is the most ventral of the four longitudinal nuclear zones of the diencephalon (see Figures 12-1, 12-2, and 12-10). It comprises the floor and that portion of the wall of the third ventricle **ventral** to the hypothalamic sulcus (sulcus limitans) [see Figure 12-10].

2. **Functional significance.** Although it weighs only a few grams, the hypothalamus is essential to life because it controls the viscera, endocrine system, vegetative functions, and homeostasis (fluid balance, body temperature, appetite, and so forth). Through limbic lobe connections, it mediates the experience and expression of emotions and the control of instinctive behaviors such as mating, feeding, aggression, and fright/flight responses.

3. **Visualization** of the hypothalamus requires:
   a. A **ventral** view of the base of the brain to see its **external** aspect
   b. **Sagittal section** through the lumen of the third ventricle to see its **medial** aspect
   c. **Coronal sections** to see its **transverse** extent

4. **Ventral aspect of the hypothalamus.** Locate the following in Figure 12-9:
   a. Optic chiasm and tract
   b. Infundibular stalk (neurohypophysis is cut off)
   c. Median and lateral eminences (the tuber cinereum or tuberal region)
   d. Mammillary bodies (the postmammillary sulcus separates the hypothalamus from the midbrain basis)

5. **Medial aspect of the hypothalamus** (Figure 12-10)
   a. The **rostral boundary** of the hypothalamus is the junction of the lamina terminalis of the diencephalon with the anterior commissure of the telencephalon.

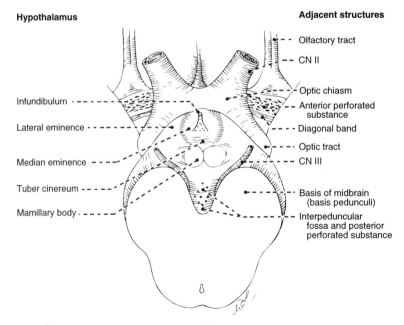

FIGURE 12-9. Gross anatomy of the ventral surface of the hypothalamus.

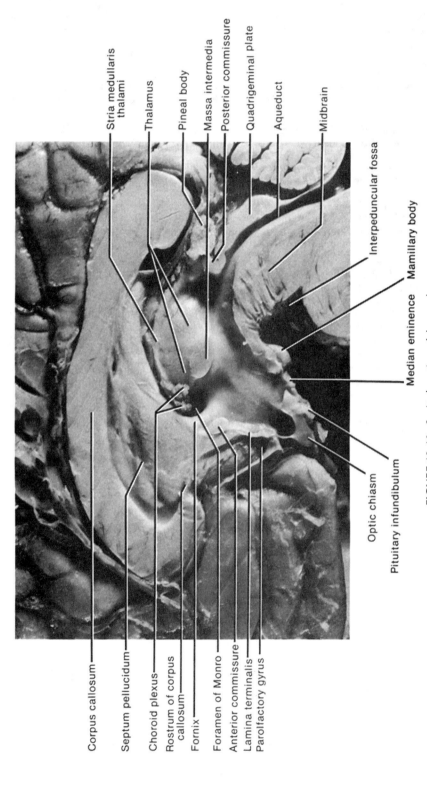

Corpus callosum

Septum pellucidum

Choroid plexus

Rostrum of corpus
callosum

Fornix

Foramen of Monro

Anterior commissure

Lamina terminalis

Parolfactory gyrus

Stria medullaris
thalami

Thalamus

Pineal body

Massa intermedia

Posterior commissure

Quadrigeminal plate

Aqueduct

Midbrain

Interpeduncular fossa

Mamillary body

Median eminence

Pituitary infundibulum

Optic chiasm

FIGURE 12-10. Sagittal section of the cerebrum.

305

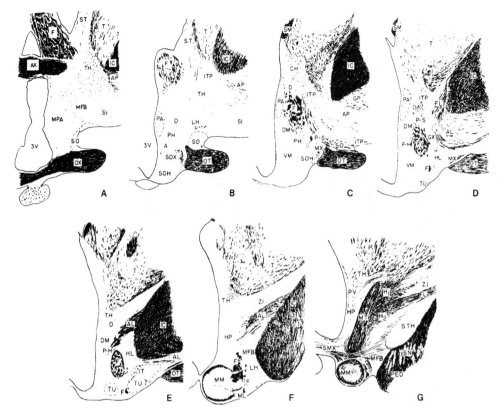

FIGURE 12-11. Myelin-stained atlas of coronal sections of the hypothalamus, anterior to posterior levels (A–G). A = anterior hypothalamic area; AL = ansa lenticularis; AP = ansa peduncularis; AX = anterior commissure; CH = corticohabenular fibers; D = dorsal hypothalamic area; DM = dorsomedial hypothalamic nucleus; F = fornix; FL = fasciculus lenticularis; GP = globus pallidus; GX = dorsal supraoptic commissure, pars dorsalis; H_1, H_2 = fields of Forel; HL and LH = lateral hypothalamic area; HP = posterior hypothalamic area; IC = internal capsule; Ic = nucleus intercalatus; IT = fibers of nucleus tuberalis; ITP = inferior thalamic peduncle; MFB = medial forebrain bundle; ML = lateral mammillary nucleus; MM = medial mammillary nucleus; MPA = medial preoptic area; MT = mammillothalamic tract; MX = dorsal supraoptic commissure, pars ventralis; OT = optic tract; OX = optic chiasm; PA = paraventricular nucleus; PED = cerebral peduncle; PH = paraventricularhypophyseal fibers; P-H = pallidohypothalamic fibers; P-S = paraventriculosupraoptic fibers; PV = periventricular system; SI = substantia innominata; SM = stria medullaris; SMX = supramammillary commissure; SN = substantia nigra; SO = supraoptic nucleus; SOH = supraopticohypophyseal tract; SOX = supraoptic commissures; ST = stria terminalis; STH = subthalamic nucleus; T = thalamus; TH = thalamohypothalamic fibers; TU = nucleus tuberis laterale; VM = ventromedial hypothalamic nucleus; ZI = zona incerta; 3V = third ventricle. (Reprinted with permission from Raven Press, NY. Originally from Ingram WR: Nuclear organization and chief connections of the primate hypothalamus. In *Proceedings of the Association for Research in Nervous and Mental Disease*, 1939.)

     b. The **dorsal boundary** of the hypothalamus is the plane of the hypothalamic sulcus, running longitudinally in the wall of the third ventricle.

     c. The **caudal boundary** of the hypothalamus is the plane of a line drawn from the postmammillary sulcus to the lip of the posterior commissure.

     d. In Figure 12-10, locate the anterior commissure. Then trace the hypothalamus ventrally and caudally through the lamina terminalis, the optic chiasm, median eminence, and mammillary body region to its midbrain junction.

  6. Lateral boundary of the hypothalamus in transverse sections (Figure 12-11)

     a. At **rostral** levels, Figure 12-11 shows that the hypothalamus is bounded laterally by the:

       (1) Ventromedial edge of the internal capsule

       (2) Medial tip of the globus pallidus and the ansa peduncularis

(3) Substantia innominata of the anterior perforated substance and the diagonal band, which belong to the telencephalon (see Figure 12-9)
   b. At **caudal** levels, the ventromedial edge of the internal capsule marks the lateral hypothalamic boundary, as the capsular fibers descend into the midbrain basis.

7. Giving the hypothalamus a name and formal boundaries may obscure a more important fact—its anatomical and functional continuity as a link or center in the circuitry that controls visceration, homeostasis, and affect.
   a. At its **caudal** end, the hypothalamus extends the periaqueductal gray matter and RF into the diencephalon.
   b. At its **rostral** end, the hypothalamus merges with basal rhinencephalic structures of the telencephalon, namely the anterior perforated substance, substantia innominata (just ventral to the caudate nucleus), and septal region.

B. **Nuclei and regions of the hypothalamus**

1. The hypothalamus displays some well-delineated nuclei and others with obscure boundaries, referred to as groups or areas (Figure 12-12 and Table 12-6).

2. **Anterior group of hypothalamic nuclei**
   a. The **preoptic** area is dorsal to the optic chiasm at the level of the lamina terminalis, where the hypothalamus meets the telencephalon.
   b. The **supraoptic** and **paraventricular** nuclei have fairly large neurons and sharp boundaries (see Figure 12-11A–D).
      (1) The **supraoptic** nuclei drape over the optic tract.
      (2) The **paraventricular** nuclei form a plate of neurons in the subependymal zone of the wall of the third ventricle (see Figure 12-11B–D).

3. **Middle group of hypothalamic nuclei.** A parasagittal plane through the fornix splits the hypothalamus into **medial** and **lateral** nuclear areas (see Figure 12-11C–E).
   a. The **medial** hypothalamic region contains two large nuclei, the **ventromedial** and **dorsomedial**, at the midhypothalamic level. A small **arcuate** nucleus (infundibular nucleus) is located in the periventricular zone, just dorsal to the median eminence.

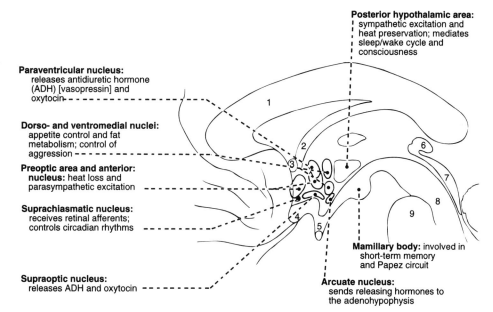

FIGURE 12-12. Nuclear regions of the hypothalamus as superimposed on a sagittal section of the cerebrum (compare with Figure 12-10). *1* = corpus callosum; *2* = fornix; *3* = anterior commissure; *4* = optic chiasm; *5* = infundibulum; *6* = pineal body; *7* = quadrigeminal plane; *8* = midbrain; *9* = pons.

TABLE 12-6. Hypothalamic Nuclei*

Dorsal group
  N. subthalamicus
  N. globus pallidus
Anterior group
  Preoptic area
  N. paraventricularis
  N. supraopticus (n. tangentialis of Cajal)
  N. praeopticus lateralis (interstitial n. of the medial forebrain bundle)
  N. hypothalamicus anterior
  N. suprachiasmaticus
Middle group
  N. hypothalamicus lateralis
  N. hypothalamicus ventromedialis
  N. hypothalamicus dorsomedialis
  N. tuberis and arcuatus of the infundibulum
Posterior group
  N. hypothalamicus posterior
  N. mammillaris medialis, pars medialis and pars lateralis
  N. mammillaris lateralis (n. intercalatus of Le Gros Clark)

N. and n = nucleus.
*Partial listing.

    b. The **lateral** hypothalamic area extends from the midhypothalamus into the posterior hypothalamus zone. It also includes the tuberal nuclei along the ventral, surface border of the hypothalamus.

  4. Posterior group of hypothalamic nuclei (see Figure 12-11F)
    a. The **mammillary nucleus**, the largest and most conspicuous of the hypothalamic nuclei (see Figure 12-10), has **medial** and **lateral** parts.
      (1) The **lateral** part receives the fornix.
      (2) The **medial** part sends mammillary efferents to the thalamus and brain stem tegmentum.
    b. The posterior hypothalamic nuclei merge with similar neurons of the posterior part of the lateral nucleus. The entire lateral zone of the hypothalamus can be thought of as a continuum from the lateral preoptic zone caudally through the posterior hypothalamic zone, to where it merges with the midbrain tegmentum.

C. **Connections of the hypothalamus**

  1. Preview
    a. Highlighting its role in the rhinencephalic, limbic, autonomic, and endocrine systems, the strongest afferent and efferent connections of the hypothalamus are with basal rhinencephalic structures of the telencephalon, including the:
      (1) Amygdala and adjacent basal frontal and temporal lobe cortex
      (2) Hippocampal formation and pyriform cortex [paleocortex and archicortex (see Figure 13-31)]
      (3) Limbic nuclei and midline nuclei of the thalamus
      (4) RF and periaqueductal gray matter of the brain stem
      (5) Retina (via optic nerve and chiasm to suprachiasmatic nucleus)
    b. To focus on the sources of hypothalamic afferents, note where they do not come from or come from in only small numbers:
      (1) Striatum
      (2) Lemniscal systems (medial, lateral, spinal, and trigeminal)
      (3) Cerebellum
      (4) Thalamus (other than midline and intralaminar nuclei and nucleus medialis)
      (5) Neocortex (projections established in lower animals, but questionable in humans)

c. In general, the hypothalamus will return efferents to its afferent sources, either directly or by feedback circuits.

d. The hypothalamus has numerous short, multisynaptic connections within itself and with neighboring structures, as well as several conspicuous, named fiber systems.

2. Fiber systems of the hypothalamus
  a. Medial forebrain bundle
    (1) The medial forebrain bundle runs longitudinally from the medial basal rhinencephalic structures of the substantia innominata, through the lateral part of the hypothalamus, and into the brain stem tegmentum and periaqueductal gray matter [see Figure 12-11 A, F, and G (the bundle is present in sections B–E, but not labeled)].
    (2) The bundle conveys afferent and efferent fibers, receiving and paying them out along its course. It is laden with interstitial neurons, forming numerous short, polysynaptic pathways.
    (3) Edinger named it the **medial forebrain bundle** to contrast it with the **lateral forebrain bundle**, which is composed of the internal capsule and the pallidal efferents.
      (a) The lateral forebrain bundle, consisting mainly of myelinated fibers, is the highway for somatic motor and sensory events and willed movements, as related to external space.
      (b) The medial forebrain bundle, consisting mainly of unmyelinated fibers, is the highway for automatic visceral control, as related to internal space.
  b. Three arching systems of fibers related to the hypothalamus
    (1) Three arching fiber systems distribute axons in the depths of the cerebrum: the **stria terminalis**, **stria medullaris**, and **fornix** (Figures 12-13 and 12-14).
    (2) These bundles interchange axons in complicated pathways. They connect the amygdala, rhinencephalon, and hippocampus of the telencephalon with the hypothalamus, thalamus, and epithalamus (habenula) of the diencephalon.

3. The **stria terminalis** arises in the amygdala and follows the tail of the caudate nucleus around the roof of the inferior horn of the lateral ventricle to occupy the thalamostriate seam in the floor of the body of the lateral ventricle (see Figure 12-2). The stria terminalis decussates in part at the anterior commissure. At this site, the fibers distribute to the:
  a. Opposite stria terminalis and amygdala
  b. Preoptic area and anterior hypothalamus

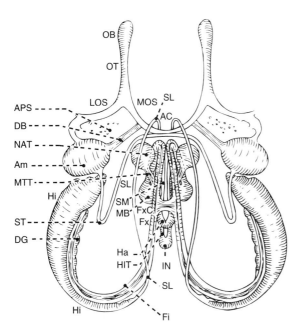

FIGURE 12-13. Dorsal stereoscopic view of the arching fiber systems related to the hypothalamus. *AC* = anterior commissure; *AM* = amygdala; *APS* = anterior perforated substance; *DB* = diagonal band; *DG* = dentate gyrus; *Fx* = fornix; *FxC* = fornix commissure; *Ha* = habenula; *Hi* = hippocampus; *HIT* = habenulointerpeduncular tract; *IN* = interpeduncular nucleus; *LOS* = lateral olfactory stria; *MB* = mammillary body; *MTT* = mammillothalamic tract; *NAT* = nucleus anterior of the thalamus; *OB* = olfactory bulb; *OT* = olfactory tract; *SL* = stria lancisii; *SM* = stria medullaris; *ST* = stria terminalis.

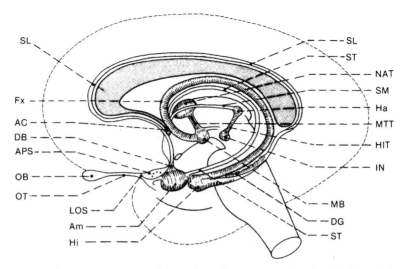

FIGURE 12-14. Lateral stereoscopic view of the arching fiber systems related to the hypothalamus. *AC* = anterior commissure; *Am* = amygdala; *APS* = anterior perforated substance; *DB* = diagonal band; *DG* = dentate gyrus; *Fx* = fornix; *Ha* = habenula; *Hi* = hippocampus; *HIT* = habenulointerpeduncular tract; *IN* = interpeduncular nucleus; *LOS* = lateral olfactory stria; *MB* = mammillary body; *MTT* = mammillothalamic tract; *NAT* = nucleus anterior of the thalamus; *OB* = olfactory bulb; *OT* = olfactory tract; *SL* = stria lancisii; *SM* = stria medullaris; *ST* = stria terminalis.

    c. Thalamus dorsalis
    d. Habenula of the epithalamus, via the stria medullaris

4. The **stria medullaris** of the thalamus runs along the dorsomedial edge of the thalamus, where it suspends the roof of the third ventricle (see Figures 12-2 and 12-14). Its fiber systems are more closely related to the habenula than the hypothalamus.

5. The **fornix** arises in the hippocampus and adjacent subiculum (see Figure 13-16).
    a. Proceeding dorsally, it forms a commissure with its mate and arches over the roof of the third ventricle to reach the anterior commissure (see Figures 12-13 and 12-14).
    b. At the anterior commissure, it splits into **precommissural** and **postcommissural** bundles.
        (1) Precommissural fornix fibers enter the basal rhinencephalic region, septum, and anterior region of the hypothalamus.
        (2) Postcommissural fibers, the bulk of the fornix, turn caudally through the hypothalamus to synapse in the lateral part of the mammillary nucleus and the lateral and posterior hypothalamic areas.
        (3) Some fornix axons reach the thalamus, particularly nucleus medialis dorsalis, and may even reach the midbrain.

6. The **mammillary fasciculus** arises in the medial nucleus of the mammillary body. It divides into two components.
    a. The **mammillothalamic** tract runs to the nucleus anterior, one of the limbic nuclei of the thalamus (see Figure 12-11G).
    b. The **mammillotegmental** tract turns caudally to enter the midbrain tegmentum just ventral to the medial lemniscus. It ends in the RF. Efferents return through the mammillotegmental tract to the mamillary nucleus from the RF.

7. The **ansa peduncularis** loops around the medial tip of the globus pallidus (see Figure 12-11A–C). It interconnects the thalamus and hypothalamus with the basal rhinencephalon, amygdala, the cortex of the temporal lobe, and the orbital surface of the frontal lobes. The fibers run in two streams.
    a. One stream, the anterior part of the inferior thalamic peduncle, conveys fibers to and from thalamic nuclei and the temporal lobe.

      b. The other component of the ansa, the ventral amygdalofugal pathway, connects the amygdala with the hypothalamus.

    8. The **dorsal longitudinal fasciculus** (of Schütz) runs from the hypothalamus throughout the length of the brain stem, in the periaqueductal gray matter, ventral to the lumen of the aqueduct and fourth ventricle. It interconnects the hypothalamus with the periaqueductal gray matter and with the dorsal motor nucleus [general visceral efferent (GVE) nucleus] of cranial nerve (CN) X.

    9. Commissures. Several commissural pathways run through the supraoptic area, midportion, and mammillary region of the hypothalamus. They interconnect the hypothalamus, basal motor nuclei, RF, and pretectal and tectal areas of the right and left sides.

   10. Chemically specified tracts. The brain stem sends catecholaminergic and serotonergic pathways to the hypothalamus and much of the rest of the forebrain (see Chapter 14 II and III).

   11. Tables 12-7 and 12-8 review the **afferent and efferent connections of the hypothalamus**.

TABLE 12-7. Summary of Afferents to the Hypothalamus

Source of Afferents	
Cerebral cortex	Pyriform cortex, hippocampal formation, and ectocortex (ectocortical projections established in lower animals, postulated in humans)
Subcortex of telencephalon	Amygdala and basal forebrain (septal nuclei, anterior perforated substance, and nucleus accumbens)
Diencephalon	Retina and numerous intrahypothalamic connections
Midbrain	Periaqueductal gray matter, reticular formation, dorsal and ventral tegmental dopaminergic and serotonergic nuclei
Pons	Parabrachial nucleus, nucleus locus coeruleus, and serotonergic raphe nuclei
Medulla	Nucleus of solitary tract and adrenergic nuclei
Spinal cord	Small projection from ascending spinal sensory systems

TABLE 12-8. Summary of Efferents from the Hypothalamus

Structures That Receive the Efferents	Specific Targets of Efferents
Cortex	Diffuse projections to the entire cortex
Subcortical telencephalon	Amygdala and basal forebrain
Diencephalon	Nucleus anterior of the thalamus, neurohypophysis, adenohypophysis, and numerous intrahypothalamic connections
Midbrain	Periaqueductal gray matter, reticular formation, and Edinger-Westphal nucleus
Pons	Parabrachial nucleus, periaqueductal gray matter, and reticular formation
Medulla	Nucleus ambiguus, nucleus solitarius, dorsal motor nucleus of CN X, medullary reticular formation
Spinal cord	Preganglionic sympathetic and parasympathetic neurons

CN = cranial nerve.

D. **Function of the hypothalamus as a receptor in relation to blood-brain barrier permeability**

1. In addition to receiving axons from numerous afferent pathways, the hypothalamus acts in a sense as its own receptor, in part because of selective permeability of the blood-brain barrier in certain hypothalamic nuclei.

2. Intrinsic mechanisms sample body temperature and the osmolality of the blood and cerebrospinal fluid (CSF).

3. Various hormones (e.g., estrogen and progesterone) and drugs become affixed to hypothalamic neurons and alter the endocrine activity and general behavior of the individual by modulating neuronal responses.

4. Certain circumventricular sites constitute areas of increased permeability where capillary walls come into direct contact with neurons or glia. These sites allow substances circulating in the blood to affect neurons directly (Figure 12-15).

   a. The vascular organ of the lamina terminalis, the **organum vasculosum**, in the preoptic area at the anteroventral end of the third ventricle, detects pyrogens. It and the **subfornical** organ detect angiotensin II, which controls blood pressure and drinking behavior.

   b. The **area postrema**, located in the floor of the fourth ventricle, detects cholecystokinins, which control feeding and gastrointestinal activity, and acts as a vomiting receptor. The pineal body, median eminence, and neurohypophysis also allow increased blood-brain barrier permeability.

E. **Pituitary body (of Vesalius)**

1. The pituitary body is only 0.5 cm high, 1.0 cm long, and 1.5 cm wide, yet it controls the endocrine system, under direction of the hypothalamus.

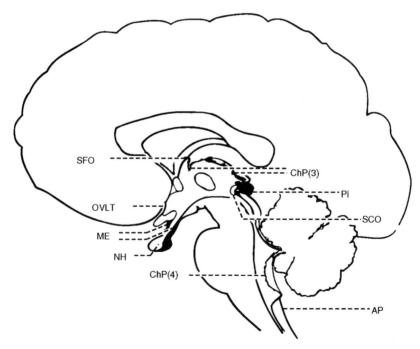

FIGURE 12-15. Midsagittal section of the brain to show the circumventricular sites of increased blood-brain permeability. *AP* = area postrema; *ChP* = choroid plexus (*3* or *4* = third or fourth ventricle); *ME* = median eminence; *NH* = neurohypophysis; *OVLT* = organum vasculosum of the lamina terminalis; *Pi* = pineal gland; *SCO* = subcommissural organ; *SFO* = subfornical organ. (Reproduced with permission from McKinley MJ, Oldfield BJ: Circumventricular organs. In *The Human Nervous System.* Edited by Paxinos G. Academic Press Inc., San Diego, Harcourt Brace Jovanovich, 1990, p 416.)

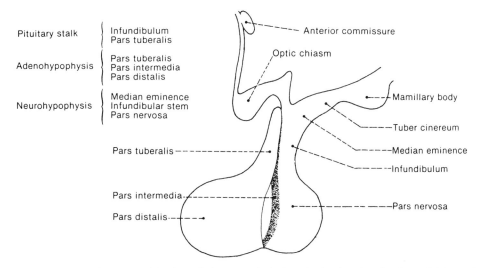

Pituitary stalk { Infundibulum / Pars tuberalis

Adenohypophysis { Pars tuberalis / Pars intermedia / Pars distalis

Neurohypophysis { Median eminence / Infundibular stem / Pars nervosa

Anterior commissure

Optic chiasm

Mamillary body

Tuber cinereum

Median eminence

Infundibulum

Pars tuberalis

Pars intermedia

Pars distalis

Pars nervosa

FIGURE 12-16. Sagittal section of the hypothalamus and pituitary body, showing the three divisions of the pituitary body: the pituitary stalk, the adenohypophysis, and the neurohypophysis.

2. The pituitary body consists of the **pituitary stalk**, the **adenohypophysis**, and the **neurohypophysis** (Figure 12-16).

3. Embryologically, the pituitary body has a dual origin (see Figure 3-5).
   a. The **neurohypophysis** evaginates from the hypothalamus, thus originating from and remaining neural tissue.
   b. The **adenohypophysis** evaginates from the oral ectoderm. Its glandular cells manufacture a number of major hormones: thyrotropin [thyroid-stimulating hormone (TSH)], adrenocorticotropic hormone (ACTH), luteinizing hormone (LH), follicle stimulating hormone (FSH), growth hormone (GH), and prolactin.

4. Control of release of hormones of the adenohypophysis
   a. The neuronal perikarya of the ventromedial, infundibular, and tuberal nuclei manufacture releasing factors that travel down the axons by axoplasmic flow. These axons form a **tuberoinfundibular** tract (Figure 12-17A).
   b. The axon tips secrete their releasing factors into capillaries, which convey them to a **portal** network around the gland cells of the adenohypophysis. The gland cells then release their trophic hormones directly into the bloodstream, which distributes them to endocrine glands and other tissues.

5. Release of hormones in the neurohypophysis. A **supraopticohypophyseal** tract conveys axons from the supraoptic and paraventricular nuclei that contact the capillary system of the neurohypophysis (see Figure 12-17B). The axons release two neurosecretory hormones into the capillaries: **antidiuretic hormone** (ADH; vasopressin) and **oxytocin** (see Figure 12-17B).
   a. **ADH** increases the absorption of water from the distal tubule of the kidney; thus, it conserves water. The supraoptic nucleus mainly produces ADH.
      (1) The release of ADH is governed in part by the osmolality of the blood circulating through the supraoptic nucleus.
      (2) Increased filling of the heart by an overload of fluid stimulates vagal receptors that reflexly inhibit ADH secretion by way of vagal afferents.
   b. **Oxytocin** causes contraction of smooth muscle of the uterus and breast. The paraventricular nucleus mainly produces oxytocin.

F. **Functions and clinical syndromes of the hypothalamus and pituitary gland**

1. A review of the adult derivatives of the hypothalamus and subthalamus will emphasize the extreme diversity of structure and function of these parts of the diencephalon (Table 12-9).

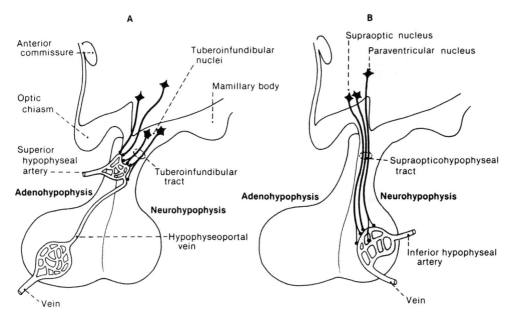

FIGURE 12-17. Sagittal section of the hypothalamus and pituitary body. (*A*) System of portal blood vessels for the transport of hormone-releasing factors from the hypothalamus to the adenohypophysis. (*B*) Supraopticohypophyseal tract and paraventricular-hypophyseal tract for the release of antidiuretic hormone and oxytocin into the systemic circulation.

TABLE 12-9. Derivatives of the Hypothalamus

Adult Derivatives	Function
Retina and optic stalk	Receptor for vision
Globus pallidus and subthalamic nucleus	Somatomotor control
Neurohypophysis (including median eminence)	Secretes antidiuretic hormone and oxytocin
Hypothalamus proper	Controls release of adenohypophyseal trophic factors for endocrine glands, influencing growth and body proportions
	Integrates and controls autonomic nervous system and limbic lobe
	Controls instinctive and cyclic behaviors and the expression of emotion: appetite for food and water, sexual development and mating, maternal responses, expression of aggression, sleep and circadian rhythms
	Role in memory and maintenance of consciousness

2. **Hypothalamic control of autonomic functions.** The anterior and posterior areas of the hypothalamus contain centers that coordinate the activities of the sympathetic and parasympathetic nervous systems.
    a. **Parasympathetic control**
        (1) The anterior and medial hypothalamus tend to produce parasympathetic discharges. Stimulation of certain sites causes pupilloconstriction, bradycardia, vasodilation, and a tendency for reduced blood pressure and increased motility of the gut and bladder.

(2) Destruction of the anterior hypothalamus results in irreversible hyperthermia. Normally, it acts as a heat loss center.

b. Sympathetic control

(1) Stimulation of the posterior and lateral hypothalamus produces a fright/flight response manifested by pupillodilation, increased heart rate and blood pressure, increased breathing, and reduced gut motility.

(2) Destruction of this hypothalamic region results in lethargy, sleepiness, and hypothermia. Normally, it acts as a heat conservation center.

(3) Both sympathetic and parasympathetic projections from the hypothalamus control pupillary size.

3. Control of appetite

a. Hypothalamic lesions may cause hyperphagia or aphagia. The most critical region appears to be the midhypothalamus. Lesions in or near the ventromedial nucleus in rats causes hyperphagia with obesity and aggressive behavior.

b. In the diencephalic syndrome of infancy, usually caused by a hypothalamic glioma, the infant shows severe cachexia and extreme emotional lability.

4. Control of water balance

a. Damage to the infundibular stalk or neurohypophysis blocks the release of ADH. The patient has polydypsia and polyuria (diabetes insipidus).

b. Disorders of the region may result in excessive or inappropriate release of ADH, resulting in oliguria and water retention.

c. The hypothalamus also may alter water balance by mediating the release of ACTH, which controls adrenal gland secretions.

5. Control of circadian rhythms and cycles

a. The suprachiasmatic nucleus, which receives direct retinal afferents, at least in lower animals, controls the sleep-wake cycle.

b. Recent evidence indicates that the paraventricular nuclei of the fetus signal the time for birth by releasing ACTH, which stimulates cortisol production that then results in uterine contractions.

6. Role in affective expression and sexuality

a. Stimulation or lesions of the hypothalamus may elicit behavioral reactions resembling fear and rage. The animal will snarl, hiss, bite, and claw in response to trivial stimuli, such as a puff of air. If the hypothalamus remains intact, removing the cerebral hemispheres rostral to the diencephalon also releases these reactions, called **sham rage**.

b. Small tumors of the hypothalamus may cause gelastic epilepsy, in which epileptiform discharges, as documented by electroencephalography, induce seizures featured by outbursts of laughter.

c. Hypothalamic or neighboring tumors may cause precocious puberty with adult sexual drives or, conversely, delayed puberty and lack of sexual development. The preoptic area controls the release of gonadotropins. It also contains a dimorphic nucleus that distinguishes males from females. Further analysis of this region could establish a biological basis for homosexuality.

7. Role in mental processes and memory

a. In Korsakoff's syndrome, the patient, usually a severe alcoholic, has hallucinations, delirium, disorientation to time and place, loss of recent memory, and confabulates.

(1) The lesion consists of hemorrhagic, necrotic foci that appear in the hypothalamus, particularly in the mamillary bodies; in the thalamus, particularly in the nucleus medialis dorsalis; and in the periaqueductal gray matter and tegmentum of the midbrain.

(2) The midbrain lesion may damage CN III and cause diplopia and pupillary abnormalities.

b. The presence of opioid receptors in the hypothalamus and its relation to affective states, such as satiety and euphoria, make it a prime region for the action of addictive and mood-altering drugs (see Chapter 14 V).

G.   **Summary of diametric syndromes of the hypothalamus and pituitary gland.** Lesions that upset the balances maintained by the hypothalamus and pituitary body may cause the following diametric syndromes:

1. Hyperthermia/hypothermia

2. Anorexia/hyperphagia leading to cachexia/obesity

3. Oliguria/polyuria

4. Precocious puberty/delayed puberty

5. Hypersexuality/hyposexuality

6. Hyperpituitarism/hypopituitarism

7. Gigantism/dwarfism

8. Lethargy/aggression

IV.   EPITHALAMUS

A.   The epithalamus is the most dorsal of the four longitudinal nuclear zones of the diencephalon (see Figure 12-1).

B.   The epithalamus consists of the:

1. Roof of the third ventricle and stria medullaris

2. Habenular nuclei and commissure

3. Pretectal nuclei

4. Pineal body

C.   **Connections of the habenula**

1. The habenular nuclei receive afferents from the stria medullaris, periventricular neurons of the third ventricle and periaqueductal gray matter, RF, and the interpeduncular nucleus of the midbrain.

2. The habenula sends efferents to the RF, periaqueductal gray matter, and interpeduncular nucleus by the habenulointerpeduncular tract (fasciculus retroflexus of Meynert).

3. A habenular commissure connects the habenular nuclei of the two sides.

D.   **Functions of the habenula.** The function of the habenular complex is uncertain. It may link the rhinencephalic, hypothalamic, and limbic control mechanisms with the rostral part of the brain stem. It is presumed to mediate olfactory stimuli and feeding behavior.

E.   **Pineal body.** The pineal body manufactures melatonin. It has a cyclic release and is thought to mediate some cyclic functions, such as the sleep cycle, and to control reproductive cycles and puberty.

■ STUDY QUESTIONS

DIRECTIONS: Each of the numbered items or incomplete statements in this section is followed by answers or by completions of the statement. Select the ONE lettered answer or completion that is BEST in each case.

1. A patient who has been losing vision and complains of excessive thirst and water drinking would most likely have a lesion affecting the

(A) lateral geniculate bodies and midbrain
(B) optic chiasm and infundibular stalk
(C) posterior hypothalamus and mamillary bodies
(D) superior colliculus, pineal body, and pretectal region
(E) medial nuclei of the thalamus and the optic tract

2. Bilateral lesions of which of the following thalamic nuclei or their thalamocortical-corticothalamic circuits would be most likely to cause a syndrome of apathy, reduced drive, and reduced reactions to various stimuli, including pain?

(A) Nucleus medialis
(B) Nucleus pulvinaris
(C) Nucleus ventralis posterior
(D) Nucleus ventralis anterior
(E) Nucleus corpus geniculatum laterale

3. As the pyramidal tract descends through the internal capsule, it shifts

(A) from the genu into the anterior limb
(B) into the external capsule
(C) posteriorly in the posterior limb
(D) from the posterior limb into the genu
(E) from the posterior limb to the inferior thalamic peduncle

4. The most important structure for designating the location of the various thalamic nuclei is the

(A) nucleus pulvinaris
(B) nucleus reticularis
(C) stratum zonale
(D) zona incerta
(E) internal medullary lamina

5. The region of the brain most important for regulation of body temperature is the

(A) habenula
(B) anterior hypothalamus
(C) mammillary body
(D) nucleus anterior of the thalamus
(E) pretectal region

6. Select the pathway that runs through the sublenticular and retrolenticular part of the internal capsule.

(A) Frontopontine pathway
(B) Parietal radiations of the thalamus
(C) Pyramidal tract
(D) Geniculocalcarine tract
(E) None of the above

7. Which thalamic nuclei connects most predominantly with limbic pathways and forms part of the Papez circuit?

(A) Nucleus pulvinaris
(B) Nucleus anterior
(C) Centrum medianum
(D) Nucleus ventralis lateralis
(E) Medial geniculate body

8. Select the INCORRECT statement about the medial forebrain bundle.

(A) It interconnects the basal telencephalic olfactory region with the hypothalamus and brain stem
(B) It consists mainly of rapidly conducting, myelinated axons
(C) It occupies the periventricular zone of the hypothalamus
(D) It conducts numerous ascending and descending short pathways
(E) It runs medial to the internal capsule

9. Select the INCORRECT generalization about the specific sensory relay nuclei of the thalamus.

(A) They occupy the posterior and ventrolateral region of the thalamus
(B) They receive a discrete afferent pathway via a lemniscus
(C) They project in a topographic way to the cerebral cortex
(D) They have discrete cytoarchitectural or laminar boundaries
(E) They do not receive myelinated fibers

10. Select the generalization about thalamic connections that is NOT true.

(A) Most efferents from the thalamus run rostrally to telencephalic targets
(B) Virtually all parts of the cerebral cortex connect with the thalamus
(C) The topography of the pathways that arrive at thalamic nuclei is preserved in the topography of the pathways that leave the nucleus
(D) Most thalamic nuclei interchange numerous efferent and afferent pathways with the hypothalamus
(E) The ascending reticular activating system (ARAS) relays through the midline and intralaminar nuclei

11. A specific thalamic nucleus relays each of the following senses to the cortex EXCEPT

(A) sight
(B) hearing
(C) smell
(D) touch
(E) taste

Questions 12–16

Match the thalamic boundary with the structure immediately related to it.

(A) Third ventricle
(B) Posterior limb of the internal capsule
(C) Thalamic fasciculus and zona incerta
(D) Stratum zonale and body of lateral ventricle
(E) None of the above

12. Lateral border

13. Dorsal border

14. Caudal pole (caudal tip of pulvinar)

15. Ventral border

16. Medial border

DIRECTIONS: Each set of matching questions in this section consists of a list of four to twenty-six lettered options followed by several numbered items. For each numbered item, select the appropriate lettered option(s). Each lettered option may be selected once, more than once, or not at all. EACH ITEM WILL STATE THE NUMBER OF OPTIONS TO SELECT. CHOOSE EXACTLY THIS NUMBER.

Questions 17–19

(A) Nucleus ventralis posterior
(B) Ansa peduncularis
(C) Superior (centroparietal) thalamic peduncle
(D) Mamillary bodies, walls of the posterior part of the third ventricle and tegmentum at the diencephalic-midbrain junction
(E) Frontal thalamic peduncle
(F) Lateral geniculate body
G) Medial geniculate body
(H) Pulvinar
(I) Internal capsule
(J) Geniculocalcarine tract
(K) Geniculotemporal tract
(L) Ventromedial nucleus of the hypothalamus
(M) Nucleus ventralis lateralis
(N) Medial forebrain bundle
(O) Stria medullaris

For each clinical finding, select the structure that, if interrupted, would cause it.

17. Acute sensory stroke with hemihypesthesia (SELECT 3 STRUCTURES)

18. Hemianopia (SELECT 2 STRUCTURES)

19. Memory loss, disorientation to time and place, hallucinations, confabulation, and double vision (SELECT 1 STRUCTURE)

ANSWERS AND EXPLANATIONS

1. The answer is B [III F 4, G 3; Figure 12-17B]. Polydipsia and polyuria in combination with loss of vision indicate a lesion of the optic chiasm and supraoptic nucleus or infundibular stalk. The supraoptic nucleus drapes over the dorsum of the optic chiasm. The infundibular stalk conveys the axons from the supraoptic nucleus that release the antidiuretic hormone (ADH) in the neurohypophysis. Absence of this hormone after interruption of the supraopticohypophyseal system will result in diabetes insipidus with excessive thirst.

2. The answer is A [II O 3 c]. In the 1930s, Egas Moniz found that lesions of the frontal lobe white matter caused a syndrome consisting of apathy, reduced drive, and reduced responsivity. The lesions interrupted the circuit between nucleus medialis and the frontal cortex anterior to the motor area. Lesions of this circuit at the nuclear, white matter, or cortical level tend to produce a similar behavioral result. Neurosurgeons have sectioned the frontal lobe white matter, an operation called prefrontal leukotomy, to reduce the response of terminal cancer patients to pain and to treat severe mental disorders.

3. The answer is C [II L 4 a, b]. Recent investigations have shown that as the pyramidal tract descends through the internal capsule, it shifts posteriorly from the region of the genu into the posterior part of the posterior limb. The older textbooks show the fibers as located only in the anterior part of the posterior limb. This relationship is true only in the superior part of the capsule. The shift in location of the pyramidal fibers is important because different arteries supply the anterior limb, genu, and posterior limb of the internal capsule.

4. The answer is E [II C 3]. Sections through the thalamus disclose a grossly visible lamina of medullated fibers, the internal medullary lamina, that roughly divides the thalamus into medial and lateral nuclear groups. This gross subdivision corresponds with the histologic and functional separation of the medial and lateral groups of thalamic nuclei.

5. The answer is B [III F 2 a, b]. The hypothalamus maintains the constancy of the internal environment by controlling temperature, circulation, and metabolism through its influence on the pituitary gland, endocrine and exocrine glands, and the cardiovascular system. Destruction of the anterior hypothalamic region causes irreversible hyperthermia by impairing the patient's ability to lose heat by sweating and vasodilation.

6. The answer is D [II L 3 a, b, c; Figure 12-6; Table 12-4]. The internal capsule conveys virtually all of the thalamocortical and corticothalamic connections, including the auditory and optic radiations from the geniculate bodies. Many tracts, such as the pyramidal tract, drop longitudinally through the posterior limb. Other pathways, such as the fasciculus lenticularis, run transversely across the capsule and connect the basal motor nuclei with each other and with the thalamus. The optic radiation, the geniculocalcarine tract, runs from the lateral geniculate body in a forward trajectory across the sublenticular part of the capsule. Part of the geniculocalcarine tract sweeps around the temporal horn and the remainder passes through the retrolenticular part.

7. The answer is B [II F 2 a, b]. The various thalamic nuclei can be classified by their afferent and efferent connections. When they are so classified, two of the nuclei have primarily limbic connections: the nucleus anterior and nucleus lateralis dorsalis, which project to the overlying cingulate gyrus. The nucleus anterior receives major afferents from the fornix and mammillothalamic tract, which are also part of the limbic circuitry.

8. The answer is B [III C 2 a]. The medial forebrain bundle contrasts with the lateral forebrain bundle, which consists of the internal capsule. The lateral bundle consists of fibers that form "capsules" (internal and external) and mainly convey myelinated somatosensory and somatomotor pathways. The medial forebrain bundle is, in analogy, a pathway of the visceral system. It consists of poorly myelinated or unmyelinated fibers running to-and-fro, mainly in short pathways, from the basal telencephalic olfactory region, through the lateral hypothalamus, to the periaqueductal gray matter and reticular formation (RF) of the brain stem. The bundle also conveys many of the axons from chemically specified nuclei of the brain stem tegmentum.

9. The answer is E [II F 1 a, b, c]. The sensory relay nuclei occupy discrete zones in the ventral and posterior regions of the thalamus, behind the somatomotor nuclei. Sensory nuclei receive discrete afferent or lemniscal pathways consisting of large numbers of myelinated fibers, and each projects in a topographic way to the cerebral cortex. The separate nuclei and pathways for sight, vision, hearing, touch, and pain corroborate the intuitive classification of sensation into different modalities.

10. The answer is D [II F 1–4; Figure 12-4; Table 12-5]. Most thalamic efferent connections run to rostral (i.e., telencephalic) targets. The thalamus sends few if any fibers caudally, or even ventrally into the hypothalamus. The sensory nuclei of the thalamus receive the optic, auditory, and somatosensory pathways in a topographical order. For example, the lateral geniculate body receives the visual fields in a point-to-point order. The relay pathway to the cortex then preserves that order as does the sensory receptive cortex itself. The midline and intralaminar nuclei and nucleus ventralis anterior are way stations in the ascending reticular activating system (ARAS). This system, in apparent contrast to the highly specific, discrete sensory pathways, works through widespread, diffuse, nonspecific connections that subserve alerting, attention, and the sleep-wake cycle.

11. The answer is C [II E 1 a, F 1 a, b, c]. The thalamus serves as a relay center interposed between almost all of the major sensory systems and the cerebral cortex. The one major sensation that lacks a known specific thalamic relay nucleus is the sense of smell. The olfactory nerve synapses directly on the olfactory bulb of the telencephalon, making it unique among all of the sensory pathways by not passing first through the thalamus.

12–16. The answers are: 12-B, 13-D, 14-E, 15-C, 16-A [II B; Figures 12-2 and 12-3]. The thalamus is bordered laterally by the posterior limb of the internal capsule, medially by the third ventricle, ventrally by the thalamic fasciculus and zona incerta, and dorsally by the stratum zonale and body of the lateral ventricle. Thus, the thalamus borders on the lateral ventricle dorsally and on the third ventricle medially. Its dorsomedial border is the stria medullaris thalami. The stria medullaris marks the junction of the dorsal and medial boundaries of the thalamus. The choroid plexus of

the third ventricle is suspended between the stria. The thalamus ends posteriorly in the tip of the pulvinar nucleus, which projects over the superior colliculus. The pineal body rests between the pulvinars of the two thalami. Depending on one's viewpoint as to the classification of thalamic nuclei, the anterior limit of the thalamus is either the tip of nucleus ventralis anterior or the shell formed by nucleus reticularis that curves forward around the rostral limit of nucleus ventralis anterior. The anteromedial limit of the thalamus is also the posterolateral border of the foramen of Monro, the passageway for cerebrospinal fluid (CSF) from the lateral to the third ventricle. The anteromedial boundary of the foramen is the fornix (see Figure 11-2).

17. The answers are: A, C, I [II F 1 b, G 3 b; Table 12-5]. The somatosensory pathways relay to the postcentral gyrus through nucleus ventralis posterior. They preserve the topographic representation of body parts from the periphery to the cerebral cortex. Small, perforating arteries irrigate discrete areas of the thalamus, basal motor nuclei, and internal capsule. Infarctions in the distribution of these small perforating arteries cause small, oval cavities in the tissue, called lacunes. A lacune may involve only one thalamic area or one discrete region of the internal capsule, the centroparietal thalamic peduncle, or the pyramidal tract that courses through the capsule. A lacune may happen to interrupt one discrete group of motor or sensory axons. Thus, the lacune may affect only the pyramidal tract region of the capsule and cause an acute "pure" hemiplegia without sensory loss. However, larger infarcts frequently affect the capsule, or the white matter itself, causing combined sensory and motor losses contralaterally. Pure motor or sensory loss contralaterally can also occur with discrete lesions of the pyramidal tract or medial lemniscus at the brain stem level.

18. The answers are: F, J [II F 1 d; Table 12-5]. Contralateral hemianopsia may follow lesions at any level from the optic tract through the lateral geniculate body, geniculocalcarine tract, and calcarine cortex. Destruction of one medial geniculate body may impair hearing to some degree, but does not cause contralateral deafness because of the bilateral dispersion of impulses from the two ears. The pathways for the senses of vision and hearing both convey point-to-point specificity—the visual field and the low-to-high frequency of sound waves—but differ dramatically in respect to lateralization. In either case, the thalamic nuclei preserve the specificity of the original input from the optic and auditory transducers.

19. The answer is D [III F 7 a]. The clinical features suggest Korsakoff's syndrome. Damage to the hypothalamus impairs a variety of mental functions, including affective experience and memory as well as instinctive behavior and homeostasis. Loss of memory for recent events and loss of orientation to time and place in Korsakoff's syndrome are thought to reflect mainly damage to the fornix-mamillary pathway. With chronic alcoholism or severe nutritional deficiencies, hemorrhagic, necrotic lesions may appear in the posterior hypothalamus. These lesions particularly appear in the mamillary bodies, which are brownish and shrunken at autopsy, and the periaqueductal gray matter and adjacent midbrain tegmentum. In addition to the changes in mental state, the patient often has diplopia and pupillary abnormalities because of damage to the nucleus of cranial nerve (CN) III.

Chapter 13

Cerebrum

I.   **GROSS EXTERNAL ANATOMY OF THE CEREBRUM**

A.   **Review the following before starting this chapter:**

1. Definition of the cerebrum (see Figure 1-3)

2. Lobes of the cerebrum (see Figure 1-4)

3. Four components of a cerebral hemisphere as seen in coronal section (see Figure 1-6)

4. Origin of the two cerebral hemispheres by evagination from a median connecting stalk (see Figures 3-4 to 3-6)

B.   **The three facies, three poles, and three margins of a hemisphere** (Figure 13-1)

1. The **three surfaces or facies** of a cerebral hemisphere are the facies lateralis, the facies medialis, and the facies inferior (inferomedial).
   a. The **facies lateralis** is strongly **convex** because it conforms to the curve of the skullcap (calvaria).
   b. The **facies medialis** is completely **flat** because it conforms to the cerebral falx, a stiff, flat fold of dura mater inserted into the interhemispheric fissure (see Figures 1-12 and 1-13).
   c. The **facies inferior of the frontal lobe** is **concave** because it conforms to the convex orbital plate of the floor of the frontal fossa.
   d. The **facies inferior of the temporo-occipital lobe** is faintly **convex** because it conforms to the floor of the middle fossa and cerebellar tentorium.

2. Three margins—superior, inferolateral, and **inferomedial—**divide the three facies.

3. The **three poles** are the **frontal, occipital,** and **temporal.**

C.   **Lobes of the cerebrum** (see Figure 1-4)

D.   **External crevices of the cerebrum: fissures and sulci**

1. Fissures versus sulci
   a. Fissures form by evagination or invagination of the entire cerebral wall and thus alter the ventricular contour.
   b. The **sulci** merely indent the outer surface of the cerebrum but do not, in general, alter the ventricular contour. Only the **calcar avis,** caused by the calcarine sulcus, significantly indents the ventricle.
   c. Nomenclature note. Some authors refer to some sulci as fissures; for example, the calcarine sulcus may be called the calcarine fissure. However, the major fissures, such as the sylvian and interhemispheric fissures, are never called sulci.

2. Fissures
   a. The **interhemispheric fissure** separates the two cerebral hemispheres as they evaginate (see Figure 1-5 and Figure 13-19B, #1).
   b. The **sylvian** or **lateral fissure** separates the frontal and parietal lobes above from the temporal lobe below as it evaginates (see Figure 13-3).
   c. The **transverse cerebral fissure** forms by invagination of the forebrain roof plate, separating the fornix, fornix commissure, and corpus callosum above from the roof of the third ventricle below (see Figure 13-19B, #2).
   d. The **choroid fissure** is an extension of the invaginated transverse cerebral fissure. It forms as the parahippocampal gyrus and hippocampal formation roll in (see Figures 13-14 and 13-19C, #9).

3. Timetable for sulcus formation
   a. After the fissures appear, the cerebral surface remains otherwise completely smooth until sulcation commences in the sixteenth to seventeenth week of gestation.

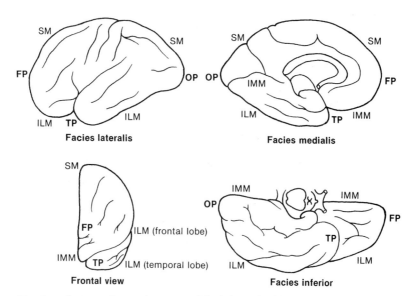

FIGURE 13-1. The three facies, poles, and margins of the left cerebral hemisphere. *FP* = frontal pole; *ILM* = inferolateral margin; *IMM* = inferomedial margin; *OP* = occipital pole; *SM* = superior margin; *TP* = temporal pole.

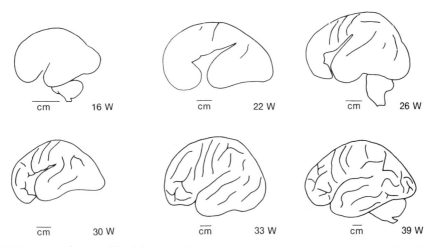

FIGURE 13-2. Lateral view of the left cerebral hemisphere showing the progressive timetable of sulcation. By 39 weeks, the sulcation is nearly complete. See Figures 13-3 through 13-5 for the names of the sulci. *W* = weeks of gestation. (Reprinted with permission from Chi JG, Dooling EC, Giles FH: Gyral development of the human brain. *Ann Neurol* 1:86–93, 1977.)

    b. From the timetable of sulcation, the pathologist can estimate the gestational age of a premature infant at autopsy (Figure 13-2).

4. The **final pattern of sulci and gyri** is shown in Figures 13-3, 13-4, and 13-5.

E. Sylvian fissure, insular region, and opercula

    1. Course of the sylvian fissure (Figure 13-6)

      a. The sylvian fissure begins at the **vallecula** ("little valley"). This space, which admits a fingertip, is located just lateral to the angle formed by the optic nerve, optic chiasm, and optic tract (see Figure 13-9). The roof of the vallecula is the anterior perforated substance.

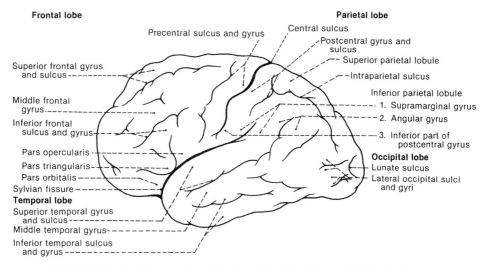

FIGURE 13-3. Sulci and gyri on facies lateralis of the left cerebral hemisphere.

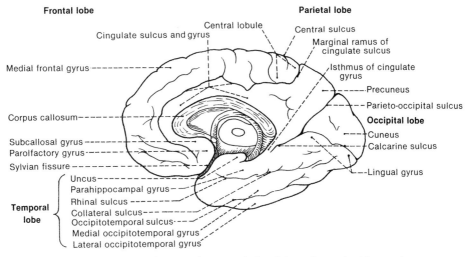

FIGURE 13-4. Sulci and gyri on facies medialis of the right cerebral hemisphere.

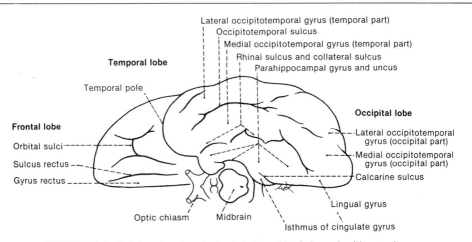

FIGURE 13-5. Sulci and gyri on facies inferior of the left cerebral hemisphere.

FIGURE 13-6. Lateral view of the left cerebral hemisphere with the parts of the sylvian (lateral) fissure and adjacent gyri labeled. *OP* = pars opercularis; *OR* = pars orbitalis; *Pcg* = postcentral gyrus; *Sgi* = supramarginal gyrus, inferior part; *Sgs* = supramarginal gyrus, superior part; *Stg* = superior temporal gyrus; *Tr* = pars triangularis. See also Figure 15-3.

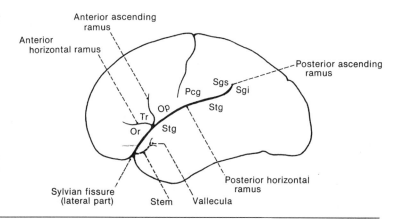

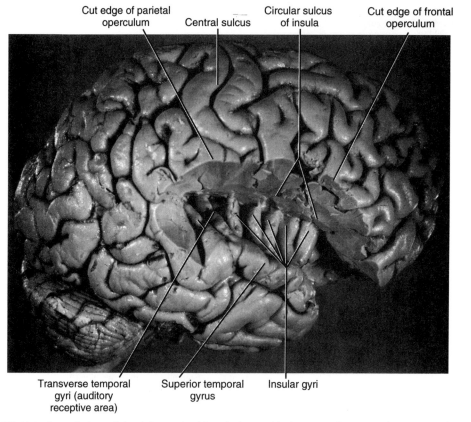

FIGURE 13-7. Lateral view of the right cerebral hemisphere with the opercula removed to expose the insular region.

b. From the vallecula, the **stem** of the sylvian fissure extends laterally. It separates the inferior surface of the frontal lobe from the temporal pole (see Figure 13-6).

c. From its stem, the sylvian fissure continues on facies lateralis as the **anterior** and **posterior horizontal rami**.

d. The posterior horizontal ramus separates the frontal and parietal lobes from the temporal lobe. It ends in an upcurved tip, surrounded by the **supramarginal gyrus**. The superior temporal sulcus often ends in a similar upcurved tip, surrounded by the **angular gyrus** (see Figure 13-3).

2. Relation of carotid and middle cerebral arteries to the sylvian fissure

a. The carotid artery ends at the vallecula by bifurcating into its terminal branches: the **middle** and **anterior cerebral arteries** (see Figures 15-14 and 15-17).

   b. From the vallecula, the middle cerebral artery courses **laterally** through the stem
   and horizontal rami of the sylvian fissure to ramify over the surface of facies lateralis.
   Similarly, the anterior cerebral artery courses **medially** to enter the interhemispheric
   fissure and ramify over facies medialis (see Figures 15-14 and 15-17).

3. Relation of the insular region and opercula to the sylvian fissure
   a. The largest enfolded cortical region, the insula (island of Reil), can be re-exposed
   by dissecting off the frontal and parietal opercula (Figure 13-7; see Figure 15-3).
   b. The dissection shows a **circular sulcus** around the insula and a radial pattern of
   insular gyri. Also exposed are the **transverse temporal gyri of Heschl**, which receive the auditory radiations from the medial geniculate body.

F.   **Surface anatomy of the rhinencephalon and basal forebrain**

1. Definition of rhinencephalon (*rhin* means nose and *encephalon* means brain, therefore nose-brain). The rhinencephalon is that part of the basal forebrain that mediates
   olfaction (the sense of smell) [Figures 13-8 and 13-9].

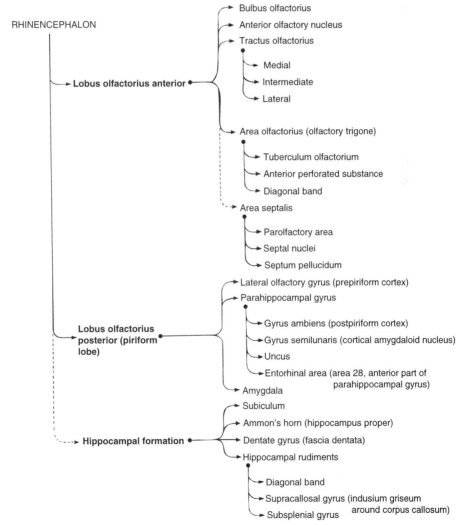

FIGURE 13-8. Dendrogram of nomenclature for the rhinencephalon. Some authors exclude the hippocampal formation from the olfactory lobe per se, as indicated by the interrupted line. (Locate the named structures in Figures 13-9 and 13-13.)

2. **Phylogenetic primacy of the rhinencephalon**
   a. The cerebrum in lower vertebrates consists largely of the rhinencephalon (Figure 13-10).
   b. In comparison to the bulk of our cerebral hemispheres, our olfactory bulbs seem to be unimportant dependencies. In fact, phylogeny indicates that the cerebral hemispheres developed as dependencies of the rhinencephalon (see Figure 13-10 and *OB* in Figure 13-20).
   c. Olfaction and its closely allied sense of taste put an organism in chemical contact with its environment. The other senses all deal with aspects of physics: light, sound, mass, gravity, heat, texture, position, and contour.
   d. We need only to smell and taste our food and smell our mates to survive and perpetuate our kind. Because a blind, deaf rat feeds and mates better than one without olfaction, chemistry serves better than physics for these instinctual behaviors, which remain much more closely linked to our nose-brain and its limbic derivatives than to our rational brain.

3. **The rhinencephalon as the hemispheric pedicle and the three concentric rings of the hemispheric wall**
   a. The cerebral hemispheres and olfactory bulbs evaginate bilaterally from a median rhinencephalic pedicle (see Figure 3-5).
   b. A **sagittal** cut through the rhinencephalic pedicle discloses it to consist of connecting **commissures**, connecting **nervous tissue**, and a connecting **membrane**.

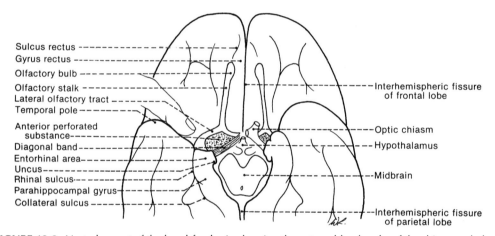

FIGURE 13-9. Ventral aspect of the basal forebrain showing the external landmarks of the rhinencephalon.

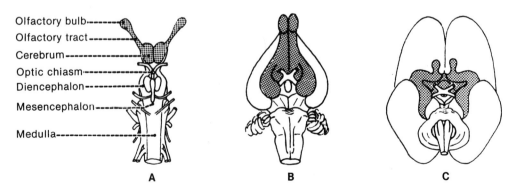

FIGURE 13-10. Ventral view of the brain of the shark (*A*), rodent (*B*), and human fetus (*C*) with the olfactory lobe shaded. (Reprinted with permission from DeMyer W: *Technique of the Neurologic Examination: A Programmed Text*, 3rd ed. New York, McGraw-Hill, 1980, p 286.)

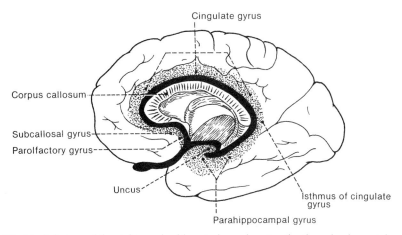

Cingulate gyrus

Corpus callosum

Subcallosal gyrus

Parolfactory gyrus

Uncus

Isthmus of cingulate gyrus

Parahippocampal gyrus

FIGURE 13-11. Medial view of the right cerebral hemisphere showing the three fundamental concentric rings, with the gyri of the limbic ring labeled. *Black area* = olfactory lobe; *dotted area* = limbic lobe; *white area* = supralimbic lobe.

    c. **Connecting commissures** consist of the:
        (1) Corpus callosum (great cerebral commissure) (see Figure 13-29)
        (2) Fornix commissure (hippocampal commissure)
        (3) Anterior commissure (rhinencephalic, temporal lobe, and amygdalar commissures) [see Figure 13-30]
        (4) Optic chiasm and **hypothalamic** commissures
        (5) Habenular commissure (commissure of the habenular nuclei)
        (6) Posterior commissure, which is located just beneath the habenular commissure and belongs to the midbrain, not the foregoing forebrain commissures
    d. **Connecting nervous tissue** consists of:
        (1) Lamina terminalis
        (2) Hypothalamic floor
        (3) Massa intermedia (variably present)
    e. **Connecting membrane.** The tela choroidea, the connecting roof plate of the cerebrum, bridges the ventricles (see Figures 12-2 and 13-19).

  4. Stretching of the rhinencephalic stalk by the corpus callosum. Huge numbers of callosal axons connect the cerebral cortex of the two hemispheres. These axons cross from one side to the other through the original median rhinencephalic stalk, stretching its wall out thin. Although thinned out, rhinencephalic rudiments still form a topologically complete **inner hemispheric ring, the first of three concentric rings** (Figure 13-11):
    a. **Olfactory lobe** (olfactory ring, rhinencephalon proper)
    b. **Limbic lobe** (limbic ring) [see Figure 13-11]
    c. **Supralimbic ring**

G. External anatomy of the limbic lobe
  1. The external surface of the limbic lobe consists of a **ring of gyri** (Table 13-1; see Figure 13-11).
  2. An **inner ring of sulci** separates the limbic lobe proper from the olfactory lobe. An **outer ring of sulci** roughly separates the limbic lobe from the supralimbic (ectocortical) ring (see Table 13-1).
  3. The enfolding of the cortex along the sylvian fissure indents the limbic ring and alters its contour.
  4. Likewise, the evagination of the olfactory bulbs and the invasion of the median pedicle of the rhinencephalon by the axons of the corpus callosum alter the contour of the olfactory ring (Figure 13-12).

TABLE 13-1. Surface Anatomy of the Limbic Ring*

Inner ring of sulci (separates limbic gyri from rhinencephalon)
 Pericallosal sulcus
 Hippocampal sulcus
 (Orbital limbus has no inner sulcus; it borders on medial and lateral olfactory stria)

Ring of limbic gyri
 Paraterminal gyrus (parolfactory gyrus of Broca)
 Subcallosal gyrus
 Cingulate gyrus
 Isthmus (connection between cingulate and parahippocampal gyri)
 Parahippocampal gyrus
 Uncus
 Gyrus ambiens (joins entorhinal area of parahippocampal gyrus to insula)
 Insula
 Orbital limbus (posterior–inferior frontal cortex) and back to paraterminal/subcallosal gyrus

Outer ring of sulci (roughly separates limbic gyri from supralimbic gyri)
 Anterior parolfactory sulcus
 Cingulate sulcus
 Subparietal sulcus
 Collateral sulcus
 Rhinal sulcus
 Circular sulcus of insula
 (Orbital limbus has no external sulcal boundary.)

*See also Figures 13-9 and 13-11.

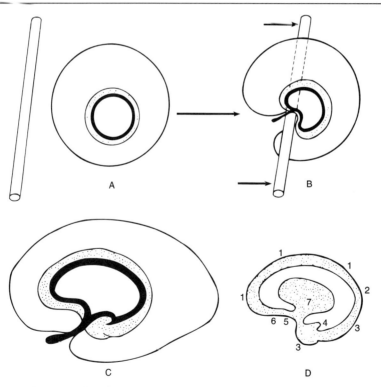

FIGURE 13-12. Medial view of the left cerebral hemisphere. (A) Conceptualization as three geometrically perfect concentric rings. (B) Indentation of the rings and evagination of the olfactory bulbs and tracts. (C) Final configuration of the medial hemispheric wall. (D) Limbic ring dissected out of the hemisphere to show its final geometry and the expansions forming the uncus (4) and insula (7). *Black area* = olfactory lobe; *dotted area* = limbic lobe; *white area* = supralimbic lobe. Limbic ring components are: *1* = cingulate gyrus; *2* = isthmus of cingulate gyrus; *3* = parahippocampal gyrus; *4* = uncus and gyrus ambiens; *5* = orbital limbus and parolfactory gyrus; *6* = subcallosal gyrus; *7* = insula (island of Reil).

II. CONNECTIONS OF THE OLFACTORY AND LIMBIC LOBES

A. Olfactory lobe connections

1. After the primary olfactory axons synapse on the olfactory bulb, **olfactory pathways**, by way of the olfactory tract, **disperse to a number of structures of the basal forebrain** around the vallecula:

   a. The **anterior perforated substance** (Figure 13-13), which forms the roof of the vallecula

   b. The **pyriform lobe**, consisting of the lateral olfactory gyrus, the uncus and ambient and semilunar gyri, and the entorhinal area (see Figure 13-35, area 28) [The pyriform cortex of the lateral olfactory gyrus constitutes the primary olfactory cortex, the entorhinal area the secondary olfactory cortex.]

   c. The **amygdala**

2. Numerous pathways connect the olfactory receptive area of basal forebrain around the vallecula with the septal region, amygdala, hypothalamus, and hippocampal formation. Although once devoted to olfaction, many of these pathways have assumed diverse roles in the limbic system.

3. **Nucleus basalis of Meynert of the anterior perforated substance.** Histologic sections through the anterior perforated substance disclose a plate of large cholinergic neurons oriented tangential to the vallecular surface. Because it projects diffusely to the cortex, the nucleus basalis, unlike many of its phylogenetically regressive neighbors, increases in size in higher animals.

   a. **Connections**

      (1) **Afferents** arrive from many of the adjacent rhinencephalic/limbic structures.

      (2) **Efferents** disperse widely to the:

         (a) Superficial layers of the cerebral cortex, particularly of the frontal and parietal lobes and hippocampus

         (b) Brain stem

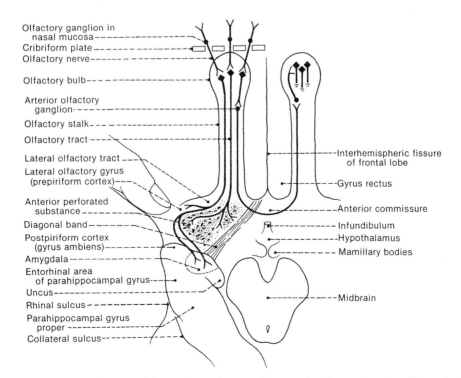

FIGURE 13-13. Basal aspect of the cerebrum showing the axonal pathways from the olfactory bulb.

b. Function. Once dismissed in textbooks as a phylogenetic curiosity, the nucleus basalis is now known to undergo severe degeneration in Alzheimer's disease, the most common dementing disease of the middle and later years of life. It is thought to augment learning, memory, consciousness, and attention span, all of which are impaired in dementia. The diffuse cholinergic projection of this nucleus, comparable to the catecholaminergic and serotonergic brain stem nuclei (see Chapter 14 II and III), suggests some type of augmenting or modulating action rather than a specific function.

B. **The amygdala and its connections**

1. **Definition.** The amygdala is a large nuclear mass located in the temporal pole, at its transition to the posterior inferior surface of the frontal lobe (see Figure 11-1). It is continuous with the uncus of the parahippocampal gyrus. Formerly classed with the basal ganglia, it is now assigned to the limbic lobe.

2. **Connections**
   a. **Afferents** come to the amygdala from the:
      (1) Anterior olfactory lobe
      (2) Pyriform, temporal, and prefrontal cortex
      (3) Hypothalamus
      (4) Nucleus medialis dorsalis of the thalamus
      (5) Brain stem tegmentum, including taste afferents via the parabrachial nucleus
   b. **Efferents** go from the amygdala to the:
      (1) Hypothalamus, septal region, thalamus, and hippocampal formation via the ventral amygdalofugal pathway and ansa peduncularis of the inferior thalamic peduncle
      (2) Opposite amygdala via the stria terminalis and anterior commissure (see Figure 13-30)
      (3) Limbic and nonlimbic cortex of all lobes
      (4) Brain stem tegmentum

3. **Functions.** Like many brain centers, the amygdala **augments, modulates, or integrates several functions**, rather than being a single center with a single function. It seems to integrate input from sensory, cognitive, and limbic pathways, leading to appropriate visceromotor and somatomotor behavioral patterns.
   a. Through its hypothalamic connections, the amygdala **modulates endocrine activity, sexuality, and reproduction**.
   b. **Destruction of the amygdala** may result in passive, defensive, or aggressive behavior.
   c. **Stimulation of the amygdala** may cause changes in mood or arrest of activity, and may activate various sympathetic and parasympathetic responses involving pupillary, cardiovascular, and visceral responses, and alterations in breathing. Breathing exemplifies the control of many such functions by three levels of the nervous system:
      (1) **Automatic** or **reflexive control** by brain stem or spinal level pathways
      (2) **Emotional control** by limbic level pathways (e.g., fright or surprise, with apnea; "It took my breath away"; or anxiety or grief with hyperventilation, sighing, and sobbing)
      (3) **Volitional control** by supralimbic and pyramidal level pathways (e.g., speech, swimming, or blowing)

C. **The hippocampal formation and its connections**

1. **Definition.** The hippocampal formation is primitive cortex along the medial aspect of the temporal lobe, rolled into the floor of the temporal horn along the choroid fissure.
   a. The hippocampal formation consists of three major regions, the **subiculum, hippocampus proper** (Ammon's horn), and **dentate gyrus** (Figures 13-14 and 13-15).
   b. Both the hippocampus and the dentate gyrus have a three-layered cortex. The subiculum is the transition zone from the three-layered to the six-layered cortex of the temporal lobe.

Hippocampal gyrus cortex   **Dentate gyrus cortex**

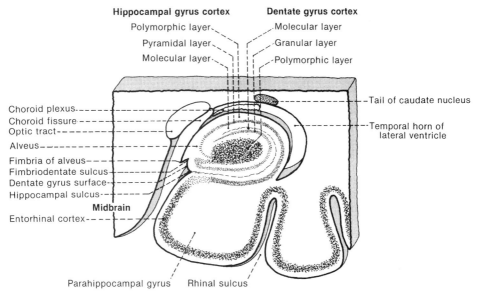

Polymorphic layer   Molecular layer
Pyramidal layer   Granular layer
Molecular layer   Polymorphic layer

Choroid plexus   Tail of caudate nucleus
Choroid fissure   Temporal horn of
Optic tract   lateral ventricle
Alveus
Fimbria of alveus
Fimbriodentate sulcus
Dentate gyrus surface
Hippocampal sulcus
Midbrain
Entorhinal cortex

Parahippocampal gyrus   Rhinal sulcus

FIGURE 13-14. Coronal section through the hippocampal formation, as seen in Nissl stain, to show laminae of neuronal perikarya (cytoarchitecture).

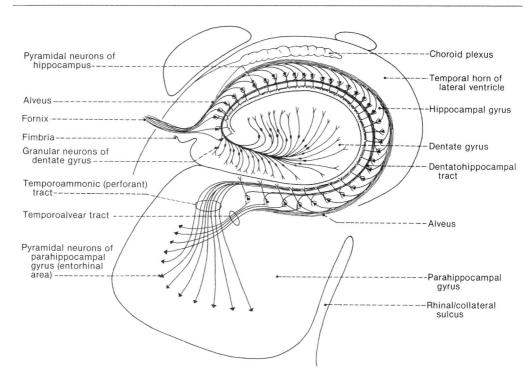

Pyramidal neurons of
hippocampus   Choroid plexus
    Temporal horn of
    lateral ventricle
Alveus   Hippocampal gyrus
Fornix
Fimbria   Dentate gyrus
Granular neurons of
dentate gyrus   Dentatohippocampal
    tract
Temporoammonic (perforant)
tract
Temporoalvear tract   Alveus
Pyramidal neurons of
parahippocampal
gyrus (entorhinal
area)   Parahippocampal
    gyrus
    Rhinal/collateral
    sulcus

FIGURE 13-15. Coronal section of the hippocampal formation showing the neuronal perikarya and their axonal connections, as seen in Golgi silver impregnation.

2. **Origins of the hippocampal formation.** Phylogenetically, the hippocampal formation originates as **rhinencephalic cortex,** but apparently retains no specific olfactory function. It does retain the primitive arrangement of a superficial layer of white matter, the **alveus,** on its ventricular surface (see Figure 13-15).

3. Connections of the hippocampal formation
  a. Afferents come to the hippocampal formation from the:
  (1) Limbic cortex and association regions of the ectocortex, which project via the uncinate fasciculus and cingulum (see Figure 13-25) to the subiculum and entorhinal region of the parahippocampal gyrus (see Figure 13-35, area 28)
  (2) Entorhinal region (area 28), which projects to the hippocampus and dentate gyrus via the **temporoammonic** (perforant) tract (see Figure 13-15)
  (3) Contralateral hippocampal formation via the fornix (hippocampal) commissure (see Figure 12-13, FxC)
  (4) Septal nuclei via the septohippocampal tract
  (5) Thalamus (nucleus anterior, lateralis dorsalis, and midline) via the inferior thalamic peduncle
  (6) Amygdala via ansa peduncularis
  (7) Gigantocellular nuclei of the basal forebrain (cholinergic), nucleus locus coeruleus (adrenergic), raphe nuclei (serotonergic), plus numerous neuropeptide pathways (see Chapter 14 VIII)
  b. Efferents of the hippocampal formation. In general, sources that send to the hippocampal formation also receive from it. Thus, impulses travel both ways in the fornix and other pathways of the hippocampal formation.
  (1) The granular neurons of the dentate gyrus synapse on the pyramidal neurons of the hippocampus but do not project beyond it (see Figure 13-15, the dentatohippocampal tract).
  (2) The pyramidal neurons of the hippocampus are the "final common pathway" out of the hippocampus proper and the dentate gyrus. Most synapse on the subiculum and entorhinal cortex but some go to the septum, thalamus, and contralateral hippocampal formation.
  (3) The cortical neurons of the subiculum are the "final common pathway" that originates most of the axons of the entire hippocampal formation. These axons, plus some from the hippocampal pyramids, enter the alveus. The alveus separates from the surface of the hippocampus. The axons then form the fornix and travel via the fornix to the:
    (a) Nucleus accumbens and septal region
    (b) Mamillary bodies of the hypothalamus
    (c) Thalamus (nuclei anterior, medialis dorsalis, and lateralis dorsalis)
    (d) Contralateral hippocampal formation
    (e) Neighboring structures of the ipsilateral temporal lobe: the entorhinal cortex and neighboring temporal lobe cortex, amygdala, and basal forebrain
    (f) Limbic and association cortex
    (g) Chemically specified nuclei of the RF and nucleus basalis (see Chapter 14)

4. Functions of the hippocampal formation
  a. The hippocampus belongs to the circuitry involved in **learning and recent memory** (see VI L and Figure 13-40). Bilateral hippocampal lesions profoundly impair recent memory. The hippocampus may also have a chemoreceptor—endocrine function.
  b. Because of its low seizure threshold, the hippocampus plays a role in the origin and propagation of **epileptic seizures**.

D. **The limbic lobe and its connections**

1. The Papez circuit. In 1937 James Papez (pronounced *Papes*, as in grapes) suggested that certain rhinencephalic and limbic pathways provided the anatomical basis for emotions and their expression through visceral and instinctual actions such as those involved in feeding, mating, mothering, and aggression (Figure 13-16). The Papez circuit, like the basal motor nuclei, consists of feed-in/feed-out pathways between cortical and subcortical centers, with a major connecting bundle in the cerebral white matter, the **cingulum** (see Figures 13-16 and 13-25, and IV E).

2. Functions of the limbic lobe. Lesions or electrical stimulation of the limbic system causes principally visceral/autonomic and complex behavioral responses. Various sites may be excitatory or inhibitory with regard to a particular function.

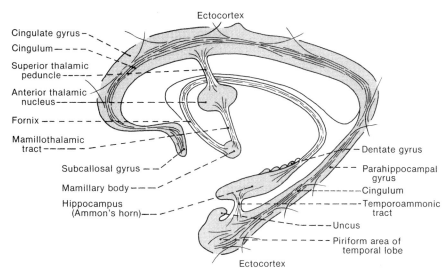

FIGURE 13-16. Lateral diagram of the circuit proposed by Papez as the anatomical basis of emotion. The cingulate gyrus connects with the parahippocampal gyrus and piriform area of the temporal lobe via the cingulum. The temporal lobe connects with the hippocampus (Ammon's horn) via the temporoammonic tract and with the fornix via the temporoalvear tract. The hippocampus connects with the mammillary body via the fornix. The mamillary body connects with the anterior nucleus of the thalamus via the mamillothalamic tract. The anterior nucleus of the thalamus connects with the cingulate gyrus via the superior thalamic peduncle, completing the circuit. Papez also included feed-in pathways to the circuit from the septal and olfactory regions and amygdala.

   a. **Visceral/autonomic responses** include changes in pupillary size, blood pressure, pulse, gastrointestinal peristalsis, bladder contraction, and breathing.
   (1) Stimulation of the cingulate gyrus can arrest breathing.
   (2) Conversely, stimulation of other sites may increase breathing.
   b. **Complex behavioral responses**. Stimulation of the limbic structures may cause a generalized arrest of activity, often accompanied by positive visceral-related actions, such as chewing, swallowing, licking the lips, or grooming. The complex behavioral reactions resulting from limbic stimulation contrast with the relatively simple contractions or twitches of the contralateral muscles following stimulation of the precentral motor cortex.
   (1) In humans, **psychomotor seizures**, which originate in or propagate through limbic connections, are characterized by an aura of fear or visceral sensation, loss of consciousness, and performance of automatic acts such as chewing or picking at the clothes. The patient may stare and show an arrest in behavior, or he may walk around and even drive a car or carry on a limited conversation. However, the patient does not remember the episode.
   (2) Reward behavior and pleasurable sensation also seem to have a limbic basis.
      (a) Animals with electrodes implanted in the septal region and connected to a bar will press the bar compulsively thousands of times, yet the only reward triggered by the bar is the electrical stimulus to the limbic structure. Such reactions suggest the septal area as a "pleasure" center.
      (b) Paul Yakovlev suggested that the posterior cingulate gyrus contained a cenesthetic center, a "feeling good" center, which might control moods of elation, but the amygdala and other limbic connections also participate.
   (3) Mental changes from midline gliomas of the limbic system and corpus callosum. Midline gliomas of the septum pellucidum and corpus callosum, which extend laterally into the limbic structures in a symmetrical, butterfly pattern, cause an organic disorder that the clinician may mistake for a functional mental illness. The patient shows changes in mood, affect, drive, and general behavior, but the neurologic examination shows no overt motor, sensory, or visual signs.

III. PHYLOGENETIC-ONTOGENETIC THEORY OF CEREBRAL MORPHOGENESIS

A. Encephalization

1. Animals can be arranged in a series of increasing intelligence in rough proportion to the increasing number of neurons in their cephalic ganglion or cerebrum, a phylogenetic process called **encephalization**.

2. Two evolutionary developments increased the number of cerebral neurons tremendously while limiting the head circumference to a manageable size:
   a. **Cortex formation**, which coats the cerebral hemispheres with layers of neurons
   b. **Fissuration/sulcation**, which enfolds the spherical surface to increase its area relative to its circumference, enabling the greatest area to fit into the smallest possible space

B. Phylogeny of the semicircular or C shape of the cerebral hemispheres

1. The cerebral hemispheres fundamentally have a semicircular shape as viewed externally and internally, and medially or laterally (Figure 13-17).

2. As seen **laterally**, a side-by-side series of animal brains shows the gradual evolution of the semicircular shape by the downward and forward evagination of the temporal lobe (Figure 13-18).
   a. Evagination of the temporal pole extends the temporal horn of the ventricle, and lengthens and increases the depth of the sylvian fissure.
   b. Similar but less extensive evagination of the frontal and occipital poles extends the ventricles in their directions (see Figure 1-7). Hence, growth vectors expand all three cerebral poles.

3. As seen **medially**, the cerebral wall **invaginates**.
   a. Figure 13-19 conceptualizes the cerebrum before invaginating as showing:
      (1) A fully exposed, membranous roof plate composed of an ependymal lining covered by pia (tela choroidea)

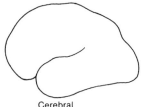

| Cerebral hemisphere | Lateral ventricle | Caudate-putamen | Fornix hippocampus | Stria terminalis-amygdala |

FIGURE 13-17. Lateral view of the left cerebral hemisphere with exploded view of its internal structures. Notice the fundamental semicircular configuration.

FIGURE 13-18. Lateral view of the left hemispheres of a series of animals. Notice the progressive phylogenetic increase in the evagination of the temporal lobe and in the length of the sylvian fissure. (*A*) Salamander. (*B*) Rodent. (*C*) Dog. (*D*) Monkey. (*E*) Human.

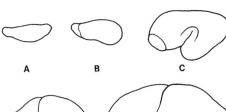

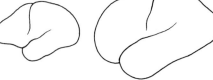

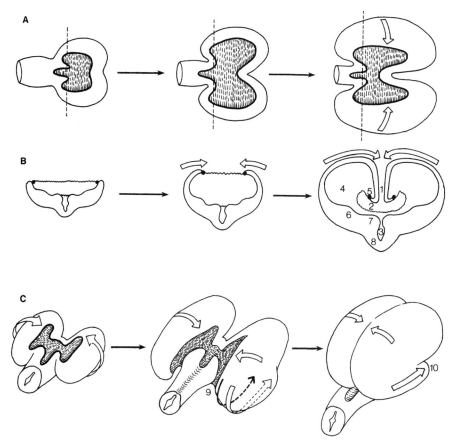

FIGURE 13-19. (*A*) Dorsal view of the developing prosencephalon. (*B*) Coronal sections of the developing prosencephalon at the level of the dashed lines in *A*. (*C*) Dorsal perspective view of the developing prosencephalon, showing the inrolling of the medial hemispheric wall and the downward and forward migration of the temporal lobe. The shaded regions of *A*, *B*, and *C* represent the membranous roof plate. The corpus callosum has not yet developed. *1* = interhemispheric fissure; *2* = transverse fissure; *3* = third ventricle; *4* = lateral ventricle; *5* = hippocampal formation (*black region*); *6* = ganglionic hillock of the corpus striatum; *7* = thalamus; *8* = hypothalamus; *9* (part *C*) = transverse fissure extending as the choroid fissure as the hippocampus originally in a dorsal position, undergoes its backward, downward, and forward migration into the evaginating temporal horn (*thin interrupted arrow*); *10* (part *C*) = completed evagination of the temporal lobe.

    (2) A fully exposed hippocampal formation, still in its primordial dorsal position, before it migrates backward, downward, and forward with the temporal lobe
  b. The initial **evagination of the cerebral hemispheres** creates an **interhemispheric fissure** (see Figure 13-19B, #1).
  c. Then, **invagination of the roof plate** and rolling in of the hippocampal formation create the **transverse cerebral fissure** (see Figure 13-19B, #2).
    (1) Growth vectors in the cerebral wall force the hippocampal formation backward, downward, and forward in a semicircular arc (Figure 13-20; see Figure 13-19), extending the transverse cerebral fissure forward on the medial surface of the temporal lobe as the **choroid fissure**.
    (2) Thus, the backward, downward, and forward semicircular migration of the hippocampal formation **medially** matches the similar configuration of the temporal lobe as viewed **laterally**.
  d. The same process draws out the tail of the caudate nucleus (see Figure 13-17).

C.   **Formation of the cavum veli interpositi and cavum septi pellucidi**

  1. The transverse cerebral and interhemispheric fissures are extracerebral spaces originally in free communication with each other (see Figure 13-19B, #1 and 2).

FIGURE 13-20. Phylogenetic migration of the hippocampal formation (*shaded area*) in a semicircular arc. From its primitive dorsal position, it undergoes a backward, downward, and forward migration, in keeping with the phylogeny of the temporal lobe (see Figure 13-18). The fornix strings out along the pathway of migration of the hippocampal formation, retaining its anchor to the anterior commissure and hypothalamus. *AC* = anterior commissure; *CC* = corpus callosum; *F* = fornix; *HF* = hippocampal formation; *MB* = mammillary body; *OB* = olfactory bulb.

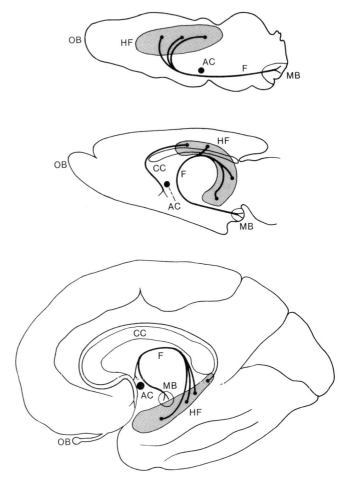

2. As the corpus callosum grows through the median stalk connecting the hemispheres, it bulges backward, with the fornix and fornix commissure clinging to its underbelly (Figure 13-21). By this shelf-like, backward extension, the corpus callosum separates the interhemispheric fissure above from the transverse fissure below.
   a. The space **beneath** the corpus callosum, fornix, and fornix commissure—the original transverse cerebral fissure—is now called the **cavum veli interpositi**.
   b. The velum interpositum, which is another name for the tela choroidea or roof of the third ventricle, extends laterally at the foramen of Monro as the roof plate of the lateral ventricles (see Figure 13-19).

3. As the two anterior pillars of the fornix stretch away from the undersurface of the genu of the corpus callosum, in concert with the migration of the hippocampal formation (see Figure 13-20), they pull out a thin membrane, the **septum pellucidum**, on each side. The cavity between the two leaves of the septum pellucidum, the **cavum septi pellucidi**, is an entirely separate space from the cavum veli interpositi, and both caves are topologically separate from the ventricles.

D. **Review of cerebral organogenesis.** In summary, the major events of cerebral organogenesis are:

1. **Closure** of the neural tube

2. **Transverse segmentation** of the prosencephalon into a telencephalon and a diencephalon

3. Evagination

   a. Evagination converts the holospheric prosencephalon into a hemispheric organ (see Figure 3-5).

   b. Evagination produces the three hemispheric poles, particularly the temporal. The temporal lobe evagination creates the sylvian fissure, and opercularization along the fissure buries the insula.

   c. The olfactory bulbs and tracts also evaginate.

4. Invagination of the medial hemispheric wall creates the transverse fissure, a lateral extension of the interhemispheric fissure that resulted from evagination of the cerebral hemispheres (see Figure 13-19B, #2).

   a. Then backward, downward, and forward migration of the hippocampal formation extends the transverse fissure as the choroid fissure.

   b. The corpus callosum enlarges backward as a shelf, forming a roof over the cavum veli interpositi.

E. **Holoprosencephaly.** In this striking malformation, the cerebrum bears an uncanny resemblance to the diagrammatic representation of the prosencephalon shown in Figure 13-19 A and B. Holoprosencephaly (Figure 13-22) can be interpreted as a total arrest in the process of evagination and invagination of the forebrain described above.

   1. The prosencephalon remains holospheric rather than proceeding to evaginate its walls laterally to become hemispheric (see Figure 3-5).

   2. The cerebrum lacks all three poles, in particular a fully evaginated temporal pole, and therefore lacks an enfolded insula and sylvian fissure.

   3. If we consider the olfactory bulb as the pole of the olfactory lobe, then all four poles of the cerebrum fail to evaginate in holoprosencephaly. The characteristic absence of the olfactory lobe (the olfactory bulbs and tracts) is called **arhinencephaly**.

   4. The prosencephalic cavity remains as a single holoventricle without a subdivision into lateral and third ventricles connected by a Y-shaped foramen of Monro.

   a. The foramen of Monro remains as a gaping communication that occupies the anterior-posterior diameter of the ventricle, rather than narrowing to a small aperture under the two columns of the fornix.

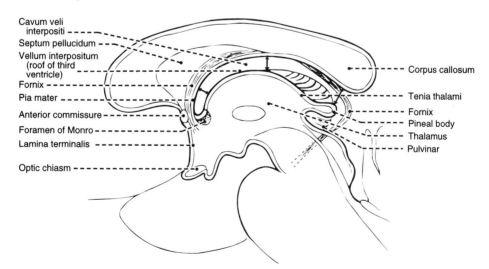

FIGURE 13-21. Sagittal section through the cavum veli interpositi (*open area* delineated by 3 *arrows*). The most posterior arrow marks the opening or mouth of the cavum by which it communicates with the rest of the subarachnoid space. Thus, the cavum is a subarachnoid recess, outside of the brain proper, created by the backward growth of the corpus callosum over the thalami and the roof of the third ventricle. The floor (*dark line*) of the cavum velum interpositum is the roof of the third ventricle. It consists of a tela choroidea, which is a membrane composed of a lining of ependyma and a covering of pia matter. Anteriorly, the pia reflects backward on the undersurface of the fornix after the tela choroidea bridges the foramen of Monro.

FIGURE 13-22. Dorsal view of a human brain showing holoprosencephaly (compare with Figure 13-19). *1* = gyrated ecocortex covering the prosencephalic holosphere, which has failed to evaginate (cleave) into hemispheres; *2* = limbic mesocortex; *3* = archicortex (hippocampal formation) with fimbria-fornix bordering the monoventricle; *4* = cavity of holoventricle (monoventricle); *5* = ganglionic hillock of the corpus striatum; *6* = thalamus, uncleft from its neighbor; hence, the two thalami are not divided by a third ventricle; *7* = cut edge of the greatly expanded roof plate, which covered the monoventricle intra vitam. The roof plate should have been folded into the transverse and choroid fissures (see Figure 13-19B); *8* = normally sulcated and hemispherized cerebellum.

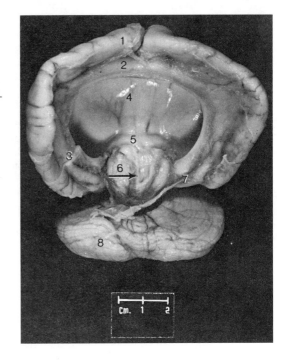

    b. Because the thalami fail to hemispherize by separating in the midline, they do not form a cleft for the third ventricle.

5. The roof plate remains totally exposed—everted, as it were—because of failure of enfolding of the medial hemispheric wall to create an interhemispheric fissure and transverse cerebral fissure.

6. The corpus callosum fails to grow back over the ventricular roof.

7. The hippocampal formation remains exposed in its primordial dorsal position (see Figure 13-22, #3) because it fails to roll into the choroid fissure and migrate backward, downward, and forward.

8. The limbic lobe occupies its familiar position as a concentric ring around the hippocampal formation and rhinencephalon of the inner ring (see Figures 13-11 and 13-19).

9. The cortex of the holosphere forms and sulcates because histogenesis is governed by laws different from those governing organogenesis.

IV. WHITE MATTER OF THE CEREBRUM

A. **Composition.** White matter consists of:

1. Axons, which run in organized tracts

2. Glia
    a. Oligodendrocytes, which provide myelin
    b. Astrocytes, which provide scaffolding

3. Blood vessels

B. **Timetable for development.** The various tracts to and from the cerebral cortex invade the cerebral wall in a definite sequence (Table 13-2) and then myelinate in a definite sequence (see Figure 3-23).

C. **Destinations of cortical axons.** Cortical axons may synapse on other cortical neurons or on infracortical neurons. Depending on the location of the **cortical** or **infracortical** target neuron, whether ipsilateral or contralateral, the developing efferent axons reach different destinations, which leads to their classification as **association fibers**, **commissural fibers**, or **projection fibers** (Figure 13-23).

1. **Association fibers.** The axons of cortical neurons, which synapse on **ipsilateral** cortical neurons, associate these neurons in their function; hence, the name **association fibers** (see Figure 13-23).

TABLE 13-2. Approximate Times during Gestation When Various Tracts Appear

End of first month	Spinal trigeminal tract
	Fasciculus solitarius
	Medial longitudinal fasciculus
During second month	Mamillotegmental tract
	Olfactory nerve
	Posterior commissure
	Transverse fibers of hindbrain
	Fasciculus retroflexus
	Crossed olivary fibers
	Thalamic peduncles
	Stria medullaris thalami
	Inferior cerebellar peduncle
	Internal capsule
During third month	Anterior commissure
During fourth month	Columns of fornix
	Corpus callosum
	Pontine fibers
During fifth month	Pyramidal fibers

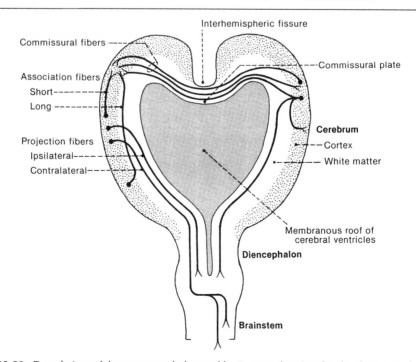

FIGURE 13-23. Dorsal view of the prosencephalon and brain stem showing the development of commissural, association, and projection fibers.

2. **Commissural fibers**
   a. Cortical axons that cross the midline to synapse on **contralateral** cortical neurons are called **commissural fibers**.
   b. Commissures differ from decussations because commissural fibers cross the midline to connect mirror-image points, whereas decussating fibers cross to connect non–mirror-image points.

3. **Projection fibers**
   a. Cortical axons that synapse on infracortical neurons "project" the cortical influence onto the lower centers, like the thalamus; hence, they are called **projection fibers**.
   b. Projection fibers may end **ipsilaterally** or **contralaterally**. In the latter case they are decussations.
   c. The term "projection fiber" may also apply to infracortical connections. Thus, the cerebellum "projects" to the thalamus.

4. Any given axon may branch to send collateral fibers to association, commissural, or projection pathways (see Figure 13-23).

D. **Association pathways of the cerebral white matter**

1. **Short association fibers**
   a. Many association axons synapse close to their neuron of origin. They remain **intracortical** and do not enter the deep white matter.
   b. Many association axons that travel for short distances arch around the depth of a sulcus. They form a visible U-shaped lamina on the undersurface of the cortex, called an **arcuate bundle** (Figure 13-24).
   c. The **uncinate** (U-shaped) **fasciculus** is one of the largest arcuate bundles (Figures 13-25 and 13-26).
   d. As the intracortical association fibers travel longer distances, they laminate in a peripheral-to-central manner.
      (1) In the cerebral white matter, the short fibers—the arcuate bundles—laminate on the **inner** surface of the cortex, and the long fibers laminate deeper in the white matter (see Figure 13-24).

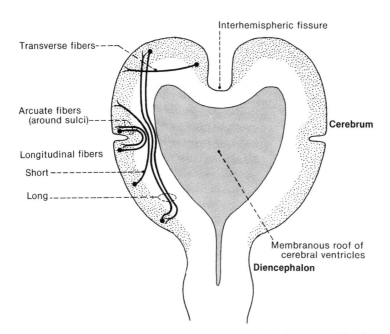

FIGURE 13-24. Dorsal view of the prosencephalon showing the development of the short, arcuate association fibers and the lamination of the long association fibers deep to them. Transverse and vertical association fibers of intermediate length crisscross the deep white matter.

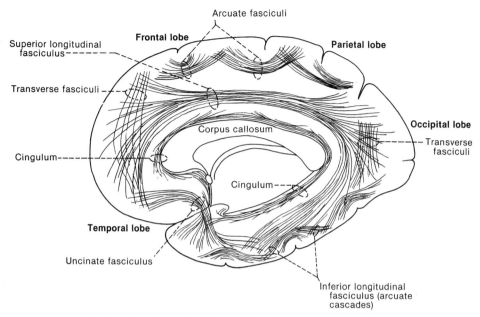

FIGURE 13-25. Sagittal section of a cerebral hemisphere showing several association pathways (see also Figure 13-26).

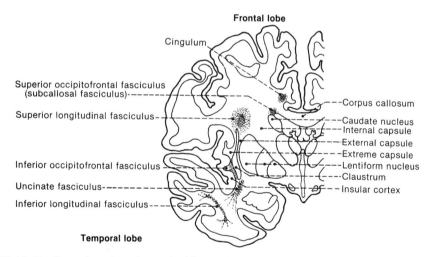

FIGURE 13-26. Coronal section of a cerebral hemisphere showing several longitudinally running association pathways (see also Figure 13-25).

           (2) In the spinal cord, in contrast, the short axons or ground bundles laminate on the **outer** surface of the gray matter, and the long fibers laminate on the periphery of the ground bundles.

  2. Long association fibers

      a. The long association fibers accumulate into more or less distinctive bundles that stand out on gross dissection (Table 13-3).

      b. The bundles continually pay out and receive axons along their course. In fact, recent studies show that a series of arcuate cascades, rather than a single inferior longitudinal fasciculus, connects the temporal and occipital regions.

TABLE 13-3. Long Association Bundles of the Cerebral Hemisphere Arranged in Medial-to-Lateral and Dorsal-to-Ventral Order*

Cingulum (supracallosal fasciculus)

Superior occipitofrontal fasciculus (subcallosal fasciculus)

Superior longitudinal fasciculus

Inferior occipitofrontal fasciculus

Inferior longitudinal fasciculus (occipitotemporal fasciculus)—now regarded as a series of arcuate cascades rather than a single bundle

*See also Figures 13-25 and 13-26.

FIGURE 13-27. Coronal section through the cerebrum at the level of the body of the corpus callosum and the genu of the internal capsule showing the distribution of axons from the cingulum. Fibers of the cingulum form dorsal and ventral lamina of the corpus callosum. The middle lamina of the corpus callosum transmits cortical commissural fibers (see also Figure 13-29). *1* = cortico-cortical fibers; *2* = lateral fibers; *3* = corticoperforant fibers; *4* = dorsal transcallosal fibers; *5* = ventral trans-callosal fibers.

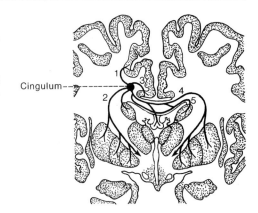

   c. In addition to the longitudinally running long bundles, pathways of intermediate length crisscross vertically and transversely between facies medialis and facies lateralis or in a superior to inferior direction in all of the lobes (see Figure 13-25).
   d. **Lesions** that interrupt the long intracortical pathways disconnect one part of the cerebrum from another and from infracortical centers, leading to varying degrees of dementia as well as sensory and motor deficits.
   e. Certain **demyelinating diseases** preferentially attack the long pathways, sparing the arcuate bundles.

E. **The cingulum**

   1. The cingulum is the **association pathway of the limbic lobe**. It conveys long and short axons. It girdles the hemisphere from the parolfactory and subcallosal regions of the frontal lobe around to the parahippocampal gyrus and temporal pole (see Figures 13-16, 13-25, and 13-26).
   a. Limbic fibers of the uncinate fasciculus then complete the limbic ring by connecting the temporal lobe to the inferior frontal region.
   b. The temporal cortex that receives the limbic connections of the cingulum and uncinate fasciculus sends axons to the hippocampus (Ammon's horn) as the temporoammonic tract (of Cajal) and into the fornix as the temporoalvear tract. These connections belong to the Papez circuit (see Figure 13-16).

   2. In addition to its cortical connections, the cingulum distributes axons from the limbic nuclei of the thalamus and from the cortex to the corpus striatum (Figure 13-27).

   3. **Cingulotomy** by stereotaxic surgery may reduce the reaction of the terminally ill patient to pain and may reduce the intensity of obsessive-compulsive neuroses.

F. **Cortical commissures** (Table 13-4)

   1. **Corpus callosum**
   a. **Development** (see III C 2 and Figure 13-20)

b. **Gross subdivisions.** The corpus callosum, the largest crossing bundle in the central nervous system (CNS), has a **rostrum, genu, body**, and **splenium** (Figure 13-28).
c. **Fiber connections.** Through its middle lamina; the corpus callosum connects mirror-image areas of the cortex of the two hemispheres. Its dorsal and ventral lamina convey axons of the cingulum (see Figure 13-27). Thus, it contains commissural and decussating fibers.
   (1) Those axons that curve around the interhemispheric fissure anteriorly comprise the **forceps minor**; they form the genu. Those curving around posteriorly comprise the **forceps major**; they form the splenium (Figure 13-29).
   (2) Regions that lack transcallosal connections include:
      (a) Primary sensory areas 1, 2, and 17 and part of the primary auditory receptive area (see Figure 13-35, area 41)
      (b) Those parts of the motor cortex (see Figure 13-35, area 4) serving the upper and lower extremities (In contrast, the motor areas for the face, shoulder, and pelvic girdle and trunk do have callosal connections.)
      (c) Anterior superior frontal region

2. **Hippocampal commissure (psalterium, lyre of David)**
   a. The hippocampal commissure connects the hippocampal formations of the two hemispheres.
   b. Moved backward by the growth of the corpus callosum and the migration of the hippocampal formations, the hippocampal commissure crosses beneath the posterior part of the body of the corpus callosum. It is part of the rhinencephalic underwall of that structure.

TABLE 13-4. The Cortical Commissures

Corpus callosum*
Gross subdivisions: rostrum, genu, body, and splenium
Radiatio corporis callosi
Tapetum
Anterior forceps (forceps minor)
Posterior forceps (forceps major)

Hippocampal commissure (psalterium)

Anterior commissure†
Interbulbar and intertubercular components from olfactory bulb and olfactory tubercle
Prepiriform, interamygdaloid, and interparahippocampal gyrus components
Ectocortical components:
   Small contingent from the superorostral frontal cortex
   Intertemporal component connecting the temporal gyri (the largest component in primates)

*See Figure 13-29.
†See Figure 13-30.

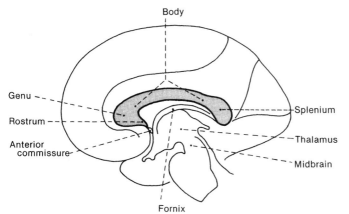

FIGURE 13-28. Sagittal section of the corpus callosum showing the division into four parts: rostrum, genu, body, and splenium.

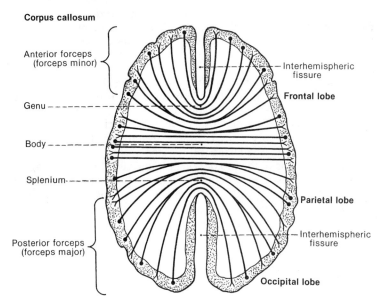

Corpus callosum

Anterior forceps
(forceps minor)

Genu

Body

Splenium

Posterior forceps
(forceps major)

Interhemispheric
fissure

Frontal lobe

Parietal lobe

Interhemispheric
fissure

Occipital lobe

FIGURE 13-29. Horizontal section through the cerebral hemispheres and corpus callosum showing the pattern of the crossing nerve fibers in the genu, body, and splenium.

FIGURE 13-30. Ventral view of the cerebral hemispheres showing the fibers of the anterior commissure. *1* = interbulbar component; *2* = intertubercular (interanterior perforated substance) component; *3* = interamygdaloid component; *4* = ectocortical component; *5* = interparahippocampal gyrus component; *6* = stria terminalis (interamygdaloid component).

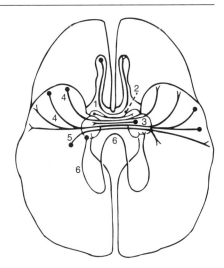

3. **Anterior Commissure**
    a. The anterior commissure crosses in the commissural plate ventral to the corpus callosum (Figure 13-30; see Figure 12-10).
    b. Phylogenetically, it originates as a noncortical or rhinencephalic commissure, linking the olfactory bulbs, the amygdala, and other basal forebrain neurons.
    c. In higher animals, ectocortical fibers linking frontal and temporal cortex predominate. The fibers laminate in the same manner as the corpus callosum (see Figure 13-30 and Table 13-4).

4. **Clinical effects of cerebral commissurotomy: the split brain.** Sagittal section of the corpus callosum, anterior commissure, and the optic chiasm disconnects the two cerebral hemispheres. The individual has a "split brain" (actually a split cerebrum) and cannot transfer information from one hemisphere to the other. Specific tests are required to demonstrate the deficits.
    a. If blindfolded, the individual cannot match an item held in one hand or seen in one visual field with what is felt or seen on the other side.

b. A right-handed patient can execute a verbal command with the right hand because the motor cortex remains connected to the language centers of the left hemisphere. The patient cannot execute the command with the left hand because the right hemisphere, disconnected from the left, does not understand language.

5. Agenesis of the corpus callosum. The fibers of the corpus callosum may fail to cross during development. The fibers then accumulate along the ipsilateral ventricular wall (Probst's bundle), rather than crossing in the commissural plate.

G. Noncortical commissures of the diencephalon

1. The hypothalamic commissures connect the globus pallidus and the subthalamus, the pretectal nuclei, the medial geniculate bodies, and the hypothalamic nuclei themselves.

2. The habenular commissure links the habenular nuclei of the epithalamus and anchors the dorsal lip of the evagination that produces the pineal body.

3. The posterior commissure, technically part of the midbrain, anchors the ventral lip of the evagination that produces the pineal body. It connects the pretectal and collicular areas of the two sides and the satellite optomotor nuclei around the nucleus of cranial nerve (CN) III.

H. **Subcortical projection pathways from the cerebral cortex** are summarized in Table 13-5.

I. **Summary of the pathways comprising the cerebral white matter**

1. Short (arcuate), intermediate, and long association bundles (see Table 13-3)

2. Commissures (see Table 13-4)

3. Cortical projection fibers (see Table 13-5)

4. Thalamic peduncles (see Table 12-5)

5. Internal (see Table 12-4), external, and extreme capsules

V. CEREBRAL CORTEX

A. **Definition.** The cerebral cortex consists of thin horizontal layers of neurons and nerve fibers, forming a brownish-gray sheet on the surface of the cerebral hemispheres. The vernacular term "gray matter" refers either to the cortex or to nuclear masses.

B. **Ontogeny of cortical lamination**

1. Ontogenetically, the cerebral wall consists of three zones: **periventricular** (germinal), **intermediate**, and **marginal**.

TABLE 13-5. Subcortical Projection Pathways from Cortical Neurons

Corticobulbar and corticospinal projections of the pyramidal system
Corticoextrapyramidal projections to basal motor nuclei
Corticotegmental optomotor projections to the reticular formation and accessory nuclei for control of volitional eye movements
Corticopretectal–tectal projections, mainly from the occipital lobe for reflex eye movements based on vision
Corticopontine projections
Corticohypothalamic projections (existence uncertain in humans)
Corticoreticular projections

2. The cortical neuroblasts start migrating from the germinal zone into the marginal zone in the second month of gestation (see Figure 3-10).

    a. After migrating to the cerebral surface, the vast majority of cortical neuroblasts direct their axons inward into the intermediate zone, expanding it to form the deep white matter.

    b. Successive waves of cortical neuroblasts leave the germinal zone at later and later times.

    c. The neurons for inner cortical layers migrate to the cerebral surface first. Then the neurons for the outer layers migrate through the inner layers to reach their terminal positions. Thus, the four outer layers of cortical neurons develop after the inner two, in an inside-out sequence.

    d. By the eighth month of gestation, the cortex shows its final six lamina.

C. **Phylogeny of the cerebral cortex: paleocortex, archicortex, and neocortex**

1. Paleocortex

    a. In primitive animals, the cerebral neurons have a nucleate-reticulate pattern that extends throughout the entire cerebral wall. This nucleate-reticulate pattern, with a hint of lamination, persists as paleocortex in all subsequent animals, including humans, in the olfactory region around the vallecula of the basal forebrain as part of the rhinencephalon.

    b. In higher submammalia, particularly reptiles, more and more neurons migrate to the cerebral surface, where they commence to laminate (see Figure 3-10).

    c. In mammalia, the cortex has three or six distinct layers, called **archicortex** and **neocortex**, respectively (Figure 13-31).

2. Archicortex

    a. The three-layered archicortex, phylogenetically intermediate between the paleo-cortex and neocortex, occurs in the hippocampal formation. Its efferent axons

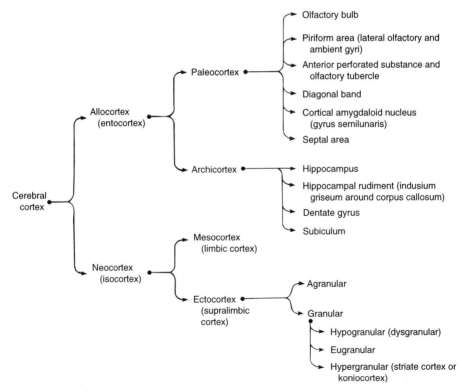

FIGURE 13-31. Dendrogram of the phylogenetic terminology for the cerebral cortex.

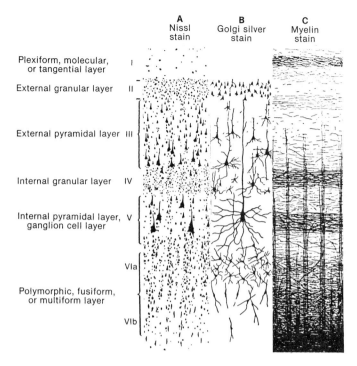

A
Nissl
stain

B
Golgi silver
stain

C
Myelin
stain

Plexiform, molecular,
or tangential layer I

External granular layer II

External pyramidal layer III

Internal granular layer IV

Internal pyramidal layer, V
ganglion cell layer

VIa

Polymorphic, fusiform,
or multiform layer

VIb

FIGURE 13-32. Histologic sections of the ectocortex. (*A*) Nissl stain. (*B*) Golgi silver impregnation. (*C*) Myelin stain. (Reprinted with permission from Brodal A: *Neurological Anatomy*. New York, Oxford University Press, 1981, p 63.)

are directed outward into the alveus, which forms a superficial rather than a deep layer of white matter (see Figures 13-14 and 13-15).

b. Archicortex, along with paleocortex and the pericallosal rudiment (indusium griseum), is the cortex of the inner of the three concentric rings of the hemispheric wall (see Figure 13-11). The median stalk, connecting the two rings on each side at the hilus of the hemispheres, is perforated and expanded by the corpus callosum.

3. Neocortex, consisting of mesocortex and ectocortex, has six layers.

    a. Mesocortex is the six-layered cortex that **covers the limbic lobe**. It covers the second of the three concentric cerebral rings (see Figure 13-11).

    b. Ectocortex is the six-layered **supralimbic cortex**. It is phylogenetically new and ascendent, covering most of the cerebral surface. Like mesocortex, it directs the vast majority of its efferent axons inward and receives subcortical afferents by way of the deep white matter.

    c. The **exuberant overgrowth of ectocortex accounts for the increasing brain size in higher animals**. It is what fulfills the process of encephalization, and leads to the need for the extensive sulcation and fissuration of the brain in higher animals.

D. Six horizontal layers of the ectocortex

1. Nissl-stained sections disclose **six horizontal layers** of neuronal perikarya and also their tendency to **align in vertical columns** (Figure 13-32A and Table 13-6).

2. Golgi-stained sections show the **full branching patterns** of the various types of cortical neurons (see Figures 13-32B and 13-33).

3. Myelin-stained sections show a **grid** of entering and exiting nerve fibers, obviously designed for **vertical and horizontal dispersion of nerve impulses** (see Figure 13-32C and Table 13-6).

    a. The larger cortical dendrites, as well as the entering and exiting nerve fibers, run in vertical columns, perpendicular to the cortical surface.

    b. When the vertically oriented nerve fibers or dendrites branch, their collaterals tend to run perpendicular to the vertical columns, thus contributing to the horizontal lamination of the cortex (Table 13-7; see Figure 13-32C).

TABLE 13-6. The Horizontal Laminae of the Neocortex As Seen in Nissl Stain*

Layer	Average Width	Synonyms	Outstanding Cellular Characteristics
I	10%	Plexiform, molecular, or tangential layer	Neuronal perikarya very sparse; contains axons and dendrites
II	10%	External granular layer	Numerous small pyramidal and stellate neurons
III	30%	External pyramidal layer	Numerous medium-sized pyramidal neurons, increasing in size from superficial to deep parts of the layer
IV	10%	Internal granular layer	Numerous small stellate (granular) neurons
V	20%	Internal pyramidal layer (ganglion cell layer)	Medium to very large pyramidal neurons with small numbers of stellate neurons
VI	20%	Polymorphic layer (fusiform or multiform layer)	Many fusiform or polymorphic perikarya; some pyramidal and stellate neurons

*See also Figure 13-32.

TABLE 13-7. Horizontal Strata of Myelinated Fibers of the Ectocortex

Layer	Name of Stripe or Plexus	Source of Fibers
I	Tangential plexus of Retzius	Horizontal neurons of layer 1
II	None present	
III	Outer main layer (line of Kaes-Bechterew)	Terminal collaterals of cortical association and commissural fibers
IV	Outer line of Baillarger (line of Gennari or Vicq d'Azyr in visual cortex)	Terminal plexus of incoming thalamocortical fibers; sometimes crowds into layer IIIc
V	Inner main layer or inner line of Baillarger	Collaterals of fibers in transit to and from the cortex
VI	Indistinct	Collaterals of fibers in transit to and from the cortex

    c. The horizontal laminae or striae of myelinated fibers (lines of Baillarger) are readily visible in the sensory receptive areas of the cortex, hence the name **striate** or **striped** cortex for all three primary sensory receptive areas.

E. **Vertical (radial) arrangement of cortical neurons**

    1. The vertical columns of the cortex create a matrix of countless vertical stacks of 100 to 300 synaptically connected neurons.

        a. These countless vertical stacks, rather than the horizontal lamination, may constitute the "functional units" of the cortex.

        b. The horizontal lamination and the vertical cylindrical arrangement of cortical neurons occur throughout the mammalia.

    2. The vertical cylinders may vary in diameter up to several hundred micra. For example, a thalamocortical relay axon ends in a cylindrical tuft with a longitudinal spread of around 300 μ.

        a. The size of a cylinder, as defined by the spread of thalamic afferents, may differ from the size defined by association fiber afferents.

        b. Dendrites and axonal collaterals may spread over radii of different lengths.

c. These arrangements provide for varying degrees of "cross talk" between the neurons **within** a vertical cylinder and **between** the vertical cylinders themselves.

3. Some cylinders, such as those in the sensory receptive cortices, might receive afferents from a restricted group of sensory neurons. The more specific the sensory topography, as in the tonotopic auditory cortex or retinotopic visual cortex, the more restricted the afferents to the cylinder.

4. Although cylinders are not as evident in the motor cortex, a vertical stack might activate only a tiny group of lower motoneurons (LMNs). However, the localization in either motor or sensory systems should not be regarded too rigidly.
   a. Destruction of one vertical zone in the motor cortex does not cause paralysis of one tiny group of LMNs. Some overlap exists, and each vertical zone might function as the maximum or modal point for a particular LMN pool rather than having the fatality of a telephone switchboard.
   b. This issue reflects an old controversy as to the degree of plasticity of the motor cortex and whether the motor cortex represents "muscles" or "movements."

F. **Five anatomical types of cortical neurons.** Cortical neurons fall into five types that differ both in the size and length of their axons and in shape (i.e., pattern of dendritic branching) [Figure 13-33]. The three most common types of neurons have a **pyramidal, stellate,** or **fusiform** perikaryon. The two less common types, the **neurons of Martinotti** and the **horizontal neurons of Cajal,** have a polygonal or fusiform perikaryon, respectively.

1. The **pyramidal neurons,** named for their pyramid-shaped perikaryon, vary in height from 10 to 100 μ.
   a. Structure
      (1) A long **apical dendrite** extends vertically from the apex of the pyramid.
      (2) Basal dendrites extend laterally in horizontal and oblique planes from the base of the pyramid. The horizontal spread of the basal dendrites and the distal branches of the apical dendrite is 50 to 300 μ.
      (3) From the base of the pyramid, an **axon** extends into the white matter (Golgi type I neuron).
         (a) Typically, the axon collateralizes into branches that form **association, commissural,** or **projection fibers.**
         (b) The recurrent axonal collaterals of the association fibers may end on other pyramidal neurons or cortical interneurons.
   b. Location and function of pyramidal neurons. The pyramidal neurons of **layer V,** along with fusiform neurons of layer VI, provide most of the efferent axons of the cerebral cortex. Two **specialized large pyramidal efferent neurons** are those of Betz and Meynert.
      (1) The **Betz neurons,** the largest neurons of the cortex, are located in layer V of the motor cortex (Figure 13-34A, area 4). The perikaryon measures as much as 100 μ in height. The Betz neurons originate the large myelinated axons of the pyramidal tract.
      (2) The **Meynert cells** are large pyramidal neurons located in layer V of the visual receptive cortex in the occipital lobe (see Figure 13-34D, area 17). They send axons to the brain stem that mediate visually directed reflex eye movements.

2. The **stellate or granular neurons** have a small round, polygonal, or triangular perikaryon, 4 to 8 μ in diameter, which reflects a very busy, more random pattern of dendritic branching (see Figure 13-33). These neurons are most numerous in layer IV of the primary sensory cortices.
   a. The **dendrites** extend only a short distance from the perikaryon, and the **axon** runs only a short distance (Golgi type II neuron) to form intracortical connections.
   b. The various types of stellate neurons and the Cajal and Martinotti neurons are **cortical interneurons** whose axons remain within the cerebral cortex.
   c. Stellate neuronal subtypes are either **excitatory or inhibitory.** Each subtype produces characteristic axodendritic and axoaxonic synapses.

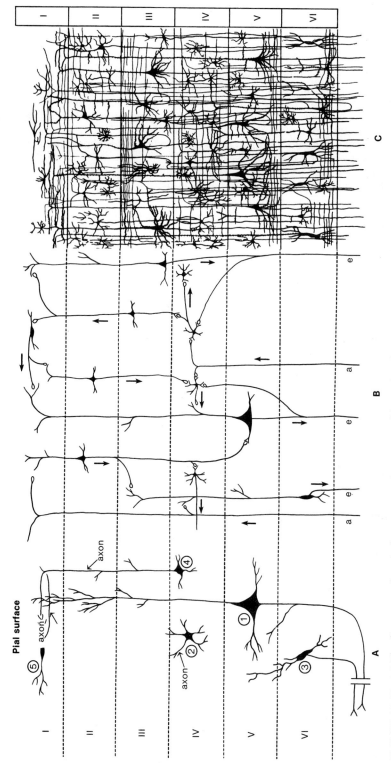

FIGURE 13-33. (A) The five types of cortical neurons as demonstrated by Golgi silver impregnation (for layer names, see Figure 13-32). 1 = pyramidal neuron; 2 = stellate neuron; 3 = fusiform neuron; 4 = neuron of Martinotti; 5 = neuron of Cajal. (B) Typical synaptic connections of cortical neurons. a = afferent; e = efferent. (C) Lateral branching of cortical dendrites and afferent and efferent axons. (C is adapted with permission from Sarkisov SA: *The Structure and Functions of the Brain*. Bloomington, IN, Indiana University Press, 1966, p 134.)

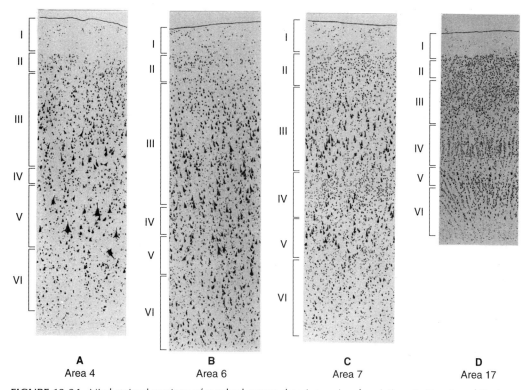

FIGURE 13-34. Nissl-stained sections of cerebral cortex showing regional variations in its cytoarchitecture (for layer names, see Figure 13-32). (*A*) Agranular, area 4. (*B*) Dysgranular, area 6. (*C*) Eugranular, area 7. (*D*) Hypergranular, area 17. (Adapted with permission from Campbell AW: *Histological Studies on the Localization of Cerebral Function.* Cambridge, University Press, 1905.)

3. The **fusiform neurons** are **most common in layer VI**. They have an elongated perikaryon, which gives off a dendrite from each end (see Figure 13-33). Their axons enter the deep white matter (Golgi type I neurons).

4. The **Martinotti neurons** occur in **all cortical layers except layer I**. They have a polygonal perikaryon with short dendrites. Their axons, directed vertically toward the cortical surface, give off collaterals to the neuronal layers as they ascend (see Figure 13-33).

5. The **horizontal neurons of Cajal** occur **only in layer I**. The long axis of their fusiform perikarya and their dendrites and axons run horizontal to the surface and remain in layer I (see Figure 13-33). Because layer I has only Cajal neurons and they are infrequent, it has the fewest neurons of any of the cortical layers.

G. **Connections and synaptic relations of the cortical neurons**

1. The outer four cortical layers, **layers I through IV**, tend to be receptive and internuncial in function. The inner two layers, **layers V and VI**, tend to be efferent, but the dichotomy is by no means strict.

2. All layers contain intracortical interneurons, and all except layer I contribute some axons to the white matter.
   a. Cortical commissural and association axons arise mainly from neurons in layers II and III.
   b. Corticothalamic axons arise in layer VI and possibly layer V.
   c. Corticostriatal, corticorubral, corticotectal, corticoreticular, corticopontine, corticobulbar, and corticospinal axons arise mainly in layer V.

3. **Sources of afferent fibers to the cortical neurons.** Major sources of afferents include other cortical neurons, thalamocortical and hypothalamocortical projections, and certain chemically specified nuclei of the brain stem.
   a. Of the synapses on cortical neurons, 95% or more come from other cortical neurons by way of association and commissural pathways.
   b. The thalamic nuclei provide perhaps 1% of the cortical input.
   c. Certain chemically specified nuclei project more or less diffusely to the entire cortex, as detailed in Chapter 14:
      (1) From the brain stem [the nucleus locus coeruleus (noradrenergic) and the ventral tegmental nucleus (dopaminergic)]
      (2) From the nuclei of brain stem raphe (serotonergic)
      (3) From the nucleus basalis of Meynert (cholinergic)

4. **Mode of termination of thalamic afferents**
   a. The **specific thalamic afferent fibers**, which carry topographic information, generally ascend to synapse in layer IV and the deeper part of layer III before branching.
      (1) On reaching these layers, the fibers branch horizontally, forming a conspicuous horizontal **outer stripe of Baillarger** in layer IV (see Figure 13-33C).
      (2) The axons end as tufts. They synapse on the dendrites of pyramidal neurons, or on granular neurons, which relay to the pyramidal neurons.
   b. **Nonspecific thalamic afferents** are thought to be collaterals of thalamostriate fibers.
      (1) They terminate diffusely in all layers, spreading over a much greater diameter than the specific thalamic tufts.
      (2) Their **role** would appear to be dispersion of ascending reticular activating system (ARAS) activity, rather than localization.

H. Areal subdivisions of the neocortex (cortical maps)

1. **Cytoarchitectural subdivisions.** Nissl-stained sections from various cortical areas show differences in the size and shape of neuronal perikarya, their density in the various layers, the thickness of the layers, and the degree of radial striation. These characteristics are spoken of as the cytoarchitecture of the cortex (see Figure 13-34).
   a. **The underlying theory that cytoarchitectural differences correlate with functional differences is only partially true.** Some cortical regions, such as the paracentral motor and sensory cortex, obviously differ in cytoarchitecture and function, but the functions overlap the cytoarchitectural boundaries even in these regions.
   b. **Even when similar in architecture, cortical regions may not function alike** because their afferent and efferent connections differ. For example, the cerebellar cortex, with its monotonous, uniform cytoarchitecture, shows localization of function because of differences in connections.

2. **Brodmann's cytoarchitectural map** (1904)
   a. The map most commonly used, Brodmann's cytoarchitectural map divides the cerebral cortex into 52 regions (Figure 13-35). Brodmann assigned the numbers arbitrarily and did not intend their sequence on the map to imply any cytoarchitectural or functional kinship.
   b. Today, authors use Brodmann's numbers in two ways:
      (1) In their original sense, to designate cytoarchitecture as such
      (2) As a shorthand system to designate some region on the cerebral surface

3. **Von Bonin and Bailey's cytoarchitectural map** (1951). After Brodmann, some authors proposed as many as 200 cytoarchitectural areas, causing Von Bonin and Bailey in 1951 to suggest that these authors had overread minor differences. Von Bonin and Bailey emphasized that most cortical areas look much alike and offered a simplified map of a dozen areas.
   a. They used color to identify the areas and gradations of color to emphasize gradual transitions between areas.
   b. They rejected Brodmann's system of numbers and stippling because it failed to reflect the degree to which a given area resembled or differed from others, and gave a false impression of the sharpness of many areal boundaries.

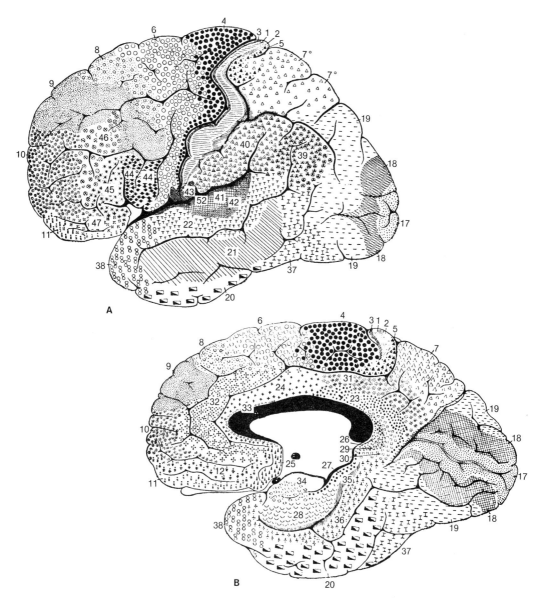

FIGURE 13-35. Brodmann's cytoarchitectural map of the cerebral cortex. (*A*) Lateral view of the left cerebral hemisphere. (*B*) Medial view of the right cerebral hemisphere. (Reprinted with permission from Brodmann K: Physiologie des Gehirns, in Die Allgemeine Chirurgie der Gehirnkrankheiten. *Neue Deutch Chirurgia*, vol. 11. Stuttgart, Ferdinand Enke Verlag, 1914, p 1.)

4. Granular layer as a cytoarchitectural criterion

    a. A glance at various cortical sections reveals great variations in the width of layer IV, which is packed with granular neurons and is receptive in function. Using this one layer allows the separation of four cortical variants:

        (1) Agranular: no distinct granular layer

        (2) Hypogranular (dysgranular): thin, discontinuous granular layer

        (3) Eugranular: average-width granular layer

        (4) Hypergranular (koniocortex or striate cortex): excessively wide granular layer

    b. The cortex in front of and behind the central sulcus aptly demonstrates the value of this criterion.

        (1) Commencing with the precentral gyrus, **area 4** of Brodmann's map is **agranular** (see Figure 13-35).

(2) Going forward into **area 6**, the granular layer appears sporadically, making this area **hypo-** or **dysgranular**.

(3) Forward of area 6, the prefrontal cortex, **and continuing through area 10** of the frontal pole, the cortex is **eugranular**.

    c. Just posterior to the central sulcus and the agranular cortex of area 4, lie **areas 3, 1, and 2**. These areas have a very wide internal granular layer, making them **hypergranular or striate** cortex.

I.   **Cytoarchitectural areas of the frontal lobe neocortex**

1. Motor cortex, areas 4 and 6

    a. Area 4 of the precentral gyrus is agranular and very thick, lacks distinct radial striations, and has huge pyramidal neurons of Betz in layer V (see Figure 13-34A).

        (1) The Betz neurons, which originate large myelinated fibers for the pyramidal tract, are largest where area 4 extends onto the medial side of the hemisphere (see Figure 13-35B). These largest fibers extend the longest distance, to the sacral cord.

        (2) Betz neurons gradually get smaller as they extend laterally over the superior hemispheric crest and ventrally down along the precentral gyrus in a triangular field (see Figure 13-35A).

    b. Identification of area 4 as part of the motor cortex rests on functional evidence, not sheer anatomy.

        (1) Electrical stimulation of the region elicits movements of the contralateral extremities.

        (2) Destruction of the region results in contralateral "pyramidal tract" signs.

    c. The correlation between function and structure is imperfect even for such distinctive cytoarchitecture. Motor responses also occur following electrical stimulation of area 6, the postcentral hypergranular sensory cortex, and the supplementary motor cortex.

    d. Area 6, forward of area 4, thins somewhat and is hypogranular. The granular neurons commence to appear in small patches. A few large neurons reminiscent of the Betz cells occur here and there.

2. Prefrontal cortex, in front of area 6, shows a well-developed internal granular layer; thus, it is eugranular.

3. Area 10, the frontal pole cortex, gets thinner, as is typical of polar cortex, but it maintains the standard six layers.

J.   **Cytoarchitecture of the parietal, temporal, and occipital neocortex** (see Figure 13-34)

1. The hypergranular (striate) cortex (see Figure 13-34D) of areas 3, 1, and 2 of the postcentral gyrus undergoes a gradual transition posteriorly to eugranular cortex (see Figure 13-34C).

2. Striate cortex characterizes the primary sensory receptive cortex of:

    a. Areas 3, 1, and 2 (somesthetic) of the parietal lobe

    b. Areas 41 and 42 (auditory) of the temporal lobe

    c. Area 17 (visual) of the occipital lobe

3. The remainder of the parietal, temporal, and occipital lobes are eugranular, resembling the eugranular cortex of the prefrontal region. While variations do exist in the cytoarchitecture in these regions, they are less striking than the differences in motor and sensory cortex.

K.   **Cytoarchitecture of the limbic lobe**

1. In the mesocortex of the limbic lobe, the granular neurons occur less frequently in layers II and IV, with more neurons being pyramidal.

2. The radial striations are less distinct than in many other areas.

3. Specific thalamic afferents tend to end in the external lamina, layers I to III, and the efferents tend to arise from the internal lamina, layers IV to VI.

a. Looked at in another way, the thalamic afferents tend to be offset a layer closer to the surface. This apparently reflects a more primitive phylogenetic feature, because in the rodent, thalamic afferents extend to layer I.
b. The dendrites of the neurons in layer II of the limbic cortex extend into layer I to receive the synaptic contacts.

VI. FUNCTIONAL LOCALIZATION IN THE CEREBRUM, AND CLINICAL SYNDROMES

A. **Representation of movement.** In the past, the criterion for designating an area as a motor area was that electrical stimulation of the area elicited movements, and lesions in the area caused paralysis. Now, new scanning techniques allow direct, noninvasive identification of the active neural tissue involved in cerebral events by radioactive measurement of neuronal metabolism [positron emission tomography (PET) scanning].

1. The old and new methods of identification confirm the existence of **three** more or less **contiguous motor areas in the frontal lobes bilaterally**: classic motor area, supplementary motor area, and frontal eye fields (Figure 13-36).
   a. The **classic motor area** occupies the precentral gyrus, areas 4 and 6, with some spillover into the postcentral gyrus. Stimulation activates the contralateral muscles through the pyramidal system in a discrete, upside-down somatotopic pattern (Figure 13-37B).
   b. The **supplementary motor area** occupies the medial hemispheric wall in area 6, just anterior to the lumbosacral representation in area 4 of the classic motor area.
      (1) **Stimulation** of the supplementary motor area produces postural movements, which are more complex and more bilateral than the discrete movements resulting from stimulation of the classic motor area.
      (2) **Unilateral destruction** of this area causes no clear motor syndrome in humans, but radioactive scanning suggests that it may be involved in motor planning. For example, when a person thinks about moving one hand, this area shows an increase in metabolism before the classic motor area shows activation.
      (3) In some patients, **infarction** of the left supplementary area causes aphasia (see VI G).

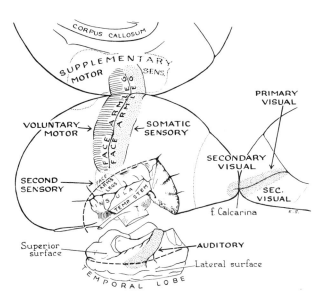

FIGURE 13-36. Map showing the location of the motor (*lined*) and sensory (*dotted*) areas of the left cerebral hemisphere. (Reprinted with permission from Penfield W, Roberts L: *Speech and Brain Mechanisms.* Princeton, University Press, 1959, p 32.)

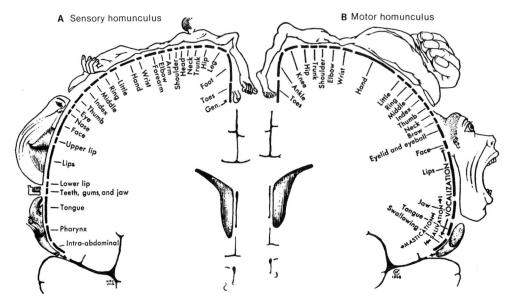

FIGURE 13-37. (A) Sensory representation in the postcentral gyrus. (B) Motor representation in the precentral gyrus. (From Penfield W, Rasmussen T: *The Cerebral Cortex of Man.* New York, Hafner Publishing, 1968, pp 44, 57.)

 c. The **frontal eye field** occupies the posterior part of the middle frontal gyrus, approximately the inferior part of area 8.
  (1) Unilateral stimulation causes conjugate contralateral deviation of the eyes. Destruction results in ipsilateral conjugate deviation of both eyes because the opposite frontal eye field acts unopposed.
  (2) An occipital eye field is located on facies lateralis of the occipital lobe. Stimulation turns the eyes contralaterally.

2. Apraxia
 a. **Definition.** Apraxia is the inability of a previously normal patient with an acquired cerebral lesion to execute a normal volitional act, even though the motor systems and mental status are relatively intact and the patient is not paralyzed.
  (1) The apraxias differ from the well-categorized LMN, pyramidal (see Table 6-3), cerebellar (see Figure 10-13), and basal motor (see Table 11-1) syndromes. The patient seems to have lost the motor engrams or templates for skilled movements.
  (2) As with the pyramidal tract, the discussion of apraxia is limited to the effects of postnatal lesions inflicted on previously normal brains. Direct transfer of the concepts and terminology of adult neurology to **children with prenatal lesions** that cause learning and motor disabilities and the congenital apraxias is fraught with scientific pitfalls.
 b. **Speech apraxia.** An area in the posterior end of the inferior frontal gyrus, approximately area 44, close to the primary motor cortex, controls the bulbar muscles to produce speech. After destruction of this area on the left side, the patient loses the ability to utter words, but the bulbar muscles are not paralyzed for other voluntary actions, such as biting, if the primary motor area is spared.
 c. **Writing apraxia (dysgraphia).** Lesions of the left angular gyrus region may cause dysgraphia. The patient loses the ability to form letters, although the arm is not paralyzed.
 d. **Dressing apraxia.** The patient cannot orient the clothes to place them on the body. Dressing apraxia usually occurs with a lesion in the posterior part of the right parietal lobe.
 e. **Gait apraxia.** The patient becomes unable to stand and walk although not paralyzed. Gait apraxia is usually associated with diffuse cerebral disease such as Alzheimer's disease.

B. **Representation of general and special somatic sensation.** Primary sensory areas are the somatosensory area of the postcentral gyrus, the visual area along the calcarine sulcus, and the auditory area of the transverse temporal gyri.

1. The **primary somatosensory area** (see Figure 13-35, areas 3, 1, and 2) has a somatotopy closely resembling that of the classic motor area (see Figure 13-37A). A **secondary sensory area** is located on the superior lip of the sylvian fissure, adjacent to the insula (see Figure 13-36).
   a. Both primary and secondary sensory areas receive relays from nucleus ventralis posterior, but, as with the classic and supplementary motor cortices, the secondary sensory area has less discrete somatotopy.
   b. No special clinical syndrome of destruction of the secondary sensory area is known in humans.

2. The **primary visual receptive area (area 17)** occupies the superior and inferior banks of the calcarine sulcus. It has a strict retinotopic representation of the macula and contralateral visual field (see Figure 10-9).

3. The **primary auditory receptive area (areas 41 and 42)** occupies the posterior-superior region of the superior temporal gyrus, in the floor of the sylvian fissure (supratemporal plane or planum temporale) [see Figure 13-7].
   a. The gyri have a strict tonotopic representation.
   b. Destruction of one auditory area reduces hearing bilaterally, with somewhat more severe loss contralaterally.
   c. Unilateral lesions do not cause complete contralateral deafness because of the bilateral connections through the lateral lemniscus.

C. **Sensory association areas.** The primary sensory receptive areas just described represent their modalities in a strict keyboard topography. The cerebrum must still interpret the symbolic significance or overall meaning of the sensory stimuli. The cortex surrounding the primary areas re-represents the sensory data to integrate, analyze, or associate it with the memories, current perceptions, and future goals of the individual, all of which are functions of the sensorium.

1. The **visual association cortex, approximately areas 18 and 19**, gives meaning to visual stimuli, either words or objects.
   a. A car speeding toward a person is a pattern of impulses that activates area 17.
   b. Areas 18 and 19 re-represent the car's configuration and associate it with data from the rest of the brain, especially the memory. Thus, the brain recognizes the impulses arriving at area 17 as a car, perceives its direction and velocity, and interprets it as a threat to survival. The sensorium decides, "Danger! Get out of the way," flashes a fear experience, and instructs the voluntary and vegetative motor systems to act appropriately for survival.

2. The **somatosensory association area, approximately area 7,** occupies the strip of cortex behind the postcentral sulcus. It gives meaning or recognition to afferent impulses from the skin and proprioceptors.

3. The **auditory association area**, approximately area 22, gives meaning to sounds and, more importantly, to spoken words.

D. **Contrasting effects of lesions of primary sensory and association areas**

1. **Destruction of primary sensory areas, or of the pathways leading to them** through receptors, nerves, the spinal cord, lemnisci, thalamus or thalamic peduncles, or primary sensory cortex, causes defects that match the topography and modality of the pathway. The patient suffers numbness, hypesthesia or anesthesia, blindness, or deafness.

2. **Irritative lesions of the respective sensory pathways or their primary sensory cortex** cause tingling or paresthesias, flashes of light, or ringing, buzzing sounds.

3. **Destructive lesions of association cortex** rob the individual of the meaning or symbolic significance of the primary sensation. Such defects constitute **agnosias**.

E. **Agnosias**

1. **Definition.** Agnosia is the inability of a previously normal person who has an acquired cerebral lesion to recognize the symbolic significance or meaning of a sensory stimulus, even though the sensory pathway and primary sensory cortex are sufficiently intact to register the stimulus, and the mental status is relatively intact.

2. **Common somatosensory agnosias caused by lesions of the parietal lobe association area**
   a. **Astereognosis** (*a* means not, *stereo* means form, *gnosia* means knowing: literally, "not form knowing") is the inability to recognize the form of an object placed in the hand. For example, a patient cannot distinguish a paper clip from a safety pin by feeling the objects.
   b. **Astatognosia** (*a* means not, *stat* means station, *gnosia* means knowing) is the inability to recognize the position of the body parts.

3. **Common visual agnosias caused by occipital lobe lesions**. Two important visual agnosias are for faces (prosopagnosia) and words (dyslexia).
   a. **Prosopagnosia** is the inability to recognize faces (face blindness) in the presence of intact visual pathways and primary visual cortex. The lesion responsible for prosopagnosia is in the association cortex of the temporo-occipital region on facies inferior (inferomedialis) of the hemisphere.
   b. **Dyslexia** is the inability to recognize written words or the meaning of words (word blindness), in the presence of intact visual pathways and primary visual cortex. The lesion responsible for word agnosia is in the association cortex of the left occipital lobe, on facies lateralis.

4. **Auditory agnosia** for spoken words (word deafness but not sound deafness) occurs as a result of lesions of the auditory association area, area 22, of the temporal lobe. It is analogous to dyslexia (word blindness).

F. **Anatomic connections of the primary cortical sensory areas and the association areas**

1. The primary areas receive their thalamocortical afferents from the sensory relay nuclei. The association areas receive their thalamic afferents from the association (ectocortical) nuclei of the thalamus.

2. The primary sensory areas connect with their association areas by means of horizontal fibers in the laminae of the cortex and arcuate fibers.

3. The more generalized meanings may come from:
   a. Numerous progressive arcuate cascades (see Figure 13-25), which extend the associations like a Huygens wave front
   b. Long association fibers
   c. Callosal connections

4. The primary sensory areas have few commissural connections through the corpus callosum. These areas are for discrete, topographic representations.

5. The association areas have rich callosal connections, in keeping with their role of dispersing their information to form the widest associations of the primary sensory data.

G. **Representation of language: the aphasias**

1. **Receiving and expressing language.** We express language through speaking or writing and receive it through auditing or reading. Thus, we speak/listen or write/read. Disorders in expressing or receiving words as symbols for communication are called **aphasias**.

2. **Definition of aphasia.** Aphasia is the inability of a previously normal person with an acquired cerebral lesion to understand or express words as symbols for communication, even though the primary sensory systems, motor mechanisms of phonation, and mental state (sensorium) are relatively intact.

3. **Anatomical basis for language reception and expression**
   a. In most normal individuals, the critical region for receiving and expressing language is the left parasylvian area (Figure 13-38), and its connections with itself

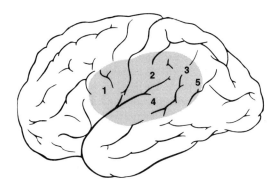

FIGURE 13-38. Lateral view of the left cerebral hemisphere, the one which is usually dominant for language. *1* = posterior-inferior frontal area of Broca; *2* = inferior parietal lobule (parietal operculum); *3* = angular gyrus; *4* = superior temporal gyrus area of Wernicke; *5* = confluence of the parietal, occipital, and temporal lobes.

by means of the **arcuate fasciculus** and with the left thalamus through the thalamic peduncles.

b. Anatomically, the left sylvian fissure is somewhat longer than the right, and the supratemporal plane is larger in area. A prominent **arcuate** fasciculus runs from the auditory association cortex (see Figure 13-38, area 4), around the posterior ramus of the sylvian fissure, and into the posterior inferior frontal region (see Figure 13-38, area 1). This arcuate fasciculus connects the centers for receptive and expressive speech.

c. Lesions of the left thalamus, which connect with the parasylvian area, give rise to syndromes of aphasia similar to those resulting from lesions of the cortex or intervening white matter of the thalamic peduncles.

d. The left supplementary motor area may also represent speech to some extent because its destruction may cause aphasia.

4. Types of aphasia and localizing significance. The types of expressive and receptive aphasia correlate with the location of the lesion within the aphasic zone (Table 13-8; see Figure 13-38).

a. Lesions in site 1 (see Figure 13-38) cause mainly a nonfluent, expressive aphasia, with relative preservation of receptive language. In this nonfluent or Broca's aphasia, the patient produces few words.

b. Lesions in sites 2 to 4 (see Figure 13-38) tend to impair language reception. The patient produces many words and speech sounds, but they are garbled and incomprehensible: so-called Wernicke's fluent aphasia.

c. Lesions at or posterior to site 5 cause dyslexia (see Table 13-8).

5. The most common causes of aphasia are infarcts in the distribution of the left middle cerebral artery and head trauma. The left middle cerebral artery supplies the parasylvian zone exclusively (see Figure 15-14).

H. **Reduction in interpreting and expressing emotions by the inflections and modulations of speech.** Lesions of the parasylvian area of the right cerebral hemisphere, mirroring those of the left hemisphere that cause aphasia, interfere with recognizing and expressing the emotional inflections of words.

1. While retaining the ability to produce the words that express emotion, the patient fails to add emotional inflections and modulations to the words. The patient's speech sounds flat and without feeling.

2. The patient also fails to interpret the emotional connotations and inflections of the speech of others, while still recognizing the actual words spoken or heard.

I. **Gerstmann's syndrome, a left posterior parasylvian area syndrome.** Lesions of the left angular and supramarginal gyrus region tend to produce Gerstmann's syndrome, consisting of dysgraphia, dyscalculia, right-left disorientation, and finger agnosia (inability to recognize and name one's own or the examiner's fingers). Some degree of aphasia, including dyslexia, is usually also present. The aphasia and other components of the syndrome vary from patient to patient.

TABLE 13-8. Types of Aphasia As Related to the Site of the Lesion*

Type	Clinical Features	Lesion Site
Global aphasia	Inability to speak/audit or read/write	Entire left parasylvian area (sites 1–5 of Figure 13-38)
Motor aphasia (speech apraxia, Broca's aphasia, nonfluent aphasia)	Inability to utter words or write (agraphia); comprehension of speech by auditing or reading remains relatively intact	Posterior part of inferior frontal gyrus (site 1 of Figure 13-38)
Agraphia (writing apraxia, without conspicuous speech apraxia)	Inability to write words, spell, or form letters correctly	Left angular–supramarginal gyrus area (site 3 of Figure 13-38); another type of agraphia may follow lesions at site 1 of Figure 13-38
"Pure" word deafness	Inability to understand spoken words	Posterior part of the superior temporal gyrus (site 4 of Figure 13-38)
"Pure" word blindness	Inability to understand written or printed words	Anterior part of the occipital lobe at its junction with the temporal and parietal lobes (site 5 of Figure 13-38)
Wernicke's aphasia (fluent aphasia)	Inability to comprehend spoken or written language; the patient makes fluent vocalizations that have the phrasing and rhythm of language but consist of parts of words mixed together—a "word salad" devoid of meaning; dyslexia may also be present	Inferior posterior part of the parietal lobe at its junctions with the temporal and occipital lobes (sites 2 to 4 of Figure 13-38)
Conduction aphasia	Similar to Wernicke's aphasia, but the patient retains understanding of written and spoken words while being unable to produce them	Interruption of the arcuate bundle that connects the parasylvian area of the frontal, parietal, and temporal lobes around the posterior end of the lateral fissure, thus disconnecting the receptive speech areas from Broca's motor area

*See also Figure 13-38.

J. **Left-sided hemineglect, a right posterior parasylvian area syndrome.** A lesion in the right hemisphere (an almost mirror-image of the lesion that produces Gerstmann's syndrome) spares language, but causes a very different set of deficits. The patient:

1. Lacks awareness of the left half of space and ignores tactile, auditory, and visual stimuli from the left side, and even ignores food on the left half of the plate

2. Is unable to draw the left half of figures or designs, and is unable to reproduce matchstick constructions (constructional apraxia)

3. Is unable to orient clothes for dressing (dressing apraxia)

4. Often fails to recognize the existence of neurologic defects, even when the lesion extends to the paracentral area, causing hemiplegia and hemianesthesia. Failure to recognize such defects is called **anosognosia** (*a* means not, *noso* means disease, and *gnosia* means knowing).

K. **A summary of syndromes of the right and left cerebral hemispheres** is presented in Figure 13-39.

L. **Representation of recent memory.** This discussion involves only recent memory, because we know more about its anatomical substrate than about memory for remote events.

1. Pure amnestic syndrome

a. **Definition.** The pure amnestic syndrome is characterized by temporal disorientation—the patient cannot remember the day, date, time, or current events but can remember previously learned information and skills. Other mental functions, along with motor and sensory functions, remain relatively intact. The patient walks around, talks normally, reads, and can calculate. The patient shows no motor or sensory loss, apraxia, or agnosia, and may do well on IQ tests.

b. **Anatomical basis of the amnestic syndrome.** Lesions that cause pure amnesia involve one or more of the following structures, usually bilaterally (Figure 13-40):

(1) Medial, inferior quadrant of the temporal lobe, including the hippocampal formation

(2) Stalk of white matter connecting it with the thalamus (inferior thalamic peduncle)

(3) Nucleus medialis dorsalis of the thalamus

(4) Fornix/mammillary bodies

c. Although the lesion frequently involves the hippocampus-fornix and mammillary body circuit, particularly in **Korsakoff's syndrome** (see Chapter 12 III F 7 a), the exact role of the individual parts of the circuit is unclear.

(1) Neurosurgical section of the anterior pillars of the fornix, as has been attempted to treat epileptic seizures, does not cause amnesia, nor do pure lesions of the mammillary bodies.

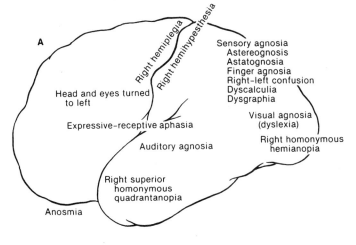

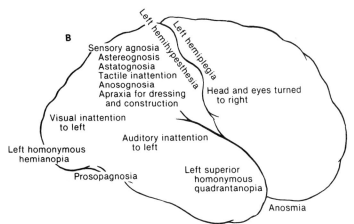

FIGURE 13-39. Summary of some of the outstanding neurologic signs and symptoms caused by focal destructive lesions in the right or left cerebral hemisphere as detected by neurologic examination. (*A*) Lateral view of the left cerebral hemisphere. (*B*) Lateral view of the right cerebral hemisphere. Notice that some signs and symptoms, such as hemiplegia, are common to both hemispheres.

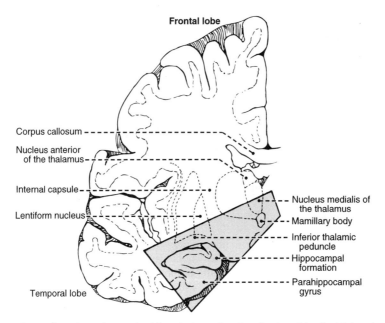

Frontal lobe

Corpus callosum

Nucleus anterior
of the thalamus

Internal capsule

Lentiform nucleus

Nucleus medialis of
the thalamus

Mamillary body

Inferior thalamic
peduncle

Hippocampal
formation

Parahippocampal
gyrus

Temporal lobe

FIGURE 13-40. Coronal section of a cerebral hemisphere showing the "corridor," which, when damaged bilaterally, causes amnesia. (Adapted with permission form Horel JA: The neuroanatomy of memory. *Brain* 101:403–445, 1978.)

> (2) However, recent work suggests that a lesion of the fornix in its commissural region may cause loss of recent memory.

2. Any diffuse cerebral disease, including the normal effects of aging, also selectively impairs recent memory before remote memory. However, as the disease process advances, the patient shows global dementia rather than pure loss of recent memory.

M. **Multi-site representation of "higher" mental functions.** This section has described clinical deficits that correlate strongly with local lesions of the cerebrum. However, the cerebrum appears to represent many so-called "higher" mental functions generally or in several sites, rather than in specific centers. Focal brain lesions may impair, but do not specifically abolish, functions such as foresight, planning, socially appropriate behavior, conscience, and cognition. Similarly, lesions of limbic circuits that alter mood and affective responses may result in hypersexuality and murderous aggression or in passivity and taming effects, but correlation of these clinical states with specific lesion sites is uncertain.

VII. **EPILOGUE.** As humans, we all share, in our brains, an ultimate common perception of life. We experience it as a process, as a series of ongoing events. From our neuronal circuits we know **who** we and others are, **where** we are, **when** it is, and **what** is happening. Answering these adverbial questions of **who, where, when,** and **what,** we arrive at a common sense of what constitutes appropriate behavior. We come in out of the rain, avoid fire, and do not try to walk through walls. We speak gently to the ill, the old, and the unfortunate, and we don't shout "Fire!" in a crowded theater. Our "common sense" tells us not to try to mount our neighbor's mate, even though our limbic system urges us on. This common sense, the **sensorium commune** as named by the ancients, depends on reticular formation, thalamic, and cortical circuitry. In the recent past, to try to specify *which* neurons and circuits were involved required an idiot's audacity. Now, with PET scanning, we can almost trace a thought in its circuits through the brain; thus, our mind emanates from specific structure. Lesions of this structure alter thought, will, and behavior—our very experiences. To understand the brain/thought/behavior trinity is the Holy Grail of neuroanatomy.

STUDY QUESTIONS

DIRECTIONS: Each of the numbered items or incomplete statements in this section is followed by answers or by completions of the statement. Select the ONE lettered answer or completion that is BEST in each case.

1. The stem of the lateral (sylvian) fissure, which contains the middle cerebral artery, extends

(A) medially from the parahippocampal gyrus
(B) laterally from the vallecula (the anterior perforated space)
(C) posteriorly from the anterior ascending ramus to the tip of the posterior ramus
(D) vertically through the inferior frontal gyrus
(E) none of the above

2. The main efferent layers of the cerebral cortex are

(A) layers IV and VI
(B) layers V and VI
(C) layers I and II
(D) layers III and IV
(E) none of the above

3. One of the greatest differences between the archicortex of the hippocampal formation and the ectocortex (neocortex) is

(A) absence of distinct lamination in archicortex
(B) lack of significant function of archicortex
(C) presence of a superficial layer of white matter in the archicortex
(D) absence of the pyramidal neurons in archicortex
(E) scarcity of the pathways between archicortex and the limbic system

4. The inferior longitudinal fasciculus connects the

(A) frontal and occipital lobes
(B) temporal and frontal poles
(C) parietal lobe and frontal poles
(D) occipital and temporal lobes
(E) limbic and temporal lobes

5. After interruption of the corpus callosum the patient would be unable to

(A) feel sensation in either of the hands
(B) execute a verbal command with the left hand
(C) maintain bladder and bowel control
(D) perform arithmetical calculations
(E) maintain consciousness

6. Anosognosia is most characteristic of which of the following lesions?

(A) Diffuse cerebral disease
(B) Left posterior parietal lesions
(C) Right posterior parietal lesions
(D) Left temporal lobe lesions
(E) Right frontal lobe lesions

7. The body part with the largest relative representation in the sensorimotor cortex is the

(A) trunk
(B) thumb
(C) neck
(D) genitalia
(E) middle finger

8. Select the feature that distinguishes the cerebellar cortex from the cerebral cortex.

(A) A surface layer of white matter
(B) Indistinct lamination of its layers
(C) Contains only two cell types
(D) Only one neuronal type originates cortifugal axons
(E) Fewer surface crevices

DIRECTIONS: Each of the numbered items or incomplete statements in this section is negatively phrased, as indicated by a capitalized word such as NOT, LEAST, or EXCEPT. Select the ONE lettered answer or completion that is BEST in each case.

9. Select the statement about the corpus callosum that is NOT true.

(A) It is the largest bundle of fibers that crosses the midline of the brain
(B) Its splenium connects cortex of the posterior parts of the cerebral hemispheres
(C) The fornix and fornix commissure run along its ventral surface
(D) It conveys most of the projection fibers from the two cerebral hemispheres to lower centers
(E) Far fewer transcallosal axons connect the hand areas than the trunk areas of the sensorimotor cortex

10. Characteristic features of the cerebral cortex include all of the following EXCEPT

(A) few sharp cytoarchitectural boundaries
(B) laminar arrangements of neurons
(C) conspicuous stripes of myelinated fibers
(D) radial or columnar arrangement of neurons
(E) numerous pyramidal neurons in all six layers

11. Which of the following statements about apraxia is NOT true?

(A) Bilateral pyramidal tract interruption would preclude testing a patient for apraxia
(B) Language apraxia implies a left hemisphere lesion
(C) Lesions of the cortex and the thalamocortical circuits can cause apraxia
(D) Dyslexia is a form of aphasic apraxia
(E) Apraxia can affect common learned actions like dressing and walking

12. The ring of limbic cortex around the hilus of the hemispheres includes all of the following structures EXCEPT

(A) angular and supramarginal gyri
(B) cingulate gyrus
(C) posterior orbital cortex of frontal lobes
(D) insular cortex
(E) parahippocampal gyrus

13. Pathways in the classic Papez (visceral brain) circuit include all of the following EXCEPT for the

(A) occipitofrontal fasciculus
(B) fornix
(C) superior thalamic peduncle
(D) mammillothalamic tract
(E) temporoammonic tract

14. Some authors restrict the term fissures to those crevices of the cerebral surface formed by the evagination of the telencephalon. Select the statement about fissures as compared to sulci that is NOT true. Fissures

(A) form earlier
(B) are longer
(C) are less numerous
(D) are deeper
(E) are not bordered by cortex

15. The following statements relate the type of aphasia to the lesion site. Select the comparison that is NOT true.

(A) Motor aphasia/left posterior-inferior frontal region
(B) Dyslexia/lateral surface of the left occipital lobe
(C) Global aphasia/left inferior parietal area
(D) Fluent aphasia/left posterior parasylvian area
(E) Auditory agnosia/left superior temporal gyrus

16. Select the statement about the surface contours of the brain that is NOT true.

(A) The medial face is the flattest surface
(B) The temporal pole is concave
(C) The lateral face is strongly convex
(D) The orbital surface is concave
(E) The temporo-occipital region of the inferomedial face is convex

DIRECTIONS: Each set of matching questions in this section consists of a list of four to twenty-six lettered options (some of which may be in figures) followed by several numbered items. For each numbered item, select the ONE lettered option that is most closely associated with it. To avoid spending too much time on matching sets with large numbers of options, it is generally advisable to begin each set by reading the list of options. Then, for each item in the set, try to generate the correct answer and locate it in the option list, rather than evaluating each option individually. Each lettered option may be selected once, more than once, or not at all.

Questions 17–21

Match the cortical areas with their identifying anatomical or cytoarchitectural characteristics.

(A) Has a conspicuous internal granular layer and an outer line of Baillarger
(B) Has very large pyramidal neurons in layer V
(C) Has three layers of neurons
(D) Is the thinnest cortex (in general)
(E) Lacks distinctive features

17. Precentral gyrus (area 4)

18. Calcarine cortex

19. Association cortex

20. Polar cortex

21. Postcentral gyrus (areas 3,1, and 2)

Questions 22–26

Match the clinical deficit with the expected lesion site.

(A) Left angular gyrus
(B) Right parasylvian area
(C) Either parietal lobe (behind areas 3,1, and 2)
(D) Inferior medial quadrants of temporal lobes
(E) Medial inferior temporo-occipital region

22. Loss of ability to recognize or express the affective connotations of speech without aphasia per se

23. Loss of recent memory

24. Dyscalculia, dysgraphia, right-left disorientation, and finger agnosia

25. Prosopagnosia

26. Astereognosis

Questions 27–31

Match the cortical cell type with the usual orientation of its axon.

(A) Directed toward the white matter
(B) Directed toward the cortical surface
(C) Directed tangential to the cortical surface
(D) More or less randomly directed, ending on nearby neurons (Golgi type II axons)
(E) None of the above

27. Pyramidal neurons

28. Stellate neurons

29. Martinotti neurons

30. Fusiform neurons of layer VI

31. Horizontal neurons of Cajal

Questions 32–36

Match each description below with the relevant fissure or space.

(A) Choroid fissure and transverse cerebral fissure
(B) Cavum veli interpositi
(C) Sylvian fissure
(D) Cavum septi pellucidi
(E) Interhemispheric fissure

32. Forms by invagination of the medial wall of the cerebral hemispheres

33. Located between the fornices and the anterior part of the corpus callosum

34. The corpus callosum, enlarging posteriorly from the commissural plate, forms its roof

35. The roof of the third ventricle forms its floor

36. Occupied by the cerebral falx after evagination of the cerebral hemispheres

Questions 37–39

(A) Cingulum
(B) Temporoammonic tract
(C) Arcuate fasciculus
(D) Hippocampal (fornical) commissure
(E) Superior longitudinal fasciculus
(F) Anterior commissure
(G) Posterior commissure
(H) Temporoalvear tract
(I) Ansa peduncularis and inferior thalamic peduncle
(J) Superior thalamic peduncle
(K) Corpus callosum
(L) Superior occipitofrontal fasciculus
(M) Dorsal and ventral transcallosal fibers
(N) Stria terminalis

For each group of sites, select the pathways that connect them.

37. Entorhinal cortex or amygdala with the ipsilateral hippocampal formation (SELECT 2 PATHWAYS)

38. Temporal lobe archicortex or amygdala on one side with the opposite temporal lobe (SELECT 3 PATHWAYS)

39. Auditory receptive region and zone of Wernicke with the inferior posterior frontal area of Broca (SELECT 1 PATHWAY)

ANSWERS AND EXPLANATIONS

1. The answer is B [I E 1 b, 2 a, b; Figure 13-6]. The lateral fissure is divided into specific parts, which correspond to branches of the middle cerebral artery and the anatomical landmarks of the cerebrum. The stem of the lateral fissure commences at the anterior perforated substance in a little depression called the vallecula and extends laterally from that region. The stem separates the temporal pole from the overlying posterior-inferior aspect of the frontal lobe. It contains the proximal part of the middle cerebral artery after it originates from the internal carotid artery in the vallecula. While in the stem, the middle cerebral artery gives off the lateral striate arteries.

2. The answer is B [V G 1, 2 b]. Some cortical layers are mainly receptive and others efferent. The superficial layers from I to IV tend to be receptive, and the deeper layers, including V and VI, tend to be efferent. The more superficial layers act more or less as cortical interneurons that receive impulses and modulate the output of neurons of layers V and VI. Layers V and VI contain the largest neurons of the cortex.

3. The answer is C [II C 1 b, 2;V C 2, 3]. Archicortex and neocortex are both distinctly laminated. Both types of cortex contain pyramidal neurons, and both have numerous connections with the limbic system. One major difference is that archicortex has a distinct superficial layer of nerve fibers or white matter in comparison to ectocortex or neocortex, which has its white matter on its inner surface and forms the deep white matter of the cerebral wall.

4. The answer is D [IV D 2 b; Figure 13-25]. The inferior longitudinal fasciculus is one of the many bundles in the cerebral white matter that connects different regions of the cerebral cortex. Although generally depicted as a single bundle of long axons, recent studies suggest that it consists of a series of arcuate cascades rather than a single pathway composed of long fibers. This pathway connects the occipital lobe, which is predominantly responsible for visual function, with the temporal lobe.

5. The answer is B [IV F 4]. The corpus callosum connects the two hemispheres and transfers information from one to the other. After interruption of the corpus callosum, the pa-

tient cannot execute a verbal command with the left hand but will do so readily with the right hand. The left hemisphere understands the command and can direct the right extremities, by means of the pyramidal tract, to execute the command. The right hemisphere does not understand the command because it lacks a center to decode the meaning of the words, information that must come across the corpus callosum from the left hemisphere. Thus, the patient will not be able to execute a verbal command with the left hand.

6. The answer is C [VI J]. Functional localization in the two hemispheres differs even though anatomically the hemispheres look almost like mirror images of each other. A large, acute destructive lesion of the right hemisphere that damages the paracentral region (pre- and postcentral gyri) will cause contralateral hemiplegia and loss of sensation. If the lesions extend to the posterior parietal or posterior parasylvian area, the patient fails to attend to stimuli from the left side and fails to recognize the left hemiparesis and sensory loss. To name this unawareness of left-sided neurologic defects after a right parietal lesion, Josef Babinski coined the term anosognosia. A lesion of the corresponding posterior parietal parasylvian area of the left hemisphere causes aphasia, not contralateral anosognosia.

7. The answer is B [Figure 13-37]. Some body parts have a larger area of cortex devoted to their motor and sensory representation than other parts. The largest representations involve the tongue, the thumb, the little finger, and the corresponding digits of the foot, as well as the hands and feet in general. Apparently, the complexity of motor actions and sensory contacts in these regions requires a larger cortical circuitry than the simpler movements and sensations mediated by the trunk.

8. The answer is D [V F 1 b]. The cerebellar cortex contains five types of neurons but only one type, the Purkinje cell, originates corticofugal axons. Different types of neurons of the cerebral cortex originate its corticofugal axons. The surface of the cerebral cortex contains far fewer crevices than the cerebellar cortex.

9. The answer is D [IV F 1 b, c (1); Figure 13-28]. The corpus callosum contains some projection fibers from the cingulate gyrus to the striatum and pallidum, but the vast majority of projection fibers (i.e., corticothalamic, corticobulbar, and corticospinal) bypass it. The corpus callosum is the largest bundle of commissural fibers in the brain. It connects mirror image points of the two cerebral hemispheres, but conveys far fewer connections for the hand areas of the sensorimotor cortex than for the trunk. Anteriorly, it has a rostrum, genu, and body; posteriorly, it has a splenium. The splenium, which connects the cortex of the posterior parts of the cerebral hemispheres, forms the forceps major.

10. The answer is E [V D 1, 3 c, E 1, F 1, b, 3; Figure 13-32]. Layer one of the cerebral cortex contains no pyramidal neurons. The neurons of the cerebral cortex show both a laminar arrangement and a radial or columnar arrangement. Several regions of the cortex contain grossly visible stripes of myelinated fibers. These are most conspicuous in the sensory receptive areas. Most cytoarchitectural boundaries are vague rather than sharply defined.

11. The answer is D [VI A 2, E 3 b]. Apraxia is the inability of a patient who is not paralyzed and not demented to perform a normal volitional act. Examples include dressing apraxia (inability to orient the clothes to put them on) or constructional apraxia (inability to copy, draw, or construct geometric figures). The expressive forms of aphasia, involving the motor actions to speak or write, can be thought of as language apraxia. Dyslexia is a defect in language reception, thus, it is not an apraxia, which means the inability of a nonparalyzed patient to execute a volitional action.

12. The answer is A [I G; Table 13-1; Figure 13-11]. The supramarginal and angular gyri belong to the ectocortex and occupy the lateral facies of a cerebral hemisphere. The limbic lobe forms a ring of structures around the hemispheric hilus on the medial and inferior aspects of each hemisphere. The rhinencephalon bounds the limbic ring internally and the ectocortex externally or peripherally. The cortical surface of the ring consists of the cingulate gyrus and its isthmus to the parahippocampal gyrus, the uncus, and insula; the posterior orbital cortex on the inferior surface of the frontal lobe; and the parolfactory and subcallosal gyri. The latter gyri lead back to the cingulate gyrus to complete the ring.

13. The answer is A [II D 1, 2; Figure 13-16]. The occipitofrontal fasciculus is an intracortical association pathway that is not part of the Papez circuit. The classic Papez circuit includes the hippocampus, fornix, mamillary bodies, mamillothalamic tract, and thalamocortical projection from the nucleus anterior to the cingulate gyrus, then through the cingulum back to the temporal lobe and hippocampus. The amygdala connects with this circuit through the ansa peduncularis. The Papez circuit mediates emotional experience and the accompanying visceromotor activities of the autonomic system. At some point in the integrative process, the limbic system programs somatomotor actions related to emotion and visceral function. The amygdala acts as one such integrative center.

14. The answer is E [I D]. The cerebral surface shows crevices of two types: fissures and sulci. Fissures form by evagination of the telencephalon, of the hemispheres per se, and of the temporal lobes. They are longer and deeper than sulci. After evagination, sulcation occurs in a definite timetable sequence. The embryologic mechanisms of sulcation are entirely different from fissuration; each can occur independently from the other. In lissencephaly, the fissures form but not the sulci. In holoprosencephaly, the fissures fail to form but the holospheric cerebrum sulcates.

15. The answer is C [VI G 4; Table 13-8; Figure 13-38]. Depending on the lesion site and size, the patient may have mainly expressive aphasia, mainly receptive aphasia, or global aphasia. The lesion that causes aphasia is usually in the left parasylvian zone in both right- and left-handed individuals. Global aphasia requires an extensive lesion of all or most of the parasylvian region. Expressive aphasia for spoken language occurs after a lesion of the posterior-inferior frontal region, an integrative area for verbal expression adjacent to the corticobulbar pathway that mediates word articulation. The more posterior lesions of the aphasic zone, adjacent to the primary auditory and visual receptive cortices, cause receptive aphasia. The patient produces numerous fluent vocalizations and intonations that resemble words but consist of garbled syllables. One theory is that the patient loses the self-corrective monitoring afforded by listening to his or her own speech, and the patient fails to perceive that the sounds produced do not express the intended words.

16. The answer is B [I B 1]. Each face of the cerebral hemisphere has a distinctive contour. By knowing these contours, the examiner may recognize and become immediately oriented to the level of coronal, sagittal, or horizontal sections on radiographic brain scans. All three poles are strongly convex. The medial face is flat because the cerebral hemispheres abut on the flat cerebral falx. The dorsolateral aspect of the cerebral hemispheres is distinctly convex, and fits into the contours of the calvarium. The bony orbital roof bulges upward, causing a concavity in the undersurface of the frontal lobe that rests on it. Facies inferior of the temporo-occipital region is convex, fitting into the contour of the tentorium cerebelli.

17–21. The answers are: 17-B, 18-A, 19-E, 20-D, 21-A [V H 4 c, I 1 a, 2, 3, J 3]. Some regions of neocortex or ectocortex have specific structural features, whereas most of the cortex, generally called association cortex, looks much the same, lacking conspicuous regional differences or distinctive or unique characteristics. Throughout the cerebral cortex, the first, and to a lesser extent, the second cortical layers show the least regional variations from site to site.

The motor and sensory cortices show the most striking regional variations. The precentral gyrus is thick and has the largest cortical neurons, the neurons of Betz in layer V. It lacks a distinct internal granular layer.

Sensory cortex (somatosensory, visual, and auditory) has a thick, distinctive layer IV (internal granular layer) and a distinct outer layer stripe of Baillarger. This stripe represents the incoming thalamic afferents from the sensory relay nuclei of the thalamus. These afferents penetrate the deeper layers of the cortex at right angles to the cortical surface and then branch horizontally to run parallel to the cortical surface as stripes of Baillarger.

The cortical association areas lack these conspicuous features, but show minor variations from site to site in the thickness of the individual layers and in the density and size of neurons in the layers. On the crests of the gyri, the cortex is thicker than where it bends around the depths of the sulci.

The cortex of the poles in general is the thinnest and has the least number of neurons per unit of volume.

22–26. The answers are: 22-B, 23-D, 24-A, 25-E, 26-C [VI E 2 a, 3 a, H 1, I, J, L 1 b]. Lesions of some areas of the cerebrum cause definite clinical syndromes with specific de-

fects, whereas lesions of the parts of the cortex known as association areas may cause some personality and behavioral changes but no specific neurologic signs. For example, lesions of the frontal lobe anterior to the motor cortex do not cause any evident hemiplegia, sensory loss, or aphasia, but will reduce the general drive of the individual and may cause subtle changes in personality.

Lesions of the left angular gyrus, in its transition to the occipital lobe, tend to cause a syndrome of dyscalculia, dysgraphia, right-left disorientation, and finger agnosia. These features usually merge with some degree of receptive aphasia. The receptive aphasias are more obvious with lesions of the posterior parasylvian area, which involve the inferior part of the parietal lobe and extend around into the posterior-superior part of the temporal lobe.

Loss of recent memory will result from lesions of the medial parts of the temporal lobe. Such individuals again will have no obvious motor, sensory, or language deficits. They tend to retain their remote memory and may score well on IQ tests.

Lesions that affect the inferomedial part of the temporo-occipital region tend to cause a peculiar agnosia for faces, a defect known as prosopagnosia. These patients cannot recognize a person's face either with the person present or in the form of a photograph. In prosopagnosia, the lesion may also encroach on the geniculocalcarine pathway and cause a contralateral visual field defect, but the visual field defect does not cause the agnosia for faces.

Lesions of the parietal lobe behind the postcentral gyrus will cause astereognosis (stereoagnosia), in which the patient fails to recognize the form of objects felt with fingers but not viewed. The patient may also have other forms of agnosia, such as the inability to recognize numbers written on the skin of the palm or the fingers. With lesions in the anterior part of the parietal lobes, which affect the postcentral gyrus and its sensory receptive area, the patient also may fail to recognize the form of objects, a condition called stereoanesthesia rather than stereoagnosia. For a sensory defect to qualify as agnosia, the sensory pathway to the cortex and the primary receptive cortex have to be intact. The lesion causing agnosia involves the so-called association areas adjacent to the primary sensory areas. The association areas of the cortex give meaning and recognition to the primary sensory stimuli.

27–31. The answers are: 27-A, 28-D, 29-B, 30-A, 31-C [V F 1 a (3), 2, 3, 4, 5]. Although the cerebral cortex consists of neurons that vary greatly in size and type, they can be classified into five fundamental groups.

Pyramidal neurons occur in layers II, III, V, and VI. Tiniest in layer II, they increase in size through layer III. They are largest in layer V and less conspicuous again in layer IV. Layer V in particular and, to a lesser degree, layer VI have large numbers of pyramidal neurons and fusiform neurons. Both types of neurons have their axons directed toward the white matter and give rise to cortical efferent pathways. The pyramidal neurons vary greatly in the size of the perikaryon, dendritic branching, and axon diameter. The large Betz cells of layer V, with their myelin sheaths, may reach 20 μ in diameter. Although providing perhaps only 25,000 of the 1,200,000 axons of the pyramidal tract, they are the fastest conducting of the corticofugal axons.

The stellate or granular neurons concentrate in layer IV, a very thick layer in the sensory receptive cortex; they have a more random orientation of both axons and dendrites. These act mainly as intracortical association neurons or cortical interneurons.

Similarly, Martinotti neurons and the horizontal neurons of Cajal are cortical interneurons. Their circuits modify the afferent input into the cortex and integrate it to modulate the efferent neurons of the cortex. The Martinotti neurons have their axons directed toward the surface of the cortex. The horizontal neurons of Cajal are confined to the first layer of the cortex. They are the only neuronal type in that layer, which has the fewest neurons of any of the six standard cortical layers.

32–36. The answers are: 32-A, 33-D, 34-B, 35-B, 36-E [I D 2 c, d; II C 1; III C 2, 3; Figure 13-19]. The anatomy of midline caves and spaces of the cerebrum can only be understood from embryology. The roof plate of the prosencephalon is a membrane that covers the lateral and third ventricles. Evagination of the medial hemispheric wall with rolling in of the hippocampal formation creates the transverse cerebral fissure. As the hippocampus migrates posteriorly and inferiorly with the evagination of the temporal lobe, the transverse cerebral fissure continues as the choroid fissure, with the hippocampal formation forming its floor in the temporal lobe.

As the corpus callosum enlarges posteriorly, it covers the fornix and fornix commissure, which constitute the immediate roof of the cavum and veli interpositi. The space above the corpus callosum is the interhemispheric fissure. The space below it and the fornix is the cavum veli interpositi. The roof of the third ventricle is the floor of this cavum. In agenesis of the corpus callosum, no cavum veli interpositi is present. The entire space between the medial walls of the cerebral hemispheres is the interhemispheric fissure. In normal individuals as well as those with agenesis of the corpus callosum, the cerebral falx occupies the interhemispheric fissure.

The cavum septi pellucidi has as its floor the anterior pillars of the fornices and as its roof the undersurface of the anterior part of the corpus callosum. Its lateral walls are membranous, the septum pellucidum per se, one leaf of which extends to the corpus callosum from each fornix. This cave is present in all normal infants at birth; then, the leaves of the two septi fuse, obliterating the cavity. Tumors of the septal region cause changes in personality and affect because the region belongs to the limbic system. Persistence of the cavum septi pellucidi is often associated with other brain defects that cause mental retardation.

37. The answers are: B, I [II B 2 b (1), C 3 a (2); Figure 13-15]. The cortex of the parahippocampal gyrus and subicular and entorhinal areas connects with the ipsilateral hippocampal formation by the temporoammonic tracts. The term temporoammonic comes from the old name Ammon's horn for the hippocampal formation. It is also called the perforant tract because it perforates the subiculum. By contrast, the temporoalvear tract conveys axons from the subiculum that bypass the hippocampus and dentate gyrus to enter the alveus and ultimately the post-commissural fornix. Limbic lobe axons run through the cingulum to the regions of temporal cortex that project to the hippocampus and alveus. Axons from the amygdala to the hippocampus run through the ansa peduncularis, which also connects the amygdala with other regions of the basal forebrain, temporal cortex, and diencephalon.

38. The answers are: D, F, N [IV F 3 b, c; Figure 13-30]. Three pathways convey interhemispheric connections between the anterior part of one temporal lobe and the same regions of the other temporal lobe. One pathway, an ectocortical component, runs from the cortex of one side to the other, straight across the anterior commissure. The amygdala sends axons by two pathways. One pathway runs directly across the anterior commissure, and another through the stria terminalis. The hippocampal commissure connects the hippocampal formation of the two sides. It bridges across from one fornix to the other under the posterior part of the corpus callosum, where the fornices approach each other in the midline.

39. The answer is C [VI G 3 a, b; Table 13-8]. The arcuate fasciculus arcs from the auditory association cortex (area 42) around the posterior end of the sylvian fissure. In company with axons from the occipital word association area, the arcuate fasciculus then runs forward through the inferior parietal region to Broca's area (area 44). Thus, it connects the language reception areas of the posterior parasylvian area with the expressive or motor speech region located anteriorly. Lesions that interrupt the arcuate fasciculus in the inferior parietal region disconnect the receptive and motor speech areas. The patient has so-called conduction aphasia, characterized by retaining the ability to understand spoken and written words, but unable to produce them.

Chapter 14

Chemical Neuroanatomy

I. **SPECIFICATION OF NEURONS AND TRACTS BY NEUROTRANSMITTER CHEMISTRY**

A. **Discovery of the chemical transmission of the nerve impulse**

1. The theory that electrical messages crossed synapses began to topple in the 1920s and 1930s when neuroscientists discovered that stimulation of peripheral nerves caused the release of chemical substances at their endings. The chemical substances, catecholamines and acetylcholine, reproduced the effects of nerve stimulation when applied directly to the postsynaptic neuron or effector.

2. In the mid-1950s, new techniques confirmed the presence of peripheral nervous system (PNS) neurotransmitters in the central nervous system (CNS) and disclosed many new neurotransmitters.
   a. The new techniques include analytic chemistry, enzyme histochemistry, immunocytochemistry, radioactive labeling of metabolites, and the use of fluorescence microscopy to demonstrate catecholamines in situ in CNS neurons.
   b. Many catecholaminergic tracts, now readily demonstrated by fluorescence microscopy, eluded the classic methods of tract demonstration because they consist of fine axons that do not readily accept silver impregnation and lack myelin sheaths. Hence, the classic myelin stains and silver impregnation methods for axons failed to disclose these pathways.

B. **Classification of neurotransmitters.** Most neurotransmitters consist of small amine molecules or peptides and can be classified as follows:

1. **Monoaminergic**
   a. **Catecholaminergic**
      (1) Adrenergic
      (2) Noradrenergic
      (3) Dopaminergic
   b. **Serotonergic**

2. **Cholinergic**

3. **Amino acids** (Quantitatively, the major transmitters of the CNS belong to this group.)
   a. Excitatory (glutamic, aspartic, cysteic, and homocysteic acid)
   b. Inhibitory [gamma-aminobutyric acid (GABA), glycine, taurine, and β-alanine]

4. **Peptidergic**

5. **Small gaseous molecules**
   a. Nitric oxide and carbon monoxide constitute a newly recognized class of CNS and PNS communicants, as yet difficult to classify functionally as neurotransmitters, neuromodulators, or second messengers. They act by diffusion rather than being secreted in packets at synapses and binding to receptor sites on membrane surfaces. Nerve impulses can activate enzymes in neurons for their synthesis.
   b. Both gases relax smooth muscle and may be involved in memory and other CNS functions. They appear to cause retrograde activation of presynaptic potentials, thus enhancing long-term potentiation at synapses.

C. **Classification of neuronal systems by neurotransmitter chemistry**

1. Modern techniques have modified Dale's original theory that each neuron releases one and only one neurotransmitter. Although one transmitter may predominate, neurons may also liberate other chemicals as cotransmitters or comodulators (see VIII C).

2. The classification of neurons by their currently recognized "major" transmitter should not obscure the newer insight that release of cotransmitters is the rule. Rapidly changing and improved techniques of study make this an ever-changing, often contradictory field.

II. CATECHOLAMINERGIC NEURONS AND THEIR PATHWAYS IN THE CENTRAL NERVOUS SYSTEM

A. Location of dopaminergic perikarya

1. Dopaminergic perikarya occur in the following regions of the CNS:
   a. **Telencephalon.** The olfactory bulb and septal region contain the only dopaminergic perikarya of the telencephalon.
   b. **Diencephalon.** Dopaminergic perikarya extend as scattered groups through the zona incerta and hypothalamus and into the retina.
   c. **Brain stem tegmentum. Dopaminergic** perikarya concentrate in the midbrain, **noradrenergic** in the pons, and **adrenergic** in the medulla, but some overlap occurs.

2. Regions of the CNS lacking dopaminergic perikarya include:
   a. Spinal cord gray matter
   b. Motor and sensory nuclei of the cranial nerves
   c. Thalamic nuclei
   d. Cerebral and cerebellar cortices

B. General distribution of dopaminergic axons. The length and distribution of dopaminergic axons correlate rather well with the location of their perikarya.

1. The **telencephalic** dopaminergic neurons of the olfactory bulb have **no** axons at all. They function as amacrine interneurons by means of dendrodendritic contacts on adjacent neurons, as do the dopaminergic interneurons of the retina (see Figure 9-4).

2. The **diencephalic** dopaminergic perikarya of the zona incerta and hypothalamus project **short** axons, mainly within the hypothalamus itself.

3. The **mesencephalic** dopaminergic perikarya, consisting of the **substantia nigra** and **ventral tegmental nucleus**, project axons for **medium** and **long** distances.
   a. These axons run principally rostrally. They go to other midbrain targets, the diencephalon, the basal ganglia, and the cerebral cortex.
   b. To signify the origin and termination of mesencephalic dopaminergic tracts, authors describe them as **mesodiencephalic, mesostriatal, mesoallocortical, mesoneocortical**, and so forth.

C. Specific distributions of dopaminergic pathways from the mesencephalon

1. The **substantia nigra**—pars compacta and pars reticulata—extends the entire length of the midbrain, from the midbrain-diencephalic junction to the midbrain-pontine junction (see Figures 7-19 to 7-21 and 11-7).
   a. **Nigromesencephalic axons** run to the superior colliculus and pedunculopontine nucleus.
   b. **The nigrostriatal (mesostriatal) tract** projects to the corpus striatum, which includes the caudate nucleus, putamen, and pallidum (Figure 14-1A). It is the largest projection of the pars compacta, which sends mainly axons of medium length.
      (1) The nigrostriatal tract turns medially from its origin to enter field H_2 of Forel, ventral to the zona incerta. At the level of the subthalamic nucleus, the axons veer into the internal capsule and fan out as they ascend to innervate all parts of the corpus striatum, including the nucleus accumbens.
      (2) Pars compacta sends dopaminergic axons and pars reticulata GABAergic axons.

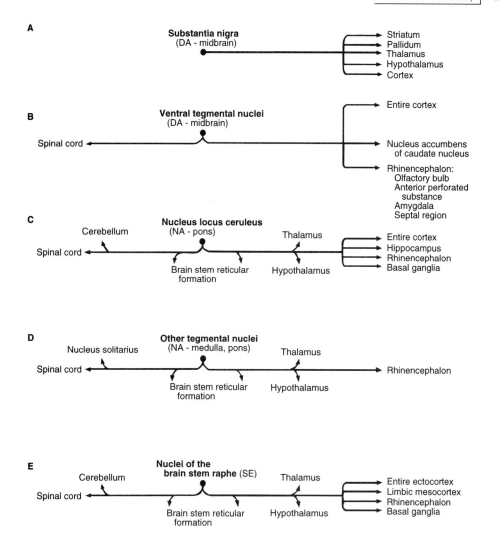

FIGURE 14-1. Distribution of dopaminergic, noradrenergic, and serotonergic pathways in the central nervous system. *DA* = dopaminergic; *NA* = noradrenergic; *SE* = serotonergic.

    c. Nigrodiencephalic axons run to the ventral thalamic motor nuclei, subthalamic nucleus, pallidum, and hypothalamus.
    d. Nigrocortical axons
        (1) In reaching the head of the caudate nucleus, many fibers run just dorsal to or in the medial forebrain bundle. Mesolimbic axons fan out from the medial forebrain bundle into the amygdala and entorhinal cortex of the temporal lobe.
        (2) Pars compacta apparently sends some dopaminergic projections to the motor cortex but more come from the ventral tegmental nucleus.
2. The ventral paramedian tegmental dopaminergic nucleus
    a. The ventral paramedian tegmental nucleus lies mediodorsal to the medial margin of the substantia nigra (see Figure 7-20). It sends longer and more extensive pathways than the substantia nigra, reaching **caudally** to the spinal cord and **rostrally** to the cerebral cortex (see Figure 14-1B).
    b. Caudally projecting dopaminergic axons from the ventral tegmental nucleus and from some dopaminergic perikarya in the hypothalamus run to the spinal cord.
    c. Rostrally projecting axons consist of **mesolimbic, mesoallocortical,** and **mesoneocortical** components. They run ventromedial to and in close association with

the nigrostriatal pathway and then continue through the hypothalamus in the medial forebrain bundle.

    d. At the retrochiasmatic level, **mesolimbic** and **mesoallocortical** pathways veer laterally into the ansa peduncularis to reach the amygdala, piriform cortex, and entorhinal area (area 28) of the limbic system (see Figure 14-1B) as well as the supralimbic cortex.

        (1) Axons, proceeding rostrally, enter the nucleus accumbens, anterior perforated substance (olfactory tubercle), and septal region.

        (2) Some extend forward to the olfactory bulb.

    e. The **mesoneocortical** pathway from the ventral tegmental nucleus runs through and around the head of the caudate nucleus to reach the cingulate gyrus and general cortex.

D. **Noradrenergic pathways**

  1. Location of noradrenergic perikarya

    a. Noradrenergic perikarya extend from the medulla through the brain stem and ventral diencephalon to the olfactory bulb and septal area, but most concentrate in the pons.

    b. The noradrenergic perikarya in the pons form two groups: the nucleus locus coeruleus and several additional nuclei.

  2. The **nucleus locus coeruleus** is a small, grossly visible, darkly pigmented area in the dorsal pontine tegmentum, lateroventral to the aqueduct and fourth ventricle.

    a. **Afferents** to the nucleus locus coeruleus come from:

        (1) Cerebral and cerebellar cortices

        (2) The hypothalamus

        (3) Reticular formation (RF)

            (a) The dorsal raphe nucleus of the midbrain is the largest serotonergic nucleus and the largest single source of afferents to the nucleus locus coeruleus.

            (b) The nucleus paragigantocellularis and the nucleus prepositus hypoglossi in the RF of the medulla also deliver afferents to the nucleus locus coeruleus.

    b. **Efferents** from the nucleus locus coeruleus disperse more widely than those of any other known nucleus (see Figure 14-1C).

        (1) In keeping with efferent RF neurons, the axons undergo a T-like bifurcation into ascending and descending branches (see Figure 7-37).

        (2) The individual axons from the nucleus locus coeruleus collateralize locally and then sprout hundreds of thousands of axonal endings that extend into all major subdivisions of the neuraxis, including the cerebral cortex, diencephalon, brain stem, cerebellum, and spinal cord.

  3. The other noradrenergic perikarya of the pontine tegmentum, apart from the nucleus locus coeruleus, distribute their axons in a similar but less extensive manner (see Figure 14-1D).

    a. Rostrally, these axons probably do not extend past the olfactory bulb and septum.

    b. Scattered noradrenergic neurons in the medulla send axons to the spinal cord and to the nucleus solitarius.

  4. Course of rostrally running noradrenergic pathways. Noradrenergic axons from the pons distribute by **periventricular** and **tegmental** pathways.

    a. The **periventricular pathway** extends in the periaqueductal gray matter from the medulla to the periventricular region of the thalamus and hypothalamus.

        (1) The periventricular pathway distributes axons from the nucleus locus coeruleus, the other pontomedullary noradrenergic nuclei, and serotonergic nuclei.

        (2) In part, it may include the dorsal longitudinal fasciculus of Schütz, located in the ventral part of the periaqueductal gray matter.

    b. The **tegmental pathway** runs through the region designated as the central tegmental tract (see Figures 7-16 to 7-19). The noradrenergic axons concentrate in the dorsomedial sector of the tract as the **dorsal tegmental bundle**. This bundle splits as the noradrenergic fibers fan out in the midbrain into **dorsal** and **ventral** components.

(1) The **dorsal** bundle, mostly from the nucleus locus coeruleus, ascends ventrolateral to the periaqueductal gray matter en route to midbrain, diencephalic, and telencephalic targets. Traversing the diencephalon in the medial forebrain bundle, it reaches the telencephalon by two routes.

(a) The majority of the fibers veer **dorsally** to enter the cingulum, internal capsule, and adjacent deep white matter to disperse diffusely and uniformly to the entire cortex.

(b) Other fibers veer **ventrolaterally** through the ansa peduncularis and inferior thalamic peduncle to reach the piriform cortex, amygdala, and hippocampus.

(c) Hippocampal fibers travel with the cingulum.

(2) The **ventral bundle**, mostly from the noradrenergic perikarya of the pons, outside the nucleus locus coeruleus, ascends through the central tegmental tract en route to its midbrain and forebrain targets. In the forebrain, it roughly follows the medial forebrain bundle.

5. **Cortical distribution of noradrenergic terminals**
   a. Noradrenergic axons from the nucleus locus coeruleus spread uniformly and diffusely to the entire cerebral cortex and hippocampus.
   b. Noradrenergic terminals end in close proximity to the membranes of the cortical neurons but do not form distinct terminal synaptic bars. In this respect, they resemble the endings of the serotonergic axons but differ from the dopaminergic endings, which are synapses.

E. **Function of catecholaminergic pathways**

1. Facile generalizations about the function of any of the chemically specified systems are difficult to make for several reasons.
   a. Some dopaminergic pathways, such as the nigrostriatal pathway, are highly organized according to body topography. Other catecholaminergic projections are more diffuse, having a less distinct topography. Presumably, they modulate or gate many general functions (e.g., mood, attention, and vigilance) rather than initiating functions or transmitting specific, point-to-point communication.
   b. The receptor as well as the transmitter determines the effect on different neurons.
   c. The state of activity of the system at the time of neurotransmitter release may alter the outcome.
   d. Some systems are linked in loops of alternating excitation and inhibition.
      (1) Stimulation of inhibitory neurons may reduce a specified behavior.
      (2) Inhibition of inhibitory neurons may increase a particular behavior.
      (3) Stimulation or inhibition of excitatory neurons produces converse effects.

2. The amacrine dopaminergic neurons of the olfactory bulb and retina may function to inhibit the lateral transfer of excitatory activity, thus increasing the signal-to-noise ratio in these systems.

3. The response of noradrenergic neurons to axonal interruption differs strikingly from that of other CNS neurons because of the tendency of the axons to regenerate, at least in lower animals. In contrast, the axons of other CNS tracts, such as the pyramidal tract or optic tract, do not regenerate.

F. **Clinical effects of dysfunction of catecholaminergic pathways**

1. The effect of catecholaminergic neurotransmitters on motor function is complex, depending on the amount of the neurotransmitter and the degree of sensitivity of the receptors.
   a. An **excess** of dopamine at synaptic terminals or **hypersensitivity** of dopamine receptors causes involuntary movements.
   b. A **decrease** in dopamine synapses, as occurs after interruption of the dopaminergic projection from the substantia nigra, results in bradykinesia and parkinsonism (see Table 11-1).

2. In schizophrenia, the limbic dopaminergic system is thought to be overactive. Drugs that block the action of dopamine improve the condition.
   a. Most of the effective medications also cause extrapyramidal syndromes such as parkinsonism or other involuntary movements because they also block dopaminergic activity in the basal motor nuclei.
   b. Patients chronically treated with dopamine blockers may show a variety of involuntary movements called **tardive dyskinesia**. Long-term blockade may cause the dopaminergic receptors in the basal motor nuclei to become hypersensitive to dopamine, resulting in the tardive dyskinesia.

3. In Alzheimer's disease and parkinsonism, the neurons of the nucleus locus coeruleus degenerate, as do neurons at other loci, including the nucleus basalis, the substantia nigra, and the cerebral cortex itself.

III. SEROTONERGIC PATHWAYS

A. Location of serotonergic neurons

1. Serotonergic perikarya extend from the caudal medulla to the rostral end of the midbrain. They occur predominantly in the median and paramedian plane of the brain stem tegmentum, within and along side of the median raphe. They form fairly distinct nuclei (see Figure 7-38). The hypothalamus contains scattered serotonergic perikarya, but except for some amacrine neurons of the retina, few or no serotonergic perikarya occur rostral to this level.

2. The raphe and paramedian zone of the midbrain contain the two largest serotonergic nuclei, the **dorsal raphe nucleus** and the **median raphe nucleus** (see Figure 7-38).

3. Although serotonergic perikarya run continuously through the raphe and paramedian zone, the pontomedullary transition zone contains the next highest density of serotonergic nuclei, the nuclei **raphe magnus** and **raphe pallidus** (see Figure 7-38).

4. The ventrolateral RF of the medulla contains scattered serotonergic perikarya.

B. Morphology of serotonergic neurons

1. Serotonergic neurons tend to have primitive, large, relatively unbranched dendrites (isodendritic) [see Figure 7-37].

2. The dendrites from the serotonergic perikarya may intertwine in bundles with the dendrites of other RF neurons and the shafts of glial cells (tanicytes) in the floor of the fourth ventricle of the medulla.
   a. These bundles run as vertically oriented shafts that extend in the median plane from the floor of the fourth ventricle to the ventral margin of the medullary tegmentum.
   b. Blood vessels frequently abut on these bundles.
   c. These arrangements presumably allow for intimate interchange of chemical communication between the raphe neurons and the cerebrospinal fluid (CSF) and blood. Perhaps these anatomic arrangements allow the dendrites to sip the blood and CSF.

C. Afferents to the serotonergic nuclei include the:

1. Sensorimotor cortex

2. Limbic periventricular and habenular systems

3. RF

4. Fastigial nucleus of the cerebellum

5. Spinal cord via spinoreticular tracts

D. **Efferents** from the serotonergic nuclei

1. The serotonergic distribution resembles the noradrenergic distribution, but provides the largest and most dense innervation to the cerebral cortex of the known neuro-chemical systems.

2. The axons of the serotonergic nuclei divide into **ascending** and **descending** branches. The serotonergic neurons at each brain stem level project strongly to surrounding RF and, ultimately, to all of the major subdivisions of the CNS (see Figure 14-1E).
   a. The **caudal serotonergic nuclei** in the medulla tend to project caudally, forming a bulbospinal tract.
   b. The **intermediate serotonergic nuclei** in the pons project caudally to the medulla and spinal cord. Some axons run rostrally to the midbrain, diencephalon, and cerebrum, and dorsally into the cerebellum.
   c. The **rostral serotonergic nuclei** in the midbrain project mainly rostrally, to the forebrain.
      (1) The **dorsal raphe nucleus** provides fine axons with small varicosities.
      (2) The **median raphe nucleus** provides axons with large spherical varicosities.
   d. The ascending axons from the serotonergic nuclei of the midbrain form two streams.
      (1) A **dorsal stream** runs through the ventral part of the periaqueductal gray matter, in the dorsal longitudinal bundle of Schütz.
      (2) A **ventral stream** runs through the midbrain tegmentum. Both streams unite in the medial forebrain bundles and disperse from there.
      (3) The serotonergic axons project to the nonspecific thalamic nuclei (i.e., those that do not relay specific pathways from basal motor nuclei, the cerebellum, or the lemnisci).
      (4) The remaining ascending serotonergic axons reach the striatum, rhinencephalon, limbic system, and then the neocortex, which they innervate diffusely and profusely.

3. Outside of the raphe nuclei themselves, the highest concentrations of serotonin in the CNS occur in the substantia nigra, substantia innominata, striatum, and hypothalamus.
   a. In the telencephalon, the limbic areas, hippocampus, cingulate gyrus, and amygdala contain especially high concentrations of serotonin.
   b. In the neocortex, sensory cortex, particularly striate cortex (area 17), receives dense serotonergic innervation.
   c. Some uncertainty exists as to the percent of endings that are true synapses. Serotonergic terminals form distinct baskets around some types of cortical neurons.

E. **Functions of the serotonergic system**

1. The widespread connections of the serotonergic system in general suggest that it plays an augmenting or modulating role rather than initiating specific behaviors or conveying highly focal, point-to-point connections.

2. As a general rule, serotonin acts as an inhibitory neurotransmitter, but it may also have excitatory functions.

3. Bulbospinal serotonergic axons make an inhibitory monosynaptic connection with sympathetic neurons of the spinal cord, establishing a link in a pathway for the control of cardiovascular responses.

4. The bulbospinal serotonergic pathway also reaches the substantia gelatinosa and may play a role in pain modulation (Figure 14-2).
   a. Electrical stimulation of the raphe, which causes serotonin release at axonal endings, produces analgesia in animals by increasing the pain threshold.
   b. Serotonin depletion decreases the pain threshold.

5. Anatomic destruction of the raphe serotonergic nuclei or pharmacologic inhibition of serotonin synthesis causes insomnia, suggesting a sleep-initiating role for the serotonergic system.

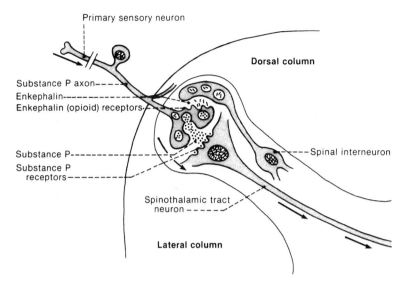

FIGURE 14-2. Simplified diagram of possible neurotransmitter interactions in the pain pathway in the dorsal quadrant of the spinal cord. *Arrows* indicate the direction of flow of pain impulses. See VIII F 2 a-c for further explanation.

6. Some serotonergic axons terminate on CNS blood vessels and ventricular surfaces, as do some noradrenergic axons. These terminals presumably control the blood-brain barrier.

7. The anatomical arrangement of the medullary dendritic bundles suggests a route by which CSF and bloodborne chemical substances might directly influence RF neurons.

8. The serotonergic nuclei of the raphe undergo extensive degeneration in chronic alcoholics, more so at medullary than mesencephalic levels. These patients exhibit signs of brain dysfunction.

9. In summary, the exact function of serotonin in the CNS remains a mystery. Stimulation or destruction of the serotonergic system alters the following visceral and behavioral functions, but may not exclusively control any:
   a. Homeostatic functions, such as water balance, blood flow, temperature regulation, and sleep
   b. Overall activity level and aggression
   c. Self-stimulation and the learning of avoidance behavior
   d. Sexual behavior
   e. Pain responses

IV. CHOLINERGIC PATHWAYS

A. Cholinergic neurons of the PNS

1. Acetylcholine is the established neurotransmitter for:
   a. Preganglionic autonomic axons
   b. Postganglionic axons of the parasympathetic nervous system
   c. Postganglionic sympathetic axons to sweat glands and the adrenal medulla
   d. Motoneurons to skeletal muscle, whether branchial or somatic (The recurrent collaterals from motoneurons to Renshaw neurons are also cholinergic.)

2. In the PNS, and presumably most of the time in the CNS, acetylcholine acts as an excitatory transmitter.

B. **Cholinergic pathways of the CNS**

1. Identification of cholinergic neurons in the CNS

   a. Current techniques do not directly localize acetylcholine itself in the CNS. The inference that a neuron acts by cholinergic transmission rests largely on demonstration of the degradative enzyme, acetylcholinesterase, or on the presence of the synthesizing enzyme, choline acetyltransferase (ChAT), which may occur in the neuronal perikarya, axons, and synaptic endings.

   b. The presence of these enzymes in neurons does not establish acetylcholine as a transmitter because it may have roles other than neurotransmission.

   c. The highest concentrations of these enzymes occur in the central segments of the dorsal roots but not in the peripheral, the interpeduncular region, the striatum, retina, hippocampus, and amygdala.

   d. In the monkey cerebral cortex, the association areas show the least ChAT activity, the sensorimotor regions show intermediate activity, and the limbic mesocortex shows the most, except for the cingulate gyrus.

2. Probable and possible cholinergic perikarya and pathways

   a. Scattered local circuit cholinergic neurons. These interneurons occur in the striatum, including the nucleus accumbens, the basal forebrain, the RF, and possibly the spinal gray matter and cerebral cortex. The presence of intrinsic cholinergic neurons in the cortex, hippocampus, amygdala, and parts of the thalamus is still unsettled.

   b. The striatum. The matrix shows very strong enzyme activity, but controversy exists as to whether it represents extrinisc or intrinsic neurons.

   c. Basal forebrain. The gigantocellular complex that extends from the septal region through the anterior perforated substance and diagonal band (see Figure 13-13), including the nucleus basalis, projects cholinergic axons diffusely to the entire cerebral cortex.

   d. Hypothalamus. The supraoptic and paraventricular nuclei stain for ChAT. Neurons of the posterior part of the lateral hypothalamus that stain for ChAT may project to the cerebral cortex.

   e. Pedunculopontine and laterodorsal nuclei of the midbrain-pontine tegmentum. Most of the pedunculopontine nucleus is on the dorsolateral margin of the superior cerebellar peduncle. But the medial part, on the medial margin of the peduncle, fades into the laterodorsal tegmental nucleus located in the periaqueductal gray matter between the aqueduct and medial longitudinal fasciculus.

   (1) Ascending projections. This complex sends ascending cholinergic projections through the midbrain tegmentum or medial forebrain bundle to the interpeduncular nucleus, hypothalamus, thalamus, basal forebrain, and a small number to the cerebral cortex.

   (a) The whole complex projects strongly to intralaminar nuclei, as do the parabrachial nuclei and contiguous RF.

   (b) The laterodorsal nucleus projects to the anteroventral and mediodorsal thalamus, and the pedunculopontine nucleus projects to the lateral tier of relay nuclei, including the lateral geniculate body.

   (2) Descending projections. These projections to the paramedian medullary RF may mediate the rapid eye movements (REM) and inhibition of muscle tone that characterize REM sleep.

   (3) The midbrain cholinergic systems may originate a series of cholinergic cascades, which play upon the thalamus, hypothalamus, striatum, rhinencephalon, and adjacent limbic structures, and ultimately the cortex. This, with other projections of the pontomesencephalic RF, may constitute, at least in part, the elusive anatomical substrate of the ascending reticular activating system (ARAS).

   f. The projections from the gigantocellular complex of the basal forebrain and the pedunculopontine-laterodorsal tegmental complex constitute the best characterized cholinergic pathways known in the CNS (Table 14-1).

TABLE 14-1. Cholinergic Pathways of the Central Nervous System*

Probable cholinergic pathways

Recurrent collaterals to Renshaw neurons from ventral motoneurons

Primary afferents for vision and hearing

Septohippocampal tract

Nucleus basalis of Meynert and gigantocellular complex of the basal forebrain

Projections of the pedunculopontine nucleus and laterodorsal tegmental nucleus to reticular formation of the medulla and to the thalamus, striatum, and cortex (ascending reticular activating system)

Paraventricular and supraoptic nuclei

Possible cholinergic pathways

Some striatal interneurons and efferents

Efferents of ventral and posteromedial thalamic nuclei

Lateral geniculate and cochlear nuclei; hence the primary and secondary neurons of the visual and auditory systems

Some hypothalamic neurons, which are cholinergic with dopaminergic and peptide cotransmitters

Some neurons of the cerebral cortex

*Many of these pathways use cotransmitters.

V. GAMMA-AMINOBUTYRIC ACID (GABA) PATHWAYS (GABAergic pathways)

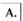

A. Location of GABAergic perikarya

1. Technically, it is easy to identify GABA-positive axonal terminals but difficult to identify the perikarya of origin. The description of the GABAergic system is based on the concentrations of GABA and gamma-aminodecarboxylase (GAD). The concentration of GAD is preferred for several reasons.
   a. Glial cells also take up GABA.
   b. Glutamic acid, a GABA precursor, itself acts as a transmitter.
   c. GABA coexists in many neurons with other neurotransmitters.

2. GABAergic neurons are confined to the CNS; axons of the PNS do not use GABAergic transmission.
   a. In general, GABAergic neurons project short axons (Golgi type II neurons) and act in the short interneuronal circuits throughout the gray matter of the entire CNS.
   b. Some intermediate length tracts (but apparently not the long tracts) use GABAergic transmission.
      (1) Most intrinsic neurons of the cerebellum, including the Purkinje neurons, are GABAergic (see Table 10-4).
      (2) The nigrostriatal projection from pars reticulata of the substantia nigra is GABAergic.
      (3) The striatonigral and striatopallidal projections are GABAergic, and the striatum contains numerous GABAergic interneurons.

3. GABA and GAD have the highest concentrations in the dorsal horns, cerebellum, collicular plate, substantia nigra, hypothalamus, pallidum, and anterior perforated substance (substantia innominata).

4. In the spinal cord, GABA and GAD concentrations are highest in the substantia gelatinosa, nucleus dorsalis of Clarke, and the nuclei gracilis and cuneatus. The remainder of the dorsal horn and the ventral horns also contain GABAergic interneurons.

5. In the telencephalon, the rhinencephalon contains GABAergic interneurons in the olfactory bulb, substantia innominata, septal region, and medial amygdalar region.

6. The cortex contains only average amounts of GABAergic interneurons, but they appear to have an even distribution. Possibly about 30% of the cortical interneurons use GABA as the primary transmitter.

7. The hippocampus contains GABAergic interneurons that synapse on its granular and pyramidal neurons.

B. **Function of the GABAergic system**

1. GABA and glycine are regarded as inhibitory transmitters.

2. GABAergic neurons act as inhibitory interneurons throughout all parts of the CNS, from spinal gray matter to cerebral cortex, although differing in numbers at various sites.

3. In Huntington's chorea, the amount of GABA in the striatum is very small; this correlates with the predominant loss of the small interneurons seen histologically and the choreiform movements seen clinically.

4. Neuropharmacologists have introduced drugs to treat epileptic seizures by manipulating the GABA metabolic pathway and GABA receptors. These efforts arise from the theory that increasing the inhibitory action of GABA will block the excessive, hypersynchronous discharge of neurons that causes seizures.

VI. **NEUROCHEMICAL PATHWAYS THAT BYPASS THE THALAMUS ON THEIR WAY TO THE CEREBRAL CORTEX**

A. Several chemically specified pathways to the cerebral cortex share common features.

1. The axons arise in discrete infracortical nuclei of the brain stem tegmentum, hypothalamus, or basal forebrain.

2. The axons bypass the thalamus and have direct access to the cortex.

3. The axons branch profusely and disperse widely and diffusely to the entire cortex.

4. Most endings form traditional synapses and release a specific, known chemical neurotransmitter, but in some cases the endings are not true synapses.

5. The pathways are thought to act as modulators of various functions rather than mediating a specific function or modality.

B. Table 14-2 summarizes these systems.

TABLE 14-2. Some Chemically Specified Diffuse Cortical Modulating Pathways That Bypass the Thalamus

Neurotransmitter	Nucleus of Origin
Acetylcholine	Gigantocellular complex of basal forebrain, including the nucleus basalis of Meynert Hypothalamus
Gamma-aminobutyric acid, histamine, and neuropeptides	Hypothalamus
Dopamine	Ventral tegmental region (midbrain)
Serotonin	Raphe nuclei (midbrain)
Noradrenaline	Locus coeruleus

VII. GLUTAMATE AND ASPARTATE PATHWAYS

A. Currently these two dicarboxylic amino acids appear to be the principal, but not exclusive, excitatory neurotransmitters in the CNS. Acetylcholine also acts centrally but predominates as the excitatory transmitter in the PNS.

B. Excitatory interneurons of spinal cord gray matter act by glutamate and aspartate transmission.

C. The majority of excitatory cortical neurons act by glutaminergic or aspartate transmission. Excitatory cortical efferents to other parts of the cortex and to the striatum and thalamus use glutamate, but the neurotransmitter of the pyramidal tract remains uncertain. The large Betz cells, at least in the monkey cortex, do not show glutaminase immunoreactivity.

D. **Excitotoxicity of aspartate and glutamate**

1. Injured neurons, as in hypoxia, liberate aspartate and glutamate. They act on N-methyl-D-aspartate (NMDA) receptors, which are most numerous in the regions most vulnerable to hypoxia—the cerebral cortex, hippocampus, striatum, and cerebellum. Release of these transmitters triggers a cascade of events that leads to cell death by causing an excessive influx of calcium and sodium.

2. Treatment of infarcts and hypoxia in infants and adults now centers on blocking NMDA receptors and may also lead to more effective treatment of the hypersynchronous discharge of neurons that results in epileptic seizures.

VIII. NEUROPEPTIDE PATHWAYS

A. **Discovery of peptides as messengers and neurotransmitters**

1. In 1931, von Euler and Gaddum isolated Substance P from the brain and gut that caused contraction of intestinal muscle and dilation of blood vessels. Forty years later the active substance was identified as a peptide. Peptides consist of 2 to 40 amino acids linked to each other.

2. Subsequently, peptides were discovered in CNS neurons and the pituitary gland. Scientists also found that the hypothalamus uses peptide messengers to control the release of pituitary hormones (see Figure 12-17A). The first hypothalamic-hypophyseal releasing peptide, thyrotropin releasing factor (TRF), was discovered in 1969.

3. A veritable explosion of interest in neuropeptides followed the discovery in the mid-1970s that opiates (e.g., morphine) localize in regions of the brain that mediate affective experiences and pain perception.

   a. Two naturally occurring endogenous neuropeptides, called **enkephalins**, were found to bind to the opioid receptors of neurons and to reproduce the action of morphine. Naloxone blocks the action of these peptides and morphine. Enkephalins are widely distributed in all regions of the CNS, except for the cerebellum, which lacks conspicuous neuropeptides.

   b. Currently, the term **endorphins** (from "endogenous" and "morphine") is either used generically for the whole class of endogenous peptide neurotransmitters that have opioid activity, or for a specific opiomelanocortin. Opiomelanocortins (opiocortins) include opioid and nonopioid peptides.

B. **Production of neuropeptides**

1. In contrast to other neurotransmitters, neuropeptides are produced by ribosomes directed by messenger ribonucleic acid (mRNA), and thus arise in neuronal perikarya

or dendrites. Proteolytic enzymes then cleave the neuropeptides from larger pro-hormones.

2. After packaging into vesicles, the neuropeptide is transported down the axon to the axon terminals where calcium-dependent mechanisms release them.

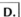 **Role of neuropeptides as cotransmitters**

1. Neuroactive peptides do not act as the sole transmitter of many axons. In the CNS and PNS they seem to function as cotransmitters that perhaps enhance or modify the action of a classic, primary transmitter, such as acetylcholine or adrenalin.

2. The type of peptide cotransmitter may provide the "unique signature" for the axons of pathways that share a common "major" neurotransmitter. For example, postganglionic parasympathetic axons act by cholinergic transmission, but the axons to salivary glands and smooth muscles, particularly sphincters, also coliberate vasoactive intestinal peptide (VIP).

3. The most numerous chemically specified cortical neurons contain VIP. These VIP neurons line up in the radial columns that characterize cortical cytoarchitecture. Thus, the central and peripheral pathways are neuropeptide-coded.

4. Neurons may alter their neuropeptide transmitter during ontogenesis and in response to internal and external contingencies. Such a capability could underlie plasticity of neuronal functions, learning, memory, and Pavlovian conditioning of reflexes.

D. **Function of neuroactive peptides**

1. Functional classes of neuropeptides
   a. The neuraxis, from the cerebral cortex to the spinal cord, except the cerebellum, has abundant excitatory and inhibitory neuropeptidergic interneurons as primary or cotransmitters.
   b. Peptides are now known that act as neurotransmitters or neuromodulators, as releasing factors for adenohypophyseal hormones, and as hormones themselves. Thus, neuropeptides fall into one of three classes: **neurohypophyseal, adenohypophyseal**, and **neurotransmitter**, but the same peptide may perform more than one of these functions.

2. Neurohypophyseal neuropeptides. These are the actual hormones released from the neurohypophysis (see Figure 12-17B) and include oxytocin and vasopressin, which arise from the supraoptic and paraventricular nuclei.

3. Adenohypophyseal releasing neuropeptides. After synthesis by hypothalamic neurons, these neuropeptides empty into an adenohypophyseal portal system of blood vessels (see Figure 12-17A) and **promote** or **inhibit** the release of hormones from adenohypophyseal cells.
   a. The arcuate nuclei of the median eminence manufacture a number of neurohypophyseal-related peptides, including adrenocorticotropic hormone (ACTH), β-endorphin, and dopamine.
   b. Neuropeptides manufactured in the hypothalamic neurons that control hormone release include:
      (1) TRF
      (2) Gonadotropin releasing factor (GRF)
      (3) Corticotropin releasing factor (CRF)
      (4) Somatostatin (SST), which inhibits the release of somatotropin (the growth hormone) and other adenohypophyseal hormones

4. Neurotransmitter neuropeptides include:
   a. Opioid neuropeptides
      (1) Opiocortins
         (a) ACTH; corticotropin
         (b) β-endorphin
         (c) Melanocyte stimulating hormone (MSH)

(2) Enkephalins

(3) Dynorphin

b. **Nonopioid neuropeptides** include the hyophyseal and endocrine-related releasing factors and hormones.

c. **Substance P and VIPs** (found in the gut and CNS)

E. **Opiocortin (β-endorphins, ACTH) neuropeptides: location of perikarya and distribution of axons**

1. **Hypothalamic opioid nuclei**

   a. Arcuate and paramedian opioid nuclei distribute their axons widely to RF (including monoaminergic groups), periaqueductal gray matter, the hypothalamus-pituitary gland, the thalamus, and rhinencephalic-limbic forebrain structures.

   b. Laterodorsal hypothalamic neurons distribute axons to forebrain structures: the olfactory bulb, hippocampal formation, and ectocortex.

2. **Medullary opioid nuclei**

   a. The perikarya are located in the commissural division of nucleus tractus solitarii and extend ventrolaterally through nucleus reticularis of the medulla into the catecholaminergic region, medial to nucleus ambiguus.

   b. Axons distribute to the RF of the medulla and to the central gray matter of the spinal cord at all levels.

   c. Medullary and arcuate opiocortin axonal terminals strongly overlap the perikarya containing CRF, giving them a unique codistribution.

      (1) CRF perikarya are scattered from the rostral level of the spinal cord to the septal region.

      (2) The codistribution is strong in the periventricular region of the hypothalamus and in the paraventricular nucleus, which has about the greatest concentration of CRF perikarya in the CNS.

3. **Function of opiocortin neuropeptides**

   a. The medullary corticotropin system is in a prime location to mediate cardiovascular, respiratory, and gastrointestinal tract reflexes of cranial nerve (CN) IX and CN X.

   b. The hypothalamic and paraventricular nuclear connections provide a pathway for regulating the release of vasopressin [antidiuretic hormone (ADH)] or oxytocin by the paraventricular nucleus.

   c. Overall, the endogenous peptide system functions in regulation of pain thresholds, blood pressure, appetite and thirst control, temperature, and reproduction.

   d. Finally, endorphins in the limbic system and hypothalamus probably mediate the "feel good" states, such as the "highs" that follow exercise.

F. **Substance P**

1. A particularly high concentration occurs in the areas devoted to pain transmission, autonomic, and limbic functions. These areas include:

   a. Small dorsal root axons and axonal terminals ending on the substantia gelatinosa of the spinal cord and on the spinal nucleus of CN V

   b. Dental pulp nerves

   c. Perikarya of small neurons in dorsal root ganglions (A high concentration occurs in approximately 20% of the perikarya.)

   d. Periaqueductal gray matter, substantia nigra, and interpeduncular region of the brain stem

   e. Medial preoptic area and habenula of the diencephalon

   f. Striatum

   g. Amygdala

   h. Cerebral cortex

2. Substance P currently appears to act as the primary neurotransmitter for pain in dorsal roots, although it may not function as a pain mediator at its other sites in the CNS.

a. Figure 14-2 illustrates one theory of the mechanism of pain control by interactions of several transmitter systems.

b. The primary sensory neuron releases substance P to excite the neurons in the substantia gelatinosa or other secondary neurons of the spinothalamic pathway.

c. Certain spinal interneurons, if activated, release enkephalin, which attaches to the enkephalin (opioid) receptors on the terminals of substance P axons. Opiate drugs such as morphine may also attach to these receptors. Activation of these receptors by enkephalin or opiate drugs blocks the release of substance P into the synaptic cleft and, hence, transmission of pain impulses through the spinothalamic tract. Such an action constitutes **presynaptic inhibition** of neurotransmission.

d. The exact way that serotonergic bulbospinal axons inhibit pain transmission is uncertain.

3. The supraspinal sites for opioid receptors that control pain transmission at spinal levels concentrate in the midbrain and medulla. Nucleus raphe magnus of the medulla sends serotonergic bulbospinal axons while others descend from nucleus gigantocellularis and the more rostral monaminergic nuclei of the brain stem.

IX. MODEL OF EXCITATORY AND INHIBITORY NEUROTRANSMITTER INTERACTIONS

A. The basal motor nuclei, which are rich in many known neurotransmitters, illustrate the complex interaction of excitatory and inhibitory neurons that characterize many CNS circuits (Figure 14-3).

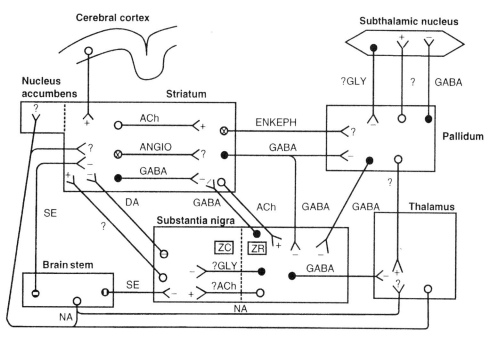

FIGURE 14-3. Simplified diagram for the conceptual understanding of the interaction of numerous neurotransmitter pathways in the motor circuits. *ACh* = acetylcholine; *ANGIO* = angiotensin; *DA* = dopaminergic pathway; *ENKEPH* = enkephalin; *GABA* = gamma-aminobutyric acid; *GLY* = glycine; *NA* = noradrenergic pathway; *SE* = serotonergic pathway; *ZC* = zona compacta of the substantia nigra; *ZR* = zona reticularis of the substantia nigra; + = excitatory; − = inhibitory.

B. As a final statement on chemical neuroanatomy, we must face the irony that the balance between excitatory and inhibitory neurotransmitter chemicals in our limbic pathways determines human drives, instinctual behaviors, our moods, and our tendency to attack or forgive. Just as wry, the balance of neurochemicals at axonal endings determines our rationality or irrationality, our perceptions, and our very mind. Instead of "How are you?" as the invitation to disclose your state of mind, the question becomes "Which of your neurochemical systems predominates today, the serotonergic, dopaminergic, cholinergic, or peptidergic?"

STUDY QUESTIONS

DIRECTIONS: Each of the numbered items or incomplete statements in this section is negatively phrased, as indicated by a capitalized word such as NOT, LEAST, or EXCEPT. Select the ONE lettered answer or completion that is BEST in each case.

1. Which of the following statements about dopaminergic neurons of the substantia nigra is NOT true?

(A) Their perikarya are large and pigmented, and the nucleus is grossly visible
(B) They project their axons mainly to structures rostral to the location of their perikarya
(C) They form distinctive nuclear groups
(D) Their perikarya are concentrated in the periaqueductal region of the midbrain
(E) They send most of their axons to the striatum

2. Which of the following statements about serotonergic neurons is NOT true?

(A) Serotonergic perikarya of the brain stem are concentrated in the median raphe and paramedian region
(B) The serotonergic perikarya extend nearly to the rostrocaudal extent of the brain stem
(C) Serotonergic neurons are large and of the isodendritic type
(D) Electrical stimulation of some serotonergic nuclei produces analgesia
(E) Few serotonergic axons reach the cerebral cortex

3. Select the INCORRECT statement about cholinergic pathways.

(A) The axons of the nucleus basalis distribute widely to the cerebral cortex
(B) The ventral motoneurons of the brain stem and spinal cord are cholinergic
(C) Cholinergic neurons of the midbrain are thought to belong to the ascending reticular activating system (ARAS)
(D) Cholinergic pathways in general tend to be inhibitory
(E) The primary and secondary neurons in the afferent pathway for hearing and vision are thought to be cholinergic

4. Which of the following statements about peptides is NOT correct?

(A) Neuropeptides act as cotransmitters at the effector endings of the lower motoneurons (LMNs) of the autonomic nervous system
(B) Hypothalamic nerve endings release neuropeptides, which release hormones from the adenohypophysis
(C) Periaqueductal gray matter receives large numbers of peptidergic nerve endings from the hypothalamus
(D) The cerebral cortex receives no peptidergic nerve endings
(E) The gut, pituitary gland, and hypothalamus contain many similar peptides

5. All of the following neurons are thought to act by GABAergic transmission EXCEPT

(A) Purkinje neurons
(B) striatal interneurons
(C) neurons of the substantia nigra, pars reticulata
(D) ganglion cell layer of the retina
(E) interneurons of the spinal gray matter and hippocampus

6. All of the following general statements about the perikarya of the noradrenergic neurons are true EXCEPT

(A) the pontomedullary tegmentum contains the largest concentration of noradrenergic neurons
(B) their axons project virtually exclusively to forebrain targets
(C) they produce small, unmyelinated axons with a tremendous number of collaterals
(D) some group neatly into the known cytoarchitectural subdivisions of the reticular formation (RF); others do not
(E) Their axonal distributions were discovered only after the development of fluorescence microscopy

DIRECTIONS: Each set of matching questions in this section consists of a list of four to twenty-six lettered options followed by several numbered items. For each numbered item, select the appropriate lettered option(s). Each lettered option may be selected once, more than once, or not at all. EACH ITEM WILL STATE THE NUMBER OF OPTIONS TO SELECT. CHOOSE EXACTLY THIS NUMBER.

Questions 7–11

(A) Pedunculopontine nucleus
(B) Raphe nuclei of the midbrain
(C) Nucleus basalis and the gigantocellular complex of the basal forebrain
(D) Ventral tegmental area of the midbrain
(E) Nuclei of motor cranial nerves
(F) Intermediolateral cell column of the spinal cord
(G) Paraventricular nuclei of the hypothalamus
(H) Ventral motoneurons of the spinal cord
(I) Substantia nigra, pars compacta
(J) Substantia nigra, pars reticulata
(K) Arcuate nucleus of the hypothalamus
(L) Laterodorsal tegmental nucleus of the midbrain
(M) Supraoptic nucleus of the hypothalamus
(N) Medullary reticular formation (RF)

For each chemically specified pathway, select the site or sites of origin.

7. Dopaminergic axons to the cerebral cortex (SELECT 2 SITES)

8. Cholinergic axons to peripheral effectors (SELECT 3 SITES)

9. Serotonergic axons to area 17 (visual cortex) [SELECT 1 SITE]

10. Peptide releasing factors or hormones to the pituitary gland (SELECT 3 SITES)

11. Cholinergic axons from the brain stem to the midline and intralaminar nuclei of the thalamus (SELECT 2 SITES)

ANSWERS AND EXPLANATIONS

1. The answer is D [II B 3 a, C 1 b, c]. In general, the neurons of the substantia nigra project rostrally in contrast to certain other catecholaminergic neurons that typically produce ascending and descending branches. Degeneration of the substantia nigra deprives the striatum of dopaminergic innervation and results in parkinsonism. The dopaminergic perikarya have a much more restricted location in the brain stem than the serotonergic perikarya. Most dopaminergic perikarya are concentrated in the midbrain, just dorsal to the basis, where they form two well-delineated and well-recognized nuclei: the ventral paramedian tegmental nucleus and the substantia nigra (pars compacta and pars reticularis). The neuronal perikarya of the substantia nigra accumulate a black pigment, which makes the nucleus grossly visible and gives it its name.

2. The answer is E [III D 2 d (4), E 4 a, b]. Serotonergic nuclei of the midbrain project strongly to most forebrain regions, including the cerebral cortex. Serotonergic neurons are concentrated in the median raphe and extend throughout the entire brain stem, but they are present in largest numbers in the dorsal raphe nucleus and median raphe of the caudal midbrain tegmentum and rostral pons. Electrical stimulation reduces the response to pain. Destruction of the raphe nuclei or pharmacologic blockade of serotonin action causes insomnia, suggesting a sleep-initiating role of the serotonergic system.

3. The answer is D [IV A 2]. Acetylcholine generally acts as an excitatory transmitter. The ventral motoneurons are cholinergic, as are many of the axon terminals in the midbrain and basal ganglia and probably the primary and secondary auditory pathways. Cholinergic axons of nucleus basalis of Meynert distribute widely to the cerebral cortex, as do other neurons of the gigantocellular complex of the basal forebrain. This nucleus degenerates in Alzheimer's disease, the most common form of dementia in older persons. Cholinergic neurons of the midbrain are thought to belong to the ascending reticular activating system (ARAS).

4. The answer is D [VIII A 3 a, C 3, D 1]. Neuropeptides act as releasing factors and neurotransmitters throughout the central nervous system (CNS), including the cortex.

Some opiocorticoid and neuropeptide perikarya in the hypothalamus project widely to the forebrain. Others, in the medulla, project widely to the reticular formation (RF) and the catecholaminergic nuclei of the brain stem. They also connect strongly with the periaqueductal and periventricular gray matter, including the central gray matter of the spinal cord.

5. The answer is D [V A 2 b; Table 14-1]. Inhibitory GABAergic interneurons occur throughout virtually all areas of the central nervous system (CNS). The Purkinje cells and the other inhibitory neurons of the cerebellar cortex are GABAergic, with only the granule neurons being excitatory. The ganglion cell layer of the retina consists of Golgi type I neurons that project a considerable distance to the lateral geniculate body and are regarded as cholinergic. Primary sensory axons and the longer tracts, such as the spinocerebellar tract, are not typically GABAergic. The neurotransmitter of the pyramidal tract remains uncertain, but is excitatory rather than GABAergic.

6. The answer is B [II D 2 b]. The axons from the pontine noradrenergic neurons have the widest distribution of any central nervous system (CNS) pathways. Each axon typically bifurcates numerous times to produce hundreds of thousands of synapses and distributes them to virtually every region of the nervous system. Despite their wide distribution, the axons, being small and unmyelinated, eluded discovery until the advent of fluorescence microscopy. Some noradrenergic perikarya, as identified by fluorescence microscopy, form discrete nuclei, such as the nucleus locus coeruleus. Other scattered dopaminergic neurons do not conform to specific known nuclear configurations of the reticular formation (RF), as determined by Nissl staining.

7. The answers are: D, I [II A 1 c, B 3]. The cerebral cortex receives innervation from dopaminergic nuclei of the midbrain, the substantia nigra (pars compacta), and the ventral tegmental nuclei. The ventral tegmental nuclei send the majority of dopaminergic axons to the cortex. The substantia nigra (pars compacta) sends most of its axons to the striatum. The ventral tegmental nuclei are located medial and dorsal to the medial part of the substantia nigra, in the rostral part of the midbrain. More caudally, the interpeduncular nucleus replaces the ventral tegmental nuclei and bears the same relation to the medial margin of the substantia nigra.

8. The answers are: E, F, H [IV A 1–2]. The efferent axons that issue from the brain stem and spinal cord to autonomic ganglia or skeletal muscle use acetylcholine as their major transmitter. They may also use cotransmitters that may be peptides or even gases, such as nitric oxide and carbon monoxide. The major transmitter is common to several axonal systems, while the neuropeptide cotransmitter provides specificity that differs with the effector innervated and with the receptors.

9. The answer is B [III A 1, D 3 b]. Most of the serotonergic innervation of the central nervous system (CNS) comes from nuclei in or alongside the median raphe. The numerous decussating axons that cross the midline form the raphe. The cerebral cortex receives diffuse serotonergic innervation with regional differences. In the neocortex, area 17, the visual receptive area receives a particularly dense network of serotonergic axons. Limbic areas and the striatum and substantia nigra also receive dense serotonergic innervation.

10. The answers are: G, K, M [VIII A 2, D 2, 3 a]. The nuclei of the hypothalamus operate by means of peptides as well as catecholamines

and acetycholine. The arcuate nucleus displays dopamine, adrenocorticotropic hormone (ACTH), β-endorphins, and β-lipotrophic hormone. It appears that the hypothalamic and limbic-related neurons will display a richer number of neuroactive substances than the long tracts. Similar peptides act as releasing factors, as hormones themselves, and act both in the central nervous system (CNS) and peripheral nervous system (PNS).

11. The answers are: A, L [IV B 2 e (1) (a), f]. A complex of cholinergic neurons occupies the dorsal part of the tegmentum in the caudal part of the midbrain, extending into the rostral part of the pons. One nucleus of the complex, the pedunculopontine nucleus, receives its name from its location on the dorsolateral and medial sides of the superior cerebellar peduncle. The medial part of this nucleus extends to the other cluster of cholinergic neurons, the laterodorsal tegmental nuclei. These nuclei may generate a cholinergic cascade that plays on the thalamus, which in turn plays on the cerebral cortex, perhaps by cholinergic transmission. This cholinergic system may represent part of, or the main component of, the ascending reticular activating system (ARAS). The exact anatomical basis of this system, which is crucial for consciousness, still has not been fully identified. Diffuse cortical projections from several hypothalamic nuclei may also participate in cortical arousal.

Chapter 15

Blood Supply of the Central Nervous System

I. EMBRYOGENESIS OF CENTRAL NERVOUS SYSTEM VESSELS

A. Surface origin of vessels

1. The vessels of the central nervous system (CNS) originate as coalescing channels in the mesenchyme that coats the surface of the neural tube and produces its meninges.

2. From the initial, almost random network of anastomoses, particular channels enlarge while others atrophy and disappear (Figure 15-1).

3. One product of coalescence—essentially a single **ventral median artery**—extends along the entire neuraxis, although it splits and reunites rostrally (see Figure 15-1C).

B. Basic pattern of cerebral arteries

1. The ventral median artery at spinal levels receives its blood from somite arteries, which branch off at regular intervals from the aorta (see Figure 15-1C). At cerebral levels, the internal carotid arteries (ICAs) and vertebral arteries bring blood to the ventral surface. The branchial arch arteries contribute to the arterial supply of the brain stem via nerve roots.

2. After receiving its blood from extracranial sources, the ventral arterial channel distributes the blood through **paramedian** and **circumferential** arteries, which then perforate the wall of the neuraxis (Figure 15-2).

   a. The **paramedian arteries** branch off at right angles to the longitudinal ventral trunk and perforate the neural tube wall just dorsal to their origin (see Figure 15-2B).

   b. The **circumferential arteries** circumnavigate the neuraxis, sending perforating branches into it. The circumferential arteries form two groups: short and long.

   (1) The **short** circumferential arteries extend around the brain stem.

   (2) The **long** circumferential arteries, after extending dorsally around the brain stem, continue around the circumference of the cerebellar and cerebral hemispheres (see Figure 15-2C). They form on the hemispheric surface before the completion of fissuration and before any sulcation commences. They then follow the contour of the cortical surfaces as the surfaces fold into crevices (Figure 15-3).

II. BLOOD SUPPLY OF THE SPINAL CORD

A. Spinal arteries

1. A spinal artery enters the intervertebral foramina with each spinal nerve and travels to the cord along each dorsal and ventral root.

   a. Although each radicular artery remains, only a few develop into major feeders for the ventral spinal artery.

   b. The largest feeder is the artery of Adamkiewicz (Figure 15-4).

2. **Paramedian branches of the ventral spinal artery** enter the cord via the ventral median sulcus. **Circumferential branches** send short perforating arteries into the peripheral part of the ventral and lateral white columns (Figure 15-5).

3. The **dorsal root arteries** coalesce into paired longitudinal dorsal spinal arteries.

   a. These dorsal arteries take a wavy, irregular course along the line of attachment of the dorsal roots rather than running straight like the ventral spinal artery, and are of lesser importance.

   b. The dorsal arteries form many circumferential anastomoses with each other and with circumferential branches of the ventral spinal artery (see Figure 15-5).

FIGURE 15-1. Ventral aspect of the developing neural tube showing the arterial pattern. (*A*) Early stage of random vascularization. (*B*) Theoretical stage of single ventral artery with segmental feeders. Branchial-arch vessels are not shown. (*C*) Final plan of arterial vessels. A few channels enlarge while others diminish or atrophy entirely.

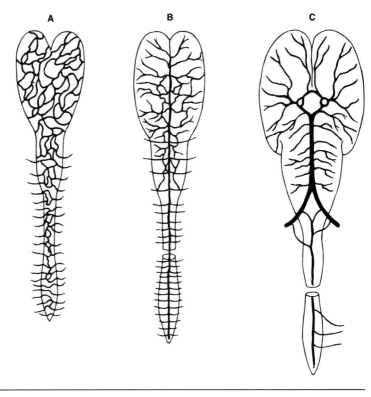

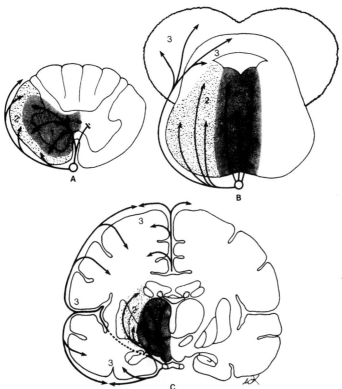

FIGURE 15-2. Transverse sections of the (*A*) spinal cord, (*B*) brain stem, and (*C*) cerebrum, showing how a ventral arterial channel provides paramedian branches and short and long circumferential branches that then perforate the wall of the neural tube. 1 = paramedian vessel (*shaded area*); 2 = short circumferential vessel (*dotted area*); 3 = long circumferential vessel (*white area*).

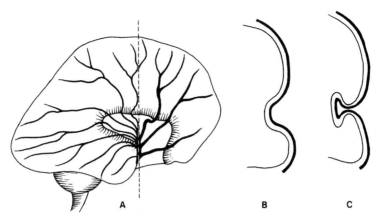

FIGURE 15-3. (*A*) Lateral view of the right cerebral hemisphere. The cerebral vessels form on the surface of the cerebrum and are then infolded into the fissures some sulci, in this case the insular region of the Sylvian fissure. (*B*) Coronal section at the level indicated by the interrupted line in (*A*). (*C*) Coronal section at the same level at a later stage, showing further infolding of the cerebral arteries as the opercula grow over the sylvian fissure.

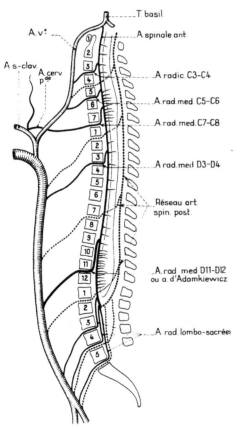

FIGURE 15-4. Lateral view of the arterial blood supply of the spinal cord. A few of the original 31 pairs of somite arteries from the aorta enlarge and provide most of the arterial blood. *A. cerv.* = cervical artery; *A. radic.* or A. rad. med. = radiculomedullary artery; A. rad. lombo-sacrées = lumbosacral radiculomedullary artery; *A. s-clav.* = subclavian artery; *A. spinale ant.* = ventral (anterior) spinal artery; *A. v.* = vertebral artery; *Réseau art. spin. post.* = network of posterior spinal arteries; *T. basil.* = trunk of basilar artery. (Reprinted with permission from Djindjian R: *Angiography of the Spinal Cord.* Baltimore, University Park Press, 1970, p 16.)

4. All in all, the ventral spinal artery irrigates approximately the ventral two-thirds of the cord; the dorsal spinal arteries irrigate approximately the dorsal one-third (see Figure 15-5).
   a. Figure 6-24C shows the classic area of spinal cord infarction resulting from occlusion of the ventral spinal artery.

FIGURE 15-5. Segment of the spinal cord showing the arterial irrigation pattern. Compare with Figure 6-24C, which shows the region infarcted by anterior spinal artery occlusion.

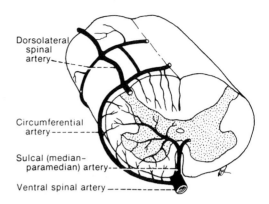

Dorsolateral spinal artery

Circumferential artery

Sulcal (median-paramedian) artery

Ventral spinal artery

      b. Because the ventral spinal artery is the main source of arterial blood, occlusion of it or one of its major feeders may infarct the whole diameter of the cord.

B. Spinal veins

    1. The blood from the spinal cord drains into three longitudinal systems, which anastomose extensively: the **spinal cord plexus** itself; the **epidural**, or **internal vertebral, plexus**; and the **external vertebral plexus**.

      a. The **spinal cord plexus** occupies the subarachnoid space. It communicates freely with the internal vertebral plexus.

      b. The **internal vertebral**, or **epidural, plexus** extends the length of the vertebral column in the epidural space. This space ends at the foramen magnum, where the dura mater becomes tightly adherent to the skull, forming its inner periosteum.

      c. The **internal vertebral plexus** communicates freely through the intervertebral foramina with the **external vertebral plexus**, which runs along the outside of the vertebral column.

    2. Because these venous systems lack valves, blood readily refluxes from one compartment to the other.

      a. Infected emboli or cancer cells may disseminate through and lodge in the plexuses.

      b. The resultant abscess or enlarging tumor in the epidural space then compresses the spinal cord or roots.

      c. Emboli in the external vertebral plexus may result in a retroperitoneal inflammatory mass or a neoplastic mass.

III. ARTERIAL BLOOD SUPPLY OF THE BRAIN

A. Metabolic requirements of the brain

    1. The brain must receive oxygen and glucose continuously to survive. Neurons commence to die within 5 minutes of complete cardiac arrest, which deprives the brain of both substrates.

    2. The brain comprises only about 2% of body weight; however, it uses about 20% of the inspired oxygen and receives about 20% of the cardiac output. Blood flow is 50 ml/100 g of brain tissue/min. Oxygen consumption is 46 ml/min.

    3. Figure 15-6 shows the tremendous volume of the CNS occupied by the arteries.

B. Four major arterial feeders for the brain

    1. The brain receives its blood from two pairs of arteries: two **vertebral arteries** (VAs) and two **ICAs**.

2. These four arteries penetrate foramina at the base of the skull to approach the brain ventrally, where they coalesce incompletely into a ventral median trunk (Figure 15-7).

3. The **ICAs** run through the neck to enter the carotid canal at the skull base. They enter the intracranial space through the foramen lacerum, located just posterolateral to the sella turcica.

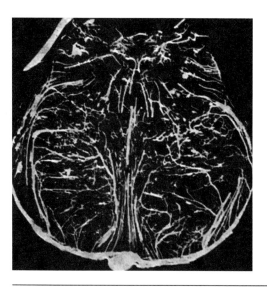

FIGURE 15-6. Transverse section of the pons with the arteries injected to show the volume of neural tissue occupied by arteries alone. (Reprinted with permission from Hassler O: Arterial pattern of human brainstem. *Neurology* 17:368–375, 1967.)

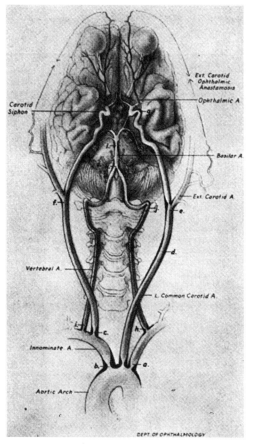

FIGURE 15-7. The four major arteries that supply the brain: two carotid arteries and two vertebral arteries. All of these approach the brain ventrally. The letters a–g indicate common sites for arteriosclerotic plaques, which may lead to insufficiency of arterial blood flow or actual arterial occlusions. (Reprinted with permission from Hoyt WF: Some neuro-ophthalmologic considerations in cerebral vascular insufficiency. *Arch Ophthalmol* 62:260–274, 1959.)

4. The **VAs** run through the transverse processes of the cervical vertebrae. They enter the skull through the foramen magnum, where they pierce the dura mater. Then they course rostrally through the subarachnoid space ventral to the medulla to unite into the **basilar artery** (BA) at the pontomedullary junction (see Figure 15-9).

C. **Arterial patterns at the base of the brain**

1. The branches of the four major arteries at the base of the brain and those of the coronary arteries are the two most important vascular patterns in the body. Study the progressogram in Figure 15-8 in relation to Figure 15-9.

2. Anterior anastomotic circle (of Willis). A bug commencing at the BA bifurcation may enter either the right or left posterior communicating artery (PComA), crawl through the PComA, cross the ICA lumen, enter the anterior cerebral artery (ACA), cross the anterior communicating artery (AComA), and return through the opposite vessels to the BA bifurcation, having negotiated the circle of Willis (see Figure 15-9).

D. **Distribution of the vertebrobasilar system (posterior circulation)** [Figure 15-10]

1. The VA on each side gives off the following vessels:
  a. Many small, unnamed paramedian perforating arteries to the medulla oblongata
  b. A posterior communicating branch as the origin of the ventral spinal artery
  c. One long circumferential branch, the posterior inferior cerebellar artery (PICA)

2. The BA commences at the pontomedullary junction where the VAs unite. It extends the length of the pons to reach the interpeduncular fossa. The BA gives off the following vessels:
  a. Numerous unnamed paramedian perforating arteries to the pons

FIGURE 15-8. Progressogram of an insect figurine representing the arterial pattern at the base of the brain. To learn it, make your own drawing as follows:
1. Draw a pair of eyes: ICAs (Figure 15-9 has the key to the arterial abbreviations).
2. Draw in the facial outline, completing the anterior anastomotic circle (of Willis): ICA, ACA, AComA, ICA, PComA, and PCA.
3. Add a trunk and a pair of hind legs: BA and VAs.
4. Add four forelegs (all insects have six legs): SCA and the extension of PCA from the basilar.
5. Add antennae (feelers): extension of ACA into the interhemispheric fissure.
6. Put a tube in each ear for MCA and striate it with hair for the lenticulostriate arteries, LSAs. Add bangs from ACA for the MSAs. Add a goatee from PCA for the PSAs (Figure 15-17).
7. Create a few irregular ribs: unnamed paramedian arteries.
8. Add a belt: IAAs and AICAs.
9. Attach some feelers to the hind legs: PCAs; add a penis, completing the posterior anastomotic circle: VSA.
10. Label the completed arteries on part 9 from Figure 15-9.
11. Transpose the arteries onto the ventral aspect of the brain, and relate them to the cranial nerves (Figure 15-9).
12. Mentally connect the two ICAs and two VAs of Figure 15-7 with those of Figures 15-8 and 15-9.
(Reprinted with permission from DeMyer W: *Technique of the Neurologic Examination: A Programmed Text*, 3rd ed. New York, McGraw-Hill, 1980, p 92.)

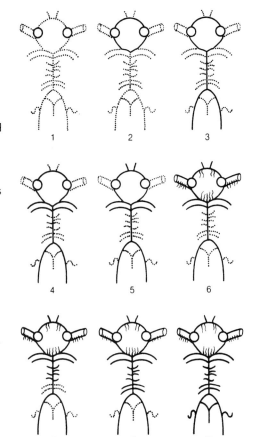

Major arteries   Cranial nerves

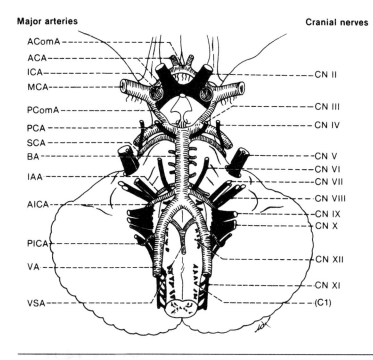

FIGURE 15-9. Ventral aspect of the brain stem and cerebrum with the arteries in place. *ACA* = anterior cerebral artery; *AICA* = anterior inferior cerebellar artery; *AComA* = anterior communicating artery; *BA* = basilar artery; *IAA* = internal auditory artery; *ICA* = internal carotid artery; *MCA* = middle cerebral artery; *PCA* = posterior cerebral artery; *PICA* = posterior inferior cerebellar artery; *PComA* = posterior communicating artery; *SCA* = superior cerebellar artery; *VA* = vertebral artery; *VSA* = ventral spinal artery.

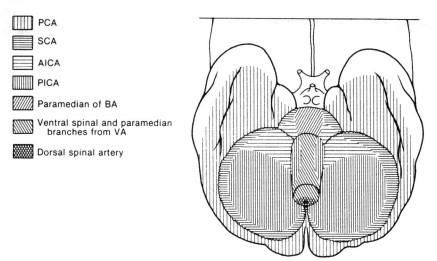

FIGURE 15-10. Ventral view of the brain stem and cerebellum showing the surface distribution of the vertebrobasilar arteries (posterior circulation).

      b. One short circumferential artery, the internal auditory artery (IAA)
      c. Three named long circumferential arteries:
          (1) Anterior inferior cerebellar artery (AICA)
          (2) Superior cerebellar artery (SCA)
          (3) Posterior cerebral artery (PCA)

    3. Embryologically, the PCA arises from the PComA. Thus, the segment that connects the BA and PCA is the true "communicating" branch. Some authors call this segment the **basilar communicating artery** or **mesencephalic artery** to acknowledge this fact (see Figure 15-19).

    4. Superficial and deep distributions of the vertebrobasilar system are illustrated in Figures 15-10, 15-11, and 15-12.

FIGURE 15-11. Sagittal view of the brain stem and cerebellum showing the distribution of the vertebrobasilar arteries (posterior circulation).

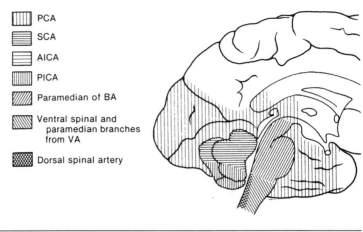

PCA

SCA

AICA

PICA

Paramedian of BA

Ventral spinal and paramedian branches from VA

Dorsal spinal artery

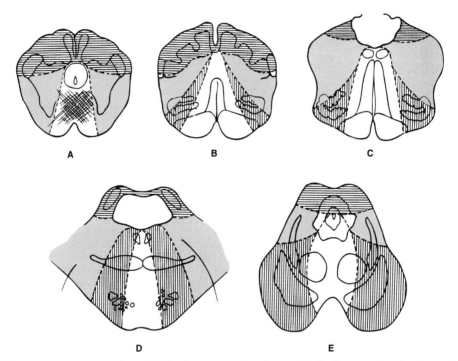

A B C

D E

FIGURE 15-12. Transverse sections of the brain stem showing the arterial distributions. See also Figure 15-2A and B. (*A*) Medullocervical junction. (*B*) Medulla oblongata, caudal level. (*C*) Medulla oblongata, middle level. (*D*) Pons. (*E*) Midbrain. *White area* indicates paramedian vessels; *vertical lines* indicate short circumferential vessels, intermediate group; *shaded area* indicates short circumferential vessels, lateral group; *horizontal lines* indicate long circumferential vessels, or in the caudal part of the medulla, dorsal spinal arteries.

E. **External and surface distribution of the internal carotid system (anterior circulation)**

1. **Cavernous and parasellar segment of the ICA.** After penetrating the foramen lacerum, the ICA enters the cavernous sinus by piercing the dural layer that forms one wall of the sinus.
   a. Traversing the split in the dura, which is the cavernous sinus, the ICA folds itself into an S-shaped carotid siphon.
   b. Piercing the dura again, the ICA emerges into the vallecular region of the subarachnoid space, where it gives off several important branches (Figure 15-13).
2. **Terminal branches of the ICA.** After entering at the vallecula, the ICA divides into two major terminal arteries: the middle cerebral artery (MCA) and the ACA,

which, along with the PCA, irrigate the cerebrum (Figure 15-14). Thus, both the cerebrum and cerebellum receive three large, long circumferential arteries— the ACA, MCA, and PCA for the cerebrum and the SCA, AICA, and PICA for the cerebellum.

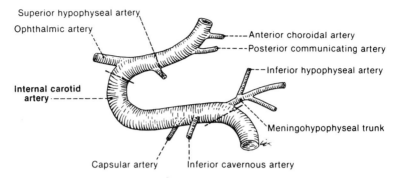

FIGURE 15-13. Lateral view of the left carotid artery at the siphon or parasellar region. The lower interrupted line is where the carotid artery enters the cavernous sinus and the upper interrupted line where it exits.

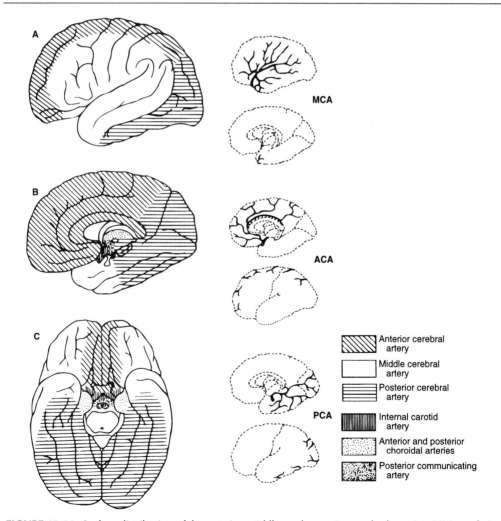

FIGURE 15-14. Surface distribution of the anterior, middle, and posterior cerebral arteries. (A) Lateral view of the left cerebral hemisphere. (B) Medial view of the left cerebral hemisphere. (C) Ventral view of the cerebrum. *ACA* = anterior cerebral artery; *MCA* = middle cerebral artery; *PCA* = posterior cerebral artery.

3. **Surface distribution of the ACA, MCA, and PICA** (see Figure 15-14)
   a. To remember the distribution of the three cerebral arteries, you need to learn only one—the MCA. Clasp your head between your hands with your fingers pointing backward: your hand exactly covers the distribution of the MCA. Notice that the curve of your thenar eminence covers the temporal pole (Figure 15-15).
   b. The three poles of the cerebrum receive blood from one of the three cerebral arteries—the **frontal (anterior) pole** from the ACA, the **occipital (posterior) pole** from the PCA, and the **temporal (middle) pole** from the MCA.
   c. Notice that **medially** the ACA and PCA meet slightly anterior to the parieto-occipital sulcus (see Figures 15-14B and 15-15B).
   d. Notice that **laterally** the junction of the ACA and MCA delineate a semicircular "basket handle" arc (see Figures 15-14A and 15-15A).
   e. Junction zones between arterial territories are sites of "watershed" infarcts that occur in hypotension and anoxia.

F. **Internal distribution of the cerebral arteries** (Figure 15-16)

1. **Paramedian and striate arteries**
   a. From the anterior spinal and vertebral arteries up through the ACAs to their AComA, the ventral arterial trunk gives off numerous small, unnamed penetrating vessels to the paramedian zone of neural tissue.
   b. In three regions—**medial, lateral,** and **posterior**—these paramedian vessels form tufts or leashes of numerous fine branches, called **striate arteries,** from their resemblance to the striations of a comb.
   c. The **medial striate arteries** arise from the ACA and perforate the medial part of the basal forebrain. The medial-most of the striate arteries and often the largest, the **recurrent artery of Heubner,** irrigates the basal third of the caudate nucleus. It may reach the anterior limb or genu of the internal capsule (Figures 15-17 and 15-18).
   d. The **lateral striate arteries** arise from the MCA.
      (1) They enter the basal forebrain by perforating the **anterior perforated substance,** which forms the roof of the vallecula. They irrigate the superior two-thirds of the caudate nucleus and the putamen and arch through them to reach the superior part of the internal capsule (see Figure 15-18B).
      (2) Because they irrigate the lentiform nucleus, they are often called **lenticulo-striate arteries** (see Figure 15-18B).
   e. The **posterior striate arteries** arise from PCA (see Figure 15-17).

2. Learn the arterial supply of the internal capsule from Figure 15-18.

3. Learn the arterial supply of the thalamus from Figure 15-19.

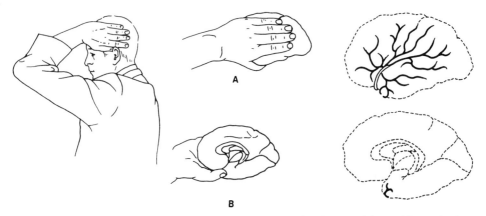

FIGURE 15-15. A "handy" method for remembering the surface distribution of the middle cerebral artery and, therefore, all three major cerebral arteries (i.e., place your palms on the sides of your head with your fingers and thumbs in a horizontal position). (A) Lateral aspect of the left cerebral hemisphere. (B) Medial aspect of the right cerebral hemisphere.

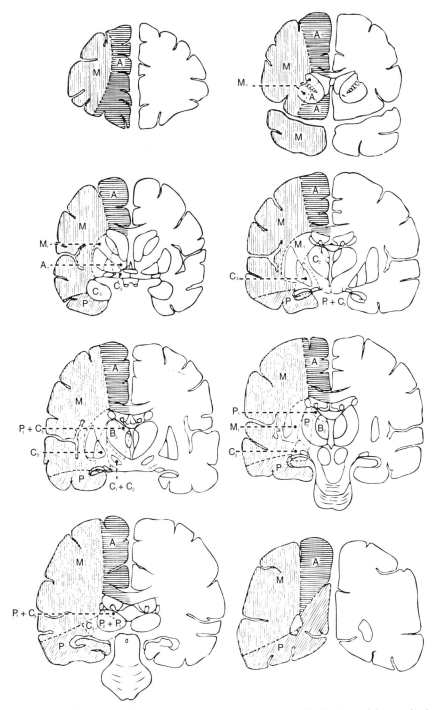

FIGURE 15-16. Coronal sections of the cerebrum showing the internal distributions of the cerebral arteries. *A* = anterior cerebral artery; *A₁* = medial striate arteries; *B* = basilar communicating artery (mesencephalic artery); *B₁* = paramedian arteries; *B₂* = thalamoperforate artery; *C* = internal carotid artery; *C₁* = paramedian perforating arteries to the wall of the third ventricle, hypothalamus, and subthalamus (ventral diencephalon); *C₂* = posterior communicating artery, including the thalamotuberal artery; *C₃* = anterior choroidal artery; *M* = middle cerebral artery; *M₁* = lateral striate arteries (lenticulostriate arteries); *P* = posterior cerebral artery (proper); *P₁* = posterior choroidal artery; *P₂* = thalamogeniculate artery.

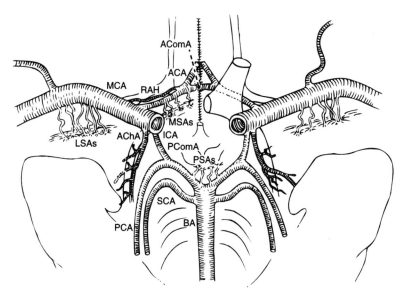

FIGURE 15-17. Ventral view of the circle of Willis showing the medial, lateral, and posterior perforating groups of arteries. *ACA* = anterior cerebral arteries; *AChA* = anterior choroidal artery; *AComA* = anterior communicating artery; *BA* = basilar artery; *ICA* = internal carotid artery; *LSAs* = lateral striate arteries; *MCA* = middle cerebral artery; *MSAs* = medial striate arteries; *PCA* = posterior cerebral artery; *PComA* = posterior communicating artery; *PSAs* = posterior striate arteries; *RAH* = recurrent artery of Heubner; *SCA* = superior cerebellar artery.

IV. VENOUS DRAINAGE OF THE BRAIN

A. Basic plan

1. The veins of the brain, unlike those of other organs, run their courses independent of the arteries. Unlike arteries, they anastomose freely, forming four interconnected systems: the **intra-axial veins**, the **superficial** and **deep venous systems**, and the **venous sinuses**.

2. The first system of venules and veins, the **intra-axial veins proper**, collect capillary blood and drain into a series of veins mostly on the external surface of the brain, called the **superficial** and **deep venous systems**. The superficial and deep systems empty into the **intradural sinuses**, which ultimately empty into the extracranial veins.

B. Intradural venous sinuses

1. The layers of the dura split to create endothelium-lined venous channels called **sinuses** (Table 15-1; Figures 15-20 and 15-21).

2. The venous sinuses empty into extracranial veins by means of several emissary veins that exit through foramina in the calvaria or the base of the skull.

3. The most important and the largest such vein, the **internal jugular vein**, exits through the jugular foramen as a continuation of the sigmoid sinus. The jugular vein travels through the neck in a sheath with the ICA and the vagus nerve.

C. Superficial cerebral veins (Table 15-2; see Figure 15-20)

1. The **lateral** and **medial superior superficial veins** drain into the superior sagittal sinus, which drains mainly into the right transverse dural sinus and right jugular vein.

2. The **inferior lateral superficial veins** drain into the superior petrosal and transverse sinuses, which ultimately drain into the jugular vein.

3. Major anastomoses of the superficial cerebral veins on facies lateralis of a cerebral hemisphere include:
  a. Anastomosis of the veins of Trolard and Labbé with each other [the vein of Trolard then empties into the superior sagittal sinus, and the vein of Labbé empties into the transverse sinus (see Figure 15-20)]
  b. Anastomosis of the vein of Trolard and Labbé with the middle cerebral (sylvian) veins
4. The superficial middle cerebral veins reach the cavernous sinuses via the sphenoparietal sinuses or via the superior petrosal sinuses.

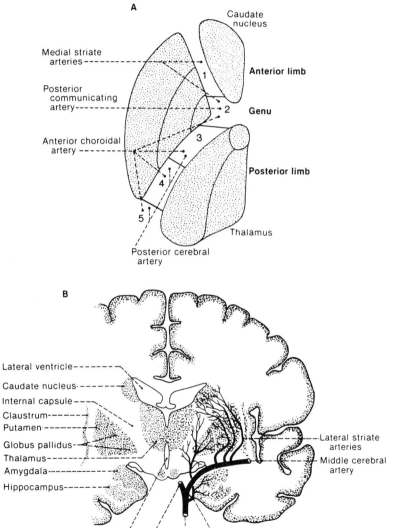

FIGURE 15-18. Arterial irrigation areas of the superior and inferior levels of the internal capsule. (*A*) Horizontal section of the inferior level of the internal capsule showing the areas irrigated by different arteries. *1* = anterior limb; *2* = genu; *3* = anterior part of posterior limb; *4* = posterior part of posterior limb; *5* = retrolenticular part. (*B*) Coronal section of the internal capsule through the genu. The superior part of the entire capsule receives blood only from the arcades of lateral striate (lenticulostriate) arteries. At the coronal level shown, the anterior choroidal artery supplies the inferior part of the internal capsule and the medial part of the globus pallidus. It may also send a small branch into the ventrolateral aspect of the thalamus, but the lateral striate arteries do not supply the thalamus.

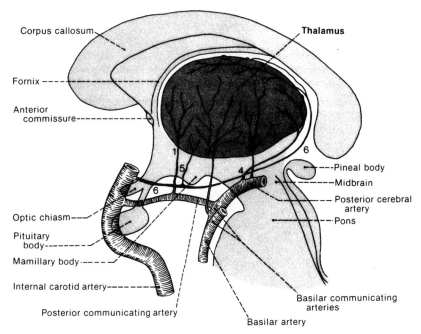

FIGURE 15-19. Sagittal section of the cerebrum showing the distribution of the thalamic arteries and their origins from the internal carotid, posterior communicating, and posterior cerebral arteries. *1* = thalamotuberal (premamillary) artery; *2* = thalamoperforant (postmamillary) artery; *3* = thalamogeniculate artery; *4* = posterior choroidal artery; *5* = lateroventral artery; *6* = anterior choroidal artery. (Adapted with permission from Plets C, et al: The vascularization of the human thalamus. *Acta Neurol Belg* 70·687–770, 1970).

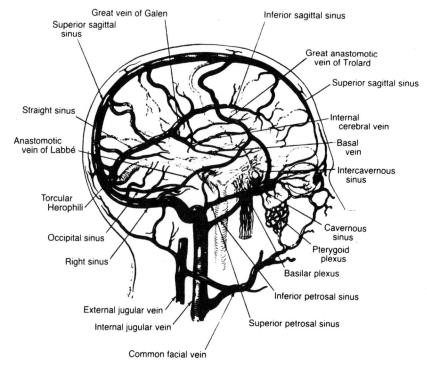

FIGURE 15-20. Lateral perspective view of the dural sinuses. (Reprinted with permission from Shenkin HA: Dynamic anatomy of cerebral circulation. *Arch Neur Psychiatry* 60:245, 1948. Original drawing by Ralph Sweet).

TABLE 15-1. Intradural Venous Sinuses

Sinus	Location	Receives	Empties Into
Superior longitudinal (sagittal) sinus	Falx, attached margin	Superior superficial cerebral veins from upper part of facies medialis and facies lateralis	Transverse sinus, mainly the right
Inferior longitudinal (sagittal) sinus	Falx, free margin	Superficial cerebral veins from inferior part of facies medialis (excepting inferior frontal lobe) and from corpus callosum	Sinus rectus
Straight sinus (sinus rectus)	Junction of falx with tentorium	Inferior longitudinal sinus and great vein of Galen	Transverse sinus, mainly the left
Transverse sinus	Margin of tentorium attached to occipital bone	Superior longitudinal sinus, straight sinus, superior petrosal sinus	Sigmoid sinus
Sigmoid sinus	Between transverse sinus and jugular vein	Transverse sinus and inferior petrosal sinus	Jugular bulb and vein
Cavernous sinus	Parasellar area	Ophthalmic vein and sphenoparietal sinus	Superior and inferior petrosal sinuses and numerous emissary veins into nasopharynx; circular (intercavernous) sinuses connect the two cavernous sinuses
Superior petrosal sinus	Margin of tentorium attached to petrous ridge of temporal bone	Cavernous sinus, superficial middle cerebral vein, adjacent temporal lobe, superior cerebellar veins	Transverse sinus
Inferior petrosal sinus	Line of petro-occipital suture	Inferior cerebellar veins, medulla, pons, middle ear	Jugular bulb

FIGURE 15-21. Deep cerebral venous system. (*A*) Sagittal section, medial aspect of the right cerebral hemisphere, showing the deep cerebral venous system. (*B*) Dorsal view of the deep venous system, in relation to the cerebral ventricles (*interrupted lines*). *1* = septal vein; *2,3* = thalamostriate branches; *4* = terminal vein; *5* = internal cerebral vein; *6* = anterior perforating veins; *7* = posterior perforating veins; *8* = basal vein of Rosenthal; *9* = vein of Galen; *10* = straight sinus; *11* = superior sagittal sinus; *12* = inferior sagittal sinus; *13* = choroid vein; *14* = confluent sinus

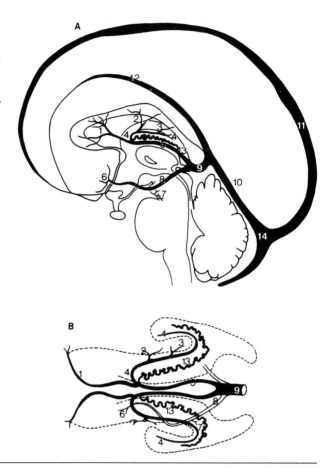

TABLE 15-2. Drainage of Cerebral Veins

Brain Region Drained	Sinus Outlet
Superficial cerebral veins	
Superior	
Upper part of facies medialis and facies lateralis	Superior longitudinal sinus
Inferior	
Facies inferior and lower part of facies lateralis and facies medialis	Superior petrosal and transverse sinuses; some superficial posterior cerebral veins enter the vein of Galen
Deep cerebral veins	
Galenic system	
Corpus striatum, dorsal thalamus, periventricular white matter, choroid plexus	Sinus rectus
Miscellaneous basal veins	
Ventral thalamus, midbrain, pons, medulla	Through galenic system to sinus rectus or basal channels

5. The superficial middle cerebral vein joins the deep middle cerebral vein, which drains the insular and opercular regions. It joins the basal vein of Rosenthal of the deep venous system (see IV D 1).

6. The numerous anastomoses of the superficial and deep systems and the sinuses allow quick shifts of blood in response to changes in intracranial pressure; such

changes may be related to intrathoracic pressure reflected via the jugular system or to intrinsic intracranial lesions.

Deep cerebral veins: the galenic system (see Table 15-2 and Figure 15-21)

1. The major tributaries of the vein of Galen are the **basal vein of Rosenthal** and the **internal cerebral vein**.
   a. The basal vein commences at the vallecula with the union of the anterior internal frontal vein, striate veins, and deep middle cerebral vein. After collecting blood from the insular region and basal forebrain, the basal vein circles the midbrain.
   b. The basal vein then joins the **internal cerebral vein** to form the **great vein of Galen**.

2. The resultant galenic vein joins the inferior sagittal sinus and then enters the **straight sinus**, which mainly empties into the left transverse sinus (see Figure 15-20).

V. CLINICAL CORRELATIONS WITH VASCULAR ANATOMY. Major forms of cerebrovascular disease are infarction and hemorrhage.

Infarction

1. Occlusion, or narrowing, of arteries leads to infarction of the territory supplied by the artery. The arterial territories are relatively constant, and the arteries act as end-arteries, with relatively little anastomosis between territories. Thus, the clinical syndromes of infarction are fairly reproducible.

2. Infarction in the **MCA distribution** leads to contralateral hemiplegia and hemisensory loss, with aphasia if it affects the left hemisphere, or loss of left-sided spatial awareness if it affects the right hemisphere.

3. Infarction in the **ACA distribution** may cause contralateral monoplegia of the leg because the ACA irrigates the "leg area" on the medial hemispheric wall. (Compare Figure 15-14 with Figures 13-36 and 13-37.)

4. Infarction in the **internal capsule** may cause contralateral motor or sensory loss, or both (see Figure 15-18).

5. Infarction in the **vertebrobasilar distributions** in the brain stem leads to alternating signs, consisting of a cranial nerve palsy on the side of the infarct and contralateral hemiparesis or sensory loss (see Figure 7-41C). Infarction of the vertebrobasilar branches to the cerebellum, namely the SCAs or PICAs, results in ipsilateral ataxia (see Figures 10-12 and 10-13).

6. **Junction zone infarcts**, inaptly called "watershed" infarcts, occur along the junction zones of major vessels if the systemic blood pressure drops or if the patient suffers anoxia.
   a. These junction zones are farthest from the origins of the vessels and have the most precarious lifeline of blood.
   b. Junction zone infarctions commonly affect the "basket handle" arc at the junction of the ACA and MCA (see Figure 15-14).

7. **Transient ischemic attacks** may affect the distributional areas of given arteries, causing transient signs of dysfunction of the ischemic neural tissue. Transient ischemic attacks in the BA distribution cause cranial nerve and long tract signs often accompanied by transient vertigo, diplopia, and loss of consciousness.

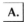

Intracranial hemorrhage (subarachnoid or intracerebral)

1. Intracranial hemorrhage, either intracerebral or extracerebral, results from rupture of an artery, vein, or an aneurysm.

2. **Intracerebral hemorrhage**
   a. Although any cerebral vessel may bleed, the lenticulostriate arteries constitute the site of predilection for hypertensive intracerebral hemorrhage.

   b. The blood may dissect through the basal ganglia to enter the ventricles. Massive intraventricular hemorrhage threatens life.

   c. In newborn infants, particularly premature infants, intraventricular hemorrhage usually occurs from rupture in the periventricular tributaries of the internal cerebral veins. The infants usually survive but may suffer neurologic complications such as hydrocephalus, cerebral palsy, and mental retardation.

3. Arterial aneurysms

   a. Aneurysms occur most frequently where the arteries of the circle of Willis branch.

   b. The aneurysm may act as a mass, compressing cranial nerves, brain tissue, the optic chiasm, or the pituitary gland. Commonly, aneurysms of the PCA or ICA compress cranial nerve (CN) III.

   c. If the aneurysm bursts, it causes subarachnoid hemorrhage or, less frequently, intracerebral or intraventricular hemorrhage.

4. Arteriovenous malformations

   a. Errors in the development of the vascular channels may leave abnormal tangles of vessels in various regions of the CNS.

   b. In the cerebrum, such lesions frequently cause seizures. They may act as arteriovenous shunts that rob the normal vessels of blood, causing ischemia of the rest of the brain.

   c. Arteriovenous malformations that empty into the galenic system may cause an aneurysmal dilation of the vein of Galen. Such a dilation may cause an output type of cardiac failure in an infant because of the large amount of blood shunted into the dilated vein.

STUDY QUESTIONS

DIRECTIONS: Each of the numbered items or incomplete statements in this section is negatively phrased, as indicated by a capitalized word such as NOT, LEAST, or EXCEPT. Select the ONE lettered answer or completion that is BEST in each case.

1. All of the following generalizations about the central nervous system (CNS) blood supply are false EXCEPT

(A) the blood vessels penetrate the CNS from the pial surface
(B) the terminal arterial distributions tend to have irregular, overlapping margins
(C) the longest brain arteries irrigate the paramedian zone of the brain
(D) the branching pattern of the major veins closely matches the branching pattern of the major arteries
(E) the thalamus receives its blood supply from the lateral striate arteries

2. Which of the following statements about the basilar artery (BA) is NOT true?

(A) It is formed by the union of the vertebral arteries (VAs)
(B) It commences at the level of the pontomedullary junction
(C) It extends from the midbrain forward to irrigate the optic nerves
(D) It terminates by bifurcating into the posterior cerebral arteries (PCAs)
(E) It sends numerous paramedian branches into the brain stem

3. All of the branches or connections listed for the following major vessels are correct EXCEPT

(A) anterior cerebral artery (ACA)/Heubner's artery of medial striate group
(B) middle cerebral artery (MCA)/lateral striate arteries
(C) galenic vein/inferior longitudinal (sagittal) sinus
(D) basilar artery (BA)/posterior inferior cerebellar artery (PICA)
(E) carotid artery/MCA

4. All of the following vessels are part of the circle of Willis EXCEPT the

(A) anterior communicating artery (AComA)
(B) posterior communicating artery (PComA)
(C) connection of the posterior cerebral arteries (PCA) with the basilar artery (BA)
(D) anterior cerebral artery (ACA)
(E) lateral striate arteries

DIRECTIONS: Each set of matching questions in this section consists of a list of four to twenty-six lettered options (some of which may be in figures) followed by several numbered items. For each numbered item, select the ONE lettered option that is most closely associated with it. To avoid spending too much time on matching sets with large numbers of options, it is generally advisable to begin each set by reading the list of options. Then, for each item in the set, try to generate the correct answer and locate it in the option list, rather than evaluating each option individually. Each lettered option may be selected once, more than once, or not at all.

Questions 5–10

For each clinical deficit, select the artery that would be most likely to cause it if occluded.

(A) Branch of basilar artery (BA)
(B) Posterior cerebral artery (PCA)
(C) Lateral striate arteries
(D) Posterior inferior cerebellar artery (PICA)
(E) Anterior cerebral artery (ACA)

5. Contralateral monoplegia of the leg

6. Contralateral hemiplegia and hemisensory loss

7. Contralateral hemianopia

8. Contralateral loss of pain and temperature and ipsilateral ataxia and Horner's syndrome

9. Medial longitudinal fasciculus (MLF) syndrome

10. Ipsilateral palsy of cranial nerve (CN) VI and contralateral hemiplegia

DIRECTIONS: Each set of matching questions in this section consists of a list of four to twenty-six lettered options followed by several numbered items. For each numbered item, select the appropriate lettered option(s). Each lettered option may be selected once, more than once, or not at all. EACH ITEM WILL STATE THE NUMBER OF OPTIONS TO SELECT. CHOOSE EXACTLY THIS NUMBER.

Questions 11–13

(A) Ventral spinal artery
(B) Vertebral artery
(C) Basilar artery (BA) per se (not the so-called basilar communicating or mesencephalic artery at the basilar tip)
(D) Posterior inferior cerebellar artery (PICA)
(E) Internal auditory artery (IAA)
(F) Superior cerebellar artery (SCA)
(G) Posterior cerebral artery (PCA)
(H) Posterior communicating artery (PComA)
(I) Internal carotid artery (ICA)
(J) Middle cerebral artery (MCA)
(K) Anterior cerebral artery (ACA)
(L) Anterior communicating artery (AComA)
(M) Anterior choroidal artery

For each of the following descriptions, select the relevant artery or arteries.

11. Arteries that directly irrigate the thalamus (SELECT 3 ARTERIES)

12. Arteries classified as long circumferential arteries (SELECT 5 ARTERIES)

13. Arteries that irrigate the poles of the cerebrum (SELECT 3 ARTERIES)

ANSWERS AND EXPLANATIONS

1. The answer is A [I A 1; V A 1]. The cerebral blood vessels penetrate the central nervous system (CNS) from the pial surface. The terminal distributions are regular in most patients, and infarcts due to occlusion of the major vessels have predictable distributions. The longest brain arteries are the long circumferential vessels.

2. The answer is C [III D 2; Figure 15-9]. The basilar artery (BA) commences with the union of the vertebral arteries (VAs) at the pontomedullary junction. It extends essentially the length of the pons, bifurcating into the posterior cerebral arteries (PCAs) at the interpeduncular fossa at the ponto-mesencephalic junction. Thus, it does not extend to the optic chiasm or nerves.

3. The answer is D [III D 1 c, 2 c]. The posterior inferior cerebellar arteries (PICAs) are usually branches of the vertebral artery (VA). The basilar artery (BA) gives rise to the posterior cerebral arteries (PCAs), the superior cerebellar arteries (SCAs), and the anterior inferior cerebellar arteries (AICAs). These are all long circumferential arteries.

4. The answer is E [III C 2; Figure 15-17]. The circle of Willis is an anastomotic circle connecting the large arteries at the base of the forebrain and midbrain. The circle commences when the anterior cerebral arteries (ACAs) and posterior communicating arteries (PComA) branch off of the internal carotid artery (ICA) at the vallecula of the sylvian fissure. The anterior communicating artery (AComA) completes the circle anteriorly, and the posterior cerebral arteries (PCAs) complete the circle posteriorly, communicating with the basilar artery (BA). The lateral striate arteries, which come from the middle cerebral arteries (MCAs), arise from the MCA distal to the circle of Willis and do not belong to it.

5–10. The answers are: 5-E, 6-C, 7-B, 8-D, 9-A, 10-A [V A]. Infarction in the distributions of the cerebral arteries produces characteristic clinical syndromes. Occlusion of the anterior cerebral artery (ACA) may cause a contralateral monoplegia of the leg because it supplies the "leg area" of the motor strip.

Occlusion of the middle cerebral artery (MCA) or lateral striate arteries generally gives rise to contralateral hemiplegia and hemisen-

sory loss, because of involvement of the pre- and postcentral gyri or the internal capsule. Extensive infarcts of the MCA distribution in the left hemisphere will also cause aphasia. When infarcts affect the right cerebral hemisphere, they may cause disturbances in the awareness of the left half of space.

Occlusion of the posterior inferior cerebellar artery (PICA) typically gives rise to ipsilateral ataxia and contralateral loss of pain and temperature. Infarction of the cerebellar hemisphere causes ataxia. Horner's syndrome is the result of interruption of descending sympathetic fibers in the dorsolateral part of the medulla, an area supplied by the PICA. That artery also supplies the lateral medullary region dorsolateral to the olivary nucleus, which conveys the pain and temperature fibers from the contralateral side of the body. Because of involvement of the descending root of cranial nerve (CN) V, the patient may also lose the corneal reflex and pain and temperature sensations over the ipsilateral side of the face. Involvement of the nucleus ambiguus or its axons, which enter CN IX and CN X, may cause paralysis of the pharyngeal and laryngeal muscles, resulting in dysarthria and dysphagia.

Occlusion of the basilar artery (BA) itself generally causes quadriplegia and loss of consciousness, because of involvement of the basis of the brain stem and the tegmentum of the midbrain or rostral pons. An infarct in the BA distribution in the basis pontis interrupts the pyramidal tracts bilaterally and causes the locked-in syndrome. If the lesion affects the pyramidal tract at the caudal end of the pons, it may also involve the CN VI fibers that run through the paramedian pontine region at that level. The patient then has an ipsilateral CN VI palsy and contralateral hemiplegia.

Restricted occlusion of the paramedian branches of the BA may cause a characteristic syndrome of contralateral hemiplegia with ipsilateral CN III palsy when the lesion affects the midbrain level. A similar lesion in the pontine tegmentum may cause the medial longitudinal fasciculus (MLF) syndrome. Occlusion of one posterior cerebral artery (PCA) results in occipital lobe infarction, causing contralateral hemianopia or complete blindness (double hemianopia) if both occipital lobes undergo infarction.

11. The answers are: G, H, M [Figure 15-19]. The thalamus receives its arterial supply from the anterior choroidal artery [a branch of the

internal carotid artery (ICA)]; the thalamotuberal artery [a branch of the posterior communicating artery (PComA)]; the thalamoperforant arteries (branches of the basilar
communicating artery); and the thalamogeniculate artery and posterior choroidal arteries
[branches of the posterior cerebral arteries
(PCA)]. Infarctions may occur in each of these
thalamic artery territories and cause different
clinical syndromes, depending on the thalamic nucleus affected. Bithalamic infarction
leads to obtundation or coma and dementia.

12. The answers are: D, F, G, J, K [I B 2; III D
2 c, E 2, 3; Figure 15-2]. The arteries of the
central nervous system (CNS) fall into three
patterns of distribution: paramedian, short circumferential, and long circumferential. All of
the long circumferential arteries start at the
base of the brain and give off penetrating
branches as they encircle the brain stem or
base of the brain. They then reach the surface
of the cerebrum and cerebellum and penetrate
from the surface to irrigate the cortex and
deep white matter.

13. The answers are: G, J, K [Figure 15-14].
Each of the long circumferential arteries of the
cerebrum irrigates one of the poles. The anterior cerebral artery (ACA) irrigates the anterior
pole, the posterior cerebral artery (PCA) irrigates the posterior pole, and the middle cerebral artery (MCA) irrigates the middle or temporal pole. Each artery irrigates other regions
on the lateral, medial, or ventral aspects of the
cerebrum.

Appendix

Standard Complete Neurologic Examination

I. INTRODUCTION TO THE NEUROLOGIC EXAMINATION

A. Detecting the neurologic manifestations of disease

1. Disease may cause changes in the mental, motor, or sensory functions of the patient.
2. The clinical neurologic examination consists of a systematic series of observations, questions, commands, and maneuvers designed to detect mental, motor, and sensory dysfunction.
3. The steps chosen for the neurologic examination, by deliberate design, test the functional circuits of the nervous system as known from the scientific study of neuroanatomy and neurophysiology.

B. The medical history

1. During the history, the clinician completes much of the neurologic examination by inspecting the patient's eyes, face, body movements, and body postures, and judging speech production. Most of the information for judging the patient's mental status also comes from the history.
2. The history and these preliminary observations determine the extent and content of the examination required for the specific patient.
3. In planning the examination for each patient, the clinician inquires specifically about actions or maneuvers that the patient suspects of triggering his or her symptoms. The clinician then reproduces these actions and performs any necessary tests.
   a. If the patient reports dizziness when standing up from a reclining position, ask the patient to move from a reclining to a standing position and then test for a drop in blood pressure (orthostatic hypotension).
   b. If the patient reports difficulty when climbing stairs, watch the patient climb stairs.

C. Equipment required for the neurologic examination (Table A-1)

II. MENTAL STATUS EXAMINATION

A. **General behavior and appearances.** Does the patient appear normal, agitated, hyperactive, or hypoactive? Note whether the patient dresses appropriately for his or her age, gender, peers, and social background.

B. **Stream of talk.** Does the patient converse normally? If not, describe the speech as rapid, incessant, and pressured, or as slow and lacking spontaneity.

C. **Mood and affective responses.** Does the patient's mood appropriately match the emotional implications of the conversation? Does the patient appear euphoric, manic, angry, inappropriately gay and giggling, or silent and weeping? Is the patient emotionally labile, histrionic, expansive, or overtly depressed?

D. **Content of thought.** Does the patient have illusions, hallucinations, delusions, misinterpretations, or obsessions? Is the patient preoccupied with bodily complaints, fears of

The appendix has been adapted with permission from the "Summarized Neurologic Examination" that appears in *Technique of the Neurologic Examination, A Programmed Text,* 4th ed. by William DeMyer, New York, McGraw-Hill, 1994.

TABLE A-1. Equipment Required for the Neurologic Examination

Instrument	Use
1. Flexible steel measuring tape scored in the metric system	Measuring occipitofrontal and other body circumferences, size of skin lesions, length of extremities, etc.
2. Stethoscope	Auscultation of the neck vessels, eyes, and cranium for bruits
3. Flashlight with rubber adapter	Checking pupillary reflexes; inspection of pharynx, and transillumination of the heads of infants
4. Transparent mm ruler	Measuring pupillary size, diameter of skin lesions, and distances on radiographic films
5. Ophthalmoscope	Funduscopy; examination of ocular media and skin surface for beads of sweat
6. Tongue blades (three per patient)	One for depressing tongue, one for eliciting gag reflex, and one (broken) for eliciting abdominal and plantar reflexes
7. Opaque vial of coffee	Testing sense of smell
8. Opaque vials of salt and sugar	Testing sense of taste
9. Tuning fork	Testing vibratory sensation and hearing (256 cps recommended)
10. Otoscope	Examination of auditory canal and drum
11. 10-cc syringe	Caloric irrigation of the ear
12. Cotton wisp	One end rolled for eliciting corneal reflex; the other loose for testing light touch
13. Reflex hammer	Eliciting muscle stretch reflexes; muscle percussion for myotonia
14. Two stoppered tubes	Testing hot and cold discrimination
15. Disposable straight pins	Testing pain sensation
16. Penny, nickel, dime, paper clip, and key	Testing stereognosis
17. Page of stimulus figures (Halstead-Reitan screening test) and table of examiner's instructions and patient's tasks	Screening for cerebral dysfunctions
18. Blood pressure cuff	Checking blood pressure and orthostatic hypotension

cancer or heart disease, or other phobias? Does the patient display delusions of persecution, surveillance, and control by malicious organizations or forces?

E. **Intellectual capacity.** Is the patient bright, average, dull or overtly retarded, or demented?

F. **Sensorium.** Assess:

1. Consciousness

2. Attention span

3. Orientation to time, person, and place

4. Memory (recent and remote)

5. Calculation ability

6. Fund of information

7. Insight, judgment, and planning

III. **SPEECH.** Is the patient's speech normal or does the patient display:

A. **Dysphonia**, difficulty in producing the voice sounds

B. **Dysarthria**, difficulty in articulating the individual sounds or the units (phonemes) of speech: f's, r's, g's, vowels, consonants, the labials [cranial nerve (CN) VII], gutterals (CN X), and linguals (CN XII)

C. **Dysprosody**, difficulty with the melody and rhythm of speech, the accent of syllables, inflections, pitch of voice, and intonations

D. **Dysphasia**, difficulty in expressing or understanding words as the symbols of communication

IV. **HEAD AND FACE**

A. **Inspection**

1. Inspect the patient's facial features to get a general impression. Look for a diagnostic facial gestalt or abnormal motility and emotional expression.

2. Inspect the head for abnormalities in shape and asymmetry.

3. Inspect the hair of the scalp, eyebrows, and beard.

4. Inspect the eyes for ptosis, width of palpebral fissures, relation of the iris to the lids, pupillary size, and interorbital distance.

5. Inspect the contours and proportions of the nose, mouth, chin, and ears for malformations.

B. **Palpate** the skull of a mature patient for lumps, depressions or tenderness, and asymmetries. In infants, palpate the skull for fontanelles and sutures. Measure and record the occipitofrontal circumference of all infants.

C. **Percuss** over the sinuses and mastoid processes for tenderness if the patient has headaches.

D. **Auscultate** for bruits over the neck, vessels, eyes, temples, and mastoid processes.

E. **Transilluminate** the sinuses if the patient has headaches. Attempt to transilluminate the head of young infants.

V. **CRANIAL NERVES**

A. **Optic group** (CN II, CN III, CN IV, and CN VI)

1. Inspect the width of the palpebral fissures, the relation of the limbus to the lid margins, the interorbital distance, and look for en- or exophthalmos.

2. Test visual acuity (central fields) by newsprint or Snellen chart (each eye separately) and test peripheral fields by confrontation. Test for inattention to simultaneous visual stimuli if a cerebral lesion is suspected.

3. Test pupillary light reflexes and record the size of the pupils.

4. Do ophthalmoscopy.

5. Test ocular motility.
   a. Test the range of ocular movements by having the patient's eyes follow your finger through all fields of gaze.
   b. During convergence, check for miosis.
   c. Do the cover-uncover test for ocular malalignment.
   d. Record nystagmus and any effects of eye movements on it.

B. **Branchiomotor group and tongue** (CN V, CN VII, CN IX, CN X, CN XI, and CN XII)

1. CN V. Inspect masseter and temporalis muscle bulk, and palpate masseters when the patient bites.

2. CN VII. Test forehead wrinkling, eyelid closure, mouth retraction, whistling or puffing out of the cheeks, and wrinkling of the skin over the neck (platysma action). Listen to labial articulations, and check for Chvostek's sign in selected cases.

3. CN IX and CN X. Listen for phonation and articulation (labial, lingual, and palatal sounds), and check swallowing, gag reflex, and palatal elevation.

4. CN XII. Check lingual articulations and midline and lateral tongue protrusion. Inspect the tongue for atrophy and fasciculations.

5. CN XI. Inspect sternocleidomastoid and trapezius contours, and test the strength of head movements and shoulder shrugging.

6. If the history raises the question of pathologic fatigability, request 100 repetitive movements (e.g., eye blinks). Consider the Tensilon (edrophonium) test.

7. Assess the rate, regularity, and depth of breathing.

C. **Special sensory group**

1. Olfaction (CN I). Use an aromatic, nonirritating substance, and test each nostril separately.

2. Taste (CN VII). Use salt or sugar. Test especially if a CN VII lesion is suspected.

3. Hearing (CN VIII)
   a. Do otoscopy.
   b. Assess threshold and acuity by noting the patient's ability to hear conversational speech and to hear a tuning fork, a watch tick, or the rustling of fingers.
   c. If history or preceding tests suggest a deficit, do the air-bone conduction test of Rinne and the vertex lateralizing test of Weber.
   d. If the history suggests a cerebral lesion, test for auditory inattention to bilateral simultaneous stimuli using finger rustling.
   e. In infants and unconscious or uncooperative patients, try the audiopalpebral reflex as a crude screening test.

4. Vestibular function (CN VIII). In selected patients, do caloric irrigation, and test for positional nystagmus.

D. **Somatic sensation of the face**

1. Testing trigeminal area sensation now obviates a return to the face after examining the patient's anogenital area and feet.

2. To determine somatic sensation of the face, test:
   a. Corneal reflex (CN V–CN VII arc)
   b. Light touch over the three divisions of CN V
   c. Temperature discrimination over the three divisions of CN V
   d. Pain perception over the three divisions of CN V
   e. Buccal mucosal sensation in selected patients

VI. SOMATIC MOTOR SYSTEMS (excluding cranial nerves)

A. Inspection

1. **Gait testing.** Assess free walking, toe and heel walking, tandem walking, and deep knee bends. Ask a child to hop on each foot and run.

2. Inspect the patient's posture and general activity level, and look for tremors or other involuntary movement.

3. Undress the patient and assess the somatotype (i.e., the build or body gestalt).

4. Observe the size and contour of the muscles, looking for atrophy, hypertrophy, body asymmetry, joint malalignments, and fasciculations.

5. Search the entire skin surface for lesions, particularly neurocutaneous stigmata such as *café au lait* spots.

B. **Palpation.** Palate muscles if they seem atrophic, hypertrophic, or if the history suggests that they may be tender or in spasm.

C. Strength testing

1. **Shoulder girdle.** Try to press the patient's arms down after he or she abducts them to shoulder height. Look for scapular winging.

2. **Upper extremities.** Test biceps, triceps, wrist dorsiflexors, and grip. Test strength of finger abduction and extension.

3. **Abdominal muscles.** Have patient do a sit-up. Watch for umbilical migration upward (Beevor's sign).

4. **Lower extremities.** Test hip flexors, abductors, adductors, knee flexors, foot dorsiflexors, invertors, and evertors. (Knee extensors were tested by the deep knee bend and plantar flexors by toe walking.)

5. Grade strength on a scale of 0 to 5 or describe as paralysis; severe, moderate, or minimal weakness; or normal. Discern whether any weakness follows a distributional pattern such as proximal-distal, right-left, or upper extremity–lower extremity.

D. **Muscle tone assessment.** Make passive movements of joints to test for spasticity, clonus, rigidity, or hypotonus and the range of movement.

E. **Muscle stretch (deep) reflex testing.** Grade 0 to 4+ and designate whether they are clonic (Figure A-1).

1. Jaw jerk (CN V afferent; CN V efferent)

2. Biceps reflex (C5–C6)

3. Triceps reflex (C7–C8)

4. Finger flexion reflex (C7–T1)

5. Quadriceps reflex (knee jerk) [L2–L4]

6. Hamstring reflex (L5–S1)

7. Triceps surae reflex (ankle jerk) [L5–S1–S3]

8. Toe flexion reflex (S1–S2)

F. **Percussion.** Percuss the thenar eminence for percussion myotonia, and test for a myotonic grip if the patient has generalized muscular weakness.

G. Skin-muscle (superficial) reflex testing

1. Abdominal skin-muscle reflexes (upper quadrants T8–T9; lower quadrants T11–T12). Do umbilical migration test (Beevor's sign) in selected cases if a thoracic cord lesion is suspected.

FIGURE A-1. Figure for recording the results of a reflex examination. The numbers represent a normal reflex pattern.

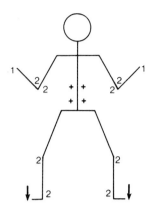

2. Cremasteric reflex (afferent L1; efferent L2)

3. Anal pucker (S4–S5) and bulbocavernosus reflexes in patients suspected of sacral and cauda equina lesions

4. Extensor toe sign or Babinski sign (afferent S1; efferent L5–S1–S2)

H. **Cerebellar system testing.** (Also see gait testing in section VI A 1 in this appendix.)

1. Finger-to-nose, overshooting and rapid alternating hand movements

2. Heel-to-knee

I. **Nerve root stretching tests.** (Do in selected patients.)

1. If disc herniation or low-back disease is suspected, do the straight-knee leg raising test (Laseague's sign) and the bent-knee leg raising test (Kernig's sign).

2. If meningeal irritation is suspected, test for nuchal rigidity and concomitant leg flexion (Brudzinski's sign), and do the straight-knee and bent-knee leg raising tests.

VII. **SOMATIC SENSORY SYSTEM**

A. **Superficial sensory modality testing.** (Include the trigeminal area if not previously tested.)

1. Light touch over hands, trunk, and feet

2. Temperature discrimination over hands, trunk, and feet

3. Pain perception over hands, trunk, and feet

B. **Deep sensory modality testing**

1. Vibration perception at knuckles, fingernails, and malleoli of ankles and toenails

2. Position sense of fingers and toes, using the fourth digits

3. Stereognosis

4. Romberg (swaying) test

5. Directional scratch test

C. **Determine the distributional pattern of any sensory loss**: dermatomal, peripheral nerve(s), central pathway, or nonorganic.

D. **Summary of dermatomal relations** (see Figure 4-12)

1. Trigeminal nerve to interaural line, where it abuts on C2 (no C1)

2. C3–C4 over "cape" area of shoulders (5-6-7-8-1 are pulled out on arms)

3. C4 abuts on T2

4. T4 is nipple level

5. T10 is umbilical level

6. L5 to big toe

7. S1 to small toe

8. S4 and S5 to the perianal zone

VIII. CEREBRAL FUNCTIONS

A. Do a complete mental status examination, emphasizing tests of the sensorium. (See section II of this appendix.)

B. If the history or mental status examination suggests a cerebral lesion, test for agraphognosia; finger agnosia; poor two-point discrimination; right-left disorientation; atopognosia; and tactile, auditory, and visual inattention to bilateral simultaneous stimuli. Test for tactile inattention to simultaneous ipsilateral stimulation of face–hand and foot–hand.

C. Have the patient do the cognitive, constructional, and performance tasks of the Halstead-Reitan screening test for cerebral dysfunction (Figure A-2 and Table A-2).

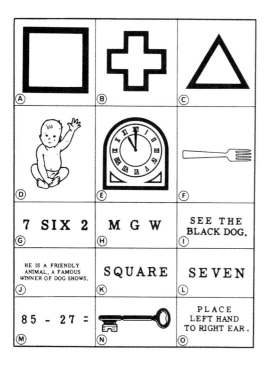

FIGURE A-2. Stimulus figures for the Halstead-Reitan cerebral function screening test.

TABLE A-2. Instructions for the Halstead-Reitan Screening Test for Cerebral Dysfunction

Patient's Task	Examiner's Instructions to the Patient
1. Copy *square* (A)	First, draw this on your paper. (Point to square, item A.) I want you to do it without lifting your pencil from the paper. Make it about the same size.
2. Name *square*	What is that shape called?
3. Spell *square*	Would you spell that word for me?
4. Copy *cross* (B)	Draw this on your paper. (Point to the cross, item B). Go around the outside like this until you get back to where you started. Make it about the same size.
5. Name *cross*	What is that shape called?
6. Spell *cross*	Would you spell that word for me?
7. Copy *triangle* (C)	Draw this on your paper. (Point to the triangle, item C.) Do it without lifting your pencil from the paper, and make it about the same size.
8. Name *triangle*	What is that shape called?
9. Spell *triangle*	Would you spell that word for me?
10. Name *baby* (D)	What is this? (Show baby, item D.)
11. Write *clock* (E)	Now, I am going to show you another picture, but do not tell me the name of it. I don't want you to say anything out loud. Just write the name of the picture on your paper. (Show clock, item E.)
12. Name *fork* (F)	What is this? (Show fork, item F.)
13. Read *7 six 2* (G)	I want you to read this. (Show item G.)
14. Read *M G W* (H)	Read this. (Show item H.)
15. Read item I	Now, I want you to read this. (Show item I.)
16. Read item J	Can you read this? (Show item J.)
17. Repeat *triangle*	Now, I am going to say some words. I want you to listen carefully and say them after me as well as you can. Say this word: *triangle.*
18. Repeat *Massachusetts*	The next one is a little harder, but do your best. Say this word: *Massachusetts.*
19. Repeat *Methodist Episcopal*	Now, repeat this phrase: *Methodist Episcopal.*
20. Write *square* (K)	Don't say this word out loud; just write it on your paper. (Point to stimulus word *square,* item K.)
21. Read *seven* (L)	Can you read this word out loud? (Show item L.)
22. Repeat *seven*	Now, I want you to repeat this after me: *seven.*
23. Repeat and explain *He shouted the warning*	I am going to say something that I want you to say after me. So listen carefully: *He shouted the warning.* Now, you say it. Would you explain what that means?
24. Write *He shouted the warning*	Now, I want you to write that sentence on the paper.
25. Compute *85 − 27* (M)	Here is an arithmetic problem. Copy it on your paper in any way you like and try to work it out. (Show item M.)
26. Compute *17 × 3*	Now, do this one in your head: *17 × 3 = ?*
27. Name *key* (N)	What is this? (Show item N.)
28. Demonstrate the use of a *key*	If you had one of these in your hand, show me how you would use it. (Show item N.)

Note: The average person with a high school education should make essentially no errors on this test and recognize immediately the impossibility of command 32. Re-test any items failed by giving tasks similar to the failed one. *continued*

TABLE A-2. Instructions for the Halstead-Reitan Screening Test for Cerebral Dysfunction

Patient's Task	Examiner's Instructions to the Patient
29. Draw *key*	Now, I want you to draw a picture that looks just like this. Try to make your key look enough like this one so that I will know it is the same key from your drawing. (Point to key, item N.)
30. Read item O	Would you read this? (Show item O.)
31. *Place left hand to right ear*	Now, would you do what it says?
32. Place left hand to left elbow	Now, I want you to place your left hand to your left elbow.

IX. CASE SUMMARY

A. Write a three-line summary of the pertinent positive historical and physical findings. (If you cannot put it in three lines, you do not understand the problem.)

B. Write down a provisional clinical diagnosis and outline the differential diagnosis.

C. Write out a list of the clinical problems.

D. Write down a sequential plan of management for:

1. Diagnostic tests to discriminate among the diagnostic possibilities

2. Therapy (state the therapeutic goals)

3. Management of the emotional, educational, and socioeconomic problems that the illness causes the patient

4. Identification of and prophylaxis for other persons now known to be "at risk" because of the patient's illness, if the illness is infectious, genetic, or environmentally induced

DIRECTIONS: Each of the numbered items or incomplete statements in this section is followed by answers or by completions of the statement. Select the ONE lettered answer or completion that is BEST in each case.

1. The level of the neuraxis that best displays the original simple, serial relationship of one spinal nerve to one dermatome is the

(A) cervical
(B) thoracic
(C) lumbar
(D) sacral
(E) coccygeal

2. Which of the following features led to the "jelly roll" hypothesis for the structure of the myelin sheath?

(A) Independence of one Schwann cell from another
(B) Indentation of the surface cytoplasm of Schwann cells by small, unmyelinated axons
(C) Encircling of axons by a lip of Schwann cell cytoplasm
(D) Enfolding of several Schwann cells by one axon
(E) Persistence of one nucleus per Schwann cell

3. Select the correct statement about the tentorium cerebelli.

(A) It is a fold of arachnoid between the cerebellar hemispheres
(B) It separates the cerebellum from the occipital lobe
(C) It is the membranous roof between the cerebellum and fourth ventricle
(D) It covers the ventral surface of the cerebellum
(E) It is composed of thin, delicate connective tissue

4. A hypertensive patient with a history of previous myocardial infarction had a sudden onset of hemiplegia, reduced touch sensation, and loss of position sense, all of which affected the left side, with bilateral preservation of pain and temperature sensation. The patient had weak muscles on the right side of the tongue but no facial weakness. The lesion, an infarct, would most likely occupy the

(A) cervicomedullary junction
(B) paramedian plane of the medulla
(C) lateral part of the pontine tegmentum
(D) dorsolateral quadrant of the medulla
(E) pontine basis

5. Destruction of the pyramidal neurons of the hippocampus (Ammon's horn) would cause severe loss of axonal projections to the

(A) nucleus ventralis lateralis of the thalamus
(B) subiculum and entorhinal cortex
(C) calcarine cortex (area 17)
(D) dorsal striatum
(E) Edinger-Westphal nucleus

6. The two cranial nerves that differ radically from the typical histology of peripheral nerves are

(A) CN I and CN II
(B) CN III and CN IV
(C) CN V and CN VI
(D) CN VII and CN VIII
(E) CN IX, CN X, CN XI, and CN XII

7. The tentorial notch provides an opening between the

(A) anterior fossa and the middle fossa
(B) right half of the supratentorial space and the left
(C) supratentorial space and the infratentorial space
(D) posterior fossa and the foramen magnum
(E) none of the above

8. The rostral-most site for a lesion that would interrupt a motor nerve to a somite or branchial muscle is the

(A) diencephalon
(B) midbrain
(C) pons
(D) medulla
(E) C1 level

9. The sublenticular and retrolenticular parts of the internal capsule convey

(A) thalamoparietal and thalamocingulate radiations
(B) thalamofrontal and thalamoparietal radiations
(C) thalamoparietal and geniculocalcarine radiations
(D) geniculocalcarine and geniculotemporal radiations
(E) none of the above

10. A fracture of the cribriform plate in the floor of the anterior cranial fossa would most likely result in which symptom?

(A) Hemianopia
(B) Diplopia
(C) Anosmia
(D) Pupillodilation
(E) Absence of the corneal reflex

11. The nucleus ambiguus supplies axons to

(A) CN IX, CN X, CN XI, and CN XII
(B) CN VII, CN IX, CN X, and CN XI
(C) CN IX and CN X
(D) CN VII, CN XI, and CN XII
(E) CN VIII, CN IX, CN X, and CN XI

12. A nerve cell process that is axonal in structure and dendritic in function is the

(A) distal process of a dorsal root ganglion neuron
(B) basal dendrites of pyramidal neurons
(C) proximal process of a bipolar ganglion neuron
(D) distal process of a motoneuron axon
(E) none of the above

13. The pyramidal tract can be described as

(A) arising only from area 4 (area gigantopyramidalis)
(B) synapsing almost exclusively directly on ventral horn cells
(C) having only small axons (less than 10 μ in diameter)
(D) having a somatotopic organization of its fibers at its origin
(E) conveying many axons from the rhinencephalon

14. The type of aphasia most likely to occur with weakness of the lower muscles of the right side of the face is

(A) dyslexia
(B) auditory word agnosia
(C) dyslexia plus dysgraphia
(D) auditory word aphasia plus dyslexia (fluent aphasia)
(E) expressive aphasia of Broca (nonfluent aphasia)

15. An elderly patient complains of severe, lightning-like jolts of pain radiating down the left side from the ear to the tip of the mandible and tongue. Touching the corner of the lip sets off the pain, but the neurologic examination is otherwise normal. The best explanation is that the pain

(A) does not follow the distribution of a sensory nerve and is therefore psychogenic
(B) results from an irritative lesion in the right postcentral gyrus
(C) results from an irritative lesion of the sphenopalatine ganglion
(D) results from an irritative lesion of the third division of CN V
(E) results from an irritative lesion of CN XII

16. Transection of which pathway would most effectively disconnect the cortex of the frontal and temporal lobes?

(A) Uncinate fasciculus
(B) Inferior longitudinal fasciculus
(C) Superior longitudinal fasciculus
(D) Cingulum
(E) Frontal thalamic radiation

17. Select the correct statement about the posterior limb of the internal capsule.

(A) It forms a large sheet that separates the thalamus from the tail of the caudate nucleus

(B) It conveys connections between nucleus ventralis lateralis and the cingulate cortex

(C) It conveys the somatosensory fibers between the thalamus and the postcentral gyrus

(D) It receives its blood supply from the anterior communicating artery

(E) It conveys few or no myelinated fibers

18. The most useful anatomical criterion to confirm the gestational age of a stillborn infant thought to be born at about 22 weeks is

(A) degree of closure of the neural tube

(B) absence of the cerebellum

(C) the pattern of the cerebral sulci

(D) degree of myelination of the association areas of the cerebral cortex and cerebral commissures

(E) the number of dorsal root ganglia

19. Communication between the cerebrospinal fluid (CSF) in the central nervous system (CNS) and the subarachnoid space occurs at which site?

(A) Lateral ventricles

(B) Third ventricle

(C) Aqueduct

(D) Fourth ventricle

(E) Spinal cord/central canal

20. The major site of neuroblast proliferation in the central nervous system (CNS) is the

(A) roof plate/tectum

(B) marginal zone of the spinal cord

(C) periventricular/pericanalicular zone

(D) white matter of the cerebrum

(E) ventral columns/basis of the brain stem

21. In which of the following ways does the epidural space of the cranium resemble the spinal epidural space?

(A) It contains a plexus of blood vessels

(B) It forms the inner periosteum of the surrounding bone

(C) It can be distended by blood or pus

(D) It contains fat cells

(E) None of the above

22. A patient brought into the hospital comatose because of a head injury initially displayed flaccid extremities. Although remaining comatose, she began to exhibit posturing in which she would extend her arms and legs, pronate and flex her wrists, plantar flex her ankles, and arch her back. The best interpretation is that the patient has

(A) bilateral spastic hemiplegia

(B) parkinsonian rigidity

(C) compression of the medullocervical junction by transforaminal herniation

(D) compression of the midbrain by transtentorial herniation

(E) an irritative lesion of the cochlear system

23. A patient presents with the recent onset of ptosis of the right eyelid and constriction of the right pupil but no ocular palsy nor diplopia. The best explanation is a lesion of

(A) CN II

(B) CN III

(C) the carotid sympathetic nerve

(D) the ophthalmic division of CN V

(E) CN VII

DIRECTIONS: Each of the numbered items or incomplete statements in this section is negatively phrased, as indicated by a capitalized word such as NOT, LEAST, or EXCEPT. Select the ONE lettered answer or completion that is BEST in each case.

24. A lesion would NOT interfere with volitional control of micturition if it occurred at which of the following sites?

(A) Medial part of motor area (area 4), in the interhemispheric fissure
(B) Transection of the ventral half of the spinal cord
(C) Pelvic splanchnic nerve
(D) Obturator nerve
(E) Pudendal nerve

25. Which of the following associations between a nerve and its function is NOT true?

(A) Median nerve/flexion of the wrist
(B) Ulnar nerve/abduction of the little finger
(C) Obturator nerve/thigh adduction
(D) Musculocutaneous nerve/elbow flexion by the biceps
(E) Common peroneal nerve/extension and flexion of the ankle

26. All of the following structures derive from the neural crest EXCEPT

(A) neuronal perikarya in the peripheral nervous system (PNS)
(B) axons of the ventral roots
(C) axons of the dorsal roots
(D) autonomic ganglia
(E) adrenal medulla

27. Which of the following statements about spinal nerves is NOT true?

(A) Each spinal nerve innervates one somite
(B) The nerve trunk is formed by the union of dorsal and ventral roots
(C) Each spinal nerve typically has one dorsal root ganglion
(D) Most spinal nerves contain parasympathetic efferent axons
(E) The spinal nerves convey axons to skeletal muscles

28. A patient complains of numbness and tingling in the thumb and index finger. A lesion responsible for this complaint could exist at any of the following sites EXCEPT

(A) the radial nerve
(B) the lower trunk or medial cord of the brachial plexus
(C) the C6 dorsal root
(D) nucleus ventralis posterior of the thalamus
(E) the postcentral gyrus

29. Which of the following areas would NOT be damaged by an infarction of a hemisphere in the territory irrigated by the anterior cerebral artery?

(A) Supplementary motor cortex
(B) Leg and genital area of the motor cortex
(C) Cingulate gyrus
(D) Genu of the corpus callosum
(E) Calcarine cortex

30. All of the following statements about dopaminergic neurons are true EXCEPT

(A) they are most numerous in the midbrain tegmentum
(B) they send their main axonal connections rostrally, in contrast to the norepinephrinergic neurons
(C) they conform to well-delineated nuclear groups
(D) they are mainly small, poorly branched, unpigmented neurons
(E) they receive strong connections from the striatum

31. Which of the following procedures would NOT reduce pain conduction or the patient's reaction to pain?

(A) Stimulation of the periaqueductal gray matter
(B) Ventrolateral cordotomy
(C) Section of the lateral division of the dorsal roots
(D) Prefrontal lobotomy or cingulotomy
(E) Section of the dorsal columns of the spinal cord

32. Which of the following statements about the reticular formation (RF) is NOT true?

(A) It widely disperses axonal connections
(B) Its perikarya use a variety of different neurotransmitters
(C) It has heterogeneous, multiple afferent connections
(D) Its output consists of a few discrete myelinated tracts
(E) It extends from the cervicomedullary junction to the diencephalon

33. Which of the following changes would NOT occur after destruction of both optic nerves?

(A) Pallor of the optic disks (optic atrophy)
(B) Dilated pupils nonreactive to light
(C) Compensatory overgrowth of oligodendroglia in the retina
(D) Wallerian degeneration of the optic tract
(E) Transneuronal degeneration of the lateral geniculate bodies

34. All of the following mucosa contain neuronal perikarya EXCEPT

(A) bladder mucosa
(B) lingual mucosa
(C) intestinal mucosa
(D) esophageal mucosa
(E) olfactory mucosa

35. Which of the following statements about the nodes of Ranvier is NOT true?

(A) A node marks the site of apposition of two adjacent Schwann cells
(B) The theory of saltatory conduction presumes that the ionic flux of the nerve impulse occurs at the nodes
(C) The internodal distance corresponds to the length of an axon myelinated by one Schwann cell
(D) The axons continue across the nodes without interruption
(E) Since the axons with the smallest diameter have the most nodes, they conduct the fastest impulses.

36. Which dermatomal level does NOT match the corresponding area of the body?

(A) C7/middle finger
(B) T4/nipple line
(C) T10/umbilicus
(D) L5/big toe
(E) S1/perianal region

37. All of the following statements about the thalamic fasciculus (field H_1 of Forel) are true EXCEPT

(A) it conveys many myelinated axons
(B) it conveys thalamofrontal axons
(C) it conveys pallidothalamic axons
(D) it forms the dorsal boundary of the zona incerta
(E) it conveys dentatothalamic axons

38. After entering the spinal cord, dorsal root axons of the spinal nerves do NOT synapse on

(A) somatic motoneurons
(B) autonomic motoneurons
(C) substantia gelatinosa
(D) amacrine neurons
(E) nucleus gracilis

39. Major sites at which large numbers of neurons lodge or accumulate after migration include all of the following EXCEPT

(A) basis pontis
(B) cerebellar cortex
(C) olivary nuclei
(D) neurohypophysis
(E) cerebral cortex

40. Which statement about the characteristics of the pia mater is NOT true?

(A) It is lined with squamous epithelium
(B) It belongs to the leptomeninges
(C) It dips into the crevices of the brain and spinal cord
(D) It intervenes between the arachnoid and the surface of the cerebral cortex
(E) It allows free permeability between the cerebrospinal fluid (CSF) and the central nervous system (CNS)

DIRECTIONS: Each set of matching questions in this section consists of a list of four to twenty-six lettered options (some of which may be in figures) followed by several numbered items. For each numbered item, select the ONE lettered option that is most closely associated with it. To avoid spending too much time on matching sets with large numbers of options, it is generally advisable to begin each set by reading the list of options. Then, for each item in the set, try to generate the correct answer and locate it in the option list, rather than evaluating each option individually. Each lettered option may be selected once, more than once, or not at all.

Questions 41–45

Match each procedure or operation with the neurotransmitter it would severely deplete.

(A) Serotonin and catecholamines in the cerebral cortex
(B) Gaba-aminobutyric acid (GABA) and glycine in the spinal cord
(C) Substance P in the dorsal horns
(D) Acetylcholine in the cerebral cortex
(E) Serotonin in the spinal cord

41. Destruction of interneurons by controlled hypoxia

42. Section of the dorsal roots

43. Section of the midbrain at the diencephalic junction

44. Destruction of the anterior perforated substance

45. Destruction of the medullary raphe

Questions 46–50

Match the cortical connections or projections with the most closely related thalamic nucleus.

(A) Nucleus ventralis lateralis
(B) Nucleus pulvinaris
(C) Nucleus anterior and lateralis dorsalis
(D) Nucleus medialis dorsalis
(E) Lateral geniculate body

46. Projects visual impulses to the calcarine cortex

47. Connects with the frontal lobe anterior to the motor cortex (prefrontal area)

48. Projects to the nonstriate areas (eulaminate isocortex) of the parieto-occipito-temporal lobes

49. Projects to the motor cortex

50. Connects with the limbic cortex of the cingulate gyrus

Questions 51–55

Match the landmarks with the cerebral lobes that they divide in full or in part.

(A) Central sulcus
(B) Lateral (sylvian) fissure
(C) Line from the superior preoccipital notch to the inferior preoccipital notch
(D) Cingulate sulcus

51. Frontal lobe from the temporal lobe

52. Parietal lobe from the temporal lobe

53. Parietal lobe from the occipital lobe

54. Limbic lobe from the frontal lobe

55. Frontal lobe from the parietal lobes

Questions 56–60

Match the characteristic property or properties of glial cells with the types of glial cells listed.

(A) Medulloblast
(B) Oligodendrocyte
(C) Microglial cell
(D) Ependymal cell
(E) Astrocyte

56. Has numerous large branches that attach to the pial surface and blood vessel walls

57. Lines the cerebral aqueduct

58. Provides support and cohesion for the central nervous system (CNS)

59. Has few processes, some of which may end on neuronal surfaces, and its nuclei line up in rows in the white matter

60. Transform into macrophages in response to injury

DIRECTIONS: Each set of matching questions in this section consists of a list of four to twenty-six lettered options followed by several numbered items. For each numbered item, select the appropriate lettered option(s). Each lettered option may be selected once, more than once, or not at all. EACH ITEM WILL STATE THE NUMBER OF OPTIONS TO SELECT. CHOOSE EXACTLY THIS NUMBER.

Questions 61–66

(A) Lateral corticospinal tract
(B) Geniculocalcarine tract
(C) Corticobulbar pathway through the medial longitudinal fasciculus to the nucleus of CN III for volitional horizontal gaze
(D) Olivocerebellar pathway
(E) Reticulospinal pathway for automatic breathing
(F) Auditory pathway from the cochlea to the lateral lemniscus
(G) Dorsal column pathway to the thalamus
(H) Retinal axons that mediate the temporal visual fields
(I) Retinal axons that mediate nasal visual fields
(J) Pupilloconstrictor pathway from the optic tract to the Edinger-Westphal nucleus
(K) Ventrolateral spinothalamic tract for pain and temperature
(L) Ventrolateral spinothalamic tract for touch
(M) Cortico-ponto-cerebello-thalamo-cortico-pyramidal pathway
(N) Corticobulbar pathway for vertical gaze to nuclei of CN III and CN IV

For each anatomic site, select the tract or pathway that decussates at that site.

61. Pretectal region–midbrain junction (SELECT 2 TRACTS/PATHWAYS)

62. Caudal midbrain or caudal midbrain–rostral pons (SELECT 2 TRACTS/PATHWAYS)

63. Optic chiasm (SELECT 1 TRACT/PATHWAY)

64. Pons (SELECT 3 TRACTS/PATHWAYS)

65. Cervicomedullary junction (SELECT 4 TRACTS/PATHWAYS)

66. All levels of the spinal cord (SELECT 2 TRACTS/PATHWAYS)

ANSWERS AND EXPLANATIONS

1. The answer is B [Chapter 4 V A 3; Figure 4-12]. Each somite of the body receives a single spinal nerve. In the thoracic region, the somites remain in their original serial order and the spinal nerves run directly into the somite derivatives rather than going through plexuses. In the arm and leg regions, the somites migrate and intermingle. Although each dermatome, sclerotome, and myotome retains its original axons, the axons meander from one nerve trunk to another in the form of plexuses in order to reach their original targets.

2. The answer is C [Chapter 3 VIII A 3, 4; Figure 3-21]. The "jelly roll" hypothesis of myelination proposes that the myelin sheath forms by a lip of Schwann cell cytoplasm that encircles the individual axons several times. A single Schwann cell can myelinate more than one axon because its cytoplasm can encircle an axon wherever it contacts the Schwann cell. So-called unmyelinated axons indent the surface of the Schwann cell but are not encircled by a lip of Schwann cell cytoplasm.

3. The answer is B [Chapter 1 VI B 2; Figure 1-13]. The tentorium cerebelli is a fold of dura mater inserted between the cerebellum and the occipital lobes and the posterior–inferior face of the temporal lobes. The tentorium forms three of the intradural venous sinuses that drain blood into the jugular vein. Along their medial margins, the two tentorial leaves attach to the cerebral falx to form the straight sinus. Along their anterolateral margins, the two tentorial leaves attach to the petrous portions of the temporal bones to form the superior petrosal sinuses. Along their lateroposterior margins, the two tentorial leaves attach to the skull to form the confluent sinus and transverse sinus.

4. The answer is B [Chapter 7 V B 1 d (5); IX A 3 a; Figures 7-13 and 7-14]. The tracts along the paramedian plane of the medulla, in dorsoventral order, consist of the medial longitudinal fasciculus, medial lemniscus, and pyramidal tract. The hypoglossal nerve also runs in the paramedian plane. The combination of weakness of bulbar muscles on one side (the tongue in this patient), contralateral hemiplegia, and hemisensory loss localize the lesion to the paramedian plane of the medulla where all three structures—the pyramidal tract, medial lemniscus, and hypoglossal nerve—are contiguous. This region receives blood from the paramedian arteries of the vertebrobasilar system and may undergo selective infarction. The face was spared because corticobulbar fibers to the facial nucleus typically depart before reaching the medulla. Pain and temperature sensations were spared because the lateral spinothalamic tracts run in the lateral part of the medulla, which the circumferential arteries supply.

5. The answer is B [Chapter 13 II C 3 b (2)]. The pyramidal neurons of the hippocampus project strongly to the subiculum and the adjacent entorhinal cortex (area 28 of Brodmann), which form the anterior part of the parahippocampal gyrus. Postmortem examination shows that hypoxia, hypoglycemia, and repeated epileptic seizures cause selective destruction of the hippocampus per se and the adjacent quadrant of the temporal lobe as well, a lesion called mesial temporal lobe sclerosis. Magnetic resonance imaging (MRI) scans document the lesion in the living patient. Acute destruction of the medial quadrant of the temporal lobe causes the pure amnestic syndrome.

6. The answer is A [Chapter 7 VIII F 1, 2]. CN I and CN II differ radically from the typical histology of peripheral nerves. CN I consists of unmyelinated axonal filaments that perforate the cribriform plate along their course from the olfactory mucosa to the olfactory bulb. CN II is actually a tract of central axons that extends from the retina to the diencephalon.

7. The answer is C [Chapter 1 VI B 2 a; Figure 1-13]. The opening in the tentorium cerebelli, the tentorial notch, separates the supratentorial space from the infratentorial space, or, more specifically, the posterior fossa from the middle fossa. The midbrain runs from the middle fossa to the posterior fossa through the tentorial notch. The superior tip of the cerebellar vermis extends slightly above the plane of the tentorial notch just dorsal to the quadrigeminal plate.

8. The answer is B [Chapter 7 VIII C 1 a, 2 a]. The myotomes of the rostral-most somites give rise to the extraocular muscles, which rotate the eyeballs. These muscles develop from somites that were originally located opposite the midbrain and receive their innervation from CN III. CN III is the rostral-most motor nerve of the central nervous system (CNS).

9. The answer is D [Chapter 12 II L 3 b (1); Figure 12-6; Table 12-4]. The sublenticular and retrolenticular parts of the internal capsule receive their name because of their relationship to the lentiform nucleus. The fibers that run under this nucleus include, among other tracts, the geniculocalcarine and geniculotemporal tracts to the occipital and temporal lobes, respectively.

10. The answer is C [Chapter 7 VIII F 1 a; Figure 7-26]. The cribriform plate, the thinnest bone of the skull, commonly fractures during head trauma. The fracture shears off the delicate axons from the olfactory ganglion, located in the nasal mucosa. After perforating the cribriform plate, these axons synapse on the olfactory bulb. The patient suffers anosmia and lack of taste because smell and taste, the two chemical senses, are closely linked in feeding behavior. Even without cribriform plate fracture, anosmia may result because the acceleration–deceleration forces cause the frontal lobe to move in relation to the skull base, shearing off the olfactory axons. With cribriform plate fracture, the meninges often rupture and cerebrospinal fluid (CSF) drips from the nose. The open access route, called a CSF fistula, then allows bacteria to enter and cause meningitis.

11. The answer is C [Chapter 7 VIII E 2 c; X D 5 a (1)]. The nucleus ambiguus is a special visceral (branchial) efferent nucleus located in the ventrolateral part of the medullary tegmentum. Although classed as visceral because the gill arches serve oxygenation, a visceral function, the nucleus in fact supplies motor axons to skeletal muscles that derive from branchial arches. CN IX and CN X deliver the axons to the muscles. These nerves deliver parasympathetic axons also, but no somatomotor axons to somite muscle.

12. The answer is A [Chapter 12 III C 3 d]. The distal (peripheral) process of a dorsal root ganglion neuron has an axonal structure but conducts impulses toward the perikaryon and, therefore, functionally acts as a dendrite. Classically, axons differ from dendrites in being long, slender processes. Dendrites tend to be short, stubby processes that receive numerous synapses. Most neurons conform to the rule that axons conduct away from the perikaryon

and dendrites toward it.

13. The answer is D [Chapter 11 IV A; Chapter 13 VI A 1 a; Figure 13-37]. The pyramidal tract arises from areas 4 and 6 and the anterior part of the parietal lobe. It consists of a mixture of axons ranging in size from small to very large. These fibers have a somatotopic organization as they originate from the cortex and, to a degree, maintain that organization as they descend through the brain stem and spinal cord.

14. The answer is E [Chapter 13 VI G 4 a; Figure 13-38]. Lesions that occupy the anterior part of the left parasylvian zone (site 1 in Figure 13-38) cause a nonfluent type of expressive (motor) aphasia. This region abuts on the motor cortex, which supplies the upper motoneuron (UMN) fibers for the contralateral facial nucleus. Thus, a patient with expressive aphasia would be more likely to have a right-sided, UMN type of facial palsy than a patient with fluent aphasia, which implies a posterior lesion in the parasylvian zone.

15. The answer is D [Chapter 7 X B 7 a; Figure 7-30]. The patient has trigeminal neuralgia, affecting the third or mandibular division of CN V. This extremely painful condition affects one or more divisions of CN V. Whether the actual lesion is in the peripheral nervous system (PNS) or the descending tract of CN V is debatable. This type of neuralgia may also affect other nerves; for example, neuralgia affecting CN IX causes glossopharyngeal neuralgia and neuralgia affecting the nerves at the back of the head causes occipital neuralgia. The key to the diagnosis in each instance is the conformity of the pain to the distribution of a sensory nerve. Lesions of the sensory cortex do not cause pain limited to peripheral nerve distributions.

16. The answer is A [Chapter 13 IV D 1 c, E 1 a; Figures 13-25 and 13-26]. A large fiber tract, the uncinate fasciculus, bends around the stem of the sylvian fissure to connect the frontal and temporal lobes. This bundle is one of the larger U-fiber systems that typically skirt around the depth of the cerebral crevices to connect adjacent gyri.

17. The answer is C [Chapter 11 I B 1; Chapter 12 II L 3 a, b; Tables 12-4 and 12-5]. The somatosensory, auditory, and visual pathways all run through the posterior limb of the internal capsule. The posterior limb separates the lentiform nucleus from the thalamus. The anterior limb of the internal capsule separates the lentiform nucleus from the caudate. The two limbs meet at a "V," around the apex of the globus pallidus of the lentiform nucleus. The capsule conveys large numbers of myelinated and unmyelinated fibers.

18. The answer is C [Chapter 13 I D 3; Figure 13-2]. A neuropathologist can estimate the gestational age by the timetable of sulcation. Before 16 weeks, the interhemispheric and sylvian fissures are present, but the general cortical surfaces of the hemispheres are smooth. At 16 weeks, the sulci begin to appear in a definite sequence. If sulcation fails, the cerebral hemispheres remain smooth, a pathological condition called lissencephaly. These infants are severely retarded because the cortex, although much thicker than normal, contains only four layers of neurons, which fail to form the proper connections. The timetable of myelination also helps to identify the maturational age of an infant, both at autopsy and by magnetic resonance imaging (MRI) scan, but the cerebral association areas and commissures do not myelinate until after birth. During the embryonic stage of development, the cerebellum has already appeared and the neural tube normally has fully closed.

19. The answer is D [Chapter 7 II B 4 a–c]. The only sites for drainage of the cerebrospinal fluid (CSF) from the ventricles into the subarachnoid space are the foramina of Lushka and Magendie. These foramina perforate the roof plate of the fourth ventricle during embryogenesis. If these foramina fail to develop, close because of scarring, or if a tumor grows in or compresses the fourth ventricle, the patient develops hydrocephalus. The ventricles balloon out and the patient requires a shunt to drain the fluid.

20. The answer is C [Chapter 3 III A 1, 2; Figure 3-10]. The major site of proliferation of neuroblasts in the developing nervous system is the periventricular/pericanalicular zone or ependymal zone. After undergoing mitosis, the neuroblasts migrate away from the ependymal zone.

21. The answer is C [Chapter 1 V B 1 a, b, 2; Figure 1-10]. At spinal levels, an actual space exists between the dura and the vertebral column. Fat and a plexus of veins occupy this spinal epidural space. At the level of the fora-

men magnum, the dura becomes adherent to the skull bones and forms the periosteum of the inner table of the skull. No actual epidural space exists, only a potential space that contains no fat or vascular plexus. Nevertheless, blood or pus may dissect the cranial dura off of the skull bones, converting the potential space to an actual space, analogous to what can happen in the pleura. The resultant epidural hematoma or epidural empyema may kill the patient by causing transtentorial or transforaminal herniation. Similarly, blood or pus may cause a subdural hematoma or empyema at spinal levels.

22. The answer is D [Chapter 7 XIV E 1 a–e; Figure 7-42]. The patient has decerebrate rigidity, a characteristic posture that follows midbrain compression or destruction. The lesion interrupts the downflow of impulses from the cerebrum through the brain stem. The vestibular system then becomes overactive and causes all of the antigravity muscles to contract, forcing the patient into the so-called decerebrate posture. In patients with supratentorial mass lesions, such as hematomas or brain edema, the cerebrum herniates downward through the tentorial notch, compressing the midbrain and often killing the patient.

23. The answer is C [Figure 5-4; Chapter 9 VI E 6 a–d]. The combination of pupilloconstriction and ptosis suggest sympathetic paralysis (Bernard-Horner's syndrome). Two muscles elevate the eyelid: the levator palpebrae, innervated by CN III, and the superior tarsal muscle of Muller, innervated by the carotid sympathetic nerve. One key to differentiation is the size of the pupil. A lesion of CN III paralyzes the levator and the pupilloconstrictor muscle. The pupil dilates because of the intact action of the pupillodilator muscle, innervated by the sympathetic nerve. In addition, the ptosis of sympathetic paralysis improves when the patient volitionally looks up because the levator is the muscle that mediates voluntary upward gaze. The lesion that causes sympathetic paralysis may occur at any site along the descending pathways from the hypothalamus, through the spinal cord, and out through the peripheral pathway along the cervical sympathetic chain and carotid artery.

24. The answer is D [Chapter 4 VI E 4 a, 5 b, c; Figure 4-14; Chapter 6 VI C 1–4; Figure 6-22]. The obturator nerve innervates the adductor muscles and overlying skin and abuts on the cutaneous area of the genitofemoral nerve. Lesions of the remaining central or peripheral sites will cause bladder dysfunction. The upper motoneuron (UMN) innervation for volitional control of the legs and external sphincters comes from the medial wall of the cerebrum. Descending motor fibers and ascending sensory fibers for the bladder run in the ventral half of the spinal cord. The pelvic splanchnic nerves convey parasympathetic visceromotor fibers for contraction of the smooth muscle of the bladder wall and vasomotor fibers for penile and clitoral erection. The pudendal nerve delivers the axons from the nucleus of Onufrowicz for the voluntary bladder and bowel sphincters.

25. The answer is E [Chapter 4 VI E 5 a; VIII B 3 a (4); Table 4-4]. The sciatic nerve divides at the popliteal space to form the common peroneal nerve and the tibial nerve. The common peroneal nerve is the extensor nerve of the foot and ankle, whereas the tibial is the flexor nerve of the foot and ankle.

26. The answer is B [Chapter 3 IV E 1; V B 2 a; Figure 3-14; Table 3-3]. Much of the peripheral nervous system (PNS) derives from the neural crest, but the ventral root axons arise from the ventral motoneurons of the gray matter of the spinal cord and brain stem. The crest derivatives include the dorsal root ganglia and their proximal and distal sensory processes, the sympathetic and parasympathetic ganglia and mucosal plexuses, and the adrenal medulla.

27. The answer is D [Chapter 3 VI C 1; Figure 3-17; Chapter 5 III B 1]. The spinal nerves typically contain four components: visceral and motor afferents and visceral and motor efferents. For most spinal nerves, the visceral efferent axon derives from the sympathetic nervous system. Only sacral nerves 2, 3, and 4 carry large numbers of parasympathetic efferent axons.

28. The answer is B [Chapter 4 VII E 3]. To analyze a sensory complaint, the clinician has to think through the sensory circuits to consider the possible sites of the lesion. To analyze numbness and tingling in one part of the body, start at the sensory receptor or peripheral nerve and think through the spinal and lemniscal pathways to the thalamus and finally the cortex. A lesion anywhere along the pathway might cause the complaint. In fact, a lesion of either the median or radial nerves could cause this patient's complaint, as could

a lesion of the upper trunk or lateral cord of the plexus or the central pathways to the somatosensory cortex in the postcentral gyrus. If the lesion had affected the lower trunk or cord, the patient would have felt the sensory disturbance on the ulnar side of the hand, not the radial side.

29. The answer is E [Chapter 15 III E 3 c; Figures 15-14 and 15-16]. Infarction in the distribution of the anterior cerebral artery destroys the tissue from the frontal pole along the superior margin of the hemisphere, extending down to and including the cingulate gyrus and corpus callosum. Because of destruction of the supplementary motor cortex and the adjacent leg and genital area of the primary motor cortex, the patient suffers contralateral monoplegia of the leg. The infarction may also destroy the postcentral sensory cortex on the medial hemispheric wall, but stops at about the parieto-occipital sulcus. Thus, the infarct stops short of the calcarine cortex, which is irrigated by the posterior cerebral artery.

30. The answer is D [Chapter 11 II H 1; Chapter 14 II B 3]. Dopaminergic neurons concentrate in the midbrain in well-delimited nuclei in the substantia nigra and ventral tegmental region. The neurons of the substantia nigra in particular are large, well branched, and become heavily pigmented as the brain matures and ages. The dopaminergic neurons project their axons to the mesencephalon or rostrally to the forebrain.

31. The answer is E [Chapter 12 II O 3; Chapter 14 VIII F 2, 3; Figure 14-2]. Dorsal column section does not interrupt pain pathways. A number of surgical procedures may reduce pain either by reducing the pain input or by reducing the patient's reaction to the pain input. Direct section of the ventrolateral quadrants of the spinal cord or of the lateral divisions of the dorsal roots will block the pain pathway. Prefrontal lobotomy and cingulotomy do not block the delivery of pain impulses but reduce the patient's reaction or response to pain. Stimulation of the periaqueductal gray matter may block pain transmission at spinal levels.

32. The answer is D [Chapter 7 XI A 1, 2, C 1 c]. The anatomical characteristics of the reticular formation (RF) include a diverse afferent input and a diverse efferent output. Many of the axons of the RF, even the long axons that leave it, lack myelin sheaths. The perikarya of the RF generally act by various neurotransmitters. Although some perikarya form denser nuclear clumps than others, the regions of the RF vary considerably in this regard. The diffuse nature of the RF and its intimate role in the control of visceral reactions, homeostasis, and postural reflexes stand in contrast to the somatic sensorimotor systems with their topographic point-to-point connections.

33. The answer is C [Chapter 9 II C 3 a (1)–(3)]. Although proliferating phagocytes remove the degenerating neurons and axons after the optic nerves are destroyed, the retina normally does not contain myelinated axons and oligodendroglia. The myelin sheaths of the optic nerve begin after the retinal axons pierce the lamina cribrosa. Transection of the optic nerves will cause anterograde and retrograde degeneration of optic nerve axons. The retrograde atrophy denudes the optic disk of axons, and it becomes pallid because the capillaries disappear. The retinal ganglion cells also die. Anterograde or Wallerian degeneration of the axons of the optic tract denudes the lateral geniculate body of afferents. The geniculate body then undergoes transneuronal atrophy. In young individuals, the calcarine cortex also atrophies. Degeneration of the geniculocalcarine tract deprives the calcarine cortex of its thalamic afferents and causes the outer line of Baillarger to disappear because it consists of myelinated fibers of thalamic origin.

34. The answer is B [Chapter 3 III D 1 a, b; Figure 3-9; Chapter 7 X C 8 a]. The lingual mucosa, although having taste buds, contains no neuronal perikarya. The geniculate ganglion of CN VII contains the perikarya that supply axons for the lingual taste buds. Neuronal perikarya arrange themselves in basically four patterns: laminae (either on external surfaces or as plexuses in the wall of viscera), nuclear masses, reticular formation (RF), and ganglia. Each of these neuronal arrangements may show a wide variety of neuronal types and degrees of concentration of neurons. The mucosa in general contain neurons, either as ganglia (e.g., the olfactory mucosa) or plexuses (e.g., the wall of the hollow viscera of the gastrointestinal or genitourinary tracts).

35. The answer is E [Chapter 4 I B 1–4; II B 2; Figure 4-4]. A node of Ranvier marks the site of apposition of two adjacent Schwann cells in the peripheral nervous system (PNS) and of oligodendroglial cells in the central nervous system (CNS). The smallest nerve fibers lack myelin sheaths and nodes, whereas all of the largest fibers are myelinated and have nodes. In the PNS, the axon and the endoneurium continue uninterrupted across the node. At each node, the naked axonal membrane allows the flux of sodium and potassium ions that depolarize the axon during the passage of a nerve impulse. Thus, the nerve impulse travels along the myelinated axons from node to node at a faster rate than if it had to travel along the entire axonal surface between the nodes.

36. The answer is E [Chapter 4 V C 1–7; Figure 4-12]. Although the clinician should not memorize dermatomal maps, knowledge of a few levels is helpful in daily practice. S1 innervates the little toe with S5 innervating the perianal region. C2 abuts on the trigeminal area. C7 innervates the index and middle fingers. T4 innervates the nipple line, and T10 innervates the level of the umbilicus. L5 innervates the big toe. From just this knowledge, the clinician can fairly well localize the common nerve root irritation syndromes and spinal cord levels without having to consult a dermatomal map.

37. The answer is B [Chapter 11 II B 3 b (1); Figures 11-7 and 11-8; Figure 12-2]. The thalamic fasciculus is medial to the internal capsule and does not convey the thalamocortical pathways. It consists of a layer or capsule of numerous myelinated axons that come from the medial lemniscus, dentatothalamic tract, and pallidothalamic tract. The thalamic fasciculus forms a myelinated layer between the thalamus and the zona incerta.

38. The answer is D [Chapter 6 III C 1–3; Figures 6-5 and 6-7; Chapter 9 II D 4 a (3), b (2), (3)]. Amacrine neurons are specialized neurons of the retina that lack axons, as originally described in the retina by Cajal. Some neurons of the olfactory bulb also lack axons. No spinal afferents terminate on these sites. When dorsal roots enter the spinal cord, they divide into medial and lateral divisions and then synapse on sensory neurons of the dorsal horn, consisting of the dorsomarginal nucleus, substantia gelatinosa, nucleus proprius (essentially in laminae 1 to 6 of Rexed), and nucleus dorsalis of lamina 7. Dorsal root axons make monosynaptic synapses with the motoneurons of lamina 9, and others travel up the dorsal columns to the nuclei gracilis and cuneatus.

39. The answer is D [Chapter 3 III D 2 a, b; Figures 3-10 and 3-11]. Although it receives axons from the hypothalamus that empty hormones into its capillaries, the neurohypophysis consists of specialized glial cells and capillaries, not neurons. In general, neuroblasts do not invade the floor plate or the roof plate per se, except in the midbrain, where they form the quadrigeminal plate. The neurohypophysis evaginates from the floor plate. Neuroblasts that migrate into the mantle zone form the nuclei of the spinal cord and brain stem. At more rostral levels, the neuroblasts of the mantle zone form the diencephalic nuclei and the basal ganglia. Neuroblasts that migrate to the surface form the cerebral and cerebellar cortices. Neuroblasts also migrate out from the ependymal zone to form the visible bumps, which include the cerebellum, basis pontis, inferior olivary eminences, quadrigeminal bodies, and mamillary bodies.

40. The answer is E [Chapter 1 V A 3, C 1–3; Figures 1-10 and 1-11]. The pia provides a protective barrier between the central nervous system (CNS) and cerebrospinal fluid (CSF) that blocks free permeability of substances dissolved in the CSF. The pia mater is the innermost of the three meningeal coverings of the CNS. With the arachnoid it constitutes the leptomeninges. A subarachnoid space that contains CSF separates the pia from the arachnoid. The pia enters the sulci, but the arachnoid bridges over the sulci. Flat epithelial cells line both the pial and arachnoid surfaces of the subarachnoid space.

41–45. The answers are: 41-B, 42-C, 43-A, 44-D, 45-E [Chapter 14 II C 1 d, D 4 b (1); III D 2 a, d (2); IV B 2 c; V B 2; VIII F 1 a]. Because we now know the neurotransmitters of many central pathways, selective section of these pathways or destruction of their perikarya will predictably deprive the brain of specific neurotransmitters. Destruction of interneurons of the spinal cord depletes gamma-aminobutyric acid (GABA) and glycine, the inhibitory transmitters produced by the interneurons. Dorsal root section reduces substance P concentration in the dorsal horns. This neurotransmitter presumably transmits pain impulses from the small fibers in the lateral division of the dorsal roots. Transection at the midbrain–diencephalic junction interrupts all of the axons that connect the catecholaminergic and serotonergic nuclei of the brain stem with the cerebral cortex, most of which run through the medial forebrain bundle. Destruction of the medullary raphe destroys the serotonergic neurons of the medulla, which project to the spinal cord. Destruction of the anterior perforated substance eliminates the perikarya of the gigantocellular complex of neurons of the basal forebrain, including the substantia innominata of Reichert and nucleus basalis. These basal neurons provide profuse cholinergic innervation to the entire cortex and to some subcortical targets as well. These neurons undergo severe degeneration in Alzheimer's disease and may account for some of the dementia and memory loss. In contrast to other rhinencephalic structures of the basal forebrain, the gigantocellular complex has increased in size and significance during phylogeny, whereas many related rhinencephalic structures have undergone phylogenetic regression.

Various drugs or chemicals can also selectively block neurotransmitters by inhibiting their formation, inhibiting their release, competing with binding sites on the postsynaptic membrane, or altering their re-uptake or degradation. By combining the evidence from anatomical lesions, chemical blockade, direct chemical analysis, and enzyme identification, neuroscientists can establish the transmitters involved in the various layers and regions of the cortex and the different nuclei and tracts of the central nervous system.

46–50. The answers are: 46-E, 47-D, 48-B, 49-A, 50-C [Chapter 12 II F, G; Figure 12-4; Table 12-5]. The thalamus and cerebral cortex reflect each other's functional organization. Functionally, the thalamic nuclei serve sensory, motor, and mental functions. The area around the calcarine fissure receives visual impulses from the geniculocalcarine tract, whereas the transverse temporal gyri on the upper surface of the temporal lobe receive the auditory impulses. Nucleus medialis dorsalis connects with the frontal lobe anterior to the motor cortex. Interruption of this connection results in apathy, indifference, and a reduced reaction to stimuli in general.

The connections from the pulvinar to the parasylvian area and the cortex behind the sensory region of the parietal lobe mediate language functions of the left hemisphere and the spatial orientation functions of the right hemisphere. Lesions of the cortex, thalamocortical and corticothalamic circuits, or nuclei that project to the particular region of the cortex tend to cause similar neurologic deficits. Thus, lesions of the left thalamus may cause aphasia, whereas lesions of the right thalamus may impair awareness of the left half of space. The thalamus also is essential for the general functions of consciousness and memory. Bilateral thalamic lesions cause varying degrees of dementia, amnesia, and obtundation, including coma.

Nucleus ventralis lateralis projects to the motor cortex after receiving the dentatothalamic tract; thus, it aids in modulating the output of the pyramidal tract to produce smooth, coordinated movements. Nucleus anterior receives the mamillothalamic tract and projects to the cingulate cortex. Papez included these connections in the limbic circuit he proposed as the anatomic substrate for the experience of emotions and their expression through behavior. Nucleus lateralis dorsalis and parts of nucleus medialis are now regarded as parts of the "limbic thalamus."

51–55. The answers are: 51-B, 52-B, 53-C, 54-D, 55-A [Chapter 1 III C 1–4; Figure 1-4]. The current boundaries of the cerebral lobes comprise a hodgepodge of natural and arbitrary landmarks. These lobar boundaries enable an observer to describe normal and pathologic variations in regions of the cerebrum and describe the exact sites of lesions. The sylvian or lateral fissure forms by the evagination of the temporal lobe from the primitive telencephalon. The sylvian fissure runs from the vallecula to the lateral face of the cerebrum, where it then forms a horizontal ramus. Anteriorly, this ramus separates the frontal lobe from the temporal lobe; posteriorly, it separates the parietal lobe from the temporal lobe. Thus, the temporal lobe forms the floor of the posterior horizontal ramus of the sylvian fissure. The opercular parts of the frontal and parietal lobes form its roof.

A line from the superior preoccipital notch to the inferior preoccipital notch arbitrarily divides the parietal and temporal lobes from the occipital lobe on the lateral face of a hemisphere. Bridging veins apparently cause these notches. A bridging vein runs from the preoccipital notch to the superior sagittal sinus and from the inferior preoccipital notch to the transverse sinus. Thus, the lobar boundaries defined by the internotch line depend on the happenstance location of veins and bear no necessary relation to the structure or function of the underlying cortex.

On the medial face of a hemisphere, the cingulate sulcus roughly divides the cingulate gyrus of the limbic lobe from the parietal and frontal lobes, which occupy the medial hemispheric wall dorsal to the cingulate sulcus.

The central sulcus, a natural crevice, separates the largest lobe of the cerebrum, the frontal lobe, from the parietal lobe. The central sulcus cuts the crest of the hemisphere just rostral to the ascending ramus of the cingulate gyrus and angles ventroanteriorly along the lateral face of the cerebrum. The central sulcus divides the motor cortex in the precentral gyrus from the sensory cortex of the postcentral gyrus.

56–60. The answers are: 56-E, 57-D, 58-E, 59-B, 60-C [Chapter 2 VI B 4 a, b; Table 2-1]. Each of the various glial cell types displays characteristic differences in morphology and function. Astrocytes are of two types, fibrous and protoplasmic. The protoplasmic astrocytes occur in gray matter and the fibrous in white matter. Astrocytes attach their end feet to the pial surface, where they form a continuous inner lining for the pia and act as part of the central nervous system (CNS)–brain barrier. Other end feet of the astrocytes abut on blood vessels and form part of the blood–brain barrier. The location and amount of extracellular space in the nervous system are in some question. Some neuroscientists suggest that the cytoplasm of astrocytes functions as the extracellular space for the CNS.

In the gray matter, oligodendrocytes form perineuronal satellites, with their perikarya near neurons and one or more processes extending to the neuronal surface. In the white matter, the perikarya of the oligodendrocytes line up in rows. Here they are called interfascicular glia because they are between the fascicles of nerve fibers. Their processes invest the CNS axons with a myelin sheath, with a "jelly roll" topology.

Microglial cells characteristically occur in gray matter. Microglia were once thought to invade the nervous system from the mesodermal coverings during embryogenesis. Current opinion holds that microglia actually derive from neural ectoderm like all other intrinsic cells of the nervous system. Microglia may transform into macrophages in response to injury. Macrophages also migrate into the CNS from the blood in response to lesions that alter the blood–brain barrier. In addition, microglia act as antigen presenters for the intrinsic immune system of the CNS.

The ependymal cells are a simple columnar epithelium that form a monolayer on the surfaces of the ventricles, aqueduct, and central canal of the spinal cord. These cells also cover the tufts of choroid plexus that project into the ventricles from the pial surface. In general, they are a rather indolent cell type that does not proliferate readily, although one tumor of the glial series, the ependymoma, does occur. As compared with medulloblastomas, ependymomas have a better prognosis because the cells do not proliferate as aggressively as medulloblasts. Both types of tumors frequently occur in the posterior fossa, where they may occupy the midline of the cerebellum or the fourth ventricle. Rarely, they occur in the cerebrum. The characteristic tumor of the oligodendrocyte is the oligodendroglioma, and of the astrocyte is a series of astrocytomas, the most malignant of which are glioblastomas.

61. The answers are: J, N [Chapter 7 XIV D 1 b; Figures 9-20 and 9-21]. Decussations at the pretectal–midbrain level in the pathway for pupilloconstriction ensure that illumination of either eye affects both pupils equally. The pathway for vertical gaze likewise decussates in the pretectal–midbrain region to ensure that the nuclei of CN III and CN IV on both sides receive equal innervation to elevate or depress the eyeballs conjugately.

62. The answers are: C, M [Chapter 7 VII E 2; Figure 9-20]. The pathway for horizontal gaze has two decussations. The corticobulbar component decussates at caudal midbrain–rostral pontine levels. The axons in the medial longitudinal fasciculus that coordinate the contraction of the lateral and medial recti during horizontal conjugate gaze then decussate at the level of the paramedian pontine reticular formation (PPRF), the so-called abducens center. This connection fulfills Hering's law of equal contraction of the muscles involved in any conjugate action of the two eyeballs. The dentatothalamic pathway decussates in the caudal part of the midbrain.

63. The answer is H [Chapter 9 III B 1 b, C 1]. The retinal axons on the nasal half of the retina that mediate the temporal fields decussate at the optic chiasm, after which the axons of the optic pathway to the calcarine cortex remain ipsilateral.

64. The answers are: C, F, M [Chapter 7 VI B 5; Figure 9-20]. The cortico-ponto-cerebellar pathway decussates in the basis pontis. In the sensory system, two decussations cause bilateral dispersion of impulses. The olfactory bulbs connect through the anterior commissure. At the superior olivary nuclei and trapezoid body, about half of the auditory axons decussate and half remain ipsilateral. Thus, unilateral destruction of the auditory pathway from the lateral lemniscus to the auditory cortex does not cause lateralized deafness.

65. The answers are: A, D, E, G, M [Figures 6-16 and 6-20; Chapter 7 V E 1–3]. The decussations at the cervicomedullary junction are the lateral corticospinal tracts, the internal arcuate axons from the nuclei gracilis and cuneatus of the dorsal columns that form the medial lemniscus, and the reticulospinal tracts for breathing. These three tracts decussate in dorsal–ventral order: the reticulospinal pathways decussate dorsally just under the obex, the lemniscal fibers of the internal arcuate decussate from nuclei gracilis and cuneatus next, and the corticospinal fibers decussate most ventrally. The olivary decussation begins at the level of the cervicomedullary junction and extends throughout the medulla. Corticobulbar fibers decussate at various levels of the brain stem. Some lower motoneurons (LMNs) of the brain stem receive mostly crossed fibers, such as the LMNs for the muscles of the lower part of the face. The upper facial muscles, the chewing and swallowing muscles, and the tongue muscles apparently receive about equal numbers of decussated and nondecussated fibers. Unilateral interruption of the corticobulbar pathways does not cause one-sided weakness of muscles because the corticobulbar fibers provide bilateral innervation. Unilateral paralysis of these muscles is almost always the result of a lesion of their LMNs or their peripheral nerves.

66. The answers are: K, L [Figure 6-15; Chapter 7 V F 3 a (2)]. The pain and temperature axons enter the central nervous system (CNS) through the dorsal roots at each segmental level of the spinal cord or through dorsal roots of the cranial nerves. The second-order neuron then decussates at or near the level of entry of the primary axon. The touch pathways through the spinothalamic tracts that ascend in the ventrolateral quadrant of the spinal cord follow the same pattern. In the dorsal columns, the primary axons ascend all of the way to the second-order neurons in the nuclei gracilis and cuneatus, which then produce the internal arcuate decussation of the medial lemniscus.

Index

Note: Page numbers in *italic* indicate illustrations, those followed by *t* indicate tables.